Master the™ PCAT®

2ND EDITION

PALM BEACH COUNTY
LIBRARY SYSTEM
3650 SUMMIT BLVD.
WEST PALM BEACH, FL 33406

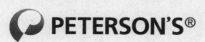 PETERSON'S®

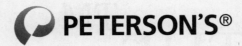

About Peterson's

Peterson's®, has been your trusted educational publisher for over 50 years. It's a milestone we're quite proud of, as we continue to offer the most accurate, dependable, high-quality educational content in the field, providing you with everything you need to succeed. No matter where you are on your academic or professional path, you can rely on Peterson's for its books, online information, expert test-prep tools, the most up-to-date education exploration data, and the highest quality career success resources—everything you need to achieve your education goals. For our complete line of products, visit **www.petersons.com**.

For more information about Peterson's range of educational products, contact Peterson's, 8740 Lucent Blvd., Suite 400 Highlands Ranch, CO 80129; 800-338-3282 Ext. 54229; or find us online at **www.petersons.com**.

© 2018 Peterson's

ISBN-13: 978-0-7689-4148-7

Printed in the United States of America

10 9 8 7 6 5 4 3 2 1   20 19 18

Second Edition

Contents

PART III: CRITICAL READING SKILLS

PART IV: BIOLOGICAL PROCESSES

PART V: CHEMICAL PROCESSES

PART VI: QUANTITATIVE REASONING

PART VIII: TWO PRACTICE TESTS

APPENDIX

Before You Begin

In 2011, the Pharmacy College Admission Test (PCAT®) became fully computer-based and is administered at Pearson VUE Test Centers in the United States and other countries. The test is not computer-adaptive, so it will not assign subsequent questions based on your answers to previous questions. The American Association of College Pharmacies (AACP) assures test-takers that the new test format presents the same "content, subtests, scoring, and reporting" as the paper-and-pencil version. Even the order of the subtests remains the same. The only thing that is different is how you take the test. You can read about this process in Chapter 1: All About the PCAT.

HOW THIS BOOK IS ORGANIZED

Peterson's Master the PCAT is divided into nine parts to facilitate your study and review for the PCAT. An Appendix provides helpful career information.

- **Part I** explains the basics about the PCAT. It covers the PCAT structure and format, registering for the test, and PCAT scoring and score reporting and provides an overview of subtests and question types.

- **Part II** offers a diagnostic test to help you identity your strengths as well as those areas where you will need to spend more time preparing. For your ease in identifying those areas, a question's category or area of focus is noted at the end of each answer explanation.

- **Part III** goes into detail about the Critical Reading passages and the types of questions you'll be answering. You'll also find strategies for selecting the correct answer.

- **Part IV** tackles the Biological Processes subtest and offers a review of important principles and concepts in General Biology, Microbiology, and Anatomy and Physiology, as well as tips and strategies for answering these test items.

- **Part V** explores concepts and principles for the Chemical Processes subtest, including topics in General Chemistry and Organic Chemistry. Tips and strategies are also presented to help you in answering Chemistry test items.

- **Part VI** reviews the topics assessed in the Quantitative Reasoning subtest of the PCAT. Part VII includes chapters on Arithmetic, Algebra, Probability and Statistics, Precalculus, and Calculus. Worked-out solutions are provided to help you identify critical steps in the problem-solving process.

- **Part VII** explains the Writing subtest, which is given in two parts during the test administration. You will learn strategies for developing well-supported and coherent responses to the prompts as you review model responses.

- **Part VIII** contains two additional Practice Tests that provide you with simulated practice in taking the PCAT under timed conditions.
- The **Appendix** provides helpful information on a variety of careers in pharmacy. In addition to listing job duties and responsibilities, each of the ten career profiles includes an explanation of the nature of the work, a projection of future job openings, and salary information compiled by the U.S. Bureau of Labor Statistics.

Each chapter in Parts III through VI contains Practice Questions to help you review what you have just learned.

SPECIAL STUDY FEATURES

Peterson's Master the PCAT has several features that will help you get the most from your study time.

Overview

Each chapter begins with a listing of the major topics in that chapter, followed by an introduction that explains what you will be reviewing in the chapter.

Summing It Up

Each chapter ends with a point-by-point summary of the main points of the chapter. It can be a handy last-minute guide to review before the test.

Bonus Information

You will find three types of notes in the margins of *Peterson's Master the PCAT* to alert you to important information about the test.

Note

Margin notes marked "Note" highlight information about the test structure itself.

Tip

A note marked "Tip" points out valuable advice for taking the PCAT.

Alert

An "Alert" identifies pitfalls in the testing format or question types that can cause mistakes in selecting answers.

Review Features

Peterson's Master the PCAT has a special feature that will help you review basic concepts and prepare for the Writing subtest:

- A Quick Review of Common Errors in Grammar, Usage, and Mechanics

USING THIS BOOK TO PREPARE FOR THE COMPUTER-BASED PCAT

There are some important things to remember as you work through this book: When taking the computer-based PCAT, you'll be entering your answers by inputting them on a keyboard or using a mouse. The Writing subtests require that you type your essay. The other subtests require that you select answer choices by clicking on them with your mouse. Since you can't answer in this fashion in a book, you'll have to fill in your answers by hand on the answer sheets provided when completing the Practice Questions and taking the Diagnostic and Practice Tests. However, be assured that the question content is similar to that found on the PCAT.

YOU ARE WELL ON YOUR WAY TO SUCCESS

You have made the decision to apply to pharmacy school and have taken a very important step in that process by registering for the PCAT. *Peterson's Master the PCAT* will help you score high on the exam and prepare you for everything you'll need to know on the day of your exam. Good luck!

GIVE US YOUR FEEDBACK

Peterson's publishes a full line of books—test prep, education exploration, financial aid, and career preparation. Peterson's publications can be found at high school guidance offices, college libraries and career centers, and your local bookstore or library. Peterson's books are now also available as eBooks.

We welcome any comments or suggestions you may have about this publication. Your feedback will help us make educational dreams possible for you—and others like you.

TOP 10 STRATEGIES TO RAISE YOUR SCORE

1. **Use the Diagnostic Test as a tool.** Taking the test and studying answers will help you identify the content that you need to spend the most time reviewing. The answer explanations include the specific content covered on the math and science questions, so you will have a quick-and-easy way to decide which topics to spend more time on.

2. **Schedule your study time.** Between now and the time you take the PCAT, plan to study at least six times a week. Try to spend the same amount of time each day. Find a place that is conducive to studying.

3. **Budget your time on the topics.** Don't move too quickly through the material, but don't get bogged down and spend too much time on one or two topics. Be sure that you are comfortable with each topic before you move on to the next one, but be aware that if you spend too much time on just a couple of topics, you will then have to rush through the rest of your review.

4. **Know the Periodic Table of Elements.** A copy of the Periodic Table is provided on the PCAT, but be sure that you know how it is organized and what this organization tells you about trends.

5. **Memorize basic math rules.** Be sure that you know basic rules of math, such as factoring and the chain rule. Though you will have access to a calculator during some portions of the test, having a firm grasp of what the basic math rules are and how to apply them will help allay some of your concerns.

6. **PRACTICE, PRACTICE, PRACTICE.** Practice may not get you a perfect score on the PCAT, but it will certainly help you score higher. Take the Diagnostic Test, complete each set of questions in each chapter, and take both Practice Tests at the back of the book.

7. **Establish a pacing schedule for taking each subtest.** Before you take the Diagnostic Test, work out what you think will be a reasonable pace for you to complete each test question. Then set the timer and take the test. After you finish, make adjustments as needed and time yourself when you take the Practice Tests at the back of the book. Whatever pacing schedule works for you, make sure you stick to it on the day of the test.

BEFORE THE TEST

8. **Find the location of the test center.** If you aren't familiar with the location of the test site, take a trial run to find it and see how long it takes you to get there. If you're driving, locate a parking lot or garage. This may seem like overkill, but who wants to arrive at the testing site with five minutes to spare and out of breath because you got lost on the way or spent 20 minutes trying to find a parking lot that turned out to be eight blocks away?

9. **Organize what you need for the test.** The night before the test, lay out on your admission ticket and the required forms of identification. You do not need anything else. Organizing ahead of time may seem like a waste of time, but you don't want to spend all morning searching for a utility bill or a library card on the day of the test.

DURING THE TEST

10. **Use the features that are given to you.** During the test, you will have access to both a calculator, for finding solutions to problems, and an erasable board, for making notes for your essays. Use them. Use the back-and-forth functions as well to bookmark a question that you can't answer easily or to review answers if you finish before timing out. But remember that your first choice is very likely to be the correct one.

PART I
PCAT BASICS

All About the PCAT

Chapter 1

OVERVIEW

- **The PCAT Structure and Testing Format**
- **Your PCAT Scores**
- **Reporting Scores to Pharmacy Schools**
- **How Pharmacy Schools Use PCAT Scores**
- **Registering for the PCAT**
- **PCAT Fees and Special Accommodations**
- **What You Should Know for Test Day**
- **Summing It Up**

The Pharmacy College Admission Test (PCAT) is developed by Pearson, with the endorsement of the American Association of Colleges of Pharmacy (AACP). Another Pearson company, Pearson VUE, administers the test at its computer testing sites in the United States and abroad. The test contains 192 multiple-choice test items and one essay prompt. According to Pearson, the "test helps identify qualified applicants to pharmacy colleges." Test items assess "general academic ability and scientific knowledge necessary for the commencement of pharmaceutical education."

THE PCAT STRUCTURE AND TESTING FORMAT

The PCAT assesses five subject areas through a series of six subtests. The subject areas are Writing, Biological Process, Chemical Process, Critical Reading, and Quantitative Reasoning. There is a 15 minute break between the third and fourth subtests. The test administration itself takes four hours, but instructions and familiarizing yourself with the machine and testing format plus the rest break adds to that time.

The Writing subtest gives you one prompt to answer, which you will do by inputting your essay. You will not have a choice of prompts from which to select. The prompts are set up as a problem-solution statement. You will be given a problem and asked to offer a solution. The statements are related to science and health issues or political, cultural, or social problems. The test-maker assures test-takers that no special knowledge is required to answer them.

The other four subtests in the subject areas are multiple-choice-only tests. There are no questions with grid-ins or highlighting. There are no questions that have more than one correct answer. The PCAT is a standard test format of a single answer choice to be selected from four possible answers.

Each of the four multiple-choice subtests has 48 questions for a total test count of 192 multiple-choice items. However, eight of the 40 items in each subtest are experimental, and you will not know which are the experimental questions. Wrong answers do not count against your score.

The PCAT is a computer-based test, but it is not computer-adaptive. The testing program does not adjust future test items based on answers to previous questions. The test is administered on special computers by Pearson Vue at Pearson Professional Centers. The computers provide functionality for word processing, marking questions to return to, pacing yourself, and moving back and forth between questions, but not subtests. You will be given an erasable board for making notes and doing calculations.

If you have taken the test in the past, you will see that the content, structure, and format of the writing prompt and 192 multiple-choice items and scoring and reporting have not changed. However, the testing calendar has changed. The PCAT is now administered in January, July, September, and October.

YOUR PCAT SCORES

The multiple-choice test items are scored by machine and trained readers evaluate the essay. The official Score Report is available online within five weeks of a test administration. This is the only official report of your score and is available online for a year. At the same time, an Official Transcript of your scores is mailed to your list of schools. The Official Transcript includes not only your latest test administration, but all scores for the past five years.

How are the individual subtest scores and composite score arrived at? The scores for the multiple-choice subtests are noted on your Score Report both as scaled scores and percentile ranks. Scaled scores range from 200 to 600 and are based on how many of the 40 nonexperimental questions in each subtest you answered correctly. Your percentile ranking from 1 to 99 shows how you performed in relation to a norm group, a group specified by certain characteristics chosen by the test-maker and held as constant.

The Writing subtest is reported as two scores, one for Conventions of Language and one for Problem Solving. The two scores are reported as Score and Mean. The former is a number from 0 to 5.0 that correlates to the rubrics used to score the essay. It is an average of the scores of the two readers for your essay. The mean score allows you to compare your performance with everyone else who took the PCAT during the same window that you did. It is the average of all these Writing scores.

REPORTING SCORES TO PHARMACY SCHOOLS

Many pharmacy schools accept applications and test scores through the Pharmacy College Application Service (PharmCAS). It is similar to the Universal College Application that you probably used when you were applying to undergraduate colleges. Candidates go online and fill out the application and indicate which pharmacy schools it should be sent to.

In addition to accepting applications through PharmCAS, many schools of pharmacy also want your PCAT scores reported through PharmCAS Code 104. Pearson reports them directly to PharmCAS and PharmaCAS sends them to your schools. Your application indicates where you want your test scores sent. You MUST include your PCAT CID (Candidate Information Number) from your registration confirmation issued by Pearson. This number is how PharmCAS matches your scores to your application.

HOW PHARMACY SCHOOLS USE PCAT SCORES

The test-maker sets no passing score or range of acceptable scores for the PCAT. Each pharmacy school sets its own policy in terms of scores and admission. Generally, the subtest and composite scores and student percentile ranking are useful tools in estimating the probability of a student's success in pharmacy coursework compared to other students. The test assesses general academic abilities and critical thinking skills, so a good score on the test is considered a good indicator of a person's success in pharmacy school. That said, pharmacy schools combine the information that the PCAT provides them with high school and undergraduate transcripts, interviews, and recommendations to make their admissions selections.

REGISTERING FOR THE PCAT

Although you apply to pharmacy school through PharmCAS, you register for the PCAT through Pearson. Pearson recommends that because seats are limited at testing sites, applicants register early for their preferred test administration date. For a better chance of getting your preferred test date, you should register by the "Register and Schedule By" deadline. Waiting for the "Late Registration and Schedule By" deadline will cost you money and may cost you your preferred test administration, according to Pearson.

The process for registering is straightforward. Once you have submitted your online request to take the PCAT, you will receive an e-mail from Pearson immediately. The e-mail details how to access your Registration Confirmation and how to schedule your seat with a Pearson VUE Test Center. Once you have your Registration Confirmation, you can schedule your seat. To get your preferred location and test date, do this as soon as possible, preferably within 24 hours of receiving your confirmation. Once you have scheduled your seat, you will receive another e-mail confirming the test date and location.

There are certain restrictions on taking the PCAT. You may not take the test more than once in any testing window, that is, within a testing month. You may not change the testing window once you have registered. You may only take the PCAT five times. If you wish to take the test a sixth time, you may need to submit documentation explaining why you want to take it again. You will not be able to

ALERT

Be sure to check to ensure that the pharmacy school(s) you are interested in accept PCAT scores through PharmCAS. If not, you will have to have them sent directly by Pearson to the schools.

ALERT

For a current list of Pearson Vue's Professional Test Centers offering the PCAT in the United States, its territories, and certain select cities abroad, visit PearsonVue.com.

register until this documentation has been received and reviewed, and you are notified that you are approved. The documentation consists of an explanation of why you want to take the test again and either a copy of your application to pharmacy school or to PharmCAS or a letter from a pharmacy school recommending that you take the test and confirming your application for the next year.

PCAT FEES AND SPECIAL ACCOMMODATIONS

The PCAT is not an inexpensive test. The registration fee is $210, which enables you to 1) take the test, 2) receive a preliminary Score Report immediately after you complete the test, 3) have access to your personal Score Report online for a year, 4) print this Score Report for a year, and 5) have three official transcripts sent to three pharmacy schools.

There are additional fees 1) to have transcripts sent to additional schools or to your first three schools if you did not designate them on your registration, 2) for late registration, 3) to have a paper version of your Score Report mailed, 4) for verifying the scores for the multiple-choice subtest should you wish to have them confirmed, and 5) if you wish your essays rescored.

However, there are no fees related to providing special accommodations for those with disabilities. A disability is described under the Americans with Disabilities Act (ADA) as a substantial impairment that "significantly limits or restricts a major life activity." Pearson requires documentation of the disability including a current letter from an appropriate professional about how the disability will affect the ability to take the test and the accommodations that will be required. A signed HIPAA Consent Form is also required. Because it can take up to 60 days to review the request, Pearson recommends submitting the necessary documentation before the "Register and Schedule by" deadline for the testing date that a candidate wishes to register for.

WHAT YOU SHOULD KNOW FOR TEST DAY

The first thing to know about taking the PCAT is that security is very tight. If you break the rules, you could be reported by the proctor and your test could be invalidated. What constitutes an infraction? Any of the following four things:

1. False ID
2. A ringing cell phone or other cell phone noise while in the testing area
3. Checking your cell phone during the break
4. Giving to or receiving any assistance from another test-taker

There are strict requirements for arriving at the test and taking the test in addition to what will get you barred outright from the test.

- You will need "two forms of valid, unexpired ID, one of which **must** contain both your photograph and your signature." A driver's license, a government-issued ID card containing a photo, and a passport are considered primary forms of valid, government-issued ID as long as they have not expired. Valid secondary ID includes credit cards, a library card, and utility bills. However, the name and address must match the information on the primary form of ID that you are submitting for proof.

- Sign-in for the test begins 30 minutes before the scheduled time of your test. It will take this long to go through the process. Arriving more than 15 minutes after your scheduled test time begins bars you from the test, and you will be ineligible to receive any refunds.

- During the sign-in process, you will be required to sign a Candidate Rules Agreement as well as have your photo taken. Depending on the facility, you will be fingerprinted or have an impression of your palm taken.

- After the sign-in, you will be given an erasable noteboard and a marker for notes and calculations and shown to your workstation. Earplugs or headphones are available from the proctor if you wish.

- Before you begin the test, you will need to read and sign an Acknowledgment page on the computer.

- The test is timed and at the appropriate time, a screen will announce your 15-minute break. This is after the Chemical Processes subtest (the third subtest). You will need to raise your hand to alert the proctor. You cannot simply get up and leave; the proctor will "escort you out of the testing room" after shifting your test into break mode. The test resumes in 15 minutes whether you are back or not.

- At the end of the test, you will receive an unofficial preliminary Score Report.

- If you do not think you did well on the test, you may choose the "No Score Option." This cancels your score, so that it is not reported to the schools on your list.

ALERT

What you cannot take to the test: food and beverages; books, notes, reference materials, and papers; highlighters and rulers; earplugs; calculators of any kind; cell phones; recording devices; cameras; and headphones or any other electronic devices.

ALERT

This cannot be repeated enough: Your first and last name must be spelled EXACTLY the same on all forms of identification that you are submitting as proof of who you are. If they do not, you will not be allowed to take the test. Just in case, take several forms of ID.

SUMMING IT UP

- The PCAT assesses five subject areas through a series of five subtests: Writing, Biological Processes, Chemical Processes, Critical Reading, and Quantitative Reasoning.

- Test administration takes four hours plus time for instructions, to familiarize yourself with the machine and testing format, and for one short break between administration of the third and fourth subtest.

- For the Writing section, there is only one prompt. No special knowledge is needed to answer this prompt.

- Each of the other subject areas has forty-eight multiple choice items for a total of 192 multiple-choice items.

- Eight of the forty-eight multiple-choice items in each section will be experimental, that is, they will not count against your score, but you will not know which are experimental.

- Wrong answers do not count against your score.

- The PCAT is a computer-based test and the testing cycle will be January, July, September, and October. The test is not computer-adaptive, however.

- The multiple-choice test items are scored by machine and trained readers evaluate the essays. The official Score Report is available online within five weeks of a test administration. This is the only official report of your score and is available online for a year.

- Scores for the multiple-choice items are reported both as scaled scores (200 to 600) and percentile rankings (1 to 99).

- The Writing subtest is reported as two scores, one score for Conventions of Language and one for Problem Solving. The report shows both a Score and a Mean.

- In addition to accepting applications through PharmCAS, many schools of pharmacy also want PCAT scores reported through PharmCAS Code 104, which is done directly by the test-maker, Pearson.

- The test-maker sets no passing score or range of acceptable scores for the PCAT. Each pharmacy school sets its own policy in terms of scores and admission.

- Generally, the subtest and composite scores and student percentile ranking are useful tools in estimating the probability of a student's success in pharmacy coursework compared to other students.

- Although application to pharmacy school is made through PharmCAS, registration to take the PCAT is made through Pearson. Pearson recommends that because seats are limited at testing sites, applicants register early for their preferred test administration date.

- Once the online request to take the PCAT has been submitted, an applicant will receive an e-mail from Pearson. The e-mail details how to download the Registration Confirmation and how to schedule a seat with a Pearson VUE Test Center.

- The registration fee enables an applicant to 1) take the test, 2) receive a preliminary Score Report immediately after the test, 3) have access to a personal Score Report online for a year, 4) enable the applicant to print this Score Report for a year, and 5) have three official transcripts sent to three pharmacy schools.

- There are no fees related to providing special accommodations, but Pearson requires documentation of a disability and has a lengthy review process.

- Security is tight at Pearson Vue Centers. Two forms of valid, current identification are required. Without them, and if they do not match the information on the initial registration, the applicant will not be allowed to take the test and the registration fee will not be refunded.

- Sign-in for the test is 30 minutes prior to the test administration time. Applicants are required to sign a Candidate Rules Agreement, be fingerprinted or have an impression of his/her palm taken, and sign an Acknowledgement.

- The test is timed with one 15-minute break between the third and fourth subtests. If the candidate is not back by the end of the 15 minutes, the computer program automatically begins the fifth subtest anyway.

- An applicant who does not think he or she did well on the test may choose the "No Score Option" at the end of the test, which cancels the score.

PCAT Questions—
A First Look

OVERVIEW

- **Format of the Test**
- **Writing Subtest**
- **Biological Processes Subtest**
- **Chemical Processes Subtest**
- **Critical Reading Subtest**
- **Quantitative Reasoning Subtest**
- **Top Test-Taking Strategies for the PCAT**
- **Summing It Up**

The PCAT is meant to help admissions committees at pharmacy colleges accept well-qualified applicants. Test items are built on principles and concepts that assess candidates' general academic ability and their knowledge of the fields of biology, chemistry, and mathematics that are the basis for coursework in pharmaceutical studies.

FORMAT OF THE TEST

The PCAT has 192 multiple-choice test items across four subtests and one writing prompt. The entire test will take four hours. However, you need to factor in time for the brief rest break and for instructions before and after the test.

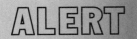

The PCAT looks like this:

PCAT TEST BLUEPRINT

Subtest	Time	Items	Content Areas	Approximate Percentages
Writing	30 min	1	Conventions of Language Problem Solving	
Biological Processes	40 min	48	General Biology	50%
			Microbiology	20%
			Anatomy and Physiology	30%
Chemical Processes	40 min	48	General Chemistry	50%
			Organic Chemistry	30%
			Basic Biochemistry Processes	20%
Critical Reading	50 min	48	Comprehension	30%
			Analysis	40%
			Evaluation	30%
Quantitative Reasoning	50 min	48	Basic Math	25%
			Algebra	25%
			Probability and Statistics	18%
			Precalculus	18%
			Calculus	14%

As you can see, the four subject area subtests all have 48 questions each. However, eight of these questions will be experimental. The experimental items are test items for Pearson and may appear in future tests as scored items. However, they will not count toward your score. But you will not know which multiple-choice items are experimental and which ones will count, so you need to give careful attention to answering each question.

Like all standardized tests, each subtest or section is timed individually. If you finish a subtest before the time is out, you may review items in that subtest, but you may not return to earlier sections, nor may you go on to the next subtest.

WRITING SUBTEST

The good news about the writing prompt is that you will not need any kind of specialized knowledge to answer it (though if you have it, use it!). The topics are highly accessible and take the form of a problem for which you must provide a solution. The topics for the prompts may be based on health; science; or social, cultural, or political issues. A writing prompt might ask you to discuss how local governments could become involved in programs to educate citizens about healthful eating. Or, you might be asked to discuss a solution to air pollution in big cities.

Your solution must be possible and well-thought out. Your writing must be organized, coherent, and concise, with well-supported reasons why your proposed solution would actually work. Scoring depends, in part, on how well writers explain their solutions. This requires an essay of "sufficient length to adequately explain a solution to the problem" according to PCAT. Sound reasoning, clarity of thought, in-depth thinking, and the relevance, specificity, and appropriateness of your supporting arguments will get you a great score.

Now here's the bad news for anyone whose never liked the editing and proofreading steps of the writing process. Your Writing subtest score will rely on the conventions of the English language more heavily than any other major standardized test with a writing section that you have ever taken. The PCAT Test Blueprint lists Conventions of Language above Problem Solving, and the official rubric also has a separate section for the Conventions of Language. According to the rubric, spelling does not seem to count, but the following are all evaluated when scoring essays:

- Essay structure (introduction, body, conclusion)
- Paragraph structure
- Sentence formation
- Variety of sentence structure
- Use of transitional words and phrases
- Usage
- Mechanics

The problem with a poor grasp of formation or structure, usage, and mechanics is that it makes it difficult for the reader to understand the writer's message—what the writer means. Tripping over incorrect grammar, ill-chosen words, and tangled sentences or sentence fragments interrupts the reader's thought process.

BIOLOGICAL PROCESSES SUBTEST

The Biological Processes subtest assesses how well test-takers understand the principles and concepts of basic or general biology, microbiology, and human anatomy and physiology. Questions may be asscociated with a short passage or they may be stand-alone questions independent of a passage. The majority of questions in both the Biological Processes and Chemical Processes subtests will require test-takers to recognize facts and apply basic principles to solve a problem. These questions involve determining the correct principle or equation behind the problem and using it to deduce the correct answer.

NOTE
You will not be given scratch paper to brainstorm and jot down ideas or outline your essay. However, you will be given an erasable board for this purpose.

TIP
Now is the time to assess your writing and identify persistent problems such as run-on sentences, dangling participles, and sentence fragments. Practice, practice, practice to avoid them on test day.

For example:

> Through which of the following mechanisms are amino acids brought to the site of protein synthesis?

In order to answer this question, you need to understand the relation, or workings, between amino acids and protein synthesis and also know what each of the four answer choices relate to. Once you determine this, you will be able to choose the correct answer.

As in the other multiple-choice sections, there are forty core questions and eight experimental questions. Some questions will require you to read diagrams or graphs to find an answer. rewrite: If you have any computations to do, you will be able to use an on-screen calculator during the Biological Processes, Chemical Processes, and Quantitative Reasoning subtests and your erasable white board to sort out your thoughts. One important thing to remember is that in almost all calculations involving temperature, the temperature must be converted from degrees Celsius to degrees Kelvin ($0°C = 273.15K$).

CHEMICAL PROCESSES SUBTEST

Knowledge of the principles and concepts of inorganic and basic organic chemistry is the subject matter of the Chemical Processes subtest. Its approach to questions is similar to the Biological Processes subtest. Questions may be associated with a short passage or they may be stand-alone questions independent of a passage. Like the Biological Processes subtest, the Chemical Processes subtest asks test-takers to recognize facts and apply principles and concepts to solve a problem. For these questions you will need to determine the correct principle or equation that the problem involves in order to select the correct answer.

For example:

> Which type of reaction is represented by the following chemical reaction?

You may never have seen the equation representing the chemical reaction. To answer the question, you need to know what happens in each type of reaction listed and how the equation relates to that type of reaction.

Math calculations may be fairly simple. Many calculations simply involve understanding proportions and will be easy to solve. The key is setting up the ratios correctly to solve for the unknown value.

You may also be asked about groups and trends on the Periodic Table of Elements. This table will be available to you for the Chemical Processes subtest by clicking on "Periodic Table" in the lower left corner of each test item related to it. This periodic table will include each element's symbol, atomic mass, and atomic number.

CRITICAL READING SUBTEST

As the PCAT Test Blueprint for the Critical Reading subtest notes, this section measures test-takers' abilities in the areas of basic comprehension, analysis, and evaluation. Passages are short and not all may be straightforward exposition. You may find some opinion pieces that contain first person narration. Recognizing this may help you in answering questions about the author's opinion and tone.

TIP

Be sure that you know the most important formulas so you can set up ratios correctly.

TIP

Be sure you are familiar with the Periodic Table of Elements. It is also a good idea to know the molecular weight of the more common elements such as O, H, etc.

The topics of the passages are likely to vary from more formal scientific articles to popular science and health topics. The important thing to keep in mind is that you do not need any background in the particular topic to read and answer the questions. All the information is in the passage.

You will find about a third of the Reading Comprehension questions are about basic comprehension and ask you to recall information or make inferences. These are easy to answer because the test questions point you back to the specific context in the passage, which often will contain direct clues. In terms of analysis questions, you may find ones that ask you to break down information in a paragraph or to select the best title for the passage (which is really a question about the main idea of the passage). The final 30 percent of the questions are evaluative and more challenging. These may take the form of question stems that ask:

> Which statement best supports the author's point in . . .
>
> Which of the following statements offers the least support . . .
>
> What additional evidence could the author have used to . . .

Reading passages quickly, but thoughtfully, will help you identify the salient information and figure out the correct answer.

QUANTITATIVE REASONING SUBTEST

According to the PCAT, the Quantitative Reasoning subtest "measures skills in mathematical processes and the ability to reason through and understand quantitative concepts and relationships." The content for this part of the test is basic math, that is, arithmetic processes and concepts such as fractions, decimals, and percents; algebra; probability and statistics; precalculus; and calculus. You may also find some trigonometry and geometry concepts embedded in some questions.

There are typically three types of math questions. 1) Most will be straightforward equations. 2) A few will be word problems that require you to figure out what is being asked. 3) There will also be some questions that require you to interpret graphics or coordinate graphs.

For example:

Evaluate $\dfrac{5^3 \left(4^2 \times 3^4\right)^{\frac{1}{2}}}{15 \times 2^{-1}}$.

What is the probability that each of four consecutive rolls of a regular, six-sided die will produce an even number?

During the Biological Processes, Chemical Processes, and Quantitative Reasoning subtests, a non-scientific standard calculator will be available by clicking on the icon in the upper left corner of each item. Alternatively, you may find using test-taking strategies more useful and less time-consuming in answering some questions than working them out using the calculator or your erasable board. Some strategies to consider are:

- Pick and plug numbers.
- Work backward from the answer choices, beginning with the third answer choice.

TIP

If you find your time running out on this section, go through and answer all the word meaning questions that you can.

TIP

While it is important to be a critical reader, do not spend too much time on each passage or question. In 50 minutes with six passages and eight questions per passage, you have about 8 minutes per passage.

TIP

Be sure you know basic rules such as the rules for factoring exponents and the chain rule.

- Simplify the complex fraction.
- Turn verbose problems into concrete language by eliminating unnecessary information.

Not all problems need to be solved; a careful reading of the answer choices may provide an answer without computation. For example, you can immediately eliminate any answer with the wrong sign.

TOP TEST-TAKING STRATEGIES FOR THE PCAT

Not all strategies will work for all questions, but there are some strategies that will work for most questions:

- Eliminate answer choices you know are incorrect.
- Use educated guessing.
- Skip and return to questions.

The more you practice these and the Quantitative Reasoning strategies, the easier they will be to remember and to apply on test day.

Eliminate Answer Choices You Know Are Incorrect

Don't overlook this time-honored strategy! It will not only help you to arrive at the correct answer, but it can also calm test jitters by helping you narrow down the answers to choose from. In the long run, this strategy may help you save time, since you only need to make educated guesses for the answer options that you did not eliminate.

Use Educated Guessing

Educated guessing builds on the above strategy, but you have to know something about the question for educated guessing to be effective. The process works with these four steps:

1. Eliminate answer choices you know are incorrect.
2. Discard any choices in which part of the answer is incorrect.
3. Reread the remaining answer choices against each other and against the question again.
4. Choose the answer that seems correct to you. More often than not, you'll be right.

Skip and Return to Questions

If at first you don't see how to answer a certain question in a reasonable amount of time, don't hesitate to skip it. After you've answered all the other questions—and before your time for the section has run out—go back to any question you have left unanswered and try to answer it. Remember: There is no wrong-answer penalty, so don't leave any questions unanswered!

SUMMING IT UP

- PCAT test items are built on principles and concepts that assess candidates' general academic ability and their knowledge of the fields of biology, chemistry, and mathematics that are the basis for coursework in pharmaceutical studies.

- The four-hour test has 192 multiple-choice test items across four subtests, and one writing prompt.

- The Writing subtest is timed for 30 minutes and the multiple-choice subtests are timed from 40 minutes for the Biological Processes and Chemical Processes subtests to 45 minutes for the Quantitative Reasoning subtest and 50 minutes for the Critical Reading subtest.

- The four subject area subtests each have 48 questions. However, eight of these questions will be experimental. They do not count toward your score, but you will not know which questions are experimental and which will count.

- Wrong answers do not count against your score.

- Like all standardized tests, each subtest or section is timed individually. If you finish a subtest before the time is up, you may review items in that subtest, but you may not return to earlier sections, nor may you go on to the next subtest.

- The essay prompt takes the form of a problem requiring a solution, but no specialized knowledge is required to answer the essay prompt, which is based on health; science; or social, cultural, or political issues.

- The solution proposed in the essay must be possible and well thought out. Writing must be organized, coherent, and concise, with well-supported reasons why your proposed solution would actually work. Scoring depends in part on how well writers explain their solutions.

- The Writing subtest score relies heavily on how well a writer applies the conventions of the English language. PCAT Test Blueprint lists Conventions of Language above Problem Solving, and the official rubric also has a separate section for the Conventions of Language.

- The Biological Processes subtest assesses how well test-takers understand the principles and concepts of basic or general biology, microbiology, and human anatomy and physiology.

- The Chemical Processes subtest seeks to assess your knowledge of the principles and concepts of inorganic and basic organic chemistry.

- The majority of questions in both the Biological and Chemical Processes subtests involve test-takers in applying basic principles to solve a problem.

- The Critical Reading subtest measures test-takers' abilities in the areas of basic comprehension, analysis, and evaluation. Passages are short and not all may be straightforward exposition; there may be some opinion pieces.

- The topics of the passages are likely to vary from more formal scientific articles to popular science and health topics.

- About 30 percent of the reading comprehension questions are basic comprehension questions, about 40 percent are analysis, and the final 30 percent are evaluative.

- The Quantitative Reasoning subtest measures skills in mathematical processes and reasoning through test items using basic math, algebra, probability and statistics, precalculus, and calculus.

- There are typically three types of math questions. 1) Most will be straightforward equations. 2) A few will be word problems that require you to figure out what is being asked. 3) There will also be some questions that require you to interpret graphics or coordinate graphs.

- A nonscientific standard calculator will be available by clicking on the icon in the upper left corner of each item during the Biological Processes, Chemical Processes, and Quantitative Reasoning subtests. Test-takers are also given erasable boards to work out problems.

- There are three basic strategies to use while taking the PCAT:
  1. Eliminate answer choices you know are incorrect.
  2. Use educated guessing.
  3. Skip and return to questions.

PART II
DIAGNOSING YOUR STRENGTHS AND WEAKNESSES

CHAPTER 3   Practice Test 1: Diagnostic

PRACTICE TEST 1: DIAGNOSTIC ANSWER SHEETS

Biological Processes

1. Ⓐ Ⓑ Ⓒ Ⓓ	11. Ⓐ Ⓑ Ⓒ Ⓓ	21. Ⓐ Ⓑ Ⓒ Ⓓ	31. Ⓐ Ⓑ Ⓒ Ⓓ	40. Ⓐ Ⓑ Ⓒ Ⓓ
2. Ⓐ Ⓑ Ⓒ Ⓓ	12. Ⓐ Ⓑ Ⓒ Ⓓ	22. Ⓐ Ⓑ Ⓒ Ⓓ	32. Ⓐ Ⓑ Ⓒ Ⓓ	41. Ⓐ Ⓑ Ⓒ Ⓓ
3. Ⓐ Ⓑ Ⓒ Ⓓ	13. Ⓐ Ⓑ Ⓒ Ⓓ	23. Ⓐ Ⓑ Ⓒ Ⓓ	33. Ⓐ Ⓑ Ⓒ Ⓓ	42. Ⓐ Ⓑ Ⓒ Ⓓ
4. Ⓐ Ⓑ Ⓒ Ⓓ	14. Ⓐ Ⓑ Ⓒ Ⓓ	24. Ⓐ Ⓑ Ⓒ Ⓓ	34. Ⓐ Ⓑ Ⓒ Ⓓ	43. Ⓐ Ⓑ Ⓒ Ⓓ
5. Ⓐ Ⓑ Ⓒ Ⓓ	15. Ⓐ Ⓑ Ⓒ Ⓓ	25. Ⓐ Ⓑ Ⓒ Ⓓ	35. Ⓐ Ⓑ Ⓒ Ⓓ	44. Ⓐ Ⓑ Ⓒ Ⓓ
6. Ⓐ Ⓑ Ⓒ Ⓓ	16. Ⓐ Ⓑ Ⓒ Ⓓ	26. Ⓐ Ⓑ Ⓒ Ⓓ	36. Ⓐ Ⓑ Ⓒ Ⓓ	45. Ⓐ Ⓑ Ⓒ Ⓓ
7. Ⓐ Ⓑ Ⓒ Ⓓ	17. Ⓐ Ⓑ Ⓒ Ⓓ	27. Ⓐ Ⓑ Ⓒ Ⓓ	37. Ⓐ Ⓑ Ⓒ Ⓓ	46. Ⓐ Ⓑ Ⓒ Ⓓ
8. Ⓐ Ⓑ Ⓒ Ⓓ	18. Ⓐ Ⓑ Ⓒ Ⓓ	28. Ⓐ Ⓑ Ⓒ Ⓓ	38. Ⓐ Ⓑ Ⓒ Ⓓ	47. Ⓐ Ⓑ Ⓒ Ⓓ
9. Ⓐ Ⓑ Ⓒ Ⓓ	19. Ⓐ Ⓑ Ⓒ Ⓓ	29. Ⓐ Ⓑ Ⓒ Ⓓ	39. Ⓐ Ⓑ Ⓒ Ⓓ	48. Ⓐ Ⓑ Ⓒ Ⓓ
10. Ⓐ Ⓑ Ⓒ Ⓓ	20. Ⓐ Ⓑ Ⓒ Ⓓ	30. Ⓐ Ⓑ Ⓒ Ⓓ		

Chemical Processes

1. Ⓐ Ⓑ Ⓒ Ⓓ	11. Ⓐ Ⓑ Ⓒ Ⓓ	21. Ⓐ Ⓑ Ⓒ Ⓓ	31. Ⓐ Ⓑ Ⓒ Ⓓ	40. Ⓐ Ⓑ Ⓒ Ⓓ
2. Ⓐ Ⓑ Ⓒ Ⓓ	12. Ⓐ Ⓑ Ⓒ Ⓓ	22. Ⓐ Ⓑ Ⓒ Ⓓ	32. Ⓐ Ⓑ Ⓒ Ⓓ	41. Ⓐ Ⓑ Ⓒ Ⓓ
3. Ⓐ Ⓑ Ⓒ Ⓓ	13. Ⓐ Ⓑ Ⓒ Ⓓ	23. Ⓐ Ⓑ Ⓒ Ⓓ	33. Ⓐ Ⓑ Ⓒ Ⓓ	42. Ⓐ Ⓑ Ⓒ Ⓓ
4. Ⓐ Ⓑ Ⓒ Ⓓ	14. Ⓐ Ⓑ Ⓒ Ⓓ	24. Ⓐ Ⓑ Ⓒ Ⓓ	34. Ⓐ Ⓑ Ⓒ Ⓓ	43. Ⓐ Ⓑ Ⓒ Ⓓ
5. Ⓐ Ⓑ Ⓒ Ⓓ	15. Ⓐ Ⓑ Ⓒ Ⓓ	25. Ⓐ Ⓑ Ⓒ Ⓓ	35. Ⓐ Ⓑ Ⓒ Ⓓ	44. Ⓐ Ⓑ Ⓒ Ⓓ
6. Ⓐ Ⓑ Ⓒ Ⓓ	16. Ⓐ Ⓑ Ⓒ Ⓓ	26. Ⓐ Ⓑ Ⓒ Ⓓ	36. Ⓐ Ⓑ Ⓒ Ⓓ	45. Ⓐ Ⓑ Ⓒ Ⓓ
7. Ⓐ Ⓑ Ⓒ Ⓓ	17. Ⓐ Ⓑ Ⓒ Ⓓ	27. Ⓐ Ⓑ Ⓒ Ⓓ	37. Ⓐ Ⓑ Ⓒ Ⓓ	46. Ⓐ Ⓑ Ⓒ Ⓓ
8. Ⓐ Ⓑ Ⓒ Ⓓ	18. Ⓐ Ⓑ Ⓒ Ⓓ	28. Ⓐ Ⓑ Ⓒ Ⓓ	38. Ⓐ Ⓑ Ⓒ Ⓓ	47. Ⓐ Ⓑ Ⓒ Ⓓ
9. Ⓐ Ⓑ Ⓒ Ⓓ	19. Ⓐ Ⓑ Ⓒ Ⓓ	29. Ⓐ Ⓑ Ⓒ Ⓓ	39. Ⓐ Ⓑ Ⓒ Ⓓ	48. Ⓐ Ⓑ Ⓒ Ⓓ
10. Ⓐ Ⓑ Ⓒ Ⓓ	20. Ⓐ Ⓑ Ⓒ Ⓓ	30. Ⓐ Ⓑ Ⓒ Ⓓ		

Critical Reading

1. Ⓐ Ⓑ Ⓒ Ⓓ	11. Ⓐ Ⓑ Ⓒ Ⓓ	21. Ⓐ Ⓑ Ⓒ Ⓓ	31. Ⓐ Ⓑ Ⓒ Ⓓ	40. Ⓐ Ⓑ Ⓒ Ⓓ
2. Ⓐ Ⓑ Ⓒ Ⓓ	12. Ⓐ Ⓑ Ⓒ Ⓓ	22. Ⓐ Ⓑ Ⓒ Ⓓ	32. Ⓐ Ⓑ Ⓒ Ⓓ	41. Ⓐ Ⓑ Ⓒ Ⓓ
3. Ⓐ Ⓑ Ⓒ Ⓓ	13. Ⓐ Ⓑ Ⓒ Ⓓ	23. Ⓐ Ⓑ Ⓒ Ⓓ	33. Ⓐ Ⓑ Ⓒ Ⓓ	42. Ⓐ Ⓑ Ⓒ Ⓓ
4. Ⓐ Ⓑ Ⓒ Ⓓ	14. Ⓐ Ⓑ Ⓒ Ⓓ	24. Ⓐ Ⓑ Ⓒ Ⓓ	34. Ⓐ Ⓑ Ⓒ Ⓓ	43. Ⓐ Ⓑ Ⓒ Ⓓ
5. Ⓐ Ⓑ Ⓒ Ⓓ	15. Ⓐ Ⓑ Ⓒ Ⓓ	25. Ⓐ Ⓑ Ⓒ Ⓓ	35. Ⓐ Ⓑ Ⓒ Ⓓ	44. Ⓐ Ⓑ Ⓒ Ⓓ
6. Ⓐ Ⓑ Ⓒ Ⓓ	16. Ⓐ Ⓑ Ⓒ Ⓓ	26. Ⓐ Ⓑ Ⓒ Ⓓ	36. Ⓐ Ⓑ Ⓒ Ⓓ	45. Ⓐ Ⓑ Ⓒ Ⓓ
7. Ⓐ Ⓑ Ⓒ Ⓓ	17. Ⓐ Ⓑ Ⓒ Ⓓ	27. Ⓐ Ⓑ Ⓒ Ⓓ	37. Ⓐ Ⓑ Ⓒ Ⓓ	46. Ⓐ Ⓑ Ⓒ Ⓓ
8. Ⓐ Ⓑ Ⓒ Ⓓ	18. Ⓐ Ⓑ Ⓒ Ⓓ	28. Ⓐ Ⓑ Ⓒ Ⓓ	38. Ⓐ Ⓑ Ⓒ Ⓓ	47. Ⓐ Ⓑ Ⓒ Ⓓ
9. Ⓐ Ⓑ Ⓒ Ⓓ	19. Ⓐ Ⓑ Ⓒ Ⓓ	29. Ⓐ Ⓑ Ⓒ Ⓓ	39. Ⓐ Ⓑ Ⓒ Ⓓ	48. Ⓐ Ⓑ Ⓒ Ⓓ
10. Ⓐ Ⓑ Ⓒ Ⓓ	20. Ⓐ Ⓑ Ⓒ Ⓓ	30. Ⓐ Ⓑ Ⓒ Ⓓ		

answer sheet

Quantitative Reasoning

1. Ⓐ Ⓑ Ⓒ Ⓓ 11. Ⓐ Ⓑ Ⓒ Ⓓ 21. Ⓐ Ⓑ Ⓒ Ⓓ 31. Ⓐ Ⓑ Ⓒ Ⓓ 40. Ⓐ Ⓑ Ⓒ Ⓓ

2. Ⓐ Ⓑ Ⓒ Ⓓ 12. Ⓐ Ⓑ Ⓒ Ⓓ 22. Ⓐ Ⓑ Ⓒ Ⓓ 32. Ⓐ Ⓑ Ⓒ Ⓓ 41. Ⓐ Ⓑ Ⓒ Ⓓ

3. Ⓐ Ⓑ Ⓒ Ⓓ 13. Ⓐ Ⓑ Ⓒ Ⓓ 23. Ⓐ Ⓑ Ⓒ Ⓓ 33. Ⓐ Ⓑ Ⓒ Ⓓ 42. Ⓐ Ⓑ Ⓒ Ⓓ

4. Ⓐ Ⓑ Ⓒ Ⓓ 14. Ⓐ Ⓑ Ⓒ Ⓓ 24. Ⓐ Ⓑ Ⓒ Ⓓ 34. Ⓐ Ⓑ Ⓒ Ⓓ 43. Ⓐ Ⓑ Ⓒ Ⓓ

5. Ⓐ Ⓑ Ⓒ Ⓓ 15. Ⓐ Ⓑ Ⓒ Ⓓ 25. Ⓐ Ⓑ Ⓒ Ⓓ 35. Ⓐ Ⓑ Ⓒ Ⓓ 44. Ⓐ Ⓑ Ⓒ Ⓓ

6. Ⓐ Ⓑ Ⓒ Ⓓ 16. Ⓐ Ⓑ Ⓒ Ⓓ 26. Ⓐ Ⓑ Ⓒ Ⓓ 36. Ⓐ Ⓑ Ⓒ Ⓓ 45. Ⓐ Ⓑ Ⓒ Ⓓ

7. Ⓐ Ⓑ Ⓒ Ⓓ 17. Ⓐ Ⓑ Ⓒ Ⓓ 27. Ⓐ Ⓑ Ⓒ Ⓓ 37. Ⓐ Ⓑ Ⓒ Ⓓ 46. Ⓐ Ⓑ Ⓒ Ⓓ

8. Ⓐ Ⓑ Ⓒ Ⓓ 18. Ⓐ Ⓑ Ⓒ Ⓓ 28. Ⓐ Ⓑ Ⓒ Ⓓ 38. Ⓐ Ⓑ Ⓒ Ⓓ 47. Ⓐ Ⓑ Ⓒ Ⓓ

9. Ⓐ Ⓑ Ⓒ Ⓓ 19. Ⓐ Ⓑ Ⓒ Ⓓ 29. Ⓐ Ⓑ Ⓒ Ⓓ 39. Ⓐ Ⓑ Ⓒ Ⓓ 48. Ⓐ Ⓑ Ⓒ Ⓓ

10. Ⓐ Ⓑ Ⓒ Ⓓ 20. Ⓐ Ⓑ Ⓒ Ⓓ 30. Ⓐ Ⓑ Ⓒ Ⓓ

SECTION 1: WRITING

1 Essay • 30 Minutes

> **Directions:** Answer the following prompt in 30 minutes.

Since 1950, 90% of the world's stocks of cod, tuna, flounder, halibut, and other fish have disappeared due to such factors as overfishing, pollution, and climate change. Discuss a solution to our having lost 90% of our fish stocks.

_____

_____

_____

_____

_____

_____

_____

_____

_____

_____

_____

_____

_____

_____

_____

_____

_____

diagnostic test

SECTION 2: BIOLOGICAL PROCESSES

48 Items • 40 Minutes

Directions: Choose the best answer for each question.

Refer to the following passage for Questions 1–6.

Nucleic acids are the biomolecule that contain all of one's genetic material. Per the central dogma of molecular biology, DNA encodes mRNA, which in turn provides the blueprint for protein synthesis. This occurs in both eukaryotic and pro-karyotic cells, with an extra splicing step between transcription and translation in eukaryotes.

1. Which of the following joins together nucleotides in a polynucleotide molecule?
   A. A hydrogen bond between a 5'OH group and a 3' phosphate group
   B. A hydrogen bond between a 5'OH group of each nucleotide
   C. A phosphodiester linkage between a 5'OH group and a 3' phosphate group
   D. A phosphodiester linkage between a 3'OH group and a 5' phosphate group

2. The 5' cap on mRNA is a
   A. modified guanine residue.
   B. polyA. tail.
   C. phosphate group.
   D. stop codon.

3. All cellular material except DNA is repli-cated during which phase of the cell cycle?
   A. G_0
   B. G_1
   C. G_2
   D. S

4. Which enzyme acts specifically to relieve the strain caused by unwinding a DNA double helix?
   A. DNA polymerase
   B. Topoisomerase
   C. DNA helicase
   D. DNA ligase

5. Which is the first transcription factor to bind DNA in order to form an initiation complex?
   A. RNA polymerase II
   B. TFIIA
   C. TFIIC
   D. TFIID

6. Which of the following is a TRUE statement about DNA replication?
   A. New DNA strands can form inde-pendent of existing DNA.
   B. New DNA strands are only synthe-sized in the 3' to 5' direction.
   C. New DNA strands are only synthe-sized in the 5' to 3' direction.
   D. DNA replication results in one new double-stranded DNA molecule.

7. The term *Homo sapiens sapiens* reveals which levels of organization in humans?
   A. Domain, kingdom, phylum
   B. Phylum, class, order
   C. Order, family, genus
   D. Genus, species, subspecies

8. Which region of a phospholipid in cell membrane bilayer faces into the cell's cytoplasm?
   - A. Phosphate group
   - B. Hydrophilic head
   - C. Hydrophobic tail
   - D. Nonpolar region

9. Which of the following best describes the function of an enzyme in a biological reaction?
   - A. Enzymes speed up a reaction by increasing the activation energy.
   - B. Enzymes alter the products of a chemical reaction.
   - C. Enzymes speed up a reaction by lowering the activation energy.
   - D. Enzymes are nonspecific and can increase the speed of a wide range of reactions.

10. Which of the following is a TRUE statement about a reaction in which $\Delta G = -2870$ KJ/mol?
   - A. The reaction requires the addition of energy to move forward.
   - B. The reaction moves spontaneously in the forward direction.
   - C. The reaction is endergonic.
   - D. The reaction is in equilibrium.

11. During the photosynthesis reaction, glucose is produced from
   - A. CO_2 and H_2O.
   - B. H_2O and O_2.
   - C. O_2 and CO_2.
   - D. CO_2 and ATP.

12. A point mutation that causes translation to stop prematurely is called a
   - A. silent mutation.
   - B. missense mutation.
   - C. nonsense mutation.
   - D. stop mutation.

13. Which of the following is an example of a physical adaptation of birds that live in an environment where the primary food source is nuts and seeds?
   - A. Long, thin beak
   - B. Strong, curved beak
   - C. Dexterous beak that can hold twigs
   - D. Small pointy beak

14. In general, bacteria that have flagella are classified as
   - A. bacilli or spirilla.
   - B. bacilli or cocci.
   - C. spirilla or cocci.
   - D. cocci or vibrio.

15. Which of the following enzymes aids the absorption of nutrients by fungi?
   - A. Fungases
   - B. Polymerases
   - C. Exoenzymes
   - D. Lysosomes

16. Which of the following statements describes what happens during the viral uncoating process?
   - A. The virus attaches to the host cell.
   - B. Genetic material is released into the host cell.
   - C. The viral genome is transcribed into mRNA.
   - D. The virus is taken into the host cell.

17. In mitosis, the nucleus dissolves and the microtubules attach to centromeres during
   - A. interphase.
   - B. prophase.
   - C. prometaphase.
   - D. metaphase.

Refer to the following passage for Questions 18–23.

Photosynthesis is a key process that allows plants, fungi, and other organisms to store energy in the form of glucose. When the energy is required for cellular processes, cellular respiration allows for its release in the form of adenosine triphosphate (ATP). Significant energy is stored within ATP, making this an ideal molecule to serve as the energetic currency for cellular processes.

18. Photoautotrophs are photosynthetic bacteria that depend upon
   A. light and H_2O.
   B. light and O_2.
   C. light and CO_2.
   D. light and N_2.

19. Which of the following statements is TRUE?
   A. As cells become more active, ATP production decreases.
   B. As cells become more active, ATP production increases.
   C. As cells become less active, ATP production increases.
   D. ATP production always occurs at a stable rate.

20. In processes of cellular metabolism, the most ATP is produced in which of the following steps?
   A. Glycolysis
   B. Krebs cycle
   C. Oxidative phosphorylation
   D. Fermentation

21. Which portion of an ATP molecule plays an important role in providing energy to a cell?
   A. Nitrogenous base
   B. Pentose
   C. Phosphate bonds
   D. Phosphate group

22. Which type of transport across the cell membrane requires ATP?
   A. Osmosis
   B. Facilitated transport
   C. Active transport
   D. Diffusion

23. Glucose molecules are broken down and oxidized to form two pyruvate molecules in
   A. oxidative phosphorylation.
   B. the citric acid cycle.
   C. photosynthesis.
   D. glycolysis.

Refer to the following passage for Questions 24–28.

Positively charged cations play critical roles in the functioning of the human body. Some roles are direct roles that involve formation of important compounds, while others are more indirect, in which ion movement or presence causes some other effect.

24. In general, a higher concentration of Na^+ ions is found
   A. inside a cell.
   B. outside a cell.
   C. inside the nucleus.
   D. inside the plasma membrane.

25. An excess of thyroxine and triiodothryonine produced by the thyroid causes
   A. high blood-calcium levels.
   B. low blood-calcium levels.
   C. hypothyroidism.
   D. hyperthyroidism.

26. Which cation is pumped across a membrane to generate ATP during chemiosmosis of cellular respiration?
   A. Na^+
   B. Ca^{2+}
   C. Mg^{2+}
   D. H^+

27. A critical cation that accounts for 2% of body mass and is essential for bone maintenance is:
    A. Na^+
    B. Ca^{2+}
    C. Mg^{2+}
    D. H^+

28. Which organelle of the cell is responsible for the capture and storage of calcium ions?
    A. Smooth ER
    B. Rough ER
    C. Ribosome
    D. Lysosome

29. A condyloid joint exhibits which of the following types of motion?
    A. Gliding
    B. Rotational
    C. Angular
    D. Hinged

30. According to the sliding filament model of muscle contraction, which part of the muscle contracts?
    A. Myosin
    B. Sarcomere
    C. Thin actin filament
    D. Thick myosin filament

31. The tempo at which the heart beats is regulated by the
    A. left atrium.
    B. right atrium.
    C. sinoatrial node.
    D. autorhythmic cells.

32. The step that occurs in the viral lytic life cycle, but not the viral lysogenic life cycle, is
    A. attachment.
    B. injection.
    C. DNA attachment.
    D. shutdown.

33. During the sexual reproduction of fungi, the fusion of the two parent cytoplasm is called
    A. plasmogamy.
    B. karyogamy.
    C. meiosis.
    D. germination.

34. Cells that provide protection against future reinfection by a particular virus are called
    A. host cells.
    B. memory B cells.
    C. T cells.
    D. B-lymphocytes.

35. Which of the following offers the best explanation as to why alveoli are formed in grape-like clusters at the ends of each bronchiole?
    A. The clusters more firmly attach to the ends of the bronchiole.
    B. The clusters cause an increase in surface area to take in O_2.
    C. The clusters allow more CO_2 into the lungs.
    D. The clusters allow for a better exchange of O_2 and CO_2.

36. Absorption of nutrients into the bloodstream mostly occurs in the
    A. stomach.
    B. large intestine.
    C. small intestine.
    D. pancreas.

37. Urine is concentrated in the
    A. juxtamedullary nephron capillary beds.
    B. peritubular capillary beds.
    C. glomerular capillary beds.
    D. corticoid nephrons.

38. An increase in estrogen levels inhibits
    A. FSH and LH.
    B. FSH and GnRH.
    C. GnRH and LH.
    D. progesterone and LH

39. Before being transported to specialized organs for processing and removal from the body, microbes or toxins at infection sites are picked up by which of the following?
    A. Lymph
    B. Blood cells
    C. Antibodies
    D. T cells

40. In a cross between two heterozygous individuals, what percentage of offspring would be homozygous for the recessive trait?
    A. 75%
    B. 50%
    C. 25%
    D. 10%

41. Which type of coenzyme links together two redox reactions?
    A. Hydrogen carrier
    B. Flavin vitamins
    C. Electron carriers
    D. Coenzyme A

42. Which of the following is the best explanation as to why the Hardy-Weinberg theorem can be used as an approximation of genotype and phenotype frequencies?
    A. The rate of evolution in a species is very fast.
    B. The rate of evolution in species is very slow.
    C. Evolution follows the bottleneck effect.
    D. Evolution follows the founder effect.

43. The inheritance pattern in which the gene at one locus alters the phenotypic expression of a gene at a separate locus is called
    A. pleiotropy.
    B. polygenic inheritance.
    C. epistasis.
    D. pedigree.

44. Variation in genetic traits is due in part to
    A. dominant alleles.
    B. recessive alleles.
    C. a large genome.
    D. homozygous alleles.

45. Bile is produced in the
    A. liver.
    B. pancreas.
    C. gallbladder.
    D. large intestine.

46. The fin of a shark that emerges from the surface of the ocean as the shark reaches the ocean surface is located on its ___ side.
    A. caudal
    B. dorsal
    C. lateral
    D. ventral

47. The metatarsals of a human would be found in his or her
  A. cranium.
  B. feet.
  C. hands.
  D. ribcage.

48. If you cracked your patella, you have hurt your
  A. ankle.
  B. knee.
  C. thigh.
  D. wrist.

SECTION 3: CHEMICAL PROCESSES

48 Items • 40 Minutes

Directions: Choose the best answer for each question.

Refer to the following passage for Questions 1–5.

Understanding orbitals and their interactions is an important step in understanding how bonds form between elements. Orbitals occupied by valence electrons interact in interesting ways, with their properties described by such models as hybrid orbitals and molecular orbital theory.

1. Which of the following shows the correct order in which electrons occupy atomic orbitals?
   A. $4p \rightarrow 4s \rightarrow 3d \rightarrow 3p \rightarrow 3s \rightarrow 2p \rightarrow 2s \rightarrow 1s$
   B. $1s \rightarrow 2s \rightarrow 2p \rightarrow 3s \rightarrow 3p \rightarrow 3d \rightarrow 4s \rightarrow 4p$
   C. $1s \rightarrow 2s \rightarrow 2p \rightarrow 3s \rightarrow 3p \rightarrow 4s \rightarrow 3d \rightarrow 4p$
   D. $4p \rightarrow 3d \rightarrow 4s \rightarrow 3p \rightarrow 3s \rightarrow 2p \rightarrow$

2. Which type of orbitals would be expected in the molecule $H - C \equiv C - H$?
   A. p, sp
   B. p, sp^2
   C. p, sp^3
   D. $sp, sp^2 \, 2s \rightarrow 1s$

3. Which quantum number indicates the shape of an atomic orbital?
   A. Angular momentum quantum number
   B. Principle quantum number
   C. Magnetic quantum number
   D. Electron spin quantum number

4. A double bond forms when which of the following bonds exist between two atoms?
   A. $2 \, \sigma$ bonds
   B. $2 \, \pi$ bonds
   C. $1 \, \sigma$ bond, $1 \, \pi$ bond
   D. $2 \, \sigma$ bonds, $2 \, \pi$ bonds

5. What is the lowest possible principle quantum number for a *d* orbital?
   A. 1
   B. 2
   C. 3
   D. 4

Refer to the following passage for Questions 6–8.

Of the three phases of matter, gases are least dense and can be most highly manipulated, as their shape and volume are not set. When performing calculations with gases, it is often assumed that gases behave ideally, which ignores certain properties of gases per the kinetic molecular theory of gases, including the fact that gas molecules have volume, among others.

6. Which of the following gases are normally found as diatomic molecules?
   A. Nitrogen and oxygen
   B. Nitrogen and ozone
   C. Oxygen and carbon dioxide
   D. Nitrogen and sulfur dioxide

7. Calculate the pressure of a 250 mL sample of 0.6 mol of gas at 298K. The gas constant is R = 0.082 L.atm/K.mol.
   A. 0.058 atm
   B. 58.6 atm
   C. 3.66 atm
   D. 3665 atm

8. According to the kinetic molecular theory of gases,
   A. gas molecules are in a fixed position in space.
   B. gas molecules do not exert attractive or repulsive forces on each other.
   C. gas molecules do exert attractive and repulsive forces on each other.
   D. the average kinetic energy of a gas molecule is independent of temperature.

Refer to the following passage for Questions 9–12.

Chemical nomenclature helps to keep chemistry universal. Consistently naming functional groups, recognizing structural formulas, and identifying patterns in chemical structures allows for chemists from a variety of backgrounds to converge and understand one another.

9. Which of the following is an example of an amine compound?
   A. $CH_3CH_2NO_2$
   B. $CH_3CH_2NH_2$
   C. $CH_3C \equiv N$
   D. $CH_3C = ONH_2$

10. What are the ionic components of the compound magnesium nitride, $Mg3N_2$?
   A. Mg and N
   B. Mg^{2+} and N_2
   C. Mg^{2+} and N^{3-}
   D. Mg^+ and N^-

11. What is the most accurate classification of the compound below?

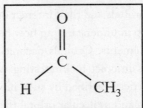

   A. Carboxylic acid
   B. Ketone
   C. Aldehyde
   D. Ester

12. Which type of functional group always contains a carbon-carbon triple bond?
   A. Alkane
   B. Alkene
   C. Alkyne
   D. Aromatic

Refer to the following passage for Questions 13–16.

Hemoglobin is a protein that carries oxygen to the cells of the human body and carbon dioxide to the lungs. Hemoglobin is composed of four symmetrical polypeptide chains and four heme cofactors that contain iron, the metal that binds oxygen.

13. The monomeric subunit that composes hemoglobin is the
   A. amino acid.
   B. fatty acid.
   C. monosaccharide.
   D. nucleotide.

14. What is the most complex level of protein structure that exists in hemoglobin?
    A. Primary
    B. Secondary
    C. Tertiary
    D. Quaternary

15. Hemoglobin is produced at the
    A. nucleolus.
    B. nucleus.
    C. ribosome.
    D. smooth endoplasmic reticulum (ER).

16. The red color of hemoglobin can be explained by:
    A. the interaction of heme's iron and oxygen.
    B. the three-dimensional shape of the protein.
    C intrinsically fluorescent residues within the protein.
    D. hydrogen bonds between heme and the protein.

Refer to the following passage for Questions 17–19

The structure of cholesterol is shown below:

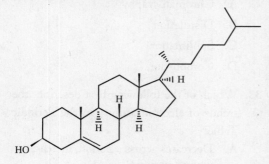

Cholesterol is a key component of animal cell plasma membranes, keeping it from becoming too fluid.

17. Based on the structure of cholesterol, which type of biomolecule is cholesterol?
    A. Carbohydrate
    B. Lipid
    C. Nucleic Acid
    D. Protein

18. Based on its structure, where on the plasma membrane would you expect the bulk of cholesterol to be located?
    A. On the internal cell surface
    B. On the external cell surface
    C. In the interior of the membrane
    D. Loosely associated with the membrane via intermolecular forces

19. The presence of cholesterol in animal cells prevents the need for a
    A. cell wall.
    B. cytoskeleton.
    C. Golgi apparatus.
    D. peroxisome.

20. The exact temperature and pressure at which a substance can exist in all three states is the
    A. melting point.
    B. critical point.
    C. triple point.
    D. freezing point

21. According to Bohr's atomic model, the energy level is greater
    A. when the energy level is constant throughout the atom.
    B. in the nucleus of an atom.
    C. in the first electron orbital.
    D. in the electron orbital farthest from the nucleus.

22. Elements that have only one valence electron are categorized as
    A. alkaline earth metals.
    B. alkali metals.
    C. transition metals.
    D. halogens.

23. If a central atom can form three covalent bonds with no lone pairs, what geometric configuration is the molecule likely to adopt?
    A. Linear
    B. Trigonal planar
    C. Tetrahedral
    D. Trigonal bipyramidal

24. What are the two main products of a neutralization reaction?
    A. Salt and water
    B. Acid and base
    C. Salt and carbon dioxide
    D. Acid and water

25. Which two types of forces cause the capillary action observed in liquids?
    A. Attraction and repulsive
    B. Surface tension and viscosity
    C. Cohesion and adhesion
    D. Intermolecular and intramolecular

26. Calculate the molarity of a solution containing 6.22 g of NaOH in 500 mL.
    A. 0.012 M
    B. 12.440 M
    C. 0.0003 M
    D. 0.311 M

27. A Lewis acid is defined as an
    A. electron pair donor.
    B. electron pair acceptor.
    C. H^+ donor.
    D. H^+ acceptor.

28. Which half-reaction is the oxidation reaction in the following chemical equation: $6Fe^{2+} + 14H^+ + Cr_2O_7^{2-} \rightarrow 6Fe^{3+} + 2Cr^{3+} + 7H_2O$?
    A. $6Fe^{2+} \rightarrow 6Fe^{3+}$
    B. $14H^+ \rightarrow 7H_2O$
    C. $Cr_2O_7^{2-} \rightarrow 2Cr^{3+}$
    D. $14H^+ + Cr_2O_7^{2-} \rightarrow 2Cr^{3+} + 7H_2O$

29. Which of the following is described as the heat content of a substance under constant pressure?
    A. Energy
    B. Enthalpy
    C. Entropy
    D. Specific heat

30. In a reaction where rate = $k[A]^2[B]$, what is the overall reaction order?
    A. −1
    B. 1
    C. 2
    D. 3

31. In which steps in a radical reaction is the product cycled back to the initial reaction to form a reaction loop?
    A. Initiation steps
    B. Propagation steps
    C. Termination steps
    D. Substitution steps

32. Which of the following methods will best separate several high boiling liquids when they are dissolved in an organic solution?
    A. Chromatography
    B. Distillation
    C. Sublimation
    D. Combustion

33. Which of the following best describes the trends of electron affinity in the Periodic Table?
    A. Decreases across a period, increases down a period
    B. Decreases across a period, decreases down a period
    C. Increases across a period, decreases down a period
    D. Increases across a period, increases down a period

34. The formation of cation radicals occurs in which method of spectroscopy?
    A. Mass spectroscopy
    B. IR spectroscopy
    C. NMR spectroscopy
    D. UV-Vis spectroscopy

35. In a high-field NMR spectroscope, which groups of highlighted protons below couple to give the highest number of multiplet peaks in the ^1H NMR spectrum?
    A. $CH_3CH_2CH_2CH_2COOH$
    B. $CH_3CH_2CH_2CH2COOH$
    C. $CH_3CH_2CH_2COOH$
    D. $CH_3CH_2CH_2COOH$

36. From what angle does an entering nucleophile attack its substrate in an S_N2 reaction?
    A. 90°
    B. 120°
    C. 180°
    D. 240°

37. Which of the following is an example of a homogenous mixture?
    A. Colloid
    B. Emulsion
    C. Solution
    D. Suspension

38. Which specific type of energy is required in the phase change from a solid to a liquid?
    A. Mechanical energy
    B. Potential energy
    C. Kinetic energy
    D. Thermal energy

39. A reaction in which a carbon-carbon double bond is formed and a functional group is removed at the same time is called a(n)
    A. E1 reaction.
    B. E2 reaction.
    C. S_N1 reaction.
    D. S_N2 reaction.

40. Determine how many moles of water are produced if 0.376 moles of methanol are burned in the reaction $2CH_3OH + 3O_2 \rightarrow 2CO_2 + 4H_2O$.
    A. 0.376
    B. 0.752
    C. 1.504
    D. 4.000

41. Which of the following describes the entropy of a system during a spontaneous reaction?
    A. $S = 0$
    B. $S < 0$
    C. $S > 0$
    D. $S = 1$

42. Which of the following is the best method for purifying a solid product from any remaining reactant material?
    A. Extraction
    B. Crystallization
    C. Chromatography
    D. Distillation

43. The relative position of shared electrons between two atoms is most dependent on the
    A. size of the atoms.
    B. number of electrons.
    C. types of hybrid orbitals.
    D. electronegativity of the atoms.

44. What type of reaction does the following potential energy diagram represent?

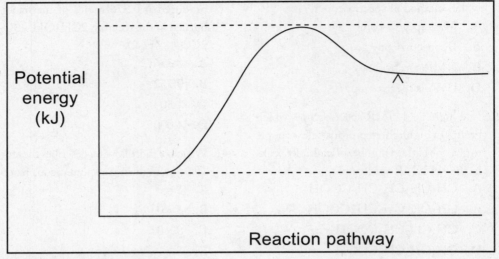

A. Exothermic reaction

B. Endothermic reaction

C. Equilibrium reaction

D. Spontaneous reaction

45. The ^{13}C NMR mode that provides the most detailed information is the
   A. gated-decoupled mode.
   B. proton noise-decoupled mode.
   C. off-resonance mode.
   D. integration mode.

46. In double-stranded DNA, guanine pairs with which base?
   A. Adenine
   B. Cytosine
   C. Thymine
   D. Uracil

47. The type of RNA that possesses anticodons for efficient protein synthesis is
   A. cDNA.
   B. mRNA.
   C. rRNA.
   D. tRNA.

48. How many monosaccharides are in an oligosaccharide?
   A. 1
   B. 2
   C. 3-6
   D. >6

SECTION 4: CRITICAL READING

48 Items • 50 Minutes

> **Directions:** Choose the best answer for each question.

Refer to the following passage for Questions 1–8.

(1)   Why is a course of antibiotics typically given over seven days? This was a question posed by Harvard psychology professor Daniel Gilbert in a 2010 opinion piece for the *New York Times*. Gilbert's article, entitled "Magic by the Numbers," attributes the seven of the seven-day course to nothing less than magic. Why? Certain numbers, according to Gilbert, have magical properties; for most of us mortals, they include the numbers related to time (such as 7, 12, and 24) and the numbers related to ten, in which, Gilbert asserts, people tend to think. (For the latter phenomenon, he boils the bulk of his explanation down to the existence of five fingers on one hand and five on the other and sums it all up with "it isn't hard to understand why an animal with ten fingers would use a base-ten counting system.")

(2)   Forgetting the magic of ten for the purposes of evaluating doctors' common recommendations, and returning to seven, why should Gilbert—or you or anyone else—receive a course of antibiotics and be told that it should be taken over seven, and not, for example, six or nine days? According to Gilbert, the answer is not just magic, but also ancient Rome. He claims the cause is the Roman emperor Constantine's reduction of the week from eight days to seven in 321 A.D.

(3)   Returning to the science of the issue, Gilbert quotes an author of a study in a respected medical journal who states that the usual recommendation of a course of antibiotics over seven to ten days for uncomplicated pneumonia is *not* based on scientific evidence. This lends credence to the number of dosage days as a cultural rather than empirical matter.

(4)   Gilbert probes further by going on to query whether, in a given seven-day course, at an assumed or typical rate of three pills per day, it might be possible that just one of those twenty-one pills is not in fact necessary. That is, what if millions of people are taking approximately five percent more medicine than they require? What are the implications of relying on the magic number seven in that case? Any reader can provide the answer on his or her own, but Gilbert spells it out. Our magical thinking may result in millions of dollars in unnecessary costs. Worse, all those pills could be our unwitting contribution to the evolution of multiple-resistant strains of bacteria that may one day allow epidemics to sweep, untreated and untreatable, through our population.

1. According to the passage, Gilbert believes that, had Constantine or anyone else not changed the number of days in a week, a typical course for antibiotics would currently be
   A. undecided.
   B. ten days.
   C. seven days.
   D. eight days.

2. The word *magic* in Gilbert's title "Magic by the Numbers" refers to
   A. dosage rates.
   B. cultural concepts.
   C. empirical evidence.
   D. ancient Rome.

3. The main point of the passage is that the number of dosage days for antibiotics may be based on
   A. magical properties of the drugs.
   B. the base-ten counting system.
   C. the numbers that people tend to think in.
   D. evidence from ancient Roman history.

4. As used in the first paragraph, the word *properties* means
   A. physical qualities or traits.
   B. things owned or possessed.
   C. attributes common to all members of a class.
   D. psychological associations.

5. The last paragraph relates to the first paragraph in that it
   A. describes possible consequences of the phenomenon introduced in the first paragraph.
   B. provides supporting evidence for the existence of the phenomenon described in the first paragraph.
   C. offers a counterargument to the thesis presented in the first paragraph.
   D. describes the worst-case scenario that could result from reliance on the base-ten number system.

6. The author's tone in paragraph 2 could best be described as
   A. amused.
   B. regretful.
   C. worried.
   D. acerbic.

7. The writer mentions the study that provides Gilbert's contention in the third paragraph in order to
   A. support the idea that seven is a typical number of dosage days for all antibiotics.
   B. clarify the difference between "magical thinking" related to time and "magical thinking" related to base-ten counting.
   C. support the idea that using seven as a typical number of dosage days is unscientific.
   D. clarify the difference between the writer's reading of Gilbert and the interpretation by a member of the scientific community.

8. Which of these adds most credibility to the information presented in the passage?
   A. The use of questions in the first, second, and fourth paragraphs
   B. The explanation of the genesis of the base-ten number system
   C. The introduction of Gilbert's credentials in the second sentence of the essay
   D. The reference to dosages for uncomplicated pneumonia in the third paragraph

Refer to the following passage for Questions 9–16.

(1)   Essential to all life on Earth, water is not only the place where the first cells evolved, but it is also pervasive. All living things are made up of approximately 70% to 90% water; the surface of the planet on which we live is approximately 70% water (97 % of which is saltwater).

(2)   What are the properties of water that make it so central and vital to living creatures? Two of them are polarity within the water molecules and hydrogen bonding, which are not unique to water, but which are key properties because they cause the molecules of water to cling together. Without hydrogen bonding, water would have extremely low melting and boiling points, and most life could not exist in the resulting steam that would cover Earth's surface.

(3)   Other properties of water are quite familiar and observable and include the facts that water expands as it freezes and that frozen water is less dense than liquid water and, therefore, can float. The ice you see on lakes, rivers, and ponds during cold weather actually serves as an insulator, enabling life below it to survive winter.

(4)   You have also observed water's ability to facilitate chemical reactions. This is evident when you mix sugar into coffee or tea, turning sugar into a solute because water is a solvent. Actually, water is called a universal solvent because of its ability to dissolve so many different substances. Yet, because some molecules are hydrophilic (from *hydro,* water, and *philic,* loving) and some are hydrophobic (from *hydro,* water, and *phobic,* afraid of), only some substances go into solution. If you have observed gasoline floating on the surface of the water near a dock or in a lake, this is evidence that water and gasoline don't mix.

(5)   Water's capacity for heat is another reason for its centrality to life on Earth. Because of its many hydrogen bonds, water is able to absorb a great deal of heat without a commensurate rise in temperature. Water also holds onto its heat; this is in evidence during the melting of ice in lakes and rivers in spring. Because water temperature changes slowly, rather than rising or dropping precipitately, organisms that live in water are able to adjust and stay alive.

(6)   Other properties of water molecules that make water vital to life include adhesion and cohesion. Even when flowing freely, water molecules cohere (due to their hydrogen bonds) rather than separate. Water also has positive and negative poles that allow it to adhere to polar surfaces. The liquid portion of your blood (and your blood is about 90% water) is the efficient transport system that it is because water coheres and adheres as it fills its vessels, allowing both nutrients and wastes to be carried. Similarly, one-celled organisms also rely on water to transport nutrients and waste molecules on which their lives rely. Of course, water's quality as a universal solvent is also at work in this and other transport: life-giving chemicals, nutrients, and minerals are carried in solution.

(7)   Water's high heat of vaporization, which allows life in hot climates to release heat efficiently, also promotes life. In addition, water has a high surface tension (which makes it sticky and elastic), which is essential for capillary action. Capillary action is involved in the movement of water through the roots of plants and also through tiny blood vessels in animals.

diagnostic test

9. According to the passage, hydrogen bonding ensures that water
   A. boils and melts easily.
   B. is less dense when frozen.
   C. is a universal solvent.
   D. has higher melting and boiling points.

10. Which of these would be the best title for the passage?
    A. "Essential to Life"
    B. "Polarity and Bonding Ensure Life on Earth"
    C. "Polarity, Bonding, Cohesion, and Adhesion"
    D. "Key Properties of Water"

11. How is the information in paragraph 4 organized?
    A. In sequence
    B. By problem and solution
    C. By main idea and details
    D. By cause and effect

12. In paragraph 4, the author mentions the Greek origins of the words *hydrophobic* and *hydrophilic* in order to
    A. transition to exceptions to universal solvency.
    B. define universal solvency.
    C. explain why gasoline and water do not mix.
    D. explain why sugar dissolves in water.

13. The author's primary purpose in this passage is to
    A. persuade readers of the importance of water to all life.
    B. compare and contrast key properties of water.
    C. entertain readers with amazing facts about water.
    D. explain how water's properties ensure life on Earth.

14. In paragraph 5, the word *precipitately* means
    A. as a result of precipitation.
    B. after precipitation.
    C. very rapidly.
    D. very slowly.

15. The author's purpose in paragraph 1 is to
    A. discuss the most important property of water.
    B. provide a structural framework for the rest of the passage.
    C. explain the purpose of the passage as a whole.
    D. make a general statement about water's importance to life.

16. Which of the following is the author's thesis statement?
    A. "Essential to all life on Earth, water is not only the place where the first cells evolved, but it is also pervasive."
    B. "All living things are made up of approximately 70% to 90% water; the surface of the planet on which we live is approximately 70% water (97 % of which is saltwater)."
    C. "What are the properties of water that make it so central and vital to living creatures?"
    D. "You have also observed water's ability to facilitate chemical reactions."

Refer to the following passage for Questions 17–24.

(1)   It wasn't until my mother was diagnosed with gastroesophageal reflux disease, also known as GERD, and sometimes referred to simply as reflux disease, that I finally learned something about this stealthy disease. GERD isn't just heartburn; nor should it be a self-treated, ongoing condition because it could have potentially very serious results. Those who frequently take medications they see advertised on TV without ever consulting a doctor may, like my mother, be doing themselves a disservice.

(2)　My introduction to this disease started with the dictionary definition: GERD is a condition in which the contents of the stomach leak backward from the stomach and into the esophagus. It is generally agreed that this occurs in most cases because a ring of muscle fibers called the lower esophageal sphincter (LES) that would normally prevent this backward movement, or reflux, has weakened or does not close well. The most <u>common</u> results of this backward movement, and the hallmark symptoms of GERD, are heartburn (a sensation in the retrosternal area) and regurgitation (the perception of flow of refluxed gastric content into the hypopharynx or mouth). My mother experienced both, though she had the former far more frequently than the latter.

(3)　One estimate of the disease's prevalence is 10% to 20% of North Americans and Europeans. It is thought that the prevalence may be higher due to the number of people who, like my mother until just recently, take over-the-counter remedies without ever consulting a doctor. Furthermore, the number of people with the disease, which is already high, is thought to be on the rise.

(4)　Symptom frequency and severity of GERD run along a continuum from, for example, occasional heartburn to non-cardiac chest pain and respiratory problems. Although they are a minority, some patients never experience heartburn and may present, instead, with symptoms such as a <u>persistent</u> cough or sore throat. Many patients, but not all, experience erosion of the esophagus caused by a higher frequency of reflux, by the contents of the reflux, or by both.

(5)　The greater the frequency and duration of heartburn and possibly other symptoms, the more likely it appears that the disease will move along a spectrum whose beginning stage is GERD without endoscopically visible esophageal injury and whose final stage is esophageal adenocarcinoma. In between those stages are esophagitis, an inflammation of the lining of the esophagus that can make swallowing difficult or painful; hemorrhage and stricture formation; and Barrett's esophagus, damage to the lining of the esophagus that is histologically confirmed (by biopsy specimen obtained during endoscopy) by the presence of columnar metaplasia.

(6)　Just as symptoms run along a continuum, so do treatments, which include <u>over-the-counter</u> antacids and classes of drugs called proton pumps inhibitors (PPIs), H-2 blockers, and promotility agents. To date, PPIs have been found most effective in curing erosive esophagitis, which, it turns out, my mother had, but which is now under control. She readily fills and refills the gastroenterologist's prescription for these meds, even though the drugs have side effects that may include increased risk of fractures and recurrent infection.

(7)　In addition to being treated with drugs, my mother, like most GERD sufferers, was counseled to make lifestyle changes, including avoidance of alcohol, tobacco, excess dietary fat, chocolate, peppermint, and caffeine. She was told to keep a healthy weight and that sleeping with the head of the bed elevated and refraining from lying down after meals may make the physical action of reflux less likely. Quite honestly, she's having a harder time with some of these changes than she is with taking her PPI every day.

17. Which of these is NOT mentioned in the passage as a recommendation for GERD sufferers?
    A. Refraining from eating peppermint
    B. Refraining from eating any fat
    C. Raising the head of one's bed
    D. Staying upright after meals

18. The author's tone could best be described as
    A. friendly.
    B. enraged.
    C. jaded.
    D. intimate.

19. Which statement from the passage best shows the author's attitude toward the disease?
    A. "GERD isn't just heartburn; nor should it be a self-treated, ongoing condition because it could have potentially very serious results."
    B. "It is generally agreed that this occurs in most cases because a ring of muscle fibers called the lower esoph-ageal sphincter (LES) that would normally prevent this backward movement, or reflux, has weakened or does not close well."
    C. "The greater the frequency and duration of heartburn and possibly other symptoms, the more likely it appears that the disease will move along a spectrum whose beginning stage is GERD without endoscopi-cally visible esophageal injury and whose final stage is esophageal adenocarcinoma."
    D. "She's having a harder time with some of these changes than she is with taking her PPI every day."

20. Which statement from the passage is an example of an opinion the author holds?
    A. "Those who frequently take medi-cations they see advertised on TV without ever consulting doctor may, like my mother, be doing themselves a disservice."
    B. "One estimate of the disease's prevalence is 10% to 20% of North Americans and Europeans."
    C. "It is thought that the prevalence may be higher due to the number of people who, like my mother, take over-the-counter remedies without ever consulting a doctor."
    D. "To date, PPIs have been found most effective in curing erosive esophagitis, which, it turns out, my mother had."

21. As stated in the passage, which of these may have similar effects on the person suffering from GERD?
    A. Not drinking alcohol and taking PPIs
    B. Taking H-2 blockers and not eating peppermint
    C. Avoiding chocolate and caffeine
    D. Not lying down after meals and raising the head of the bed

22. Which point from the passage best supports the author's suggestion that GERD should not be self-treated?
    A. Proton pumps inhibitors are most effective in treating GERD.
    B. GERD involves a leakage of stomach contents into the esophagus.
    C. People who suffer from GERD must make lifestyle changes.
    D. There is a high mortality rate among those who self-treat GERD.

23. What can be concluded from the passage about the use of PPIs for GERD?
    A. They are most effective for heartburn sufferers.
    B. They should be abandoned if the GERD sufferer has Barrett's esophagus.
    C. They are not prescribed when someone presents with a cough or sore throat.
    D. They may reverse inflammation in the lining of the esophagus.

24. Which word or term from the passage reveals a connotation bias on the part of the author?
    A. Stealthy (paragraph 1)
    B. Common (paragraph 2)
    C. Persistent (paragraph 4)
    D. Over-the-counter (paragraph 6)

Refer to the following passage for Questions 25–32.

(1)   The efficacy of drugs currently used to treat patients with Alzheimer's disease has long been a subject of debate. While no company, organization, or credible individual suggests that the drugs can in any way cure or even stop the progression of the disease, various arguments are made for their ability to ameliorate symptoms. Questions about if and when to prescribe and how long to continue the use of such drugs arise naturally not only from the agreed limitations on what the drugs may or may not do, but also from the nature of the disease and its diagnosis, or lack of diagnosis—many patients are assumed to have Alzheimer's disease without actually ever having been tested. Others who are diagnosed with dementia may be treated as if actually diagnosed with Alzheimer's disease.

(2)   The two classes of drugs currently in use to treat the symptoms of Alzheimer's disease and also, perhaps, to effect desired behavioral changes, work in different ways; for example, one widely used drug blocks the toxic effects—or brain cell death—associated with excess glutamate. This drug is widely prescribed for the moderate to severe stages of the disease. On its website, the Alzheimer's Associaton notes that the drug may temporarily delay the worsening of symptoms for some people but does not specify any percentages. It is generally agreed that the glutamate regulator has few side effects; those that it does have may be considered minor, such as headaches, confusion, constipation, and dizziness.

(3)   The second class of drugs, cholinesterase inhibitors, may effectively ameliorate symptoms—or simply reduce unwanted behaviors—at early to moderate stages of the disease, but the National Institute on Aging, an arm of the National Institutes of Health, notes that no one actually understands "how cholinesterase inhibitors work to treat Alzheimer's disease, " although it is currently assumed that the drugs assist in the breakdown of acetylcholine." (ACh is a neurotransmitter. While it plays a role in the peripheral as well as the central nervous system, the supposition of its role in learning and memory has led to the development of drugs that inhibit it in a reversible manner.) With the progression of Alzheimer's disease, however, less and less acetylcholine is produced, making these drugs ineffective eventually, though no one is sure at precisely what point. Yet, the FDA has approved at least one of the cholinesterase inhibitor to treat all stages of Alzheimer's—beginning to mild, moderate, and severe. These stages can progress over a timeline ranging from just a few years to many years, with twelve being considered an average. The Alzheimer's Association reports on its website that cholinesterase inhibitors may "delay the worsening of symptoms" for six to twelve months for about half the

people who take them. It also notes, as the drug producers themselves do, that the side effects are generally "well tolerated"; indeed, the side effects are relatively minor, at least in comparison with those of many drugs, and include nausea and loss of appetite. Therefore, cholinesterase inhibitors is the preferable treatment, but an ideal long-term solution remains tragically out of reach.

(4)　　As with the research on all Alzheimer's drugs, changes in behavior cannot be quantified, and accurate self-reporting within the patient group is not possible. Reports on drug efficacy have depended on the anecdotal reporting of caregivers.

25. In the final two sentences of paragraph 1, the author suggests that people with Alzheimer's are
   A. a large subset of those with dementia.
   B. a small subset of those with dementia.
   C. often treated for the disease without being diagnosed with it.
   D. often treated for the symptoms of dementia rather than for those Alzheimer's disease.

26. Information in the passage suggests that glutamate regulators and cholinesterase inhibitors are widely prescribed because
   A. while they make little changes in symptoms, they have no serious side effects.
   B. while they are not well tolerated, they do make the lives of caregivers easier.
   C. they may help decrease symptoms and they have relatively minor side effects.
   D. they can be depended upon to decrease symptoms in most patients and they may cure a small percentage of patients.

27. At the end of paragraph 3, what does the author conclude?
   A. The lack of a cure for Alzheimer's disease is tragic.
   B. Treating Alzheimer's disease with cholinesterase inhibitors is pointless.
   C. There will never be a cure for Alzheimer's disease.
   D. Cholinesterase inhibitors will be used to cure Alzheimer's disease some day.

28. The author implies a contradiction in the FDA's
   A. recommendation for use of cholinesterase inhibitors in the early/mild stages.
   B. recommendation for use of cholinesterase inhibitors in the severe stage.
   C. failure to regulate cholinesterase inhibitors.
   D. approval of a class of drugs based on cholinesterase.

29. The author's primary purpose in this passage is to
   A. present readers with the two classes of drugs currently used to treat Alzheimer's disease.
   B. inform readers about the limitations of the two classes of drugs currently used to treat Alzheimer's disease.
   C. argue that glutamate regulators are a superior class of drugs to cholinesterase inhibitors for treating Alzheimer's disease.
   D. explain how much progress has been made in the development of pharmaceuticals for treating Alzheimer's disease.

30. The author's purpose in the final paragraph is to

- **A.** summarize the main points made in paragraphs 2 and 3.
- **B.** create a link to the behaviors discussed in the first paragraph.
- **C.** persuade readers to participate in clinical trials for drug discovery.
- **D.** add a final "clincher" in support of the main ideas of the passage.

31. How is the information in paragraph 2 organized?

- **A.** By comparison
- **B.** By contrast
- **C.** By main idea and details
- **D.** By chronology

32. The author of the passage would most likely agree that

- **A.** Alzheimer's disease is the most devastating disease currently known to medical science.
- **B.** there are credible drug companies that claim to have a cure for Alzheimer's disease.
- **C.** treatment of Alzheimer's disease should occur as soon as the first signs of the disease are detected.
- **D.** cholinesterase inhibitors are better than the drug that blocks the toxic effects of Alzheimer's disease.

Refer to the following passage for Questions 33–40.

(1)   When I was growing up, I lived across the street from someone I used to call Snakeman, a term of reverence that carried overtones, for me, of Superman, as well all the glamour and attraction I had already invested in the creepiest of crawling things, snakes. My neighbor, Dr. Messuri, a rheumatologist by day, was, it turned out, a dedicated though amateur herpetologist by night and weekend.

(2)   From Dr. Messuri, I learned some amazing facts about snake adaptations, which are multiple and various, and which were often somewhat beyond the limits of my understanding when I learned them so long ago. He started by introducing me to the snake's senses, beginning with what may be the second-most obvious and alarming part of every snake's anatomy, the tongue. This tongue has not a single tastebud; nevertheless, the tongue is a conveyor of both taste and smell. Part of its function is to bring smell and taste into the mouth. Receptors on two pits on the roof of the snake's mouth, called Jacobson's organs, transmit information about smell and taste to the snake's brain.

(3)   Dr. Messuri also noted that some snakes have special sensory pits between their nostrils and eyes, whereas other snakes have them in the scales of their lip line. "For snakes," he explained, "these pits are the name of the hunting game. What they do is detect changes in heat, and heat means prey. A rattlesnake knows when a tiny mouse is more than a foot away simply by sensing the most minute alteration in ambient temperature!"

(4)   Holding the head of his pet boa constrictor at eye level for me to examine, Dr. Messuri also pointed out how snakes have no visible ears. (Actually, while snakes famously do not respond to loud noises, they do have an internal middle ear to which sound waves may travel.) He explained that no snake was ever charmed by the music of a snake charmer, although a snake might possibly respond to the movement of a snake charmer and his flute.

(5)   Next, Dr. Messuri had me study the snake's eyes. "Where is the snake's eyelid?" he asked, which caused me to observe that there wasn't any. He told me approvingly that

I was thinking like an evolutionary biologist when I asked how snakes, who crawl on the ground through debris, keep dangerous things out of their eyes, and pointed out the protective cap of epidermis covering one of the boa's eyes.

(6)   As for dentition, Dr. Messuri explained that that depends on the snake and its diet. Egg-eating and burrowing snakes may have just a few teeth. Others require more teeth for their far more chewy meals.

33. Information in the passage suggests that
   A. everything the author learned from Dr. Messuri was accurate.
   B. Dr. Messuri created the author's own love of and interest in snakes.
   C. Dr. Messuri preferred his nighttime hobby to his profession.
   D. Dr. Messuri nurtured the author's fascination with snakes.

34. Based on the passage, it is possible to infer that, for the author, the most riveting anatomical part of a snake was the
   A. tongue.
   B. fang.
   C. tail.
   D. eyes.

35. The mention of special receptors in paragraph 3 would most logically lead to the conclusion that
   A. a snake's specific adaptations vary according to its environment.
   B. a snake's ability to hunt prey may be hobbled by the location of special receptors.
   C. the lip line is a superior location because it is most likely closest to any prey.
   D. the lip line scales of a snake are, in most cases, vestigial.

36. Which of these is NOT mentioned in the passage as a sensory characteristic of snakes?
   A. Protective epidermal caps over the eyes
   B. Internal ears
   C. Receptor organs for conveying smell
   D. Complex dentition in multiple jaws

37. Which of the following conclusions is most effectively supported by information in the passage?
   A. A snake's tongue is the repository of adaptations most necessary to its survival.
   B. A snake's head is most likely more highly adapted to its environment than its body is.
   C. A snake's sensory adaptations are related to environment and predation.
   D. A snake's most important sensory adaptations are related to predation.

38. The ideas in the first and second sentences of paragraph 3 relate to each other by
   A. topic and restriction.
   B. analogy.
   C. contrast.
   D. thesis and antithesis.

39. Which of these statements about a snake's hearing is supported by the passage?
   A. A snake can detect at least some auditory signals.
   B. A snake's external ears evolved and changed over time.
   C. A snake cannot use its vision for defense or hunting.
   D. Auditory response in snakes is slowed by the lack of external ears.

40. Which statement from the passage is an example of an opinion the author holds?

 A. "From Dr. Messuri, I learned some amazing facts of snake adaptations, which are multiple and various…"

 B. "My neighbor, Dr. Messuri, a rheumatologist by day, was, it turned out, a dedicated though amateur herpetologist by night and weekend."

 C. "Dr. Messuri also noted that some snakes have special sensory pits between their nostrils and eyes…"

 D. "He told me approvingly that I was thinking like an evolutionary biologist…"

Refer to the following passage for Questions 41–48.

(1)   If, like me, you've experienced some difficulty wading through that deep morass of often incorrect and sometimes conflicting information about the regulation of supplements, the amorphous muck of your confusion might eventually reduce itself into the single dirty question of whether supplements are or aren't regulated. Some websites and other sources will state flatly that there is no regulation; others will cite the FDA's involvement in the arena of dietary supplements but call the regulation lax. In fact, as the FDA explains on its own website, the FDA does regulate supplements, but not in the same way it regulates foods and drugs. One example of this difference is that the FDA takes action against unsafe supplements after they reach the market. Manufacturers are to police themselves, making sure that all labeling is truthful and accurate as required by the FDA. In addition, all manufacturers must comply with certain "good" practices, as stipulated by a different U.S. regulatory agency, in their manufacturing operations. To a jaundiced eye, the holes in this regulation are as wide as the state of Nebraska.

(2)   Combine these facts with the generally accepted advice that it is better to get your nutrients from dietary sources, and the simple act of popping a vitamin into your mouth suddenly makes little sense. Or does it? The example of taking supplements for the sake of increasing bone density may be instructive.

(3)   Large amounts of calcium daily are widely recommended for women of all ages. In part, this is because the average recommended amount of 1200 mg is difficult to get in the typical diet. Even if women do get that much calcium on a daily basis (by, for example, drinking four eight-ounce glasses of milk or eating six ounces of shredded cheese each and every day), they also need vitamin D in order to absorb that calcium, and sufficient D appears even more elusive to obtain through dietary and sun sources than calcium is. Therefore, a calcium-plus-D supplement does seem to make sense for most women.

(4)   Still, when selecting that supplement, know that the government has left you pretty much on your own, so bring your lucky rabbit's foot along when you purchase it. More reasonably, you might also heed this supplement advice from the Dana Farber health library: Avoid taking more than you need. For calcium, this means assessing what you need meal by meal, since the body can absorb only so much calcium at a time. If you've ingested a large amount of calcium at a meal, skip the supplement you might otherwise have taken with it. For D, get a blood level test; then find out how much vitamin D your doctor recommends based on the findings. Obtain that D from your diet and the sun first and use a supplement for the rest. As for supplements for other conditions or maladies, be informed and seek the best dietary sources first.

41. The tone of this passage suggests that the author views the FDA's role in the regulation of supplements as
    A. admirable.
    B. laughable.
    C. somewhat lacking.
    D. highly unpredictable.

42. What can be concluded from the passage about the use of calcium-plus-D supplements for building bone density?
    A. All women should take them, though dosage may vary.
    B. All women should take them at every meal.
    C. Most women should take them, but in an informed and careful way.
    D. Women should beware of these largely unregulated supplements.

43. How does the author's advice in the final paragraph to "bring your lucky rabbit's foot" relate to the fact provided in the first paragraph that "the FDA takes action against unsafe supplements after they reach the market"?
    A. It provides supporting evidence.
    B. It emphasizes the importance.
    C. It offers contradiction for the sake of humor.
    D. It creates a transition to a new topic.

44. According to the passage, the FDA's role in the regulation of supplements is
    A. nonexistent.
    B. minimal.
    C. objective.
    D. increasing.

45. The author of this passage ties the introduction and conclusion together by
    A. advising the reader to exercise care in the use of supplements.
    B. calling on the reader to seek a doctor's advice before taking any supplement.
    C. reminding the reader that supplement labeling may not be accurate.
    D. calling on the reader to get necessary nutrients from dietary sources.

46. According to the passage, the FDA
    A. tests supplements before they are sold to the public.
    B. establishes and oversees manufacturing practices for supplements.
    C. requires that labels on supplements are truthful, but does not verify their truth.
    D. regulates supplements more closely than it regulates drugs.

47. Which of these would be the best title for the passage?
    A. "How the FDA Lets Consumers Down"
    B. "Know the Facts About Supplements"
    C. "The Pros and Cons of Taking Supplements "
    D. "Why We Need More Regulation of Supplements"

48. What evidence could the author have included that would best support the main point?
    A. Recent studies suggest that most supplements do not contain toxic fillers, colors, or other additives.
    B. Recent studies suggest that vitamin D supplements may play a role in cancer prevention and survivorship.
    C. Tablet binders affect the speed and the way in which supplements disintegrate.
    D. The transfer of supplement manufacture to big pharma may ensure higher standards of manufacture.

SECTION 5: QUANTITATIVE REASONING

48 Items • 50 Minutes

> **Directions:** Choose the best answer for each question.

1. If $f(x) = \ln(x^2 + 1)$, what is $f'(3)$?

   SHOW YOUR WORK HERE

   A. $\dfrac{1}{10}$

   B. $\dfrac{1}{5}$

   C. $\dfrac{3}{5\ln 3}$

   D. $\dfrac{3}{5}$

2. Kendall is developing a workout consisting of squats and box jumps. His total number of movements must be 300. A squat burns 1.2 calories and a box jump burns 1.5 calories, and he wants the entire workout to burn 400 calories. Which of the following systems of equations can be used to determine the number of squats, s, and the number of box jumps, b, that should be incorporated into the workout?

   A. $\begin{cases} s + b = 400 \\ 1.5s + 1.2b = 300 \end{cases}$

   B. $\begin{cases} s + b = 300 \\ 1.2s + 1.5b = 400 \end{cases}$

   C. $\begin{cases} s + b = 300 \\ 1.5s + 1.2b = 400 \end{cases}$

   D. $\begin{cases} s + b = 400 \\ 1.2s + 1.5b = 300 \end{cases}$

3. If x, y, and z are positive integers such that $x > 2y$ and $2y - 3z > 0$, then which of the following is true?

   A. $3z > x$

   B. $y - x > 0$

   C. $x - 3z > 0$

   D. $x + 2y < 0$

4. An upstart company has received funding to develop a new video gaming console. The profit based on selling x hundred consoles is described by the function $p(x) = 4x^2 - 12x - 16$, where $p(x)$ is measured in ten thousands of dollars. How many consoles must the company sell to break even?

   A. 4

   B. 10

   C. 100

   D. 400

5. What is the value of $\ln \sqrt{e}$?

   A. $\frac{1}{2}$

   B. $\frac{1}{2}e$

   C. e

   D. e^2

6. The membership at a local gym increased from 50 members to 80 members over the past 6 months. Which of the following represents its percent increase in membership?

   A. $\frac{50}{80} \times 100\%$

   B. $\frac{80 - 50}{80} \times 100\%$

   C. $\frac{80 - 50}{50} \times 100\%$

   D. $\frac{80 - 50}{50}\%$

SHOW YOUR WORK HERE

7. The cost of concessions at a movie theater are listed below:

Item	Cost
Matinee Admission Ticket	$10.50
Large Soda	$6.25
Bucket of Popcorn	$5.90
Bag of Candy	$3.75

If the theater charges 5% sales tax, what is the total cost of two matinee admission tickets, two large sodas, 1 bucket of popcorn, and three bags of candy?

A. $27.72

B. $50.65

C. $53.18

D. $55.65

8. If $f(x) = \sin x$ and $g(x) = \cos x$, what is $\left(\dfrac{f}{g}\right)(\pi)$?

A. −1

B. 0

C. $\dfrac{\sqrt{2}}{2}$

D. 1

9. What is $\dfrac{7}{3} + \dfrac{3}{4} - \dfrac{1}{\frac{3}{2}}$?

A. $\dfrac{13}{4}$

B. $\dfrac{35}{12}$

C. $\dfrac{29}{12}$

D. $\dfrac{7}{3}$

SHOW YOUR WORK HERE

10. If you pluck a guitar string, the resulting vibrations are waves traveling along the string very quickly. The speed, v, of such a wave is described by the formula $T = \dfrac{mv^2}{L}$, where m is the mass of the string, T is the tension of the string, and L is the length of the string. If the tension is 82.6 $\dfrac{\text{m} \cdot \text{kg}}{\sec^2}$, the length of the string is 0.95m, and the mass is 63g, which expression represents the speed at which the wave travels along the string?

SHOW YOUR WORK HERE

   A. $\sqrt{\dfrac{82.6 \times 95}{63}}$ meters per second

   B. $\sqrt{82.6 \times 0.95 \times 63}$ meters per second

   C. $\sqrt{\dfrac{82.6 \times 0.95}{0.63}}$ meters per second

   D. $\sqrt{\dfrac{82.6 \times 0.95}{0.063}}$ meters per second

11. If next year Tino is the manager of baseball team A, then there is a 70% probability that Carlos will sign a contract to play for the team. If Tino is not the manager, then there is a 30% probability that Carlos will sign with team A. If the probability that Tino will be the manager is 60%, what is the probability that Carlos will sign with team A?

   A. 0.12

   B. 0.42

   C. 0.50

   D. 0.54

12. A javelin thrower's score at a decathlon is the average of the distances of her four throws. Sue's distances are 55.3 m, 56.2 m, 48.7 m, and 61.4 m. What is her score?

   A. 48.7

   B. 55.4

   C. 61.4

   D. 73.9

13. If $\log_4 16 = \log_a x$, what is a?

    A. x^2

    B. x

    C. $\sqrt{x}$

    D. $-\sqrt{x}$

14. What is the equation of the line that is tangent to the graph of the function $f(x) = x^3$ at $x = 2$?

    A. $y = 12x - 16$

    B. $y = 12x$

    C. $y = 12$

    D. $y = 8x - 16$

15. A widget-producing machine produced 60 widgets on Monday, 40 on Tuesday, and 50 on Wednesday. On Thursday, it increased its rate of production so that its Monday-to-Thursday daily average number of widgets produced was 10 widgets greater than its Monday-to-Wednesday daily average number of widgets produced. How many widgets did the machine produce on Thursday?

    A. 60

    B. 70

    C. 80

    D. 90

16. What is the domain of $f(x) = \sqrt{2|x-1|-5}$?

    A. $\left(-\infty, -\frac{3}{2}\right) \cup \left[\frac{7}{2}, \infty\right)$

    B. $\left(-\infty, -\frac{3}{2}\right) \cup \left(\frac{7}{2}, \infty\right)$

    C. $\left[-\frac{3}{2}, \frac{7}{2}\right]$

    D. $\left(-\infty, \frac{3}{2}\right] \cup \left[\frac{7}{2}, \infty\right)$

SHOW YOUR WORK HERE

diagnostic test

17. If a sofa was sold for $368, and this price reflected a 20% markdown from the sofa's original price, what was the original price?

A. $294.40

B. $441.60

C. $460.00

D. $1,840.00

18. At a raffle with a single prize, Dina bought 4 tickets. If 13 other people bought an average of 6 tickets each, what is the probability that Dina will win the prize?

A. $\frac{1}{78}$

B. $\frac{2}{41}$

C. $\frac{2}{39}$

D. $\frac{1}{13}$

19. A trail map through the Rocky Mountains uses a fractional scale of 1:18,000, meaning 1 unit of distance on the map is equal to 18,000 units on the actual ground. You are hiking to a lookout post that measures 15.4 inches from your current location on the map. Approximately how many miles must you hike to get to the lookout post?

A. 3.4 miles

B. 4.4 miles

C. 13.1 miles

D. 52.5 miles

20. Which of the following is equal to $\log_3 \frac{x}{9y}$?

A. $x \log_3 9y$

B. $\log_3 \frac{x}{y} - 2$

C. $2 \log_3 \frac{x}{y}$

D. $\log_3 \frac{x}{y} + 2$

SHOW YOUR WORK HERE

21. The loudness of a sound is measured in decibels and is described by the formula $dB = 10 \cdot \log\left(\dfrac{I}{I_0}\right)$, where I_0 is the intensity of a sound that can be barely perceived by the human ear. If a large dog's bark is approximately $400 \times I_0$, which of the following is the number of decibels of such a dog's bark?

   A. $20 \cdot \log(4)$

   B. $2 + 10 \cdot \log(4)$

   C. $\log(40)$

   D. $20 + 10 \cdot \log(4)$

22. For what values of the domain is the function $f(x) = -x^3 - x$ concave up?

   A. $x < -6$

   B. $x < 0$

   C. $x > 0$

   D. $x \geq 0$

23. What is $\dfrac{dy}{dx}$ if $x^2 + x \cos y = x$?

   A. $\dfrac{\cos y + 2x - 1}{x \sin y}$

   B. $\dfrac{1}{\sin y}$

   C. $\dfrac{\cos y - 2x + 1}{-x \sin y}$

   D. $\dfrac{x}{\sin y}$

24. If the average of p and q is x, and the average of r, s, and t is y, what is the average of p, q, r, s, and t?

   A. $\dfrac{2x + 3y}{5}$

   B. $\dfrac{3x + 2y}{5}$

   C. $2x + 3y$

   D. $5(2x + 3y)$

SHOW YOUR WORK HERE

diagnostic test

25. If $4 - \sqrt[3]{2x} = 0$, what is x?

SHOW YOUR WORK HERE

    A. $\dfrac{\sqrt[3]{4}}{2}$

    B. 4

    C. 32

    D. 64

26. What is $\dfrac{7}{2}$ of 0.6 of $\dfrac{6}{9}$?

    A. $\dfrac{35}{4}$

    B. $\dfrac{143}{30}$

    C. $\dfrac{35}{9}$

    D. $\dfrac{7}{5}$

27. A city's population is dependent on time, t, and is given by the function $f(t) = 2t^{\frac{1}{2}}$. After 9 years, at what rate is the city's population changing?

    A. 6

    B. $\dfrac{1}{3}$

    C. $\dfrac{1}{6}$

    D. $-\dfrac{1}{54}$

28. The fastest commercial train in the world travels at 268 miles per hour. Which of the following expressions can be used to convert this speed to feet per second?

    A. $\dfrac{268 \times 60 \times 60}{5,280}$ feet per second

    B. $\dfrac{268 \times 5,280}{60}$ feet per second

    C. $\dfrac{268 \times 5,280}{60 \times 60}$ feet per second

    D. $\dfrac{268 \times 60}{5,280}$ feet per second

SHOW YOUR WORK HERE

29. What is the value of $\sum_{n=1}^{4} \left(3 - n^2\right)$?
    A. −13
    B. −15
    C. −18
    D. −20

30. Bowl A contains 4 marbles numbered a, $a + 1$, $a + 2$, and $a + 3$. Bowl B contains 4 marbles numbered $2a$, $2(a + 1)$, $2(a + 2)$, and $2(a + 3)$. If someone picks at random one marble from bowl A, and then at random one marble from bowl B, what is the probability that the number on the marble picked from bowl B will NOT be twice the number on the marble picked from bowl A?

    A. $\frac{15}{16}$

    B. $\frac{3}{4}$

    C. $\frac{1}{4}$

    D. $\frac{1}{16}$

31. What is $\frac{2.6}{0.65}$?

    A. 4,000
    B. 400
    C. 40
    D. 4

32. While assembling an entertainment center, you discover that a cylindrical metal connector is missing. The diameter of this piece should be 0.6 inch, with an allowable error of at most 0.04 inch. The diameters of four potential replacement parts sold by a hardware store are listed below. Which should you purchase?
    A. 0.53 inch
    B. 0.55 inch
    C. 0.63 inch
    D. 0.65 inch

33. If a and b are vectors such that $a = (-3,1)$ and $b = 2i$, what is $a - b$?

    A. $-i + j$

    B. $-5i - j$

    C. $-5i + j$

    D. $-i - 3j$

34. The mosquito population has exploded in a southern state during the summer months. Public health officials modeled this population using the function $P(t) = 2 \cdot e^{t/10}$, where t is measured in weeks and $P(t)$ is measured in millions. How many weeks does it take for the mosquito population to reach 4 million?

    A. $\ln(20)$ weeks

    B. $\ln(1{,}024)$ weeks

    C. $\dfrac{20}{e}$ weeks

    D. $2 \cdot e^{1/10}$ weeks

35. The figure below shows the box plots for two different data sets.

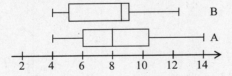

    Which of the following statements must be correct?

    A. The median of set B is greater than the median of set A.

    B. The range of set B is greater than the range of set A.

    C. The mean of set B is greater than the mean of set A.

    D. The mean of set A is greater than the mean of set B.

36. The number of handstand push-ups members of a training gym completed during a 15-minute workout are listed in the following stem-and-leaf plot.

Stem	Leaves
3	1
4	0 2
5	3 3 4 4 8 8
6	1 1 2 4 6 6 8 8
7	0 0 0
8	3 4
9	5

Here, 3|1 means 31. What is the median and mode number of push-ups completed?

A. The median is 61 and the mode is 95.

B. The median is 58 and the mode is both 66 and 68.

C. The median is 66 and the mode is 70.

D. The median is 62 and the mode is 70.

37. Ron can mulch the leaves in his yard in 3 hours. If Frank helps him using his own mower, the mulching job can be completed in 2 hours. Which equation can be used to determine the number of hours, x, it would take Frank to mulch the leaves working alone?

A. $\dfrac{1}{x+3} = \dfrac{1}{2}$

B. $\dfrac{1}{x} + \dfrac{1}{3} = \dfrac{1}{2}$

C. $\dfrac{1}{x} + \dfrac{1}{3} = 1$

D. $x + 3 = 2$

SHOW YOUR WORK HERE

38. Which of the following is the reciprocal of $\dfrac{6}{\sqrt{3}}$?

   A. $\dfrac{1}{2\sqrt{3}}$

   B. $\dfrac{2}{\sqrt{3}}$

   C. $\dfrac{\sqrt{3}}{2}$

   D. $\dfrac{6\sqrt{3}}{3}$

SHOW YOUR WORK HERE

39. Asher works 40 hours per week at a clothing store. He earns a base salary of $180 per week, plus a 2.5% commission on weekly sales exceeding $3,500. Using the functions $F(x) = 1,800 + x$, $G(x) = 0.025x$, and $H(x) = x - 3,500$, which of the following functions gives Asher's salary for a week when he sells more than $3,500 worth of merchandise?

   A. $(F \circ G \circ H)(x)$

   B. $(H \circ G \circ F)(x)$

   C. $(F + G + H)(x)$

   D. $F(x) + (G \circ H)(x)$

40. The number of sightings of black bears reported by tourists in Banff ebbs and flows seasonally. The function $S(t) = 120 \sin\left(\dfrac{\pi}{6} t\right)$, $0 \leq t \leq 11$, where $t = 0$ corresponds to March, $t = 1$ corresponds to April, etc. is used to model the number of sightings. In what month(s) is/are the minimum number of sightings reported?

   A. March and August

   B. December

   C. May

   D. December and September

41. The Johnson family is making homemade apple cider. They have purchased a trailer full of apples, which is enough to make 20 batches of cider using their apple press. The number of gallons of cider each batch produces are listed below:

2.6	3.1	4.0	3.2	2.2
2.1	1.6	2.1	1.8	2.1
1.9	1.6	1.8	1.8	2.8
1.7	2.3	2.4	2.4	2.0

What is the range of the data set?
A. 1.6
B. 2.1
C. 2.4
D. 4.0

42. A taxi charges a flat rate of $3.25 plus an additional $0.55 per mile. Janet has at most $12 to spend on a taxi ride. How many full miles could she travel?
A. 4
B. 5
C. 15
D. 16

43. Mick's tractor trailer gets approximately $12\frac{3}{4}$ miles per gallon. If there are $6\frac{1}{3}$ gallons of gas in his tank, how far can he travel with his tractor trailer?

A. $19\frac{1}{2}$ miles

B. $60\frac{1}{3}$ miles

C. $72\frac{1}{4}$ miles

D. $80\frac{3}{4}$ miles

44. For which values of x is the expression $x^2 + 2x - 3$ negative?
A. $x > -3$
B. $x < 1$
C. $-3 < x < 1$
D. $-3 \leq x \leq 1$

SHOW YOUR WORK HERE

45. Which of the following is the graph of $f(x) = -e^x$?

SHOW YOUR WORK HERE

A.

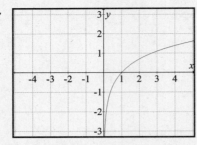

B.

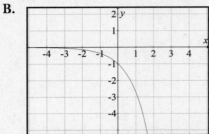

C.

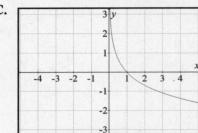

D.

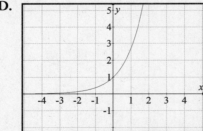

46. Vector $\overrightarrow{AB}$ has coordinates (−5,8). Vector $\overrightarrow{CD}$ is a scalar multiple of $\overrightarrow{AB}$, and the sum of the coordinates of $\overrightarrow{CD}$ is −21. What is the second coordinate of $\overrightarrow{CD}$?

A. 56

B. 35

C. −7

D. −56

47. What is the value of $\int_{-1}^{4} 3x^2 - 3x^{-2}dx$?

    A. 0
    B. 4
    C. 8
    D. This integral cannot be computed.

48. Which of the following is NOT a solution of the equation $\dfrac{\left(x^2 - 9\right)\left(x^2 - 4\right)}{x - 3}$?

    A. 3
    B. 2
    C. −2
    D. −3

ANSWER KEYS AND EXPLANATIONS

Section I: Writing

Sample of a Superior Response

The best and only realistic answer to the problem of depletion of fish stocks is well-managed and environmentally sound aquaculture. Just as agribusiness has been the answer to the problem of supplying grain and other staple food items to a hungry world, aquaculture is the answer to supplying fish to people who not only need it as a major food source, but who are also used to eating fish as a component of their cultures.

Because of the scale on which these operations can occur, farming aquatic resources, including shellfish and seaweed as well as fish, is the best answer to the problem of massive depletion of fish stocks. Only aquaculture can hope to yield the equivalent of the two-ton catch of tuna of days past. With the world's population at approximately seven billion, and many of those seven billion hungry for or accustomed to fish as a regular part of their diets, only aquaculture can continue to yield such huge amounts of fish and related foods month after month and year after year.

Of course, any aquaculture practices must be well managed and environmentally sound. We cannot risk degrading the marine environment by concentrating large populations of farmed fish, along with their feed and waste, in small areas. We have learned how some practices of agriculture are environmentally degrading to our land, our fresh water, and our oceans; as with agriculture, we must learn to control and surmount the problems of concentrating large-scale farming or cultivation efforts in a small freshwater or saltwater space.

Any new aquaculture methods should be as clean as possible. In fact, studies often cite pollution as a factor that has combined with over-fishing to deplete fish stocks around the world. Therefore, research efforts must immediately be concentrated on finding and farming those fish and other aquatic species that can be raised with the least amount of pollution.

Some may suggest that the answer to the problem of depleted fish stocks is the natural rehabilitation of those fish stocks, with long periods of time when people experience fishing moratoriums or near moratoriums. To that argument, the simple counterargument is, "Who can—or will—wait?" People are now illegally taking blue-fin tuna, despite all the laws against it. While such aquatic resources exist, there will always be some people who continue to exploit them.

Because aquaculture is the only practical and sustainable answer to the problem of depleted fish stocks, research into new fish stocks for aquaculture must begin now. Similarly, all nations should be making the development of environmentally friendly, well-managed aquatic farms a top priority. If we expect to keep eating fish throughout the twenty-first century and beyond, we cannot start acting on these goals soon enough.

This essay earns a 5.0 score for the following reasons:

- In the introductory paragraph, the writer offers a solution to the problem ("The best and only realistic answer to the problem of depletion of fish stocks is well-managed and environmentally sound aquaculture."), which will be fleshed out in the proceeding paragraphs.

- Each of the first body paragraph deals with a facet of the solution: farming (paragraph 2), environmentally sound agricultural practices (paragraph 3), clean aquaculture methods (paragraph 4), and the effectiveness of farming versus natural rehabilitation (paragraph 5). That facet is made clear at the beginning of each paragraph in a clear topic sentence.

- The transitional words and phrases *Of course*, *Therefore*, and *To that argument* guide the reader through the explanation in a clear, systematic way.

- Many details (such as the prevalence of fish in diets and studies related to the loss of fish stocks) make the writing cogent and work toward supporting the main idea. Nothing is repeated. There are no digressions.

- The reasoning throughout the essay is logical.

- The conclusion ends with an appropriate call for more research as well as a restatement of the effectiveness of aquaculture.

- There are no errors in sentence structure, and the sentences are varied and fluid.

- Words are used correctly and well.

- The essay is persuasive; the tone is appropriately serious; the voice of the writer is clear and engaged; and the second person is avoided.

- There are no mechanical errors.

Sample of a Weak Response

Here's the thing everyone has to do right away. You have to put a stop to all fishing of endangered or limited or disappearing fish stocks right now. That is the only way to make the populations of fish come back to there pre-1950 numbers. If we make laws that say no one can fish cod or tuna, flounder, or halibut, then, slowly, over some years, theres going to be more and more of those fish in the water. We will once again have our pre-1950 numbers.

The problem is that we have lost about 90% of our fish stocks since 1950, so we must do what we can do right now in order to be bringing back those fish, the cod, tuna, flounder, halibut, and more. people in the world need these fish to live, some people are bound to go hungry if we do not protect them immediately.

Some might say that its better to farm more fish, they are overlooking the problems of pollution that farming fish brings. In addition to there being problems with how some farmed fish taste because they are also fattier than other fish and eat things that fish in the wild don't eat.

This essay earns a 1.0 score for the following reasons:

- This essay is inadequate in terms of supporting details and problem solving. The writer introduces only one idea to support his or her solution and does not explain it in a cogent way.

- While the writer shows some insight in the idea selected for analysis, the idea is not explained and developed.

- The solution of outlawing the fishing of certain fish is overly simplistic.

- The essay lacks organization. The first paragraph functions as both an introductory paragraph and a body paragraph. The second paragraph is redundant. The concluding paragraph introduces counterarguments against the writer's thesis but does not even attempt to rebut them, thus weakening her or his main argument.

- There are numerous errors in sentence construction. The second paragraph is a run on sentence.

- There are numerous mechanical and usage errors.

Section 2: Biological Procesess

1. D	11. A	21. C	31. C	41. A
2. A	12. C	22. C	32. D	42. B
3. B	13. B	23. D	33. A	43. C
4. B	14. A	24. B	34. B	44. B
5. D	15. C	25. D	35. B	45. A
6. C	16. B	26. D	36. C	46. B
7. D	17. C	27. B	37. A	47. B
8. B	18. C	28. A	38. A	48. B
9. C	19. B	29. C	39. A	
10. B	20. C	30. B	40. C	

1. **The correct answer is D.** In a polynucleotide, adjacent nucleotides are joined together by a phosphodiester linkage between the –OH group on the 3' carbon of one nucleotide and the phosphate on the 5' carbon on another nucleotide. This specific bonding creates what is called a sugar-phosphate backbone of DNA. Choice A is incorrect because hydrogen bonding holds together the two strands of DNA that form the double helix, but phosphodiester linkages hold together each individual strand. Choice B is incorrect because hydrogen bonding does not hold together the nucleotides on each strand of DNA, but rather links two strands together to form a double helix. Choice C is incorrect because the phosphodiester linkages in each DNA strand occur between the OH group of the 3' carbon of one nucleotide and the phosphate on the 5' carbon of another nucleotide.

2. **The correct answer is A.** Precursor mRNA has a modified guanine nucleotide at its 5' end, which is called a 5' cap. Choice B is incorrect because the 3' end of the mRNA is also modified by the addition of a string of A bases. This is called a poly(A) tail. Choice C is incorrect because there is not a phosphate group at the 5' end of mRNA, instead there is a modified guanine. Choice D is incorrect because a stop codon is found within an mRNA strand to signal the stop of a polypeptide chain.

3. **The correct answer is B.** G_1 is a portion of the interphase of cell division. During this 5- to 6-hour time period, all cellular materials except for DNA are replicated. Choice A is incorrect because cells are at rest during the G_0 phase. Choice C is incorrect because during G_2, cells repair any errors made during DNA replication. Choice D is incorrect because the S phase is the time period in interphase in which DNA is replicated.

4. **The correct answer is B.** The enzyme topoisomerase helps to relieve the strain caused by untwisting the DNA. This enzyme catalyzes a reaction that causes gaps in the DNA to alleviate the strain the unwinding causes on the helical DNA structure. Topoisomerase breaks the DNA and then joins it back together. Choice A is incorrect because DNA polymerase is responsible for synthesizing new DNA strands. Choice C is

incorrect because DNA helicase unwinds the double-stranded DNA, but does not relieve the strain caused by this unwinding process. Choice D is incorrect because DNA ligase joins together the ends of newly synthesized DNA fragments along a template strand to form a new daughter strand.

5.　**The correct answer is D.** The first protein of the transcription initiation complex, TFIID, recognizes the TATA sequence, TATAAAA, and binds to DNA. This triggers the formation of the initiation complex and the start of transcription. Choice A is incorrect because RNA polymerase II is not a transcription factor, but an enzyme, and it cannot bind to DNA until the transcription initiation complex is formed. Choice B is incorrect because TFIID is the first transcription factor to bind to DNA. After TFIID is bound to the DNA, other transcription factors are then recruited to the promoter sequence. TFIIA can join the initiation complex after the binding of TFIID, and TFIIA acts to stabilize the transcription complex. Choice C is incorrect because TFIID is the first transcription factor to bind DNA and start the formation of the initiation complex. TFIIC is not a type of transcription factor in eukaryotic cells; it is a transcription factor involved in transcription by RNA polymerase III.

6.　**The correct answer is C.** The enzyme DNA polymerase III can continuously synthesize a new complementary strand in the mandatory 5' to 3' direction. This is possible on the strand running in the 3' to 5' direction. This strand is called the leading strand. The antiparallel strand that runs 5' to 3' is referred to as the lagging strand. DNA polymerase III still synthesizes DNA in the 5' to 3' direction, but the synthesis is not continuous on the lagging strand. Instead, short segments of DNA (about 100 to 1,000 nucleotides long) called Okazaki fragments

are synthesized and then joined. Choice A is incorrect because all new DNA strands are synthesized on a parent template strand. Choice B is incorrect because new DNA strands can only be synthesized in the 5' to 3' direction. Choice D is incorrect because DNA replication results in two identical daughter strands, not one.

7.　**The correct answer is D.** *Homo* is the genus for humans. *Sapiens* is the species that humans belong to, and *sapiens* is also the subspecies. Choice A is incorrect because humans are in the domain Eukarya, the kingdom Animalia, and the phylum Chordata. Choice B is incorrect because humans are classified in the phylum Chordata, the class Mammalia, and the order Primate. Choice C is incorrect because humans are in the order Primate, the family Hominidae, and the genus *Homo*.

8.　**The correct answer is B.** The hydrophilic heads of the phospholipids face outward into the aqueous regions both inside and outside of the cell. Choice A is incorrect because phosphate groups are found on ATP, not phospholipids. Choice C is incorrect because the hydrophobic tail ends of the phospholipids face each other in the interior region of the cell membrane. Choice D is incorrect because the nonpolar region of the phospholipid is the hydrophobic tail; the hydrophilic head is a polar region of the phospholipid.

9.　**The correct answer is C.** Enzymes are proteins that speed up metabolic reactions by lowering the activation energy barrier without affecting the overall free energy of the reaction. Choice A is incorrect because enzymes do not increase the activation energy of a reaction, they decrease it. Choice B is incorrect because enzymes speed up a reaction without being consumed by the reaction; therefore, they do not alter the products of a reaction. Choice D is incorrect because enzymes are specific to certain substrates and, therefore, each type of enzyme can catalyze only certain reactions.

10. **The correct answer is B.** Processes that have a negative ΔG value will occur spontaneously. Because of the way ΔG is dependent on entropy in the equation $\Delta G = -2870$ KJ/mol, it can be determined that every spontaneous reaction decreases a system's free energy. Choice A is incorrect because a reaction that requires an input of energy to move forward would have a positive ΔG value. Choice C is incorrect because an endergonic reaction has a positive ΔG value. Choice D is incorrect because a reaction at equilibrium would have a ΔG value close to zero.

11. **The correct answer is A.** The production of glucose during photosynthesis is carried out by the following reaction: $6CO_2 + 12H_2O$ + light energy $\rightarrow C_6H_{12}O_6 + 6O_2 + 6H_2O$. Thus, glucose is produced by the reaction of CO_2 and H_2O. Choice B is incorrect because water and oxygen do not provide the carbon atoms necessary to form glucose. Choice C is incorrect because carbon dioxide and oxygen do not provide the necessary hydrogen atoms to form glucose. Choice D is incorrect because light energy, not ATP, is required for the formation of glucose.

12. **The correct answer is C.** A point mutation can result in a nonsense mutation in which the mutation causes a stop codon to be put in the incorrect place. The result is a shortened polypeptide chain that produces an incomplete protein. Choice A is incorrect because a silent mutation is one in which the change still results in an alternate codon for the same amino acid, so the mutation is not realized. Choice B is incorrect because a missense mutation is a point mutation in which the mutation changes the amino

acid codon and that changes the resulting protein structure. Choice D is incorrect because there is no such point mutation as a stop mutation; the mutation that causes premature termination of an amino acid chain is a nonsense mutation.

13. **The correct answer is B.** Certain adaptations of a species are specific to their environment. Therefore, there are different phenotypic traits of similar organisms, depending on where they live. In an environment in which the primary food source is nuts and seeds, a bird species is likely to adapt a strong curved beak for cracking nut shells. Choice A is incorrect because a long, thin beak might be adapted in an environment in which probing for insects is the primary mechanism for finding food. Choice C is incorrect because birds that have dexterous beaks that can hold twigs have adapted this quality in order to probe for insects. Choice D is incorrect because a small pointy beak would not be a useful adaptation for cracking nuts.

14. **The correct answer is A.** There are three main bacterial shapes. Bacilli are rod-shaped bacteria that have flagella for movement, and spirilla are spiral-shaped bacteria that also have flagella. Choice B is incorrect because cocci are spherical-shaped bacteria that do not have flagella to aid in movement. Choice C is incorrect because cocci are spherical-shaped bacteria that do not have flagella to aid in movement. Choice D is incorrect because cocci are spherical-shaped bacteria that do not have flagella to aid in movement.

15. **The correct answer is C.** Fungi ingest nutrients by secreting hydrolytic enzymes called exoenzymes into their surrounding environment. The exoenzymes break down complex molecules into simple organic molecules that fungi can absorb and use. Choice A is incorrect because there are no

enzymes classified as fungases. Choice B is incorrect because polymerases are enzymes that facilitate replication of DNA or the transcription of RNA. Choice D is incorrect because lysosomes are eukaryotic cellular organelles that are sacs filled with enzymes responsible for digesting macromolecules in the cell.

16. **The correct answer is B.** The process of viral uncoating releases the viral genome from the capsid. The host cell digests the capsid proteins. When the viral capsid is destroyed, the viral genetic material (DNA) is released into the cell. Choice A is incorrect because the virus attaches to the host cell before the uncoating process. Choice C is incorrect because the viral genome is transcribed into mRNA during the process of viral replication, which occurs after the uncoating step, and after viral DNA is transported into the nucleus of the host cell. Choice D is incorrect because the virus is taken into the host cell during the process of penetration, which occurs prior to the uncoating of the virus.

17. **The correct answer is C.** During prometaphase, the nuclear envelop disintegrates, and the microtubules of the spindle can extend into the nuclear area of the cell and interact with the condensed chromosomes. The long microtubules extend from the centrosomes (still moving to opposite sides of the cell) toward the middle of the cell. Choice A is incorrect because interphase is the period during the cell cycle before mitosis occurs. Choice B is incorrect because during prophase, the nucleolus disappears. The chromatin in the nucleus become more tightly coiled and condense into discrete chromosomes. Choice D is incorrect because during metaphase, the chromosomes align at the middle of the cell.

18. **The correct answer is C.** Photosynthetic bacteria that use light as an energy source and depend upon carbon dioxide to produce their own food are called photoautotrophs. Choice A is incorrect because photoautotrophs depend on carbon dioxide to produce their own food, not water. Choice B is incorrect because CO_2, not O_2, is required for photoautotrophs to produce food. Choice D is not correct because CO_2, not nitrogen, is required for photoautotrophs to produce food.

19. **The correct answer is B.** Each cell produces its own supply of ATP as it is needed. As a cell becomes more active, ATP production increases, and as a cell becomes inactive, ATP production decreases. Choice A is incorrect because ATP production decreases when cells are less active because less energy is required to maintain cellular functions. Choice C is incorrect because as a cell becomes less active, ATP production decreases because less energy is needed to maintain cellular function. Choice D is incorrect because ATP production is regulated by the activity level of the cell, and it changes as cellular activity increases or decreases.

20. **The correct answer is C.** Together, glycolysis and the citric acid cycle produce 4 molecules of ATP. The process of oxidation phosphorylation produces the bulk of ATP molecules. Depending on which shuttle transport system is used, oxidative phosphorylation produces 32 or 34 ATP molecules. Choice A is incorrect because glycolysis only produces 2 ATP molecules, and oxidative phosphorylation produces 32 or 34. Choice B is incorrect because the Krebs cycle only produces 2 ATP molecules compared to oxidative phosphorylation, which produces 32 or 34. Choice D is incorrect because fermentation is similar to glycolysis, but occurs in the absence of oxygen.

21. **The correct answer is C.** ATP provides energy for the cell because of its phosphate bonds. These are highly unstable covalent bonds that are easily broken by hydrolysis. The hydrolysis of ATP is an exergonic process that yields ADP and P_i. ATP releases a lot of energy as these phosphate bonds are broken, and this provides energy to cells for many metabolic processes. Choice A is incorrect because the nitrogenous base does not provide energy for the cell; it combines with the ribose to create a nucleoside molecule. Choice B is incorrect because the pentose (ribose) sugar in the ATP molecule does not provide cellular energy. Choice D is incorrect because it is the breaking of the phosphate bonds, not the phosphate groups, that provides energy for the cell.

22. **The correct answer is C.** During active transport, energy in the form of ATP (adenosine triphosphate) is required to move molecules across the cell membrane and across the concentration gradient. Choice A is incorrect because osmosis is a form of passive transport across the cell membrane and is defined as the diffusion of water across the membrane. It does not require that energy be added to the cell. Choice B is incorrect because facilitated transport is another form of passive transport that relies upon the concentration gradient. Certain proteins within the cell membrane can assist in transporting molecules across the membrane. Choice D is incorrect because diffusion is a type of passive transport. Therefore, this type of movement does not require added energy. Diffusion describes a gradual change in concentration of a molecule either with or along a concentration gradient.

23. **The correct answer is D.** Glycolysis occurs in the cytoplasm of cells and is the breaking down of glucose molecules from a six-carbon sugar into two three-carbon sugars. These smaller sugars are oxidized and their atoms are rearranged to form two pyruvate molecules. Choice A is incorrect because during oxidative phosphorylation, chemiosmosis couples an electron transport system (ETS) to ATP synthesis. It does not involve the formation of pyruvate. Choice B is incorrect because the citric acid, or Krebs, cycle is the process that occurs after the formation of pyruvate in glycolysis. If there is oxygen present in the cell, the pyruvate molecules enter the mitochondrion and the enzymes involved in the citric acid cycle complete the oxidation process and release the stored energy. The goal of the Krebs cycle is to completely oxidize the remnants of the original glucose molecule. Choice C is incorrect because pyruvate molecules do not form during photosynthesis in plant cells.

24. **The correct answer is B.** In general, the concentration of Na$^+$ ions is greater outside the cell, and the concentration of K$^+$ ions is greater inside the cell. This is due to the fact that sodium channels allow for very little sodium ion to diffuse into the cell. In addition, sodium potassium actively pumps transport Na$^+$ out of the cell and K$^+$ into the cell. Choice A is incorrect because in general, the concentration of sodium ions is greater outside the cell. Choice C is incorrect because the concentration of sodium ions is greatest in the extracellular environment as compared to the cytoplasm or any organelles inside the cell. Choice D is incorrect because the plasma membrane contains channels through which sodium ions can pass either into or out of the cell, but the highest concentration of sodium ions is generally found outside the cell.

25. **The correct answer is D.** The thyroid produces thyroxine (T4) and triiodothryonine (T3), which stimulate and maintain metabolic processes. An excess of T3 and T4 can

cause hyperthyroidism. Choice A is incorrect because high blood-calcium levels are caused by the parathyroid hormone. Choice B is incorrect because blood-calcium levels are lowered by calcitoninc in the parathyroid gland. Choice C is incorrect because hypothyroidism is caused by a deficit of T3 and T4.

26. **The correct answer is D.** ATP synthase is essentially a proton pump that uses the H+ buildup in the intermembrane space of the mitochondrion to produce ATP by pumping the protons back inside the matrix. Choices A, B, and C are incorrect because their only roles in respiration are as enzymatic cofactors.

27. **The correct answer is B.** Ca2+ is also important in blood clotting, muscle contraction, and nerve signal transmission. The other ions noted in A, C, and D do not play this role in bone maintenance.

28. **The correct answer is A.** The smooth ER also captures calcium ions from the cytosol and stores them. In muscle cells, a specialized smooth ER membrane pumps calcium ions from the cytosol into the ER lumen. Choice B is incorrect because the rough ER is directly associated with the synthesis of many proteins because of the ribosomes attached to its surface. Choice C is incorrect because ribosomes are organelles within the cell that carry out protein synthesis. Choice D is incorrect because lysosomes are thought of as "cellular garbage cans" because they are responsible for getting rid of all cellular debris.

29. **The correct answer is C.** In a condyloid joint, there is angular motion in two planes and circumduction; the radiocarpal joint of the wrist moves in a condyloid fashion. Choice A is incorrect because gliding occurs in plane joints. Choice B is incorrect because rotational movement occurs in neck and limb rotation; ball-and-socket joints and pivot joints exhibit rotational motion. Choice D is incorrect because hinged is a type of joint that also exhibits angular motion.

30. **The correct answer is B.** According to the sliding filament model of muscle contraction, a sarcomere contracts, or shortens, when the thin filaments slide across the thick filaments. When the muscle is fully contracted, the thin actin filaments overlap in the middle of the sarcomere. Thus, the contraction shortens the sarcomere, but does not change the length of the microfilaments. Choice A is incorrect because myosin is the component that makes up the thick filaments, and it hydrolyzes ATP in order to provide energy for the sliding motion of the filaments. Choice C is incorrect because the thin actin filaments slide past the thick filaments, but they do not contract. Choice D is incorrect because the thick myosin filaments slide past the actin filaments, but they do not contract.

31. **The correct answer is C.** A specialized region of the heart called a pacemaker, or sinoatrial node (SA node), sets the pace, or rate, at which all heart muscles contract. The pacemaker is located in the upper wall of the right atrium in the heart. It generates an electrical signal similar to the signal produced by nerve cells. Choice A is incorrect because the left atrium is the chamber in the heart into which oxygen-rich blood flows. Choice B is incorrect because the right atrium is the chamber in the heart into which oxygen-poor blood flows. Choice D is incorrect because autorhythmic cells are cells that do not contract. They keep the heart moving at a steady pace, but the sinoatrial node sets the pace.

32. **The correct answer is D.** In the lysogenic life cycle, there is no shutdown of the host cell. The viral DNA is copied every time the

bacteria reproduce and replicate their DNA. The bacteriaphage genome is integrated into the host genome and creates what is called a prophage. The bacteria continue to grow and reproduce unharmed until something triggers the start of the lytic life cycle. Choice A is incorrect because both life cycles have the attachment stage. Choice B is incorrect because both life cycles have an injection stage. Choice C is incorrect because both life cycles have the DNA attachment stage.

33. **The correct answer is A.** During sexual reproduction, the joining together of the cytoplasm of the two parent mycelia is called plasmogamy. Choice B is incorrect because during karyogamy, the haploid nuclei from each parent fuse together to produce a diploid cell. Choice C is incorrect because during meiosis, the fungal cells divide to form new haploid cells. Choice D is incorrect because germination is the growth of the fungal spores.

34. **The correct answer is B.** Memory B cells, produced by B-lymphocytes in the immune system, provide antibody protection against future infections of the same virus. Memory B cells are only produced in cells that are undergoing an active viral infection. Choice A is incorrect because the host cell does not prevent against future infection; it is the body's immune system and the production of memory B cells that do. Choice C is incorrect because T cells are part of the immune system, but they do not act to prevent reinfection of a particular virus. Choice D is incorrect because B-lymphocytes are responsible for producing the memory B cells, but it is the memory B cells themelves that help to prevent reinfection.

35. **The correct answer is B.** The ends of each bronchiole contain grape-like clusters of air sacs called alveoli. The clusters of alveoli have a surface area 50 times greater than skin. The inner surface of the alveoli is lined with a thin layer of epithelial cells. Oxygen is dissolved on a film of moisture on the epithelium, and it diffuses into the blood capillaries that surround each alveolus. Thus, the grape-like structures allow more O_2 to pass into the lungs. Choice A is incorrect because the grape-like structure does not cause the alveoli to more firmly attach to the bronchiole. Choice C is incorrect because CO_2 diffuses out through the alveoli, but not into the lungs. Choice D is incorrect because the cluster-like structures do not allow for a more efficient exchange; they just allow more oxygen in and carbon dioxide out of the lungs.

36. **The correct answer is C.** Absorption of nutrients from food into the blood stream occurs mostly in the small intestine. Some nutrients are absorbed by simple diffusion, and others are pumped against concentration gradients into epithelial cells. Choice A is incorrect because the breakdown of food into nutrients takes place in the stomach, but absorption occurs in the small intestine. Choice B is incorrect because the large intestine is responsible for ridding the body of waste products. Choice D is incorrect because the pancreas functions to neutralize chime and break down starch, lipids, and nucleic acids.

37. **The correct answer is A.** The juxtamedullary capillary beds help to concentrate urine. They are capillary beds that have vasa recta. Vasa recta are straight arteries in the kidneys that are ordered and perpendicular to the loop of Henle. Choice B is incorrect because the peritubular capillary beds pick up solutes that have been filtered out in the glomerular bed and reabsorb them. Choice C is incorrect because the glomerular capillary beds are where filtrate is formed from blood. It is the highest pressure capillary bed in the body because the diameter of the afferent

arteriole is larger than that of the efferent arteriole. Choice D is incorrect because this specific type of nephron is found mostly in the cortex of the kidney (although some are in the loop of Henle), and about 85 percent of all nephrons are corticoid nephrons.

38. **The correct answer is A.** An increase in estrogen inhibits FSH and LH. This prevents the development of more follicles. Choice B is incorrect because GnRH is secreted from the hypothalamus and stimulates the release of LH and FSH. Choice C is incorrect because GnRH is secreted from the hypothalamus and stimulates the release of LH and FSH. Choice D is incorrect because progesterone levels drop due to the degeneration of the corpus luteum, not because of an increase in estrogen.

39. **The correct answer is A.** As lymph cycles through the lymphatic organs, it picks up and carries microbes or toxins picked up from a site of infection in the body to lymphatic organs such as the lymph nodes. Choice B is incorrect because blood cells are not responsible for ridding the body of toxins. Choice C is incorrect because antibodies are specific to fight viral infections, but lymph carries invaders to the lymphatic organs. Choice D is incorrect because T cells help to fight infection, but lymph carries the microbes and toxins to the lymph organs.

40. **The correct answer is C.** The mating of two heterozygous individuals is called a monohybrid cross. In this type of cross, 75% of the offspring would show the dominant trait, and 25% would be homozygous for the recessive trait and would show that trait. This can be determined by setting up a Punnett square to represent the cross.

	B	b
B	BB	Bb
b	Bb	bb

Choice A is incorrect because in a cross between two heterozygous individuals, 75% of the offspring would show the dominant trait. Choice B is incorrect because in a heterozygous cross, 50% of those offspring showing the dominant trait would be heterozygous dominant. Choice D is incorrect because none of the genotypes possible show up in a 10% ratio.

41. **The correct answer is A.** Hydrogen carriers link together two different redox (oxidation-reduction) reactions. They deliver protons (H+) to many different enzymes. Choice B is incorrect because flavin vitamins are coenzymes that play an important role in the Krebs cycle. Choice C is incorrect because electron carriers accept electrons and then transfer them to another molecule. Choice D is incorrect because coenzyme A is a cofactor that carries a small organic acid needed for cellular respiration.

42. **The correct answer is B.** Because the rate of evolution is so slow, it is possible to use the Hardy-Weinberg theorem to approximate allele and genotype frequencies. Choice A is incorrect because the rate of evolution in a species is generally a very slow process occurring over generations. Choice C is incorrect because the bottleneck effect is an evolutionary effect that invalidates the Hardy-Weinberg theorem. Choice D is incorrect because the founder effect is an evolutionary effect that invalidates the Hardy-Weinberg theorem.

43. **The correct answer is C.** In inheritance patterns involving epistasis, a gene at one locus on the chromosome alters the phenotypic expression of a gene at a different locus. Even though the genes are on different loci, they may be tightly linked. Choice A is incorrect because pleiotropy is the property of a gene in which it affects multiple phenotypes. Pleiotropic alleles of a gene are

responsible for the multiple symptoms associated with certain hereditary disease. Choice B is incorrect because polygenic inheritance involves the variation of a specific trait due to multiple genes acting to express one phenotypic trait. Choice D is incorrect because pedigree is a term used to describe the inheritance patterns of a family over many generations.

44. **The correct answer is B.** Genetic variation is due in part to the passing on of recessive alleles in heterozygous individuals. This latent variation is only exposed to natural selection when an individual is homozygous for a recessive trait. Choice A is incorrect because the expression of dominant traits due to the passing on of dominant alleles does not introduce variation in a species. Choice C is incorrect because a large genome only imparts genetic variation if there is more than one type of allele for each gene. Choice D is incorrect because homozygous alleles are the same and, therefore, do not introduce variability in the traits of a species.

45. **The correct answer is A.** Bile is produced in the liver and aids in digestion in the small intestine. Choice B is incorrect because the pancreas helps to regulate blood sugar and is involved in endocrine function. Choice C is incorrect because the gallbladder stores bile. Choice D is incorrect because the large intestine is involved in nutrient absorption from liquid.

46. **The correct answer is B.** The dorsal side of an animal is its back. Choice A is incorrect because it refers to the animal's posterior. Choice C is incorrect because it refers to the outer side of a body part on an organism. Choice D is incorrect because it refers to the underside of an animal or organism.

47. **The correct answer is B.** The metatarsals are found in the feet. Choices A and D are unrelated to the metatarsal bones, and Choice C is incorrect because the hands are where the metacarpals, not the metatarsals, are found.

48. **The correct answer is B.** Your patella is your knee bone. The other choices are incorrect because they do not refer to the knee.

Section 3: Chemical Procesess

1. C	**11.** C	**21.** D	**31.** B	**41.** C
2. A	**12.** C	**22.** B	**32.** A	**42.** B
3. A	**13.** A	**23.** B	**33.** C	**43.** D
4. C	**14.** D	**24.** A	**34.** A	**44.** B
5. C	**15.** C	**25.** C	**35.** B	**45.** C
6. A	**16.** A	**26.** D	**36.** C	**46.** B
7. B	**17.** B	**27.** B	**37.** C	**47.** D
8. B	**18.** C	**28.** A	**38.** D	**48.** C
9. B	**19.** A	**29.** B	**39.** B	
10. C	**20.** C	**30.** D	**40.** B	

1. **The correct answer is C.** The rules of electron configuration state that electrons are added to the allowable orbitals for each atom starting with the lowest energy level and increasing in energy levels until all the electrons occupy an orbital. Electrons fill the orbitals in the following order: $1s \rightarrow 2s \rightarrow 2p \rightarrow 3s \rightarrow 3p \rightarrow 4s \rightarrow 3d \rightarrow 4p$. None of the other answer choices show the correct order.

2. **The correct answer is A.** In an sp orbital, two p orbitals are used to form a triple bond between the carbon atoms, and the third p orbital hybridizes with the s orbital to form two sp orbitals between the C and H atoms. Choice B is incorrect because the triple bond takes up two of the p orbitals, leaving only one p orbital to hybridize with the s orbital. Choice C is incorrect because the triple bond takes up two of the p orbitals, leaving only one p orbital to hybridize with the s orbital. Choice D is incorrect because the orbitals only form one type of hybridization orbital in this molecule.

3. **The correct answer is A.** The angular momentum, l, indicates the shape of the orbital. The values of l depend on the value of the principle quantum number. For a given value of n, l has possible values from 0 to $n-1$. Therefore, if $n = 1$, the only possible value of l is 0. Choice B is incorrect because the principle quantum number, n, is an integer (1, 2, 3…) whose value determines the energy level of the orbital. The principle quantum number also relates the average distance of the electron from the nucleus in a particular orbital. Choice C is incorrect because the magnetic quantum number, ml, describes the orientation of the electron orbital in space. For each value of l, in a subshell there are $(2l + 1)$ integral values of ml. For example, if $l = 1$, then there are $[(2 \times 1) + 1]$, or three values of ml. These values are -1, 0, and 1. The number of ml values indicates the number of orbitals in a subshell of a particular l value. Choice D is incorrect because the electron spin quantum number, m_s, takes into account that there are two possible spinning motions (rotations) of an electron; clockwise or counterclockwise. Thus, m_s has a value of either $+1/2$ or $-1/2$.

4. **The correct answer is C.** When both a sigma and a pi bond exist between two atoms, a double bond is formed. Choice A

is incorrect because two sigma bonds do not form a double bond between atoms. Choice B is incorrect because two pi bonds do not form a double bond. Two pi bonds and a sigma bond between atoms form a triple bond. Choice D is incorrect because only one sigma bond and one pi bond are needed to form a double bond.

5. **The correct answer is C.** The lowest possible n value for a d orbital is 3. There are five possible d orbitals: $3dxy$, $3dyz$, $3dxz$, $3dx^2-y^2$, and $3dz^2$. Choice A is incorrect because the minimum n value for a d orbital is 3. Choice B is incorrect because for d orbitals, the lowest n value is 3. Choice D is incorrect because the lowest principle quantum number for a d orbital is 2.

6. **The correct answer is A.** Nitrogen and oxygen gas are most commonly found as diatomic molecules, N_2 and O_2. Choice B is incorrect because ozone is a polyatomic molecule, O_3. Choice C is incorrect because carbon dioxide exists as a polyatomic molecule, CO_2. Choice D is incorrect because sulfur dioxide exists as a polyatomic molecule, SO_2.

7. **The correct answer is B.** The ideal gas law can be expressed by the equation $PV = nRT$, and pressure can be determined by the equation $P = nRT/V$. Therefore, for the given gas:

    P = (0.6 mol)(0.082 L.atm/K.mol)(298K)/(0.250L)

    P = 58.6 atm

    Choice A is incorrect because this value is produced if the volume is not converted from milliliters to liters. Choice C is incorrect because this is the value calculated if the equation is incorrect: $P = nRTV$. Choice D is incorrect because this is the value given by the incorrect equation and failure to convert the volume into liters.

8. **The correct answer is B.** The kinetic molecular theory of gases states that gas molecules do not exert attractive or repulsive forces on one another, because they are separated by a distance larger than their own dimensions. Choice A is incorrect because the kinetic molecular theory of gases states that gas molecules are in constant motion. Choice C is incorrect because it is the opposite of the kinetic molecular theory of gases, which states that gas molecules do not exert attractive or repulsive forces on one another. Choice D is incorrect because the average kinetic energy of a gas molecule is proportional to a gas' temperature.

9. **The correct answer is B.** Amines are organic molecules with properties of a base. They have the general formula, R_3N, where R is an H atom or a hydrocarbon group. The simplest amine is NH_3. Choice A is incorrect because the NO_2 group makes this compound a nitro compound. Choice C is incorrect because the $C \equiv N$ bond makes this a nitrile. Choice D is incorrect because a compound with the basic formula RC = ONR'R" is an amide compound.

10. **The correct answer is C.** The ionic compound magnesium nitride is formed from the ions Mg^{2+} and N^{3-}. The formula Mg_3N_2 combines the ions in the right ratio, so that the overall compound is neutral. Choice A is incorrect because these are the elements in the compound, while they are not in the correct ionic form. Choice B is incorrect because the compound forms by combining the ions Mg^{2+} and N^{3-}. Choice D is incorrect because the compound forms by combining the ions Mg^{2+} and N^{3-}.

11. **The correct answer is C.** An aldehyde is formed when at least one of the R groups attached to the carbon atom is an H atom. Choice A is incorrect because carboxylic acids contain a carboxyl group, COOH.

Choice B is incorrect because in a ketone, the carbon atom of the carbonyl group is bound to two hydrocarbon groups, but if one of those functional groups is a single H atom, then the compound is classified as an aldehyde. Choice D is incorrect because esters have the general formula R'COOR. R' can be either an H or a hydrocarbon, and R is a hydrocarbon group.

12. **The correct answer is C.** Alkynes are hydrocarbons that contain at least one carbon-carbon triple bond. Choice A is incorrect because alkanes are hydrocarbons that contain a carbon-carbon single bond. Choice B is incorrect because alkenes are hydrocarbons that contain a carbon-carbon double bond. Choice D is incorrect because in an aromatic, every C-C bond in the ring exists as an intermediate between a double and a single bond.

13. **The correct answer is A.** Amino acids compose proteins. Choice B is incorrect because fatty acids are a subunit of lipids. Choice C is incorrect because monosaccharides are the monomeric subunit of carbohydrates. Choice D is incorrect because nucleotides are the monomeric subunit of nucleic acids (i.e.,DNA and RNA).

14. **The correct answer is D.** Because hemoglobin is made up of four separate polypeptide chains, it has quaternary structure, which is the most complex level of protein structure. Choice A is incorrect because the protein is not simply an unfolded polypeptide chain. Choice B is incorrect because the protein is a complex of folded polypeptides. Choice C is incorrect because tertiary structure would only be the most complicated level of protein structure if the protein was composed of one single polypeptide chain.

15. **The correct answer is C.** Proteins are produced via translation at ribosomes. Choice A

is incorrect because the nucleolus is responsible for ribosome production. Choice B is incorrect because the nucleus houses genetic material. Choice D is incorrect because the smooth ER produces lipids.

16. **The correct answer is A.** Iron in heme gives blood a red hue, which gets brighter with oxygen bound. Choice B is incorrect because the 3D shape of a protein does not influence its visible color. Choice C. is incorrect because fluorescence is not the same as visible color. Choice D is incorrect because the iron in heme, not hydrogen bonding, is the cause of the observed color.

17. **The correct answer is B.** Cholesterol is a derivative of a steroid, so it is a lipid. Choice A is incorrect because the C:H:O ratio is not that of a carbohydrate, and it is not composed of monosaccharides. Choice C is incorrect because cholesterol is not composed of nucleotides. Choice D is incorrect because the molecule is not composed of amino acids.

18. **The correct answer is C.** Cholesterol is largely hydrophobic, like the interior hydrocarbon tails of the phospholipids that comprise the membrane, so cholesterol should largely be located internally within the plasma membrane. Only the hydroxyl group interacts with the polar head groups of the membrane. Choices A and B are incorrect because cholesterol would have to be largely hydrophilic for this to be a favorable structure. Choice D is incorrect because this association would also require hydrophilicity, and it would not serve to increase the rigidity of the membrane if cholesterol is not integrated within the membrane.

19. **The correct answer is A.** By providing rigidity to animal cell membranes, membrane integrity is maintained, and no cell wall is needed. Choice B is incorrect because

a cytoskeleton would maintain organelle positions and provide mechanical support; animal cells have cytoskeletons. Choice C is incorrect because the Golgi apparatus is the packing and shipping center of the cell, which is unrelated to structural integrity. The same goes for Choice D. which is incorrect because animal cells still have peroxisomes, which break down fatty acids.

20. **The correct answer is C.** The unique point on a phase diagram that indicates the exact temperature and pressure at which all three phases, or states, can exist simultaneously is called the triple point. Choice A is incorrect because the melting point is the temperature and pressure at which a solid can transform into a liquid. Choice B is incorrect because the critical point is the temperature and pressure above which a substance can no longer condense into a liquid. Choice D is incorrect because the freezing point is the temperature and pressure at which a substance can change from a liquid to a solid.

21. **The correct answer is D.** The ground state refers to the lowest energy state of a system. The stability of an electron decreases as the value of n increases. Each of these levels ($n = 2, 3, 4…$) is called an excited state, or excited level. Each of these levels is higher in energy level than the ground state, and energy increases as electrons move farther from the nucleus, Choice D. Choice A is incorrect because the energy level increases with increasing distance from the nucleus. Choice B is incorrect because the region of the atom closest to the atom has the lowest energy level and is the most stable. Choice C is incorrect because the first electron orbital has the lowest energy of the system.

22. **The correct answer is B.** The first column of elements is considered Group 1 and these elements are called alkali metals. They all have one valence electron in an s orbital.

This single valence electron can be easily removed, which makes alkali metals highly reactive elements. Choice A is incorrect because the alkaline earth metals all have two valence electrons in an s orbital. Because there is an electron pair filling the s orbital, these elements are much less reactive than alkali metals. Choice C is incorrect because transition elements, or transition metals, all have valence electrons in the d orbitals. The five d orbitals hold their electrons very loosely, and most of these elements are characterized by high melting points, high electrical conductivity, low ionization energies, and many oxidation states. Choice D is incorrect because halogens have seven valence electrons (s^2p^5). Because there is an unpaired electron in the valence shell, these are highly reactive elements.

23. **The correct answer is B.** Molecules with a central atom that have no lone pairs adopt certain geometrical structures. Those with three electron pairs form a trigonal planar structure. Choice A is incorrect because molecules with two electron pairs are linear. Choice C is incorrect because molecules with four electron pairs form a tetrahedral structure. Choice D is incorrect because molecules with five electron pairs form a trigonal bipyramid.

24. **The correct answer is A.** A neutralization reaction is a specialized reaction that involves acids and bases. In this type of reaction, an acid and base combine to form a salt and water. Choice B is incorrect because an acid and a base are the reactants in a neutralization reaction, not the products. Choice C is incorrect because carbon dioxide is not a product of a neutralization reaction; the products formed are salt and water. Choice D is incorrect because acid is one of the reactants of a neutralization reaction, not a product.

25. **The correct answer is C.** The two types of forces that cause capillary action are cohesion (attraction between like molecules) and adhesion (attraction between unlike molecules). Choice A is incorrect because capillary action is caused by the attractive forces adhesion and cohesion. Choice B is incorrect because capillary action is a type of surface tension caused by adhesion and cohesion. Choice D is incorrect because intermolecular forces occur between two molecules, and intramolecular forces occur between atoms in a molecule.

26. **The correct answer is D.** The molarity of a solution is determined by the equation $M =$ moles solute/liters solution. The molecular weight of sodium hydroxide is 40 g/mol, so the number of moles in the reaction is 0.155 mol. Calculating the molarity of the solution gives the value 0.311 M. None of the other choices are correct.

27. **The correct answer is B.** The Lewis acid-base concept defines acids and bases in terms of electrons. A Lewis acid is an electron pair acceptor, and a Lewis base is an electron pair donor. Choice A is incorrect because an electron pair donor is defined as a Lewis base. Choice C is incorrect because the Brønsted-Lowry concept defines acids as donors of H^+ ions and bases as acceptors of H^+ ions. Choice D is incorrect because the Brønsted-Lowry concept defines acids as donors of H^+ ions and bases as acceptors of H^+ ions.

28. **The correct answer is A.** An oxidation reaction involves the loss of electrons by a substance. In the given reaction, Fe^{2+} loses an electron to become Fe^{3+}. Therefore, the half-reaction $6Fe^{2+} \rightarrow 6Fe^{3+}$ is the oxidation reaction. Choice B is incorrect because this is only part of the reduction reaction. The reaction shown in Choice B is not a balanced reaction. Choice C is incorrect because this

reaction is a portion of the reduction reaction. It is not representative of a complete, balanced reaction. Choice D is incorrect because $14H^+ + Cr_2O_7^{2-} \rightarrow 2Cr^{3+} + 7H_2O$ is the reduction half-reaction, not the oxidation half-reduction.

29. **The correct answer is B.** Enthalpy is defined as the heat content of a substance at a constant pressure. The enthalpy change, ΔH, is defined by the change in heat content from the initial to the final state of a substance. Choice A is incorrect because energy is defined as the capacity of a system or substance to do work. Choice C is incorrect because entropy is defined as a measure of the randomness and disorder of a system. Choice D is incorrect because specific heat is the amount of heat required to raise the temperature of 1 gram of a substance by 1 degree Celsius.

30. **The correct answer is D.** The rate law is expressed by the equation rate = $k[A]^x[B]^y$, where k is the rate constant, $[A]$ and $[B]$ are the concentrations of the reactions, and the exponents correspond to the order of the reaction. The reaction is second order for A and first order for B. The overall reaction order is equal to the sum of the reaction orders for each reactant; and, therefore, the reaction order for the overall equation is 3. Choices A, B, and C are incorrect because the sum of the reaction orders in this reaction is 3.

31. **The correct answer is B.** In the propagation steps of a radical reaction, the radical formed in the second step is the same as the radical reactant in the first step, so this radical cycles back to the first propagation step, forming a reaction loop. Choice A is incorrect because the initiation step consists of a single reaction step to form the first radical reactants for the propagation steps. Choice C is incorrect because the termination steps are a single

step in which a stable product between radicals forms. Choice D is incorrect because the radical reaction does not contain a substitution step.

32. **The correct answer is A.** Chromatography is one of the simplest and most frequently used methods of compound purification. A mixture of organic compounds is dissolved into a minimum amount of liquid. This solution is then adsorbed on to the stationary phase packed into a column. At different times and using different concentrations of solvent, the organic compounds are removed from, or eluted off, the stationary phase packed column in their pure form. Choice B is incorrect because distillation is used to separate a volatile liquid from high boiling liquids and nonvolatile solids. Choice C is incorrect because the process of sublimation is used when it is necessary to separate a volatile solid substance from substances that do not readily vaporize. Choice D is incorrect because combustion analysis is not a method of separation but rather a form of analysis, and can only be performed on substances containing carbon, hydrogen, and oxygen.

33. **The correct answer is C.** The electron affinity, E_{ea}, of an element is the energy change when an electron is added to an atom in its gaseous state to form an anion (negatively charged ion). Conversely, the electron affinity also represents the energy that is needed to pull an electron away from a negatively charged anion. Electron affinity increases across a period, and it decreases down a period. In general, nonmetals have a higher electron affinity than metals. Choice A is incorrect because electron affinity increases across a period and decreases down a period. Choice B is incorrect because electron affinity increases across a period and decreases down a period. Choice D is incorrect because electron affinity increases across a period and decreases down a period.

34. **The correct answer is A.** A small amount of sample is needed for mass spectroscopy. This sample is placed into the spectrometer and bombarded by a stream of high-energy electrons. When a high-energy electron hits an organic molecule, it dislodges a valence electron from the sample molecule, which produces what is called a cation radical (positively charged, odd number of electrons). Choice B is incorrect because in IR spectroscopy, molecules absorb infrared radiation without forming an intermediate. Choice C is incorrect because intermediates are not formed in NMR spectroscopy. Choice D is incorrect because absorbance of a compound at different wavelengths are measured without the formation of an intermediate.

35. **The correct answer is B.** Using the $n + 1$ rule, in Choice A the highlighted CH_3 protons are coupled just to one adjacent CH_2 and so give only a triplet. In Choice B, the highlighted CH_2 sits between a CH_3 and a CH_2 and so would give 4 triplets or 3 quartets (potentially a 12 peak multiplet), although not all may be resolved. In Choice C, the CH_2 sits between a CH_2 group and a carbonyl carbon (which has no protons) so it will give just a triplet. Choice D has a proton that is not adjacent to any other protons, so it would be a singlet.

36. **The correct answer is C.** The entering nucleophile attacks the substrate (electrophile) in an S_N2 reaction from a position that is 180° from the leaving group on the electrophile, and the reaction takes place all in one step without any intermediates formed. In the reaction process, as the leaving group departs from the electrophile, the remaining three groups change their orientation around the carbon atom. Choices A, B, and D are incorrect because a nucleophile attacks a substrate from a 180° angle during an S_N2 reaction.

37. **The correct answer is C.** A solution is a homogeneous mixture in which the solvent and the solute are indistinguishable because the solute is uniformly dissolved in the solvent. Choice A is incorrect because a colloid is an example of a heterogeneous mixture. Choice B is incorrect because an emulsion is another example of a heterogeneous mixture. Choice D is incorrect because a suspension is an example of a heterogeneous mixture.

38. **The correct answer is D.** The transition from a solid to a liquid requires the addition of thermal energy usually in the form of heat. This increase in temperature increases the kinetic energy of the molecules, and the substance transforms from a solid to a liquid. Choice A is incorrect because thermal energy, not mechanical energy, is required for the phase change from solid to liquid. Choice B is incorrect because the specific type of energy required for the solid-to-liquid phase change is thermal energy. Choice C is incorrect because although there is an increase in kinetic energy during the phase change from a solid to a liquid, thermal energy must be added to the substance to make the change.

39. **The correct answer is B.** In the generalized E2 reaction, a nucleophile base, $B:$, attacks a neighboring C–H bond and starts to remove the H atom from the neighboring molecule. At the same time, a double bond starts to form, and the functional group X starts to leave the molecule. Choice A is incorrect because in an E1 reaction, the dissociation of the leaving group is the first step in the reaction, and then the C–H bond breaks in the next step. Choice C is incorrect because the S_N1 reaction is an addition reaction in which a double bond is not formed. Choice D is incorrect because an S_N2 reaction is an addition reaction in which no double bond is formed.

40. **The correct answer is B.** The molar ratio of methanol to water in the balanced chemical equation is 1:2. Therefore, if 0.376 mol of methanol is burned, 0.752 mol of water will be produced. Choice A is incorrect because there is not a 1:1 ratio of methanol to water. Choice C is incorrect because there is no 1:4 ratio of methanol to water. Choice D is incorrect because the stoichiometric coefficient is 4 for the water produced, but there are twice as many moles of water produced than moles of methanol reacted, so the ratio is 1:2 methanol to water.

41. **The correct answer is C.** The second law of thermodynamics states that the entropy of the universe increases in a spontaneous process and remains unchanged in a process that is at equilibrium. Therefore, in a spontaneous reaction, the entropy is greater than zero. Choice A is incorrect because the entropy of a system is zero only at equilibrium. Choice B is incorrect because in a spontaneous reaction the entropy is always increasing, and it is greater than zero. Choice D is incorrect because the entropy of a spontaneous system is always increasing. It is not a constant value.

42. **The correct answer is B.** Crystallization is a straightforward and effective way of purifying a solid. A crude sample of the reaction product is dissolved in a minimal amount of liquid solvent and heated to boiling. The impurities are left behind in the solution, and the pure crystals are isolated through a process of filtration. Choice A is incorrect because the process of extraction involves the separation of a substance from a solution or matrix. This method can be used to extract a liquid or a solid. Choice C is incorrect because chromatography can be used to separate liquids and gases primarily. Solids can be separated by dissolving them in solution and then crystallizing the isolated product. Choice D is incorrect because the

process of distillation is a simple and effective method of purifying a volatile liquid.

43. **The correct answer is D.** The relative position of the shared electrons is dependent upon the electronegativity of the atoms. Electronegativity is the physical property of an atom that describes its relative attraction of the shared electrons in a covalent bond. The electronegativity of an atom is related to the octet rule and the propensity of an atom to fill any unfilled orbitals in its valence shell. Choice A is incorrect because although the size of an atom is dependent on electronegativity, it is the electronegativity that determines the proximity of the shared electrons to each atom. Choice B is incorrect because although the number of electrons in an atom influences its electronegativity, it is the electronegativity that determines the position of shared electrons between two atoms in a covalent bond. Choice C is incorrect because it is the electronegativity, not the type of hybrid orbital, that most influences the position of the shared atoms.

44. **The correct answer is B.** The potential energy diagram shows the relationship between the potential energy of the reactants and the products. In this diagram, the potential energy of the products is greater than the potential energy of the reactants. Therefore, this diagram represents an endothermic reaction. Choice A is incorrect because in an exothermic reaction, the potential energy of the reactants is higher than the potential energy of the products. Choice C is incorrect because the potential energy diagram does not represent an equilibrium reaction. Choice D is incorrect because the diagram indicates that the reaction is not spontaneous, because the potential energy of the products is greater than the potential energy of the reactants.

45. **The correct answer is C.** When more detailed information is needed, the ^{13}C NMR spectrometer can be operated in an off-resonance mode. In this mode, single carbon resonance lines can be split into multiple lines. This phenomenon is known as spin-spin splitting and is due to the fact that the nuclear spin of one atom can interact with nearby atoms and is affected by any electron shielding and neighboring nuclei. Choice A is incorrect because in the gated-decoupled mode, the information obtained is the relative number of carbons in a sample by measuring the area under each peak. This is not the most detailed method. Choice B is incorrect because in the proton noise-decoupled mode, obtaining a spectrum provides a carbon count of the sample molecule and gives information about the environment of each carbon, but spin-spin splitting is not observed. Choice D is incorrect because there is no integration mode on the spectrometer. The area under the peaks can be determined in the gated-decoupled mode.

46. **The correct answer is B.** Cytosine and guanine pair up in DNA. Choices A and C are incorrect because adenine and thymine pair up in DNA. Choice D is incorrect because uracil is found in RNA only, not in DNA.

47. **The correct answer is D.** Transfer RNA (tRNA) delivers amino acids to the ribosome during translation. Choice A is incorrect because complementary DNA (cDNA) is not RNA but can be produced from RNA via reverse transcriptase. Choice B is incorrect because messenger RNA (mRNA) is produced during transcription and contains codons, not anticodons. Choice C is incorrect because ribosomal RNA (rRNA) is involved in ribosomal production.

48. **The correct answer is C.** An oligosaccharide consists of 3-6 monosaccharides. Choice A is incorrect because it describes a monosaccharide. Choice B is incorrect because it describes a disaccharide. Choice D is incorrect because it describes a polysaccharide.

Section 4: Critical Reading

1. D	11. C	21. D	31. C	40. A
2. B	12. A	22. A	32. D	41. B
3. C	13. D	23. D	33. D	42. C
4. C	14. C	24. A	34. B	43. B
5. A	15. D	25. C	35. A	44. B
6. A	16. A	26. C	36. D	45. A
7. C	17. B	27. A	37. C	46. C
8. D	18. D	28. B	38. A	47. B
9. D	19. A	29. B	39. A	48. B
10. D	20. A	30. D		

1. **The correct answer is D.** Choice D is correct because Gilbert suggests that dosage over seven days is a result of our attributing "magic" to the number seven because it is a number related to time. Seven, he implies, has significance for us as a number that sums up the days of the week; had Constantine not made this change, we might have attributed "magic" to the number eight. Choice A is incorrect because, even though the passage suggests that the exact number of days over which a course of antibiotics should be given may be unknown, the question refers to Constantine, who changed the number of the days of the week from eight to seven. Choice B is incorrect because the references in the passage to Constantine have nothing to do with ten. Choice C is incorrect because seven is now our "magic" number precisely because Constantine changed the number of days in the week to seven.

2. **The correct answer is B.** Choice B is correct because the passage clearly says that our attributing magic to certain numbers is a cultural construct based on associations with time and our own ten fingers. Choice A, while tempting, is incorrect. First, it refers to dosage rates, not the number of dosage

days. Second, it is not the best answer because Gilbert is suggesting that the "magic" does not have to do with anything scientific or modern. Choice C should be eliminated because "magic" and empirical evidence are diametrically opposed; the passage does not link them in any way. Choice D, while partially correct for the "magic" of seven, is, nevertheless, not the best answer because Gilbert suggests that the "magic" we invest in certain numbers has to do both with numbers related to time and numbers related to our base-ten counting system.

3. **The correct answer is C.** Gilbert says we think in numbers related to time and the base-ten counting system; seven, a typical number of dosage days, is a number related to time. Choice A must be ruled out because the passage does not discuss or allude to magical properties of drugs. Choice B is not the best choice because Gilbert says we think in numbers related to time and the base-ten counting system; seven, a typical number of dosage days, is a number related to time, not the base-ten counting system. Choice D is nearly correct, but must be eliminated because there is a better choice; Gilbert suggests that something more

fundamental than even history is at work in the way people think and the associations that certain constructs carry.

4. **The correct answer is C.** Choice C is correct because *properties* is used in the first paragraph in the sense of attributes. Choice A is incorrect because *properties* is modified in the target sentence as magical; therefore, they are not actual physical qualities or traits. Choice B is incorrect; these properties are not owned or possessed. Choice D is incorrect because, while the magical properties may include psychological associations, they go well beyond that according to Gilbert.

5. **The correct answer is A.** Choice A is the correct answer because it describes both possible monetary and public health consequences of relying on the "magic" number seven. Choice B must be ruled out because the final paragraph is about possible consequences of relying on the "magic" number seven. Choice C must be ruled out because no counterarguments are offered to the thesis anywhere in the passage. Choice D is incorrect because the final paragraph has nothing to do with the base-ten number system.

6. **The correct answer is A.** Choice A is the correct answer because the author is clearly amused by blaming the phenomenon not just on magic, but also on ancient Rome. This detail, of course, does not have to appear to make the meaning clear. Its addition is a bit of a laugh on the author's part. Choice B must be ruled out because the author does not use any word choices or select any details that express regret. Choice C is not correct because the author does not use any word choices or select any details that express worry. Choice D must be ruled out because the author does not use any word choices or select any details that create a sharp, biting, or acerbic tone.

7. **The correct answer is C.** Choice C is correct because the author of the study clearly states that the seven- to ten-day course of antibiotics for uncomplicated pneumonia is not based on scientific evidence. Choice A is incorrect. No support is needed for the idea that antibiotics are often given over a course of seven days; furthermore, the author of the study makes a pronouncement about that number rather than just validating the number. Choice B is incorrect because, even though the study author mentions both seven and ten, there is no mention of or allusion to the difference between the two types of "magical" thinking. Choice D must be ruled out because the writer's reading of Gilbert is consistent with the ideas presented by the study's author.

8. **The correct answer is D.** Choice D is correct because, even though Gilbert has authoritative credentials, his assertion about magic does need some scientific evidence to support it when it comes to discrediting seven, or ten for that matter, as reasonable numbers of dosage days. Choice A must be ruled out because questions, which, by their very nature, are most unlikely to add any kind of credibility, do not do so in this case. Choice B is not the best choice because the explanation of where the system comes from does not lend support for the idea that seven is nothing better than "magical thinking" when it comes to determining a number of days for dosing antibiotics. Choice C is incorrect because, while Gilbert does have authoritative credentials, his assertion about magic does need some scientific evidence to support it.

9. **The correct answer is D.** Choice D is correct because the passage states that "without hydrogen bonding, water would have extremely low melting and boiling points." Choice A is incorrect because hydrogen bonding ensures the opposite. Choice B is

incorrect: nothing in the passage states that frozen water is less dense than water in its liquid state as a result of hydrogen bonding. Choice C is incorrect because nothing in the passage states that hydrogen bonding plays a role in universal solvency.

10. **The correct answer is D.** Choice D is the correct answer because each and every paragraph, except the first, discusses the properties of water. Choice A must be ruled out because, while water is essential to life and the passage says that directly, the passage is first and foremost about the properties of water. Choice B is not correct because polarity and bonding are the main subject of just one of the seven paragraphs of this essay. Choice C is incorrect because other properties of water, including universal solvency are discussed in the passage; all of these qualities can and should be subsumed under the summary term of *properties.*

11. **The correct answer is C.** Choice C is correct because the main idea of the paragraph is that water is a solvent. All other details help support or lead into that topic. Choice A should be ruled out because there is no time order or other logical sequence order in the paragraph. Choice B is incorrect; there is no statement of a problem or a solution. Choice D is tempting but incorrect; while there are causes and effects in the paragraph, they are stated in service of supporting and explaining the main idea of water's solvency.

12. **The correct answer is A.** Choice A is correct because the sentence leads away from the topic of universal solvency and into the exceptions. Choice B is incorrect; only *hydrophilic*, not *hydrophobic*, bears relation to universal solvency. Choice C should be eliminated; only *hydrophobic*, not *hydrophilic*, bears relation to why oil and gas do not mix. Choice D is incorrect; only *hydrophilic* relates to the dissolving of sugar in water.

13. **The correct answer is D.** Choice D is correct because the author's purpose is to explain or inform. Choice A is incorrect; the writer is not proving the importance of water's properties or convincing the reader of them, but simply stating them. Choice B is incorrect; the writer is listing properties, but not comparing or contrasting them. Choice C should be eliminated; while some readers may conceivably be entertained, this is expository, not literary or expressive, writing.

14. **The correct answer is C.** Choice C is correct because the word *precipitately* is never related to precipitation, and the sentence sets up a contrast with water temperature changing slowly. Choices A and B are incorrect because the word *precipitately* is never related to precipitation. Choice D is incorrect because the sentence sets up a contrast with water temperature changing slowly.

15. **The correct answer is D.** Choice D is the correct answer because the paragraph is about the relationship and importance of water to life. Choice A must be ruled out because no specific properties of water are discussed in this paragraph. Choice B is not correct because a structural framework would have to provide an ordered or organizational overview of main ideas to come, and this paragraph does not do that. Choice C is incorrect because the purpose of the passage as a whole is to explain some important properties of water, and this paragraph, while it leads into that purpose, certainly does not fulfill it.

16. **The correct answer is A.** The thesis statement sums up the author main goal in writing a particular passage, and in the case of this passage, choice A sums up the author's goal of proving that water is essential to life on Earth and pervasive. Choice B supports

that statement, but it does not lay out the overall goal of the passage in a clear, summarizing statement. Choices C and D are both the topic sentences of their respective paragraphs, and though a topic sentence serves a function similar to a thesis statement, a topic sentence does not capture the goal of an entire passage as a thesis statement does.

17. **The correct answer is B.** Choice B is correct because the passage mentions avoiding excess dietary fat, not avoiding all fat. Choice A is incorrect because the final paragraph mentions avoiding, or refraining from eating, peppermint. Choice C should be eliminated because the final paragraph mentions sleeping with the head of the bed elevated. Choice D is incorrect because the final paragraph mentions refraining from lying down after meals.

18. **The correct answer is D.** In this passage, the author is discussing something very personal: his or her mother's experience with gastroesophageal reflux disease. By opening up about something that is affecting his or her family, the author achieves an intimate tone despite the statistics and other factual information about the disease in this passage. While friendliness is a form of intimacy, it also suggests a happy tone that is not present in this passage, so choice A is not the right answer. While seeing a loved one deal with a disease is likely to make someone feel angry or even enraged, choice B does not reflect the tone of this particular passage accurately. Someone might also feel jaded under the circumstances the author describes, but choice C is not an accurate reflection of this passage's tone either.

19. **The correct answer is A.** Choice A is correct because it is one of only two choices that show an attitude; of those two choices, only Choice A shows an attitude toward the disease. Choices B and C are incorrect because they both reflect facts, not a personal attitude. Choice D is incorrect because, while it reflects the author's personal attitude, it does not comment on the disease specifically, but rather on the behavior of the author's mother.

20. **The correct answer is A.** Choice A is the correct answer because the opinion stated is that people who just go ahead and take over-the-counter remedies are doing themselves a disservice. Choice B must be ruled out; it states a fact. Choice C is not correct. It states an opinion held by others and not necessarily by the author. Choice D is incorrect because it states facts.

21. **The correct answer is D.** Choice D is correct because the passage states that refraining from lying down after meals and sleeping with the head of the bed elevated may make the physical action of reflux less likely. Choice A is incorrect; the passage does not directly state that not drinking alcohol and taking PPIs will have the same or similar benefits. The same is true for choices B and C.

22. **The correct answer is A.** This question is challenging because the author says that GERD should never be self-treated without immediately explaining why. Not until the sixth paragraph does the author explain the effectiveness of PPIs and imply that these are prescription drugs, and since one cannot get prescription drugs without a doctor's diagnosis, choice A is the best answer. Choice B merely explains what GERD is; this statement does not necessarily support the idea that the disease should not be self-treated. Choice C is not the best answer since someone can make lifestyle changes without a doctor's diagnosis. Choice D is incorrect because the author never suggests that there is a high mortality rate among those who self-treat GERD.

23. **The correct answer is D.** Because the author's mother got her erosive esophagitis under control after taking PPIs, it can be inferred that PPIs can reverse inflammation, Choice D. Choice A must be ruled out because nothing suggests that PPIs are only, or specifically, for those who present with heartburn. Choice B is not the best choice because nothing in the passage suggests this. Choice C is incorrect because nothing in the passage suggests that PPIs will not help those who present with a sore throat or a cough.

24. **The correct answer is A.** Choice A is correct because *stealthy* is the only word among the four choices that shows an attitude toward the disease; it suggests sneakiness. Choice B is incorrect; no particular attitude is conveyed by the word *common* in this context. Choice C is incorrect; no particular attitude is conveyed by the word *persistent* in this context. Choice D is incorrect; no particular attitude is conveyed by the term *over-the-counter* in this context.

25. **The correct answer is C.** Choice C is correct because the sentences stress the lack of diagnosis for Alzheimer's: many patients are just assumed to have it; others who are diagnosed with dementia are treated as if they have Alzheimer's. Choices A and B must be ruled out because, while some may regard Alzheimer's disease as a subset of dementia, the target sentences do not imply either a large or a small subset. Choice D is incorrect because the sentences stress the lack of diagnosis for Alzheimer's and not a confusion in the treatment of symptoms.

26. **The correct answer is C.** Choice C is correct because the passage says that cholinesterase inhibitors may effectively ameliorate or lessen symptoms and the glutamate blocker may delay the worsening of symptoms for some people. The passage also makes it clear that both drugs have only minor side effects. Choice A is incorrect because claims are made throughout the passage for how the drugs may "delay" or lessen the worsening of symptoms. No effect on caregivers is mentioned, so Choice B can be eliminated easily. Choice D is incorrect because the drugs only decrease the symptoms, when they work, and they do not cure anyone.

27. **The correct answer is A.** At the end of paragraph 3, the author states, "Therefore, cholinesterase inhibitors may be the preferable treatment, but an ideal long-term solution remains tragically out of reach," which supports the conclusion in choice A. The author would not state that the treatment is "preferable" if it were completely pointless, so choice B is not the best answer. Although the author does conclude that the current lack of a cure for Alzheimer's disease is tragic, she or he never expresses the fatalistic opinion in choice C. The author does not express the optimistic conclusion in choice D either.

28. **The correct answer is B.** Choice B is correct. The passage states that the drugs that assist in the breakdown of acetylcholine are ineffective at some point, implying that, as the disease progresses, the drugs lose their efficacy (and total time of efficacy is only six to twelve months). Therefore, the drugs should not be approved for use over a long course of time, and should probably not be approved for use in the final or severe stage of Alzheimer's disease. Choice A must be ruled out because cholinesterase inhibitors may be effective earlier in the disease's progression. Choice C is not the best choice because the passage does not say or imply that the FDA fails to regulate cholinesterase inhibitors. Choice D must be eliminated because nothing in the passage suggests that cholinesterase inhibitors, which may be effective for six to twelve months and which

assist in the breakdown of acetylcholine at some stages, should not have been approved.

29. **The correct answer is B.** Choice B is correct because most details in the passage are about how the drugs fall short: by being prescribed to people they may not have been meant for, for working for only a short period of time, by reports of efficacy based on anecdotal rather than empirical evidence, and so on. Choice A is tempting because the passage does most certainly present readers with two classes of drugs used to treat Alzheimer's disease, but the majority of details are about the shortcomings of these drugs, including how they may treat unwanted behaviors instead of the disease itself. Choice C is incorrect because no claim is made for the greater efficacy of one class of drugs over the other. Choice D is incorrect because the passage doesn't report much progress at all. In fact, both classes of drugs do little more than, perhaps, treat symptoms.

30. **The correct answer is D.** Choice D is the correct answer because the passage as a whole is about the shortcomings of the drugs, and the final paragraph dramatically reinforces that by adding the sobering information that the efficacy of the drugs is based on the anecdotal evidence supplied by caregivers. Choice A must be ruled out because the final paragraph does not summarize; it adds new information. Choice B must be ruled out because the first paragraph does not even mention behaviors. Choice C is incorrect; the passage informs and has no persuasive purpose.

31. **The correct answer is C.** Choice C is the correct answer because the topic of the paragraph is glutamate regulators; the main idea is the use of that particular drug class and its effects. Although the first sentence of the paragraph does little more than lead into the topic, almost all the details in the

passage are used to support the main idea of the drug's use and effects. Choice A must be ruled out because, while the first sentence of the paragraph might suggest that two classes of drugs will be compared or contrasted in the paragraph, they are not. The focus is strictly on glutamate regulators. Choice B is not correct because, while the first sentence of the paragraph might suggest that two classes of drugs will be compared or contrasted in the paragraph, they are not. The focus is strictly on glutamate regulators. Choice D must be ruled out because there is no chronological order in the passage.

32. **The correct answer is D.** The author describes the suggestion that the drug that blocks the toxic effects of Alzheimer's disease may temporarily delay the disease's worsening symptoms as "fairly dubious" while concluding that cholinesterase inhibitors are "the preferable treatment," so choice D is the best answer. Although the author is apparently concerned about Alzheimer's disease enough to write this passage, there is no implication of the extreme conclusion in choice A in this passage. The author actually states the direct opposite of choice B in the first paragraph. The author mentions the questions regarding when treatment for Alzheimer's disease should begin but offers no personal opinion on this matter at all, so choice C is not the best answer.

33. **The correct answer is D.** Choice D is correct because the author had already "invested" snakes with glamour and attraction before he met Dr. Messuri. The phrase "it turned out" is a clue to the sequence. For the same reason, Choice B can be ruled out. Choice A must be ruled out because the fourth paragraph suggests that the snake charmer information given by Dr. Messuri may be of questionable accuracy. Choice C is incorrect because there are no facts in the passage on which to base such a conclusion.

34. **The correct answer is B.** In paragraph 2, the author refers to the second-most alarming part of a snake's body. This may suggest that the author is terrified by the mouth of the snake; at any rate, because there is nothing else mentioned in the passage that appears to scare the author, the answer must be unstated in the passage, which leaves, among these choices, only the fang. Choice A is incorrect; in paragraph 2, the author refers to the tongue as the second-most alarming part of a snake's body. Choice C is incorrect because nothing in the passage states or suggests that the author feels afraid of the snake's tail. Although the passage mentions rattlesnakes, which of course bear rattles on their tails, the tails of snakes are never discussed. Choice D is not correct because nothing in the passage states or suggests that the author feels afraid of the snake's eyes.

35. **The correct answer is A.** Choice A is the only possible correct answer; it is suggested by the fact that the receptors can be in two different places, which most likely depends on the specific environment. Choice B must be ruled out because the passage is very clear about the fact that the receptors enable the snake to hunt and catch its prey. There is nothing in the passage about the ability to hunt being hobbled. Choices C and D are incorrect because nothing in the passage leads to or supports either conclusion.

36. **The correct answer is D.** Choice D is correct because, of all the choices, only complex dentition in multiple jaws is not discussed in the passage. Choice A should be ruled out because protective epidermal caps are discussed in paragraph 5. Choice B is incorrect; internal ears are discussed in paragraph 4. Choice C is incorrect because receptor organs for conveying smell are discussed in paragraph 2.

37. **The correct answer is C.** Choice C is correct because the author either suggests or directly states information related to environment or predation in relation to almost all of the senses. Choice A should be eliminated; the passage makes no claim about which senses most help the snake to survive. Choice B is incorrect because the passage does not state or imply a comparison between the adaptation of head or body to the environment. Choice D is tempting but incorrect; certainly, the snake's adaptations for hunting prey are very important, but nothing in the passage suggests they are most important aspect of its ability to hunt prey.

38. **The correct answer is A.** Choice A is correct because the first sentence introduces and speaks broadly about special sensory pits; the second sentence restricts this topic to their use in sensing prey. Choice B is incorrect; the sentences do not form or suggest an analogy. Choice C is incorrect; the second sentence names a specific aspect of the topic of the first sentence, not a contrast. Choice D should be eliminated; the two sentences do not state a thesis and antithesis.

39. **The correct answer is A.** Choice A is correct because the passage clearly states that snakes have an internal middle ear to which sound waves may travel. Choice B is incorrect; the passage does not say that snakes ever had external ears. Choice C makes some sense, but it is not the best answer because the passage does not discuss the possible uses a snake might have for its sight. Choice D is incorrect because the passage neither makes nor implies any such claim.

40. **The correct answer choice is A.** Whether or not something is amazing is a matter of personal opinion, so choice A is the best answer. Words such as *dedicated* and *amateur* may seem like opinions since they are descriptive, but in the context of choice

B, they are facts. Choices C and D are facts, since the things that Dr. Messuri said are not reflections of the author's personal opinions.

41. The correct answer is B. Choice B is the correct answer; the last sentence in paragraph 1 in which the author mocks the FDA's regulation best reveals the answer. Choices A, C, and D can all be ruled out because the last sentence of paragraph 1 reveals an extremely critical attitude toward the FDA in relation to the regulation of supplements. Choice A, *laughable,* is the opposite of critical, and Choice C, *somewhat lacking,* tends toward a slightly favorable attitude. Choice D, *highly unpredictable,* is not supported by the passage.

42. The correct answer is C. Choice C is correct because the passage makes it clear that most women cannot get the amount of calcium-plus-D that they need from dietary sources and, therefore, must take supplements. Yet, even then, careful choices are to be made based on circumstances and information. Choice A is a cautionary tale in reading all the choices carefully; not only is it not the best answer, but the passage makes it clear that some women might possibly be able to get what they need through dietary sources, and that is best. Choice B should be eliminated because the passage specifically states that women should consider what they've taken in at a meal before adding a supplement. Choice D is accurate, but far from the best choice. The passage does say that there are reasons to be wary of supplements, but at the same time, the passage argues that there can be special issues, such as those related to bone density, that may necessitate the taking of supplements.

43. The correct answer is B. Choice B is correct. The import of the idea stated in the first paragraph is that no one knows which supplements that come to market are safe and unsafe, and, therefore, you'll be lucky to choose the right one. The idea of luck or chance emphasizes this. Choice A must be ruled out. The advice to carry a rabbit's foot is not supporting evidence. Choice C is incorrect because there is no contradiction in this advice. The first paragraph suggests that getting a good or bad supplement is a matter of luck because the FDA's regulation for safety occurs, if it occurs at all, after the supplements are marketed. Choice D is incorrect because even though the sentence that follows the rabbit's foot statement in the final paragraph creates a transition, the sentence about the rabbit's foot does not.

44. The correct answer is B. Choice B is correct because facts in the passage tell you that the FDA is involved in supplement regulation, but does very little relative to what it does with food and drugs. Choice A is incorrect because paragraph 1 tells ways in which the FDA does undertake some regulatory functions. Choice C is incorrect because nothing in the passage discusses objectivity; even if it were true, there would be a better answer. Choice D is incorrect because nothing in the passage suggests an increasing role or the possibility of an increased role for the FDA.

45. The correct answer is A. Choice A is the correct answer because the first paragraph exposes what the FDA does not do in terms of the regulation of supplements and the final paragraph spells out ways in which the reader can exercise intelligence and care in the use of supplements. Choice B must be ruled out because the passage does not say this. Choice C is not correct. This information is implied by the first paragraph, but not the last paragraph. Choice D is incorrect. While the last paragraph does say this, the information establishes no specific link to the first paragraph.

46. **The correct answer is C.** Choice C is correct because this information is stated directly in paragraph 1. Choice A is incorrect because paragraph 1 states that the FDA takes action against unsafe supplements after they reach the market and does not state whether that means testing or not. Choice B is incorrect because the first paragraph states that "certain 'good'" practices are established by a different regulatory agency. Choice D is incorrect because paragraph 1 says that the FDA regulates food and drugs more closely than it regulates supplements.

47. **The correct answer is B.** Choice B is correct because the passage suggests an informed use of supplements in some cases. Choice A should be ruled out because the passage is more about taking supplements than it is about the FDA. Choice C is tempting, but incorrect because the author goes beyond an objective listing of pros and cons to dispense advice. Choice D is incorrect because, while the author might well be in favor of more regulation, the bulk of the passage is about using supplements in an informed and careful manner.

48. **The correct answer is B.** Choice B is correct because the author's main point is that, even though supplements are poorly regulated and may be unsafe, there are some cases when they must be taken because of their benefits. Choice B states possible and important benefits. Choice A must be ruled out because it contradicts the author's contention that supplements may be unsafe. Choices C and D are incorrect because neither supports the main idea that even though supplements are poorly regulated and may be unsafe, there are some cases when they must be taken because of their benefits.

answers diagnostic test

Section 5: Quantitative Reasoning

1. D	11. D	21. D	31. D	41. C
2. B	12. B	22. B	32. C	42. C
3. C	13. C	23. A	33. C	43. D
4. D	14. A	24. A	34. B	44. C
5. A	15. D	25. C	35. A	45. B
6. C	16. A	26. D	36. D	46. D
7. C	17. C	27. B	37. B	47. D
8. B	18. B	28. C	38. A	48. A
9. B	19. B	29. C	39. A	
10. D	20. B	30. B	40. B	

1. **The correct answer is D.** Apply the chain rule, using $u = x^2 + 1$:

$$\frac{d}{dx}\left[\ln\left(x^2 + 1\right)\right] = \frac{d}{du}\left(\ln u\right)\frac{d}{dx}\left(u\right)$$
$$= \frac{1}{u}\frac{d}{dx}\left(x^2 + 1\right)$$
$$= \frac{2x}{x^2 + 1}$$

Evaluating this at $x = 3$, the answer is $f'(3) = \frac{3}{5}$.

2. **The correct answer is B.** The total number of movements is $s + b$, which must equal 300. This yields the equation $s + b = 300$. The number of calories s squats burns is $1.2s$, and the number of calories b box jumps burns is $1.5b$. The sum, $1.2s + 1.5b$, must equal 400 calories. This leads to the equation $1.2s + 1.5b = 400$. So, the system in B is correct.

3. **The correct answer is C.** The second inequality implies that $2y > 3z$. Since $x > 2y$, you have $x > 2y > 3z$. Concentrating on x and z, you get $x > 3z \Rightarrow x - 3z > 0$.

4. **The correct answer is D.** Observe the following:

$$p(x) = 4x^2 - 12x - 16$$
$$= 4\left(x^2 - 3x - 4\right)$$
$$= 4(x - 4)(x + 1)$$

Set this equal to zero and solve for x. Doing so yields the solutions $x = 4$ and $x = -1$. Since x is the number of consoles, -1 cannot be a solution. Using $x = 4$, we conclude that 400 consoles must be sold to break even.

5. **The correct answer is A.** Perform the

calculations: $\ln \sqrt{e} = \ln e^{\frac{1}{2}} = \frac{1}{2} \ln e = \frac{1}{2}$.

6. **The correct answer is C.** The percent increase is computed by subtracting the two values, dividing that difference by the *original* value, and multiplying by 100%. This is precisely what is computed in C.

7. **The correct answer is C.** The total, before tax, is calculated as follows:

   2($10.50) + 2($6.25) + 1($5.90) + 3($3.75) = $50.65

   The sales tax of 5% is equal to $50.65(0.05) = $2.53. So, the total bill is $50.65 + $2.53 = $53.18.

8. **The correct answer is B.** By definition,

   $\left(\dfrac{f}{g}\right)(x) = \dfrac{f(x)}{g(x)} = \dfrac{\sin x}{\cos x} = \tan x$. At $x = \pi$,

   the tangent function equals zero (the sine is zero and the cosine is 1).

9. **The correct answer is B.** First, simplify the complex fraction, and then convert all three fractions so that they have the same denominator:

$$\frac{7}{3} + \frac{3}{4} - \frac{\frac{1}{3}}{2} = \frac{7}{3} + \frac{3}{4} - \frac{\frac{1}{3}}{\frac{2}{1}}$$

$$= \frac{7}{3} + \frac{3}{4} - \frac{1}{3} \times \frac{1}{2}$$

$$= \frac{7}{3} + \frac{3}{4} - \frac{1}{6}$$

$$= \frac{28}{12} + \frac{9}{12} - \frac{2}{12}$$

$$= \frac{35}{12}$$

10. **The correct answer is D.** Identify the values of each parameter appearing in the formula, and make certain the units all match. Here, $m = 63g = 0.063kg$, $L = 0.95m$, and $T = 82.6 \dfrac{kg \cdot m}{sec^2}$. Substitute these into the formula and solve for v:

$$82.6 = \frac{0.063 \, v^2}{0.95}$$

$$82.6 \times 0.95 = 0.063 \, v^2$$

$$\frac{82.6 \times 0.95}{0.063} = v^2$$

$$\sqrt{\frac{82.6 \times 0.95}{0.063}} = v$$

The units for the speed are meters per second.

11. **The correct answer is D.** Tino's managing the team and Tino's not managing the team are mutually exclusive events. Further, Carlos' signing with the team depends on whether Tino is the manager. There are a lot of words here, describing two different cases. Simplify things by considering each case on its own before you combine the two. First, the probability that Tino will manage and Carlos will sign is:

   (60%) × (70%) = 0.6 × 0.7 = 0.42

   Next, the probability that Tino will not manage and Carlos will sign is:

   (40%) × (30%) = 0.4 × 0.3 = 0.12

   Thus, the overall probability that Carlos will sign is:

   0.42 + 0.12 = 0.54 = 54%

12. **The correct answer is B.** Sum the four distances and divide by 4:

$$\frac{55.3 + 56.2 + 48.7 + 61.4}{4} = \frac{221.6}{4} = 55.4$$

13. **The correct answer is C.** Start by evaluating $\log_4 16$: $\log_4 16 = y \Rightarrow 4^y = 16 \Rightarrow y = 2$. This means that $\log_a x = 2$, as well. Therefore, $\log_a x = 2 \Rightarrow a^2 = x \Rightarrow a = \sqrt{x}$. (Recall that both a and x are positive by definition, so a cannot equal $-\sqrt{x}$.)

14. **The correct answer is A.** The line that is tangent to the graph of the function $f(x) = x^3$ at $x = 2$ has slope equal to $f'(2)$. Therefore, start by calculating this derivative. The derivative of $f(x) = x^3$ is $f'(x) = 3x^2$, so $f'(2) = 12$. Next, recall that the formula for the slope of a line that goes through points (x_1, y_1) and (x_2, y_2) is $m = \dfrac{y_2 - y_1}{x_2 - x_1}$. In this problem, the line in question goes through the point $(2,8)$—since the value of $f(x)$ at $x = 2$ is 8. Let (x_1, y_1) be the point $(2,8)$ and manipulate the formula of the slope, so that you get the equation of the line you're looking for:

$$m = \frac{y_2 - y_1}{x_2 - x_1}$$
$$12 = \frac{y - 8}{x - 2}$$
$$12(x - 2) = y - 8$$
$$12x - 24 + 8 = y$$
$$y = 12x - 16$$

15. **The correct answer is D.** Whenever you see a verbose question like this one, break down the situation into simpler, concrete parts in order to get an overview of the issue. In this case, on Monday through Wednesday, the machine produced a total of 150 widgets, or an average of 50 per day. If its Monday-to-Thursday daily average was greater by 10 widgets, then it was equal to 60 widgets per day. Let x be the number of widgets the machine produced on Thursday. Then:

$$\frac{60 + 40 + 50 + x}{4} = 60$$
$$\frac{150 + x}{4} = 60$$
$$150 + x = 240$$
$$x = 90$$

16. **The correct answer is A.** The function is defined for all x such that the quantity under the radical sign is nonnegative. Thus, you need:

$$2|x - 1| - 5 \geq 0 \Rightarrow 2|x - 1| \geq 5 \Rightarrow |x - 1| \geq \frac{5}{2}$$

Case 1: If $x - 1 \geq 0$, that is if $x \geq 1$, then $|x - 1| = x - 1$, and the inequality becomes:

$$|x - 1| \geq \frac{5}{2}$$
$$x - 1 \geq \frac{5}{2}$$
$$x \geq \frac{5}{2} + 1$$
$$x \geq \frac{7}{2}$$

This result is consistent with—and even more restrictive than—the requirement that x be greater than or equal to 1, so this case yields $x \geq \frac{7}{2}$.

Case 2: If $x - 1 < 0$, that is if $x < 1$, then $|x - 1| = -(x - 1)$, and the inequality becomes:

$$|x - 1| \geq \frac{5}{2}$$

$$-(x - 1) \geq \frac{5}{2}$$

$$-x + 1 \geq \frac{5}{2}$$

$$-x \geq \frac{3}{2}$$

$$x \leq -\frac{3}{2}$$

This result is consistent with—and even more restrictive than—the requirement that x be less than 1, so this case yields $x \leq -\frac{3}{2}$. Overall, the inequality holds true when $x \leq -\frac{3}{2}$ or $x \geq \frac{7}{2}$, so the domain of the function is $\left(-\infty, -\frac{3}{2}\right] \cup \left[\frac{7}{2}, \infty\right)$.

17. The correct answer is C. First, notice that since the sofa's sale price of $368 reflects a markdown from the sofa's original price, choice A, which features a price less than $368, cannot be correct. Eliminate it immediately. Next, set up a proportion. If $368 is 20% lower than the original price, then $368 is 80%, or $\frac{4}{5}$, of the original price. Therefore:

$$\frac{4}{5} = \frac{368}{x}$$

$$4x = 368 \times 5$$

$$x = \frac{368 \times 5}{4}$$

$$x = 460$$

So, the original price was $460.

18. The correct answer is B. You do not know how many tickets each of the other 13 people bought, but since they averaged 6 tickets each, then in total the other 13 people bought 13×6 tickets. Be careful, though: this is not the total number of tickets bought. To these 13×6 tickets, you must add the 4 that Dina bought. Thus, the total number of tickets bought is 82, 4 of which are Dina's. So, Dina's probability of winning is $\frac{4}{82}$, or $\frac{2}{41}$.

19. The correct answer is B. The number of inches on the ground corresponding to 15.4 inches on the map is $18,000(15.4) = 277,200$ inches. To convert this to miles, use the fact that 1 foot = 12 inches and 1 mile = 5,280 feet:

$$277,200 \text{ in.} \times \frac{1 \text{ ft.}}{12 \text{ in.}} \times \frac{1 \text{ mi.}}{5,280 \text{ ft.}}$$
$$= 4.375 \text{ mi.}$$

20. The correct answer is B. Simplify the logarithm:

$$\log_3 \frac{x}{9y} = \log_3 \frac{\frac{x}{y}}{9} = \log_3 \frac{x}{y} - \log_3 9$$

$$= \log_3 \frac{x}{y} - 2$$

21. The correct answer is D.

$$dB = 10 \log\left[\frac{400 I_0}{I_0}\right]$$

$$= 10 \log[400]$$

$$= 10 \log[4 \times 100]$$

$$= 10\left(\log[4] + \log[100]\right)$$

$$= 10\left(\log[4] + 2\right)$$

$$= 20 + 10 \log[4]$$

22. **The correct answer is B.** A function is concave up whenever its second derivative is greater than zero. For $f(x) = -x^3 - x$, $f'(x) = -3x^2 - 1$ and $f''(x) = -6x$. Let $f''(x) > 0$ and solve:

$$f''(x) > 0$$
$$-6x > 0$$
$$x < 0$$

23. **The correct answer is A.** Use implicit differentiation on $x^2 + x \cos y = x$, making sure you use the product rule on the second term:

$$2x + \cos y + x(-\sin y)\frac{dy}{dx} = 1$$
$$-x \sin y \frac{dy}{dx} = 1 - 2x - \cos y$$
$$\frac{dy}{dx} = \frac{1 - 2x - \cos y}{-x \sin y}$$
$$\frac{dy}{dx} = \frac{\cos y + 2x - 1}{x \sin y}$$

24. **The correct answer is A.** If the average of p and q is x, then $\frac{p+q}{2} = x \Rightarrow p + q = 2x$.

If the average of r, s, and t is y, then $\frac{r+s+t}{3} = y \Rightarrow r + s + t = 3y$. Therefore, the average of all five equals $\frac{(p+q)+(r+s+t)}{5}$, that is, $\frac{2x+3y}{5}$.

25. **The correct answer is C.** Isolate the root on one side, and then remove it by raising both sides of the equation to the third power:

$$4 - \sqrt[3]{2x} = 0$$
$$4 = \sqrt[3]{2x}$$
$$4^3 = \left(\sqrt[3]{2x}\right)^3$$
$$64 = 2x$$
$$x = 32$$

Indeed, substituting $x = 32$ into the original equation yields the correct answer:

$$4 - \sqrt[3]{2 \times 32} = 0 \Rightarrow 4 - \sqrt[3]{64} =$$
$$0 \Rightarrow 4 - 4 = 0$$

26. **The correct answer is D.** *Of* means you should multiply, so you have the product of three numbers. Turn the decimal into a fraction and, as you go along, see what factors are common to a numerator and a denominator (even across fractions) and cancel them in order to make it easier to solve:

$$\frac{7}{2} \times 0.6 \times \frac{6}{9} = \frac{7}{2} \times \frac{6}{10} \times \frac{2}{3}$$
$$= \frac{7}{2} \times \frac{3}{5} \times \frac{2}{3}$$
$$= \frac{7}{5}$$

27. **The correct answer is B.** The rate of change of the city's population with respect to time is the first derivative of the function of the city's population with respect to time. So, find $f'(t)$:

$$f(t) = 2t^{\frac{1}{2}}$$
$$f'(t) = 2\frac{1}{2}t^{-\frac{1}{2}}$$
$$f'(t) = \frac{1}{\sqrt{t}}$$

At $t = 9$:
$$f'(9) = \frac{1}{\sqrt{t}} = \frac{1}{\sqrt{9}} = \frac{1}{3}$$

28. **The correct answer is C.** To convert the units, use the facts that 1 mile = 5,280 feet, 1 hour = 60 minutes, and 1 minute = 60 seconds, as follows:

$$\frac{268 \text{ miles}}{1 \text{ hour}} \times \frac{5,280 \text{ feet}}{1 \text{ mile}} \times$$
$$\frac{1 \text{ hour}}{60 \text{ minutes}} \times \frac{1 \text{ minute}}{60 \text{ seconds}} =$$
$$\frac{268 \times 5,280}{60 \times 60} \text{ feet per second}$$

29. The correct answer is C. This expression represents the sum of all $\left(3 - n^2\right)$ when n equals 1, 2, 3, and 4:

$$\sum_{n=1}^{n=4}\left(3 - n^2\right) = \left(3 - 1^2\right) + \left(3 - 2^2\right) + \left(3 - 3^2\right) + \left(3 - 4^2\right)$$
$$= 3 - 1 + 3 - 4 + 3 - 9 + 3 - 16$$
$$= 12 - \left(1 + 4 + 9 + 16\right)$$
$$= 12 - 30$$
$$= -18$$

30. The correct answer is B. Consider first that the number on the marble picked from bowl B is twice the number on the marble picked from bowl A. For every marble in bowl A, there is exactly one marble in bowl B such that the number on the B marble equals twice the number on the A marble. So, the probability that the B number equals twice the A number is $\frac{1}{4}$. The probability you're asked to find is for the complementary event to this one: the probability that the B number does NOT equal twice the A number. Thus, this probability is $1 - \frac{1}{4}$, that is $\frac{3}{4}$.

31. The correct answer is D. Working backward from the answer choices may help you save some time. Look for the answer choice that, when multiplied by 0.65, yields 2.6. Choices A through C look too large to be correct, so start with choice D: 4 × 0.65 is an easy enough operation to perform, and it does, indeed, yield 2.6. So, choice D is correct. For the record, here's an efficient way to perform the division directly:

$$\frac{2.6}{0.65} = \frac{26 \times 10^{-1}}{65 \times 10^{-2}}$$
$$= \frac{26}{65} \times 10$$
$$= \frac{2 \times 13}{5 \times 13} \times 10$$
$$= \frac{2}{5} \times 10$$
$$= 4$$

32. The correct answer is C. Let x be the diameter of the part. This measurement must satisfy the inequality $|x - 0.6| \le 0.04$. Solve for x as follows:

$$-0.04 \le x - 0.6 \le 0.04$$
$$0.6 - 0.04 \le x \le 0.6 + 0.04$$
$$0.56 \le x \le 0.64$$

33. The correct answer is C. Convert the two vectors to the same notation and calculate:

$$a - b = (-3i + j) - 2i = -5i + j$$

34. The correct answer is B. Solve the equation $4 = 2\,e^{\frac{t}{10}}$ for t:

$$4 = 2e^{\frac{t}{10}}$$
$$2 = e^{\frac{t}{10}}$$
$$\ln 2 = \frac{t}{10}$$
$$10 \ln 2 = t$$
$$\ln\left(2^{10}\right) = t$$
$$\ln 1,024 = t$$

So, it takes $\ln(1,024)$ weeks.

35. The correct answer is A. Go straight to the answer choices to see what kinds of statements they present, and then evaluate them one by one. Luckily, you get a correct statement right away. The vertical line inside the rectangle in a box plot indicates the median of the data set. Thus, you can see from the graph that set B has the greater median. Set A has the greater range—indicated by the distance between the endpoints of the whiskers. You cannot tell anything about the means of the two sets, since we do not know what all the data points are. Thus, choice A is correct.

36. The correct answer is D. There are 23 data values listed in increasing order (from top to bottom in the stem-and-leaf plot). So, the median is the data value in the 12th position, which is 62. The mode is the most frequently occurring data value, which is 70.

37. **The correct answer is B.** Let x be the number of hours it takes Frank to complete the job by himself. Then, he completes $\frac{1}{x}$ of the job in 1 hour. Similarly, Ron completes $\frac{1}{3}$ job in 1 hour. If you add these two expressions together, you get the amount of the job Frank and Ron complete, working together, in 1 hour. Since it takes them 2 hours to complete the job, this sum equals $\frac{1}{2}$. So, the desired equation is $\frac{1}{x} + \frac{1}{3} = \frac{1}{2}$.

38. **The correct answer is A.** The obvious answer would be $\frac{\sqrt{3}}{6}$, but this is not listed among the answer choices, so you have to look for an alternative way to write this fraction. Start by multiplying both numerator and denominator of $\frac{6}{\sqrt{3}}$ by $\sqrt{3}$ in order to remove the square root from the denominator; then simplify the resulting fraction:

$$\frac{6}{\sqrt{3}} = \frac{6 \times \sqrt{3}}{\left(\sqrt{3}\right)\left(\sqrt{3}\right)} = \frac{6 \times \sqrt{3}}{3} = 2\sqrt{3}$$

Now the reciprocal of this number is $\frac{1}{2\sqrt{3}}$, which is the fraction listed in choice A.

39. **The correct answer is A.** The amount earned in commission on the amount beyond $3,500 is $0.025(x - 3,500)$ dollars. This is given by $G(H(x)) = (G \circ H)(x)$. The weekly salary is $180 +$ commission $= 180 + (G \circ H)(x)$ dollars. But, this is precisely $F(G(H(x))) = (F \circ G \circ H)(x)$.

40. **The correct answer is B.** The minimum population occurs when $\sin\left(\frac{\pi}{6}t\right) = -1$. The value of t for which this is true satisfies $\frac{\pi}{6}t = \frac{3\pi}{2}$. Solving for t yields $t = \frac{3\pi}{2} \cdot \frac{6}{\pi} = 9$. The month to which this corresponds is December.

41. **The correct answer is C.** The range of a data set is the difference between the maximum and minimum values, or $4.0 - 1.6 = 2.4$.

42. **The correct answer is C.** Let x be the number of miles of the taxi ride. The cost for x miles is $3.25 + 0.55x$. Since this cost cannot exceed $12, we must solve the inequality $3.25 + 0.55x \le 12$. Doing so yields $0.55x \le 8.75$, so that $x \le \frac{8.75}{0.55} \approx 15.90$. So, Janet can travel at most 15 full miles.

43. **The correct answer is D.** Multiply: $12\frac{3}{4}$ miles/gallon $\times 6\frac{1}{3}$ gallons $= \frac{51}{4}$ miles/gallon $\times \frac{19}{3}$ gallons $= \frac{323}{4}$ miles.

44. The correct answer is C. Set up and solve an inequality:

$$x^2 + 2x - 3 < 0$$
$$x^2 + 3x - x - 3 < 0$$
$$x(x + 3) - (x + 3) < 0$$
$$(x - 1)(x + 3) < 0$$

The two factors on the left are zero when x equals 1 and -3, respectively. Set up a table and see how each factor behaves for values of x to the left and right of these two values:

	$x < -3$	$-3 < x < 1$	$x > 1$
$(x - 1)$	Negative	Negative	Positive
$(x + 3)$	Negative	Positive	Positive
$(x - 1)(x + 3)$	Positive	Negative	Positive

The expression is negative when one of the factors is negative and the other is positive, that is, when x is between -3 and 1, exclusive.

If you're stuck, you can also try to plug in a few numbers in order to eliminate certain answer choices. For instance, you can easily eliminate choice D by picking $x = 1$ or $x = -4$. In both cases, the quadratic equals 0, which is not negative. Then, you can pick a number greater than 1 in order to test choice A or less than -3 in order to test choice B. In both cases, you will get a positive result, so you can eliminate these answers.

45. The correct answer is B. Check what the value of $f(x)$ is when x equals 0: $f(0) = -e^0 = -1$. So, the graph of the function passes through the point $(0, -1)$. Only Choice B features such a graph, so it is the correct answer.

46. The correct answer is D. Let c be the scalar by which $\overrightarrow{AB}$ is multiplied to produce $\overrightarrow{CD}$. Then, the coordinates of $\overrightarrow{CD}$ are $(-5c, 8c)$, and their sum is $-5c + 8c$. Set this equal to -21 and solve for c:

$$-5c + 8c = -21 \Rightarrow 3c = -21 \Rightarrow c = -7$$

Thus, the second coordinate of $\overrightarrow{CD}$ is -7×8, which equals -56.

47. The correct answer is D. This is a trick question. Instead of evaluating the definite interval, note that x^{-2} is undefined at $x = 0$, so the function is not continuous at that point. Recall that in order to be able to evaluate a function's definite integral on an interval $[a, b]$, the function must be continuous on that interval. Thus, the answer to this question is choice D: this integral cannot be computed.

48. The correct answer is A. You do not need to solve the equation. Rather, notice that since the denominator cannot be zero, x cannot be 3. Thus, choice A is the correct answer.

PART III
CRITICAL READING SKILLS

Critical Reading Skills

Chapter 4

OVERVIEW

- **The Passages**
- **Reading the Passages**
- **The Question Types**
- **A Critical Reading Study Plan**
- **Critical Reading Strategies for the PCAT**
- **Sharpening Your Critical Reading Skills Every Day**
- **Practice Questions**
- **Answer Key and Explanations**
- **Summing It Up**

As with every other part of the PCAT, the optimal way to prepare for the Critical Reading subtest is by learning about and practicing the test before you take it. The following strategies for success with Critical Reading items will help you maximize your score—and minimize your stress.

THE PASSAGES

Let's get started by getting familiar with the kinds of materials you'll be using to answer questions on the Critical Reading subtest. The topics of Critical Reading passages are pretty varied and each relates to issues pertaining to natural sciences, social sciences, or humanities. You may read:

1. **Historical Topics:** Passages that discuss events of the past.
2. **Contemporary Topics:** Passages that discuss current events.
3. **Cultural Topics:** Passages that discuss the behaviors, beliefs, and traditions of peoples throughout the world.
4. **Ethical Topics:** Passages that relate to matters of right and wrong.
5. **Political Topics:** Passages that relate to world governments and events.
6. **Technical Topics:** Passages that relate to technological developments.

That may seem like a lot, but the good news is that you won't have to study any of these topics in advance because the Critical Reading subtest only tests your ability to comprehend, analyze, and evaluate the information in the given passages.

The ways these passages may be written are equally varied. They may be:

1. informative: an objective presentation of information

2. persuasive: an attempt to persuade the reader to agree with a particular position

3. speculative: a presentation of a theory that has yet to be proven

PCAT passages aren't terribly long; they average between 400 and 600 words in length—that's about four to six paragraphs long. But you will need to read each passage carefully since each of the eight questions that follow each passage relates to that passage as a whole or a part of the passage. Here are some strategies for reading the passages effectively.

READING THE PASSAGES

Some test prep books and websites will suggest ALWAYS reading the questions first and the passage second, but a careful examination of this advice might lead you to a more logical conclusion. How many questions can you absorb while also reading some fairly sophisticated material? And how much time should you spend reading questions before you even begin the central task of reading the passage?

Furthermore, most PCAT Reading Comprehension questions require fairly sophisticated critical thinking. If you think you can scope out a half dozen or more of these questions in a minute or two, and then keep them all straight as you wade through a challenging passage, think again. You could end up focusing on the wrong information entirely. Reading the passage first makes a lot more sense.

A Sample Passage

Now that you have some information about Critical Reading passages, it's time to actually read one. Here's a model passage you'll be using to answer sample questions sprinkled throughout this chapter.

(1)   Mechanical structures are often patterned on the bodies of organic beings, and this is particularly true of robots intended to perform human functions. Robots may perform such tasks as building, serving, or even teaching or problem solving. However, robots do not always take their inspiration from human beings. In fact, researchers are currently experimenting with a new synthetic skin intended for robots that is patterned after octopus skin.

(2)   Octopus skin is unique in its ability to change both color and texture. Almost instantaneously, an octopus can reshape its skin to mimic the appearance of seaweed or coral. This rather fascinating ability is imperative to the creature's survival since it is such an effective form of camouflage. This experimental form of synthetic cephalopod (the class to which octopuses belong) skin would also give soft robots—robots covered with a malleable, silicon, skin-like material—the ability to morph from a flat, two-dimensional appearance to a textured three-dimensional one. They would then be able to hide from predatory animals in natural habitats just as the octopus does.

(3)   The skin's ability is currently dependent on the division of silicon bubbles with fiber-mesh frames. When scientists reinforce the mesh, the bubbles inflate and the skin reshapes. However, electric currents may also be used to modify the skin's appearance. During this prototype phase, scientists have already figured out how to make robots reproduce the appearances of round river stones and plants with leaves arranged in spiral patterns, among other shapes.

(4)   The obvious question is: why would a robot benefit from this particular ability? One potential use would be during military maneuvers that require a robot to move undetected over dangerous ground. Furthermore, robots that require inflated skin when in use could be deflated with this new skin to make them more compact when stacked during transportation to their destinations. The skin also has the potential for industrial, academic, and even hobby uses. Consequently, the team of scientists developing synthetic cephalopod skin is intent on ensuring the skin's ease of use despite the skin's inherent complexity.

(5)   Developers even intend the skin to have the ability to reproduce the appearance of an environment on site, just as an octopus does, and they have already been successful in creating skin with an octopus's ability to change color to blend in with its surroundings. Regardless of these incredible strides, synthetic cephalopod skin is still very much in the development phase. Yet developers remain optimistic that this marvelous technology that will no doubt revolutionize robotics will be reliable enough to cover soft robots in the near future. According to Robert Shepherd of Cornell University (as quoted in *Live Science*), "We're just at the beginning, and we have great results…"

This sample passage involves a technical topic—*robotics*—that relates to natural science—*cephalopod biology*—and it is speculative because this technology has yet to be perfected. However, there are also enough interjections in which the author expresses personal preferences in the passage for it to have elements of the persuasive passage.

Chances are you knew little about robotics or octopuses before reading this passage, but as you will see, that will not affect your ability to answer the Critical Reading questions that relate to this passage. You just need to comprehend the information in this particular passage, and that's just what you're going to learn to do now.

Before rereading our passage, we'll start with a quick rundown of the kinds of questions you'll need to answer on the Critical Reading subtest so that you'll know what to look out for while reading any PCAT passage.

Critical Reading questions fall into one of three categories: 1) Comprehension, 2) Analysis, and 3) Evaluation.

1.   <u>Comprehension</u> questions require you to recognize and understand information in a passage. Comprehension questions include:

- **Words in Context** questions (defining vocabulary words)
- **Main Idea** questions (identifying or inferring the most important idea in the passage)
- **Supporting Details** questions (identifying facts and details stated explicitly in the passage)
- **Drawing conclusions** questions (making inferences based on information stated explicitly in the passage)

TIP

Don't give up on any passage, no matter how hard it may be. A third of the questions about that passage are likely to be easy for you to answer.

TIP

Although a passage may fit into one category, such as *speculative*, as a whole, it may still have some elements of other categories, such as *persuasive* or *expository*.

2. <u>Analysis</u> questions require you to make inferences based on information in the passage or interpret that information. Analysis questions include:

   - **Relationship Between Ideas** questions (analyzing and identifying how one idea in a passage relates to another idea in it)

   - **Author's Purpose** questions (analyzing the author's main reason for making a particular statement or writing the passage as a whole)

   - **Author's Tone** questions (analyzing the author's attitude and method of conveying information)

   - **Facts/Opinions** questions (distinguishing between objective facts and subjective opinions in a passage)

   - **Rhetorical Strategies** questions (analyzing the methods the author uses to convince the reader of a particular position or belief)

3. <u>Evaluation</u> questions require you to make a judgment based on sound reasoning. Evaluation questions include:

   - **Bias** questions (evaluating the author's viewpoint, preference, or position)

   - **Support in an Argument** questions (evaluating the information the author uses to support an argument)

   - **Author's Conclusion/Thesis** (identifying the main point the author makes in a passage and evaluating its effectiveness)

While reading a passage, look out for details that seem particularly important; they could be used as the bases of questions.

Keeping these potential question types in mind, let's reread that passage about Synthetic Cephalopod Skin and take note of details that may be useful for answering questions.

(1)   Mechanical structures are often patterned on the bodies of organic beings, and this is particularly true of robots intended to perform human functions. Robots may perform such tasks as building, serving, or even teaching or problem solving. However, robots do not always take their inspiration from human beings. In fact, researchers are currently experimenting with a new synthetic skin intended for robots that is patterned after octopus skin.

Potential detail for a Main Idea question: The fact that researchers are currently experimenting with a new synthetic skin intended for robots that is patterned after octopus skin is the main idea of this passage.

(2)   Octopus skin is unique in its ability to change both color and texture. Almost instantaneously, an octopus can reshape its skin to mimic the appearance of seaweed or coral. This rather fascinating ability is imperative to the creature's survival since it is such an effective form of camouflage. This experimental form of synthetic cephalopod (the class to which octopuses belong) skin would also give soft robots—robots covered with a malleable, silicon, skin-like material— the ability to morph from a flat, two-dimensional appearance to a textured three-dimensional one. They would then be able to hide from predatory animals in natural habitats just as the octopus does.

Potential detail for a Relationship Between Ideas question: The first paragraph discussed robotic technology based on human functions and this second paragraph discusses robotic technology based on octopus functions.

Potential detail for a Supporting Details question: Seaweed and coral are two things the octopus uses its morphing skin to mimic.

Potential detail for a Words in Context question: Any unfamiliar words could be used as the bases for Words in Context questions. In this paragraph, such words include "imperative" and "malleable."

(3)   The skin's ability is currently dependent on the division of silicon bubbles with fiber-mesh frames. When scientists reinforce the mesh, the bubbles inflate and the skin reshapes. However, electric currents may also be used to modify the skin's appearance. During this prototype phase, scientists have already figured out how to make robots reproduce the appearances of round river stones and plants with leaves arranged in spiral patterns, among other shapes.

Potential detail for a Supporting Details question: The facts that both fiber-mesh and electrical currents can be used to cause synthetic cephalopod skin to morph could be used in Supporting Details questions.

Potential detail for a Words in Context question: Any unfamiliar words could be used as the bases for Words in Context questions. In this paragraph, such words include "prototype" and "modify."

(4)   The obvious question is: why would a robot benefit from this particular ability? One potential use would be during military maneuvers that require a robot to move undetected over dangerous ground. Furthermore, robots that require inflated skin when in use could be deflated with this new skin to make them more compact when stacked during transportation to their destinations. The skin also has the potential for industrial, academic, and even hobby uses. Consequently, the team of scientists developing synthetic cephalopod skin is intent on ensuring the skin's ease of use despite the skin's inherent complexity.

Potential detail for a Facts/Opinions question: Not everyone may read the first three paragraphs of this passage and ask, "why would a robot benefit from this particular ability?" yet the author thinks this question is obvious. Therefore, the opening sentence of this paragraph expresses the author's personal opinion rather than a fact. This detail may be the subject of a Facts/Opinions question.

Potential detail for a Tone question: As we shall see, the author subtly expresses some personal preferences in this passage, but overall, it is written in an informative tone intent on presenting facts. Take note of that in the event you are expected to answer a Tone question.

Potential detail for a Words in Context question: Any unfamiliar words could be used as the bases for Words in Context questions. In this paragraph, such words include "inherent."

(5)   Developers intend the skin to even have the ability to reproduce the appearance of an environment on site, just an octopus does, and they have already been successful in creating skin with an octopus's ability to change color to blend in with its surroundings. Regardless of these incredible strides, synthetic cephalopod skin is still very much in the development phase. Yet developers remain optimistic that this marvelous technology that will no doubt revolutionize robotics will be reliable enough to cover soft robots in the near future. According to Robert Shepherd of Cornell University (as quoted in *Live Science*), "We're just at the beginning, and we have great results…"

TIP

Unfamiliar words will often be used in Words in Context questions. Pay particular attention to such words and take notes of how they are used in the context of the passage.

TIP

Evidence of the author's personal opinions will often be used in facts/opinions, bias, or rhetorical strategies questions.

Potential detail for an Author's Purpose question: The author subtly expresses support for the development of this new soft skin technology by using positive words such as "incredible" and "marvelous," so you can infer that championing this technology is among the author's purposes.

Potential detail for a Rhetorical Strategies question: The author's use of positive words is a rhetorical strategy intended to get the reader to see synthetic cephalopod skin in a positive light.

Potential detail for a Bias question: Those positive words such as "incredible" and "marvelous" also reveal the author's bias in favor of that technology.

Potential detail for a Support in an Argument question: A Support in an Argument question will ask you to find elements the author uses to support a position, and you can use the various uses of the technology and its unusual nature to support the author's position that it is "marvelous."

Potential detail for an Author's Conclusion/Thesis question: It is always important to pay particular attention to the final paragraph of a passage, since this is where the author's conclusion/thesis will usually appear. In the case of this passage, the author concludes that the technology is "marvelous" and will "revolutionize" robotics.

THE QUESTION TYPES

Now we're going to take a closer look at each of the question types to get a clearer idea of how they look and how to answer them. Each of the following sections will also include a sample question that relates back to that passage about synthetic cephalopod skin we've already read and analyzed.

Comprehension

We'll start with the most basic Critical Reading question types you'll encounter on the PCAT. Chances are if you've ever taken a standardized reading test before, you've answered comprehension questions. These are the most basic questions that test your overall understanding of a reading selection. There are four types of comprehension questions.

1. Words in Context

It probably goes without saying that all reading selections are made up of words, and if you do not understand the meanings of those words, you will have a tough time comprehending the meaning of the selection as a whole. That means Words in Context questions are among the most essential of comprehension questions.

Words in Context questions will merely ask you to identify the meaning of an unfamiliar word in the passage. The key to answering such questions is the word *context*. Context refers to how the word is used in the particular passage. By using context clues, you should be able to define the meaning of any word. We're so confident of this fact, that we're going to ask you to define a word that doesn't even exist!

Read this sentence:

> The morning was so *zabdab* that Rex needed to wear his wool hat and heavy coat.

You've probably never heard the word *zabdab* before. That's to be expected since it isn't a real word. Yet you can probably still figure out its meaning by using context clues, such as the fact that the morning required Rex to put on his wool hat and heavy coat. When does one wear such items? When it's cold out, of course. So, using our context clues, we can conclude that *zabdab* means *cold*.

On the PCAT, Words in Context questions may ask you to identify totally unfamiliar words or technical terms, but they may also ask you to figure out how a more familiar word is used in a particular context. For example, the word *cold* has a number of meanings. It can be used like our fake word *zabdab* above: to mean a low, chilly temperature. However, *cold* can also mean an illness that makes you cough and sneeze, like a head cold. Once again, using context clues should help you figure out the definitions of such multiple-meaning words. For example:

> I spent the morning sneezing and coughing because I had a cold.

Does *cold* mean a chilly temperature in this sentence? Probably not since one might feel that kind of *cold*, but they would not *have* it. Also the consequences of *cold* in this sentence are sneezing and coughing, and we all know that these are the consequences of that illness called a *cold*.

On the PCAT, Words in Context questions may be asked in a number of ways, such as:

- As used in the first paragraph, the word *X* means…
- Based solely on the information in this passage, the best definition of *X* is…
- In the context in which it appears, *X* means…

Now try this sample Words in Context question using the following paragraph from the synthetic cephalopod skin passage:

> The skin's ability is currently dependent on the division of silicon bubbles with fiber-mesh frames. When scientists reinforce the mesh, the bubbles inflate and the skin reshapes. However, electric currents may also be used to modify the skin's appearance. During this prototype phase, scientists have already figured out how to make robots reproduce the appearances of round river stones and plants with leaves arranged in spiral patterns, among other shapes.

As used in the paragraph, the word *prototype* means
A. technology.
B. change.
C. first version.
D. robot.

In the paragraph, *prototype* is used to describe a particular phase in a process. The synthetic cephalopod skin will be a form of technology throughout the entirety of the process, so *technology* would be a weak word to describe a particular phase, so you can eliminate choice A. A process may change from phase to phase, but this paragraph does not indicate that a change is particular to this phase of the process of developing synthetic cephalopod skin; in fact, every phase of the process will involve change since that skin's main purpose is to change shape and color. Eliminate choice B. Choice C, however, makes sense since the paragraph describes a phase that involves a technology that has not been perfected yet, a technology that still may undergo changes, such as using electrical currents instead of fiber-mesh frames. So far, choice C is the best answer. But let's first make sure choice D is not a great answer before settling on C. Well, once again we have a word that will relate to

TIP

The correct answer to a Words in Context question will always be the same part of speech as the vocabulary word in question. For example, never choose an adjective when the word that must be defined is clearly a noun.

TIP

When answering Words in Context questions, try using each answer choice in place of the unfamiliar word in the original sentence. Answer choices that do not make any sense in that context can be eliminated.

synthetic cephalopod skin throughout its entire process of being perfected: it will always be intended for robots, so its not like there will be a robot phase and a non-robot phase. Eliminate choice D and select choice C with confidence. After all, it is the correct answer.

2. Main Ideas

TIP

Trying to identify the topic of a passage as you read can help you to answer any main idea questions that follow it.

The most basic elements of any reading selection may be words, but those words will have no purpose if they aren't used to convey a singular, main idea. The main idea is the topic of the passage as a whole. In essence, it's what the passage is about. Main Idea questions tend to be pretty straightforward, and often simply require you to distinguish between the most important ideas and the ones that merely support them. Occasionally they may attempt to trip you up with answer choices that include information that is not actually present in the given passage.

On the PCAT, Main Idea questions will expect you to identify the topic of the passage as a whole or a particular paragraph within the passage. However, they may be a little cagey about getting you to identify that topic. For example, a question may ask you to choose the best title for a particular passage. Make no mistake: these are main idea questions, and you are expected to choose the title that best sums up the main idea of the passage you just read.

On the PCAT, Main Idea questions may be asked in a number of ways, such as:

- The main point of the passage is that…
- What main point from the passage is supported by…
- Which of these would be the best title for the passage?

Now try this sample Main Idea question using the synthetic cephalopod skin passage:

Which of these would be the best title for the passage?
A. "A Future with Robots"
B. "The Biology of Octopus Skin"
C. "Silicon Bubbles and Fiber-Mesh Frames"
D. "Synthetic Cephalopod Skin"

This a pretty easy one since we keep referring to the passage as "the synthetic cephalopod skin passage," but before choosing choice D, let's just make sure it's better than the other answer choices. Yes, the passage is about robots, but choice A is too general: it makes no indication of why the robot technology in this passage is special. Choice B does refer to that special quality: octopus skin is the basis of this new robot skin. However, the passage is more about robots than octopuses, and there is nothing about the title "The Biology of Octopus Skin" that indicates this important detail. Eliminate choice B. Choice C actually isn't a terrible title since synthetic cephalopod skin is currently made of silicon bubbles and fiber-mesh frames, but that may change if electrical currents turn out to be more effective, and it is too specific to capture the main idea of the passage as a whole. So we were correct from the start: choice D is the best answer.

3. Supporting Details

If the Main Idea is the roof of a passage, then the Supporting Details are the walls that hold it upright. A topic would have no power if it were not backed up with facts. Supporting Details are those facts, and as far as Critical Reading questions go, Supporting Details questions are the easiest. Basically, you will just have to identify the facts authors use in passages. This merely requires careful reading of the passage to make sure those facts are represented accurately in the questions.

On the PCAT, Supporting Details questions will either be straightforward requests to find information in the passage or slightly trickier requests to identify information that is not present in the passage. In either case, you should go back to the passage to try to locate necessary information. Scan the passage for mentions of each answer choice in the question to find out if it is or is not present in the passage.

On the PCAT, Supporting Details questions may be asked in a number of ways, such as:

- According to the passage…
- Which of these is not mentioned in the passage?
- The word "*X*" refers to…

Now try this sample Supporting Details question using the following paragraph from the synthetic cephalopod skin passage:

> Octopus skin is unique in its ability to change both color and texture. Almost instantaneously, an octopus can reshape its skin to mimic the appearance of seaweed or coral. This rather fascinating ability is imperative to the creature's survival since it is such an effective form of camouflage. This experimental form of synthetic cephalopod (the class to which octopuses belong) skin would also give soft robots—robots covered with a malleable, silicon, skin-like material—the ability to morph from a flat, two-dimensional appearance to a textured three-dimensional one. They would then be able to hide from predatory animals in natural habitats just as the octopus does.

According to the passage, an octopus can reproduce the appearance of

A. robots.
B. cephalopods.
C. seaweed.
D. silicon.

The only tricky thing about this question is that it does not directly copy the language used in the passage. Instead of the word "mimic," it uses the synonym "reproduce." Otherwise, it's pretty straightforward. The first sentence of the paragraph states: "Almost instantaneously, an octopus can reshape its skin to mimic the appearance of seaweed or coral," which confirms that choice C is the correct answer. While skin for robots can mimic octopus skin, according to this passage, there is no indication that octopus skin can mimic robot skin, so choice A is not the right answer. "Cephalopods" are the class to which octopuses belong, so choice B is a bit redundant; it would be like saying that an octopus can mimic an octopus. Synthetic cephalopod skin is made of silicon in part, but there is no indication that octopus skin can mimic the appearance of silicon, as choice D would suggest. Choice C remains the best answer.

TIP

Comprehension questions usually focus on small, specific pieces of the passage. You don't have to understand the entire passage to get them right.

ALERT

Don't dismiss any question as a trick question: every single question is answerable.

4. Drawing Conclusions

Supporting Details questions expect you to identify information that is stated directly in the passage. Drawing Conclusions questions are not quite so straightforward. To answer such questions, you need to make inferences—which isn't quite a fancy word for "guesses"—based on suggestive information in the passage. Now these guesses are by no means random guesses. They are very logical conclusions supported by concrete information. It's just that the information does not involve explicitly identifying results.

For example, if someone said to you that Rasa stepped on a patch of ice and ended up breaking her arm, you can conclude that she probably slipped on the ice even though that detail is not stated directly. You will be expected to draw similar conclusions on the Critical Reading subtest. As you did when answering Words in Context questions, you will base your conclusions on context clues. You will never be expected to make a guess that has no information to support it.

On the PCAT, Drawing Conclusions questions may be asked in a number of ways, such as:

- The passage suggests that…
- What can be concluded from the passage?
- The author implies that…
- According to the passage, the most likely outcome is that…
- Paragraph 1 suggests that…
- On the basis of the last paragraph of the passage, it is possible to conclude that…

Now try this sample Drawing Conclusions question using the following paragraph from the synthetic cephalopod skin passage:

> Developers intend the skin to even have the ability to reproduce the appearance of an environment on site, just an octopus does, and they have already been successful in creating skin with an octopus's ability to change color to blend in with its surroundings. Regardless of these incredible strides, synthetic cephalopod skin is still very much in the development phase. Yet developers remain optimistic that this marvelous technology that will no doubt revolutionize robotics will be reliable enough to cover soft robots in the near future.

The passage suggests that synthetic cephalopod skin could

- **A.** change the way robots are used.
- **B.** make robots obsolete some day.
- **C.** cause of the extinction of octopuses.
- **D.** never became remotely possible.

We'll tackle this question by evaluating each answer choice in order. Choice A reaches the conclusion that synthetic cephalopod skin could change the way robots are made. Is there any support for this conclusion in the paragraph? Well, the author does state that the skin "will no doubt revolutionize robotics" and the rest of the passage suggests that the skin has capabilities that no other current

TIP

Return to the specific part of the passage, if listed in the question, and reread it.

feature of robotics does. All of that suggests that synthetic cephalopod skin could, indeed, change the way robots are used in the future. Let's save that answer. Choice B, however, reaches the opposite conclusion, and it does so without any real support from the passage. Why would adding a new feature to robots make them obsolete? Choice B is a conclusion that simply does not make sense, so you can go ahead and eliminate it. Choice C is similarly unrealistic. The purpose of synthetic cephalopod skin is to give robots an ability of octopuses, not to replace octopuses or run them into extinction. Eliminate choice C. Choice D is a bit trickier since synthetic cephalopod skin has not been perfected yet. However, the passage explains that enough strides have been made in its development that it is already more than remotely possible. Choice D is not the best answer. Choice A is.

Analysis

While Comprehension questions are fairly straightforward recognitions of a passage's contents, Analysis questions require deeper thought. Such questions require you to consider how ideas in a passage relate to each other, why an author wrote a particular passage, the differences between facts and opinions, and others matters beyond what is directly stated in a passage. Let's now think deeper about Analysis questions.

TIP

Analysis questions ask you to break information down in order to figure out the correct answer.

1. Relationships Between Ideas

All passages are made up of various ideas, but all ideas in a particular passage work toward a singular goal: supporting the main idea. Consequently, all ideas in a well-constructed passage are related in some way. On the PCAT, it will be one of your admittedly many jobs to understand how different ideas in a particular passage relate to each other. You might have to draw a connection between two different paragraphs, two different statements, or two different ideas in a passage.

There are several common kinds of relationships you will likely encounter on the PCAT. These relationships include:

Sequential Relationships, the relationship in which one thing follows another in order of how they occur:

Example: To drive to work I first opened my car door (*first step in sequence*), then I sat on the seat (*second step in sequence*), then I put the key in the ignition (*third step in sequence*), etc.

Cause/Effect Relationships, the relationship in which one thing causes another to happen:

Example: Turning the key in the ignition (*cause*) caused the car to start (*effect*).

Problem/Solution Relationships, the relationship in which a solution is found for a particular problem:

Example: I could not start my car (*problem*), so I brought it to the auto repair shop (*solution*).

Compare/Contrast Relationships, the relationship in which two or more things are described in order to point out how they are the same or different from each other:

Example: My car is the same color as Enid's (*compare*), but it is a totally different model from hers (*contrast*).

TIP

Parts of a passage will sometimes seem as though they have more than one relationship since, for example, a problem/solution relationship must always be sequential since a solution must always follow a problem sequentially. However, you must choose the strongest relationship.

Analysis questions ask for a deeper level of inference than required to answer the basic comprehension questions. They also require you to analyze relationships, such as cause and effect.

On the PCAT, Relationship Between Ideas questions may be asked in a number of ways, such as:

- The last paragraph relates to the first paragraph in that it…
- How does the author's statement that X relate to X?
- According to the passage, the relationship between X and X is that…
- The ideas in paragraphs 1 and 2 are mainly related by…

Now try this sample Relationships Between Ideas question using the following paragraphs from the synthetic cephalopod skin passage:

(1)   Mechanical structures are often patterned on the bodies of organic beings, and this is particularly true of robots intended to perform human functions. Robots may perform such tasks as building, serving, or even teaching or problem solving. However, robots do not always take their inspiration from human beings. In fact, researchers are currently experimenting with a new synthetic skin intended for robots that is patterned after octopus skin.

(2)   Octopus skin is unique in its ability to change both color and texture. Almost instantaneously, an octopus can reshape its skin to mimic the appearance of seaweed or coral. This rather fascinating ability is imperative to the creature's survival since it is such an effective form of camouflage. This experimental form of synthetic cephalopod (the class to which octopuses belong) skin would also give soft robots—robots covered with a malleable, silicon, skin-like material— the ability to morph from a flat, two-dimensional appearance to a textured three-dimensional one. They would then be able to hide from predatory animals in natural habitats just as the octopus does.

The second paragraph relates to the first paragraph in that it
A. explains the differences between biological life forms.
B. discusses robotic technology based on a biological life form.
C. shows how robotic technology works.
D. describes ways sea creatures protect themselves.

TIP

Reserve your slowest reading rate for the question stem. Read it with extra care and laser-like focus.

This question is essentially asking you to find a compare/contrast relationship between the two paragraphs, but it is not merely asking you to identify that relationship. You must identify precisely how the paragraphs are similar and different. Start by thinking about what they have in common. They are both about robotic technology based on biological life forms: paragraph 1 is about robotic technology based on humans and paragraph 2 is about robotic technology based on octopuses. Therein also lies the contrast since humans and octopuses are very different life forms with very different abilities. Therefore, choice B is already looking like the correct answer.

Choice A may seem like a good answer since the two paragraphs focus on different biological life forms, but their purpose is not really to highlight the differences between humans and octopuses. Because it fails to take the robot component into account, choice A is not a better answer than choice B. Eliminate it. Choice C does take robots into account, but it fails to describe the paragraphs accurately since neither explains how anything works. Choice D only describes information in paragraph 2, and since the question asks you to find a relationship between both paragraphs, it cannot be the correct answer. Choice B remains our best answer.

2. Author's Purpose

Author's usually don't write simply because they enjoy typing. There's generally a purpose behind their work. Perhaps that purpose is as simple as the desire to entertain readers with a fun story, but a purpose may be more complex than that. Perhaps authors want to convey a message, explain how to perform a process, or get the reader to side with the author on a particular issue. Sometimes authors will be very up front about their purposes, but the cagiest authors will be subtler about getting their messages across. Such approaches may force you to be a bit of a detective when taking the Critical Reading subtest as you search for clues to help you decode the author's purpose.

Let's start by looking at the most common purposes behind pieces of writing. For example, authors may want to:

- **entertain** readers, though considering the scientific nature of the passages on the PCAT, this will be the least common purpose you'll encounter

- **inform** readers of something (informative writing), which will involve a neutral description of an issue, event, or idea

- **describe** something to readers (descriptive writing), which will also be neutral but will rely heavily on descriptions of purpose or appearance

- **explain** something to the reader (expository writing), which will be neutral and explain the steps in how to perform a process, how something works, or why something exists, etc.

- **persuade** readers to believe something (argumentative writing), which will be more biased, with wording that implies the author's personal preferences and attempts to get the reader to share the author's opinions

Then, no matter what the topic, ask yourself the following:

Is the author

- arguing for a particular point of view.

    OR

- informing the reader by
  a. explaining a concept,
  b. retelling a history, or
  c. describing someone or something?

Knowing whether a passage is argumentative or expository tells you a great deal and will help you get ready for the questions that follow. For example, an argumentative essay is going to argue a single point of view (even if it acknowledges counterarguments) and it will likely have weaknesses such as bias. You will have to infer those weaknesses on your own. After reading the sample paragraph above, you might reasonably expect the contributions of others to be emphasized and those of Mendeleev to be, at least relatively speaking, downplayed.

Some passages on the PCAT may be written in the first person; these passages are more likely to be persuasive. They do not just argue a point of view, but act to persuade you to agree with that point of view. As you read them, be alert to opinions, as well as words that signal bias.

TIP

From time to time, analysis questions will ask you to interpret the meaning of a given word in the specific context.

NOTE

To determine tone, think of how the words sound when read aloud (in your head) and the feelings they carry. You may hear, for example, certainty or uncertainty, bold commands or humble requests, sarcasm or sincerity.

Typically, questions on the PCAT will ask you to identify bias, as well as tone, which is the author's attitude toward the subject. In fact, you can expect *many* questions on the PCAT that are related to author's purpose and its elements.

On the PCAT, Author's Purpose questions may be asked in a number of ways, such as:

1. The author's primary purpose in this passage is to…

2. The writer mentions X in order to…

3. The primary purpose of this passage is to…

Now try this sample Author's Purpose question based on the synthetic cephalopod skin passage:

The author's primary purpose in this passage is to

A. explain how synthetic cephalopod skin works.

B. persuade the reader to use synthetic cephalopod skin.

C. inform the reader of synthetic cephalopod skin.

D. describe how octopuses look after changing shape.

One thing to be aware of when answering Author's Purpose questions is whether the question is asking you to identify the purpose of a particular part of the passage or the passage as a whole. This particular question is asking you to identify the purpose of the passage as a whole, so you must be sure your answer takes the entire passage into account. Does the entire passage explain how synthetic cephalopod skin works or is this only explained in one paragraph? It is only explained in paragraph 2, so choice A cannot be correct. Is the author mostly concerned with persuading you to believe something? Well, the author does interject with a few personal opinions here and there—describing the technology as "marvelous" and suggesting that it will definitely be revolutionary—but as a whole, the author does not make a sustained argument, so choice B is not the best answer. So is the author mainly concerned with neutrally informing the reader of synthetic cephalopod skin? Yes, for the most part, that is what is happening throughout all five paragraphs of this passage. If choice D doesn't work—and it doesn't since it only describe a minor detail in paragraph 2—choice C is the best answer.

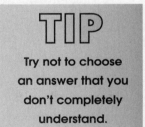

TIP

Try not to choose an answer that you don't completely understand.

3. Author's Tone

Authors help get their messages across with the ways they write those messages. Maybe they attempt to gain the reader's trust with humor or friendly language. Maybe they try to assert their authority with a serious approach that makes them come across as experts or teachers. The way an author uses language to create a feeling to reach a particular audience is known as tone, and you will have to identify the author's tone on the Critical Reading subtest.

There are many different tones an author can potentially adopt. A piece of writing can be absurd, accusatory, admiring, aggressive, ambivalent, amused, angry, apologetic, arrogant, assertive, or awe-struck—and that's just the A's! So instead of memorizing every kind of possible tone in preparation for the PCAT, it is more important to simply use your experiences as a human being who probably communicates with others on a regular basis to decode the author's tone since authors use words in much the same way as we all do in everyday speech—they just tend to choose their words more carefully. So just as you are probably capable of understanding when another person is being sincere or sarcastic based on the way that person uses words, you should be able to tell when an author is using a particular tone as well. For example, does the author use words and phrases such as "disgusted," "infuriated," and "beside myself" in an emotionally charged piece of writing? Well, then you can probably identify the tone of that piece as "angry." Does a piece of writing make you laugh? Then it likely strives for a humorous tone. You see, identifying the author's tone is not just dependent on recognizing key words—it also requires you to tune in to your own emotions and reactions. If a piece about environmental activism makes you feel like getting out there and fighting for the environmental cause too, then you can probably conclude that the author achieves an "inspirational" tone.

On the PCAT, Author's Tone questions may be asked in a number of ways, such as:

- The author's tone could best be described as…
- Which word best describes the author's overall tone in the passage?

Now try this sample Author's Tone question using the synthetic cephalopod skin passage:

The author's tone could best be described as

A. celebratory.

B. amused.

C. solemn.

D. informative.

Answering Author's Tone questions requires keen attention to word use and emotional response. A celebratory piece will likely use a lot of extreme language: *Stupendous! Incredible! Marvelous!* However, the author of this passage does not overly indulge in such language, so *celebratory* is a bit extreme to describe the passage's tone accurately, and choice A is not likely the best answer. Does the author ever seem to view synthetic cephalopod skin as something funny or charming? The author does seem to appreciate the technology, but she or he never uses language or draws on emotions indicating that she or he finds synthetic cephalopod skin to be particularly amusing. Choice B is not a great answer. Choice C goes too far in the other direction. *Solemn* indicates a grave, deadly serious tone, and it usually adopted when discussing something of terrible purpose, like nuclear war or global warming. Synthetic cephalopod skin is somewhat serious due to its military applications, but it is not really worthy of a solemn tone and the author certainly does not use a solemn tone in this passage. Choice C is wrong. As we already noticed in our sample Author's Purpose question, the author is mainly concerned with conveying information about synthetic cephalopod skin in a neutral manner, so choice D, informative, is our best answer.

4. Facts/Opinions

Facts/Opinions questions are the most straightforward analysis questions because they generally just require you to distinguish between the concrete details in a passage and the things the author personally feels and believes. Essentially, if you can recognize when the author says something with which everyone may not agree, then you can ace Fact/Opinions questions.

Example: The harp is a musical instrument.

That's a fact. No one can convincingly argue that a harp is not a musical instrument.

The harp is the most beautiful-sounding musical instrument.

ALERT

You may find qualifiers such as never and always in a question stem; these words should serve as a warning that some answers to the question may be very close, or even that more than one answer may be correct in limited ways.

Might someone not think the sound of a piano, guitar, or oboe is more beautiful? This is not a fact—it is the author's personal opinion.

On the PCAT, Facts/Opinions questions may be asked in a number of ways, such as:

- Which words from the passage reflect the author's opinion?
- Which statement from the passage is an example of an opinion the author holds?

Now try this sample Facts/Opinions question using the preceding paragraph from the synthetic cephalopod skin passage:

Which words from the passage reflect the author's opinion?

   A. "Octopus skin is unique in its ability to change both color and texture."

   B. "This rather fascinating ability is imperative to the creature's survival since it is such an effective form of camouflage."

   C. "The skin's ability is currently dependent on the division of silicon bubbles with fiber-mesh frames."

   D. "The skin also has the potential for industrial, academic, and even hobby uses."

So, once again, you are looking for a statement with which not everyone may agree even if the author presents it as unquestionable. Choice A may seem like such a statement because of its use of the word *unique*, but even though *unique* is descriptive, it is not subjective in this case: it is an objective fact that the octopus possesses a unique or individual ability, so choice A reflects a fact, not an opinion. Choice B is a different story because not everyone may necessarily find the octopuses ability "fascinating." A word like *fascinating* is never objective since different people are fascinated by different things. The personal opinion embedded in this sentence makes choice B a likely candidate for the correct answer. Choice C is straight-up factual information without any descriptive wording at all that might even be confused for a personal opinion. Eliminate it. The same is true of choice D, which uses a particularly neutral phrase in the form of "has the potential for" (as opposed to, say, "would be great for"). Facts tend to be neutral. Choice B is the right answer.

5. Rhetorical Strategies

Rhetoric is the art of making an argument. An argument is not just a hostile exchange or fight—in writing, it is any piece that attempts to persuade the reader to believe something by arguing in favor of or against something. Merely stating "I want you to believe my position" is a rather clumsy approach to rhetoric, so authors tend to use subtler strategies for getting their positions across and convincing readers that those positions are the right ones. On the Critical Reading subtest, you will have to recognize a variety of those rhetorical strategies.

Writers may use an **appeal to reason** that uses logic to convince the reader of something.

Example: If you go out in a storm without proper rain gear, you will get wet.

They may also use a more **emotional** approach that attempts to manipulate the readers' feeling in order to win support.

Example: You would feel terrible about yourself if you did not donate some of your pay to charity.

An **ethical** approach appeals to the readers' sense of right and wrong.

TIP

Watch for signal words in the question stems. Signal words may include qualifiers, like *primary*, *most*, and *best*.

TIP

Argumentative writing does not have to be hostile; it merely needs to be persuasive.

Example: It is simply unfair to gorge oneself during every meal when so many throughout the world are starving.

Personal anecdotes may be useful for personalizing an argument.

Example: Only after I got cancer did I realize the absolute necessity of universal health coverage.

Quoting an expert can lend credence to a piece of rhetorical writing.

Example: As renowned genius Albert Einstein said, "The world is a dangerous place to live not because of the people who are evil but because of the people who don't do anything about it."

Referring to **studies or other data** is an effective rhetorical strategy.

Example: A recent study by Chicago University reveals that older people tend to be happier than those under 18.

On the PCAT, Rhetorical Strategies questions may be asked in a number of ways, such as:

- Which strategy does the author use to support the overall thesis?
- Which of these adds most credibility to the information presented in the passage?

Now try this sample Rhetorical Strategies question using the following paragraph from the synthetic cephalopod skin passage:

> Developers intend even the skin to have the ability to reproduce the appearance of an environment on site, just an octopus does, and they have already been successful in creating skin with an octopus's ability to change color to blend in with its surroundings. Regardless of these incredible strides, synthetic cephalopod skin is still very much in the development phase. Yet developers remain optimistic that this marvelous technology that will no doubt revolutionize robotics will be reliable enough to cover soft robots in the near future. According to Robert Shepherd of Cornell University (as quoted in *Live Science*), "We're just at the beginning, and we have great results…"

Which strategy does the author use in this paragraph to support the overall thesis?
A. Adding personal anecdotes to show the effectiveness of synthetic cephalopod skin.
B. Referring to a specific school that supplied additional facts and statistics.
C. Listing specific results of from prestigious studies to add credibility.
D. Quoting an expert in a particular field to add credibility.

In this passage, the author's primary goal is to inform the reader of synthetic cephalopod skin, but the author also subtly tries to convince the reader that it is a worthwhile technology. In this paragraph, one strategy that works toward that agenda is the author's use of a quotation. The quote itself does not say anything specific that adds essential information to this paragraph. It is not a personal anecdote about the effectiveness of synthetic cephalopod skin (choice A), a supply of facts or statistics (choice B), or a list of results from studies (choice C). It is merely a quotation about how the results of the experiment are "great," which only has any credence at all because of the researcher's impressive credentials: he's a representative of Cornell University. Therefore, choice D is the best answer.

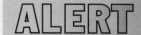

ALERT

Remember that some questions will require you to understand the passage as a whole. No matter how hard you look, you won't find the answer, or sufficient clues to it, in a single spot.

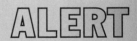

Evaluation

Matters of tone, opinion, and rhetoric are not only relevant when answering Analysis questions on the Critical Reading subtest. Such things will also be relevant when answering Evaluation questions.

Evaluation questions do not just ask you to identify when an author uses a particular rhetorical strategy in a piece of writing; they expect you to evaluate the effectiveness of those strategies. Is the author guilty of bias? Does the author include sufficient support for a statement or argument? Does the author reach a sensible conclusion or present a clear thesis? These are the kinds of things you'll have to think about when answering Evaluation questions.

1. Bias

We all have our biases—our personal opinions and feelings about particular matters. You may be biased in favor of people with particular political leanings or biased against others because of what they like to do in their spare time. Naturally, having biases can be a problem and this is especially true when it comes to rhetoric. Obvious biases can undermine an argument by making the author seem prejudiced or guilty of giving preferential treatment.

On the Critical Reading subtest, you may either have to identify an author's biases or draw conclusions about the author based on those biases. For example, if an author expresses a strong preference for technology, you may have to guess what the author would most *likely* feel about a particular technology.

You might also have to find particular words that reveal the author's biases. Such words will likely be descriptive words unnecessary for mere informative purposes.

For example:

> "That movie opens on Friday."

This is a straight-forward sentence informing the reading of when a particular movie is opening.

> "That awful-looking movie opens on Friday."

The sentence now becomes more than informative as the descriptive phrase "awful-looking" suggests the writer's bias against the movie, probably based on the way it looks in advertisements.

On the PCAT, Bias questions may be asked in a number of ways, such as:

- Which statement from the passage best shows the author's attitude toward X?
- Which word or term from the passage reveals a connotation bias on the part of the author?
- Information in the passage suggests that the author views X as…
- The author of the passage would most likely agree that…
- Which word or phrase from the passage best reveals the author's bias?

Now try this sample Bias question using the following paragraph from the synthetic cephalopod skin passage:

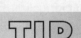

Developers even intend the skin to have the ability to reproduce the appearance of an environment on site, just an octopus does, and they have already been successful in creating skin with an octopus's ability to change color to blend in with its surroundings. Regardless of these incredible strides, synthetic cephalopod skin is still very much in the development phase. Yet developers remain optimistic that this marvelous technology that will no doubt revolutionize robotics will be reliable enough to cover soft robots in the near future. According to Robert Shepherd of Cornell University (as quoted in *Live Science*), "We're just at the beginning, and we have great results…"

Which word from the paragraph best reveals the author's bias?

A. successful

B. development

C. reliable

D. marvelous

Several of the words in these answer choices could be used to reveal bias. The key factor is finding out what these words describe. Are any used without an expressly informative purpose? Choice A, *successful*, is used to describe the progress of a process, and the sentence would not make sense without it. It is not used to indicate the author's bias for or against synthetic cephalopod skin. Choice B, *development*, is not descriptive at all, so it can be eliminated. Choice C, *reliable*, refers to a goal in the development of synthetic cephalopod skin and it is essential for understanding part of the paragraph. Choice D, *marvelous*, is not. It is the author interjecting with a personal bias in favor of the technology, and the sentence would read perfectly well without this unnecessary bit of bias. Choice D is the correct answer.

2. Support in an Argument

An argument is like a tent. The thesis is the canvas and the supporting details are the poles that hold up that canvas. Without those poles of supporting detail, the thesis would collapse. The same is true of supporting details that do not do their jobs effectively. If supporting details do not link up to the thesis logically, if they are based on conjecture or bias rather than facts and research, they may as well not exist at all.

On the Critical Reading subtest, you won't just identify supporting details; you will evaluate how they support the thesis and how effectively they do their jobs. A number of factors can render supporting details weak, such as their basis in bias rather than fact or their lack of relevance. Most often, though, you will be expected to locate the evidence that best supports the thesis. In some cases you may even have to think of evidence that is not present in a passage but would have made the passage stronger if it had been included.

On the PCAT, Support in an Argument questions may be asked in a number of ways, such as:

- Which point from the passage best supports the author's suggestion that…

- Which of the following conclusion is most effectively supported by information in the passage?

- What evidence could the author have included that would best support the main point?

- Which statement from the passage leads most credibility to the idea that…

TIP

Instead of focusing on small bits of information, Evaluation questions are likely to test your understanding of the passage as a whole.

ALERT

Saying that something is "great" does not support the idea that it is "great." Strong support will be specific about what makes the thing great.

Now try this sample Support in an Argument question using the synthetic cephalopod skin passage:

(1)   Mechanical structures are often patterned on the bodies of organic beings, and this is particularly true of robots intended to perform human functions. Robots may perform such tasks as building, serving, or even teaching or problem solving. However, robots do not always take their inspiration from human beings. In fact, researchers are currently experimenting with a new synthetic skin intended for robots that is patterned after octopus skin.

(2)   Octopus skin is unique in its ability to change both color and texture. Almost instantaneously, an octopus can reshape its skin to mimic the appearance of seaweed or coral. This ability is imperative to the creature's survival since it is such an effective form of camouflage. This experimental form of synthetic cephalopod (the class to which octopuses belong) skin would also give soft robots—robots covered with a malleable, silicon, skin-like material— the ability to morph from a flat, two-dimensional appearance to a textured three-dimensional one. They would then be able to hide from predatory animals in natural habitats just as the octopus does.

(3)   The skin's ability is currently dependent on the division of silicon bubbles with fiber-mesh frames. When scientists reinforce the mesh, the bubbles inflate and the skin reshapes. However, electric currents may also be used to modify the skin's appearance. During this prototype phase, scientists have already figured out how to make robots reproduce the appearances of round river stones and plants with leaves arranged in spiral patterns, among other shapes.

(4)   The obvious question is: why would a robot benefit from this particular ability? One potential use would be during military maneuvers that require a robot to move undetected over dangerous ground. According to Cecilia Laschi, a professor of biorobotics at the BioRobotics Institute of the Sant'Anna School of Advanced Studies (as quoted in *Live Science*), "Camouflaged robots may hide and be protected from animal attacks and may better approach animals for studying them in their natural habitats." Furthermore, robots that require inflated skin when in use could be deflated with this new skin to make them more compact when stacked during transportation to their destinations. The skin also has the potential for industrial, academic, and even hobby uses. Consequently, the team of scientists developing synthetic cephalopod skin is intent on ensuring its ease of use despite the skin's inherent complexity.

(5)   Developers even intend the skin to have the ability to reproduce the appearance of an environment on site, just an octopus does, and they have already been rather successful in creating skin with an octopus's ability to change color to blend in with its surroundings. Regardless of these incredible strides, synthetic cephalopod skin is still very much in the development phase. Yet developers remain optimistic that this marvelous technology that will no doubt revolutionize robotics will be reliable enough to cover soft robots in the near future. According to Robert Shepherd of Cornell University (as quoted in *Live Science*), "We're just at the beginning, and we have great results…"

Which point from the passage best supports Robert Shepherd's suggestion that the synthetic cephalopod skin experiment has yielded "great results"?

A. Mechanical structures are often patterned on the bodies of organic beings, and this is particularly true of robots intended to perform human functions.

B. Almost instantaneously, an octopus can reshape its skin to mimic the appearance of seaweed or coral.

C. During this prototype phase, scientists have already figured out how to make robots reproduce the appearances of round river stones and plants with leaves arranged in spiral patterns, among other shapes.

D. Yet developers remain optimistic that this marvelous technology that will no doubt revolutionize robotics will be reliable enough to cover soft robots in the near future.

The correct answer needs to provide very specific support for Shepherd's rather general statement. Choice A is general in essence and has nothing to do with Shepherd's statement, so it can be easily eliminated. Choice B may include specific information about an octopus's abilities, but Shepherd's quote is not about octopuses; it is about a technology inspired by octopuses. Eliminate choice B on grounds of irrelevance. Choice C, however, is both specific and relevant; it indicates some of the "great results" of which Shepherd speaks. Choice D is relevant, since like Shepherd's quote, it places the development of synthetic cephalopod skin in a positive light, but it lacks specifics to support that positive attitude. Choice C is best.

3. Author's Conclusion/Thesis

As we've already established while discussing Author's Purpose questions, any piece of writing needs to have a purpose. However, purpose is not enough. The piece of writing also needs to achieve the author's intended purpose by establishing a strong thesis and reaching a convincing conclusion. If a piece of writing does not do so, it will not be very strong.

A **thesis** explicitly lays out both the main idea and the author's purpose in a passage in a concise statement.

A **conclusion** summarizes the findings of the passage in a concise statement at the end of the passage.

The thesis and conclusion of a passage must be very clear. If readers miss the thesis or conclusion, they will likely miss the point of the passage and its effectiveness as a piece of rhetoric will be dissolved. On the Critical Reading subtest, you will need to identify authors' theses and conclusions in an effort to evaluate the effectiveness of the given passages.

On the PCAT, Author's Conclusion/Thesis questions may be asked in a number of ways, such as:

- Which of the following is the author's thesis statement?
- At the end of the passage, what does the author conclude?

Now try this sample Author's Conclusion/Thesis question using the following paragraph from the synthetic cephalopod skin passage:

(5)   Developers even intend the skin to have the ability to reproduce the appearance of an environment on site, just an octopus does, and they have already been rather successful in creating skin with an octopus's ability to change color to blend in with its surroundings. Regardless of these incredible strides, synthetic cephalopod skin is still very much in the development phase. Yet developers remain optimistic that this marvelous technology that will no doubt revolutionize

robotics will be reliable enough to cover soft robots in the near future. According to Robert Shepherd of Cornell University (as quoted in *Live Science*), "We're just at the beginning, and we have great results…"

At the end of the passage, what does the author conclude?

A. Researchers have achieved great results in developing synthetic cephalopod skin.

B. Researchers are optimistic that synthetic cephalopod skin will become a reliable and revolutionary technology in the future.

C. Researchers have made synthetic cephalopod skin with the ability to change color or match environment.

D. Synthetic cephalopod skin is still very much in the development phase and will take years to perfect.

Here's a hint: the final sentence of a passage is not necessarily the concluding statement. That's the case in this passage, which ends with a supporting quote from someone other than the author. That quote is paraphrased in choice A, so that answer can be eliminated. Choice B paraphrases the second-to-last sentence of the passage, which actually summarizes the main findings of the passage and serves as its concluding statement. Choice C is just an isolated detail from the paragraph, and its failure to summarize any of the passage's findings. Choice D makes the mistake of reaching a conclusion that is not actually present in the passage, which never implies that synthetic cephalopod skin "will take years to perfect." Choice B is our answer.

A CRITICAL READING STUDY PLAN

After taking the diagnostic Critical Reading subtest at the beginning of this book and examining a sample passage and sample questions for each question type in this chapter, you should have a clearer idea of the kinds of material you'll be expected to deal with on test day. Our Critical Reading subtest preparation is not over yet, though. You will need to a lot plenty of time to study for the subtest between now and test day, and this section will help you to maximize that time with a customized 3-step Critical Reading study plan. Let's get to work.

Study Plan Part 1: Get Familiar

Believe or not, you're already on your way to accomplishing part 1 of our study plan if you've done the diagnostic test, read all the material in this chapter thus far, and answered all of the sample questions in this chapter. After all that, you should be pretty familiar with PCAT-type Critical Reading passages and PCAT-type Critical Reading questions. This is crucial because you will perform better on the test if you are familiar with the exact types of reading passages and questions that are on the test. By being familiar with what's on the test, you won't waste your time studying what isn't on the test. So let's do another quick review just to make sure you are completely familiar with all of the PCAT Critical Reading material you will encounter on test day.

TIP

Creating a study plan will help you make the most of the time you have between now and test day.

TIP

Try not to study too hard the night before test day. You want to be well rested.

- **Passages** average between 400 and 600 words in length and cover the following:
  - Historical Topics
  - Contemporary Topics
  - Cultural Topics
  - Ethical Topics
  - Political Topics
  - Technical Topics
- Passage topics relate to issues pertaining to **natural sciences, social sciences**, or **humanities**
- Passages may be **informative, persuasive**, or **speculative**
- **Critical Reading** questions fall into one of three categories: 1. Comprehension, 2. Analysis, and 3. Evaluation
- **Comprehension** questions include:
  - **Words in Context** questions (defining vocabulary words)
  - **Main Idea** questions (identifying or inferring the most important idea in the passage)
  - **Supporting Details** questions (identifying facts and details stated explicitly in the passage)
  - **Drawing conclusions** questions (making inferences based on information stated explicitly in the passage)
- **Analysis** questions include:
  - **Relationship Between Ideas** questions (analyzing and identifying how one idea in a passage relates to another idea in it)
  - **Author's Purpose** questions (analyzing the author's main reason for making a particular statement or writing the passage as a whole)
  - **Author's Tone** questions (analyzing the author's attitude and method of conveying information)
  - **Facts/Opinions** questions (distinguishing between objective facts and subjective opinions in a passage)
  - **Rhetorical Strategies** questions (analyzing the methods the author uses to convince the reading of a particular position or belief)
- **Evaluation** questions include:
  - **Bias** questions (evaluating the author's viewpoint, preference, or position)
  - **Support in an Argument** questions (evaluating the information the author uses to support an argument)
  - **Author's Conclusion/Thesis** (identifying the main point the author makes in a passage and evaluating its effectiveness)

> **TIP**
>
> Slow your reading rate for the question. If you're not sure you know what the question is asking, reread it.

Study Plan Part 2: Practice, Practice, Practice

Getting familiar with passage and question types and how to answer them will get you comfortable with the kind of material on the PCAT Critical Reading test, but nothing will sharpen up your skills for actually taking the test like practice. You will practice by taking the diagnostic test and the practice tests at the end of the book—and then taking them again and again. That may sound like a waste of time or a recipe for answering questions through memorization rather than critical reading, but there are so many questions and passages on these tests that you probably won't actually remember the answers to all the questions each time you take them. And even if you do remember some of the questions, retaking them will still help you sharpen your skills, especially if you read the explanations for why answer choices are right and wrong every time.

These explanations are key as well because they will help you to understand why those sneaky test creators choose the particular wrong answers that they choose. Maybe they are trying to distract you into choosing an answer that almost seems correct because it contains some accurate information or they are misdirecting you to the wrong spot in the passage. Perhaps an answer choice may actually be correct from a certain point of view but it is still not the very best answer among all four choices. By understanding why answer choices are incorrect, you will get a better idea of how to select the correct answer choices.

Study Plan 3: Keep Track of Errors

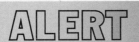

You can understand the passage perfectly and still come up with the wrong answer—if you don't pay careful attention to each word of the question stem.

Feel free to give yourself a big pat on the back every time you answer a question correctly while practicing for the Critical Reading subtest. However, you really need to pay attention to the questions you answer incorrectly. Doing so will alert you to the spots that require more intense practice. Perhaps you are a vocab whiz who always answers Words in Context questions correctly, but you always seem to stumble over Rhetorical Strategies questions. Then you should spend more time reviewing the Rhetorical Strategies section of this chapter.

Perhaps it is not a particular question type that trips you up but a particular kind of incorrect answer. If you recognize a pattern that points to difficulty with a particular kind of question, try to really tune in to those kinds of questions when retaking a practice test so you're ready to leap over those stumbling blocks. Here are a few common problems to look out for when weeding out incorrect answer choices:

> **A. Too extreme.** Answer choices that are too extreme—as in they contain a phrase such as "this always happens" when in fact the thing in question only happens *sometimes*—are wrong unless the passage specifically supports that extremism. Key words indicating an answer choice that is too extreme include *always*, *never*, and *impossible*.
>
> **B. Mistakes a part for the whole and vice versa.** If a question is asking you to indentify something that pertains to the entire passage, do not make the mistake of selecting answer choice that is only relevant to one paragraph in the passage. Similarly, a question that asks you to identify something that pertains to only one paragraph probably won't have a correct answer that relates to the entire passage in a general way. Make sure to read the question carefully and do exactly what the question expects you to do.
>
> **C. True but still wrong.** An answer choice might be true in itself, but that does not necessarily make it the correct answer to the specific question being asked. An answer choice is only correct if it fulfills the requirements of the question completely.

D. Major assumptions. Answer choices that make too many assumptions outside of the information directly stated in the passage are probably wrong. Remember that an answer choice needs sufficient support.

E. Partially correct. An answer choice is either right or wrong. It cannot be partially correct. If a choice contains any information that does not match up with what you read in the passage, then that answer choice is incorrect.

Choose the Right Plan

Now it's time to choose the best way to use this customized Critical Reading study plan because there are two basic options.

Option 1: Skills-Based Plan: This option involves really paying attention to those errors and constructing your study plan around turning your weak spots into strong spots. With this plan, you will focus your energy on figuring out why you keep making the same errors in an effort to stop making those errors. It involves retaking the practice tests and examining the explanations for each answer choice as many times as it takes to iron out your problem spots.

Option 2: Time-Based Plan: If you do not notice any particular problem areas and merely want to make the most of the time you have to study between now and test day, then a Time-Based Plan is probably best for you. This involves making a study calendar, setting a specific task for each night, and sticking to your schedule.

1. **Make a study calendar** by scheduling nights that you are available to work for a certain amount of time. 2 hours of concentrated, undistracted study time that includes room for a 15-minute break can be a very effective use of your time.

2. **Set a specific task** for each night on your schedule. For example, let's say you have twenty nights to study before test day. Then you can make a schedule that looks something like this:

Night 1	Take the diagnostic Critical Reading subtest and read each answer explanation carefully.
Night 2	Read the Critical Reading chapter and answer each sample question in it.
Night 3	Take the practice test at the end of the Critical Reading Chapter.
Night 4	Study the questions you answered incorrectly and try to figure out why you answered them incorrectly.
Night 5	Review the Critical Reading chapter.
Night 6	Retake the diagnostic test.
Night 7	Review the Critical Reading chapter again.
Night 8	Retake the practice test at the end of the Critical Reading Chapter.
Night 9	Take the Critical Reading subtest in Practice Test 2 at the end of this book.
Night 10	Study the questions you answered incorrectly and try to figure out why you answered them incorrectly.

TIP

Eliminate as many wrong answers as you can, not just the most obvious one or two. With each wrong choice you eliminate, your chance of getting the answer right increases.

Night 11	Take the Critical Reading subtest in Practice Test 3 at the end of this book
Night 12	Study the questions you answered incorrectly and try to figure out why you answered them incorrectly.
Night 13	Review the Critical Reading chapter, focusing on the sections that discuss your weak spots.
Night 14	Retake the Critical Reading subtest in Practice Test 2 at the end of this book
Night 15	Study the questions you answered incorrectly.
Night 16	Retake the Critical Reading subtest in Practice Test 3 at the end of this book.
Night 17	Study the questions you answered incorrectly.
Night 18	Retake both Critical Reading Practice Tests, allowing yourself only 50 minutes to complete each.
Night 19	Review your answers.
Night 20	Retake the diagnostic test in 50 minutes and review your answers.

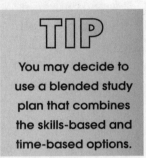

You may decide to use a blended study plan that combines the skills-based and time-based options.

3. **Stick to your plan.** This may seem obvious, but you know what they say about the best laid plans. However, you really must do whatever it takes to stick to your study plan. There can be a lot of temptations that might draw you away from the night's scheduled task, such as a fun opportunity to go out for the night with a friend. Well, there will be plenty of time to have fun after test day. For now, show some self-discipline and stick to your schedule. You will be happy you did when you get your test results, even if studying is not your favorite way to spend a couple of hours (don't worry—it isn't anyone's favorite way to spend a couple of hours).

CRITICAL READING STRATEGIES FOR THE PCAT

As you study, try applying some of the following strategies to help you navigate Critical Reading passages and the questions that accompany them.

Outline the Passage

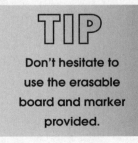

Don't hesitate to use the erasable board and marker provided.

Because you will be given an erasable board and marker to use during the test, you have the option of jotting down the thesis as well as the main idea of each paragraph as you read. That is, you have the option of outlining. If you do, make your outline simple and brief by using words and phrases, not sentences. To save time, use abbreviations and symbols such as arrows and plus signs. Stick to the main points only.

When you finish reading the passage, read your outline. Get a sense of how the passage moves from beginning to end. You might even notice a pattern of organization, such as cause and effect or chronology. Understanding the main ideas and structure will help you answer the questions that follow.

You can also mentally outline without writing. As you finish each paragraph, ask yourself if you got the main idea. Maybe you read the paragraph in too much of a rush; maybe you blanked out from nervousness. Go back and be sure you understand the main point of the paragraph you're reading before moving on to the next paragraph. Then, put it all together in your head.

Read Between the Lines

If there is one thing you can bank on during a Reading Comprehension subtest, it is that you will be asked to make inferences. As you come up with the main idea for each paragraph, also think about what is unstated, but absolutely implied in the paragraph.

For example, if a passage mentions a drug for Alzheimer's disease that is approved by the FDA for use at all stages of the disease, but the author also tells you that research suggests the drug is effective only at the beginning and middle stages of the disease, you might infer that the author believes that the FDA's ruling falls short of reality. At the very least, you can read between the lines that some people are likely taking a drug for nothing.

Decide Which Terms Matter

Some questions are going to focus on specific concepts and terms. Words that help retell or recast the main idea or thesis matter the most. On the other hand, some terms barely matter at all. There's a good chance that Reading Comprehension questions will NOT focus on the most technical terms. Instead, questions may ask you to identify or work with terms related to the main idea or the most significant supporting details. As you read, separate out the terms that matter from those that do not.

Chances are also good that you are NOT going to be asked about information that appears in parentheses or is stated as an appositive. For example, you may be reading a passage about Lyme disease that mentions that only certain ticks (*I. scapularis* and *I. pacificus*) carry the disease. In this case, the scientific names of the ticks are shown in parentheses, and you may assume that these terms are not crucial.

Unless they are essential to the main idea or are repeated, don't bother with technical or parenthetical terms as you read. If you do get a question on them, you can return to the specified paragraph or context.

Similarly, the titles of studies and the names of their authors are unlikely to be tested. After all, the makers of the PCAT, and pharmacy colleges, aren't evaluating your ability to parrot, or even identify, a minor detail. Everyone already assumes you can do this. Instead, the test is about understanding, interpreting, and evaluating information.

Know When to Stop Reading

Obviously, you can't race through the passage, nor can you keep going back, hoping that multiple readings will clarify something you didn't get the first or even, possibly, the second time. Remember that you're going to earn points by answering the questions, not by understanding every last detail of the passage. If you've read carefully once, that should be sufficient most of the time. Switch your

TIP

To read between the lines, ask yourself why certain information appears. Ask yourself how one idea relates to the next.

TIP

Focus on the terms that are most closely related to the topic and the angle or specific focus.

NOTE

Parentheses are like green traffic lights: They contain extra info that you can speed through. Dashes, on the other hand, amplify. Think of them as a yellow light, and use caution.

focus to the questions. A good approach is to read once, and then reread *parts* of the passage on a need-to basis as you answer questions.

You may hear the advice that if you can answer a question from memory, or without looking back at the passage, you spent too much time reading. That's ridiculous! A better indicator of time well spent is that you can answer *some* questions without looking back; for the rest, in general, you at least know where in the passage to look.

For the most part, the PCAT makes it easy for you to find the answers in passages. Many questions specify the exact paragraph or sentence that gives or suggests the answer. A typical question may say, "The statement about specific immunotherapy in paragraph two suggests that . . . ." In most cases, rereading the whole passage is unnecessary. You just reread the specified paragraph or sentence as needed.

SHARPENING YOUR CRITICAL READING SKILLS EVERY DAY

So you know what's on the PCAT Critical Reading subtest. You've made a study plan and a study schedule to help you prepare for test day. However, there are also ways to prepare off the schedule and ensure your critical reading skills are sharp not just for test day but for every day. After all, you will find out that having strong critical reading skills will come in handy in your everyday life. A great way to do this is to apply the strategies you've learned in this book to your everyday reading. For example, try reading your daily newspaper or online news site as if it were a Critical Reading passage. Root out the main idea of an editorial. Consider whether or not it is well supported with details and evidence. Keep an eye out for evidence of bias that weakens the author's position. Look out for unfamiliar words that you can define to build your vocabulary and strengthen your Words in Context skills.

You might even want to pretend you're a PCAT test maker by taking that editorial—or a novel you're reading or even a lengthy email from a friend—and sketching out some PCAT-type questions that relate to it. These are just some simple ways to make you even more comfortable with the material on the PCAT. Doing so may help reduce any anxiety you have about taking the test. After all, it is very natural to feel anxious before taking any test, but being well prepared and getting very familiar with a test's contents should make you feel a little less anxious.

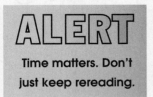

ALERT

Time matters. Don't just keep rereading.

NOTE

Applying your critical reading skills to everything you read will not only help you on test day, it will also help you to be a more effective reader every day of your life.

PRACTICE QUESTIONS

(1)   Common knowledge once suggested that ingesting less than 3,500 calories per day was the key to shedding a pound of fat. However, relatively recent developments challenge this long held notion. These developments are the work of brilliant physicist and obesity researcher Kevin Hall, Ph.D, and his colleagues at the National Institutes of Diabetes and Digestive and Kidney Diseases. As a 2011 *Lancet* paper describes, Hall and the team have at last devised a convenient mathematical model that more realistically predicts weight loss than anything else to date.

(2)   In the past, a kind of gross accounting of reduced calories tended to suggest unrealistic and overstated weight loss. This was the result of assuming that everyone's baseline characteristics are the same and that changes in metabolism have not taken place as a person has gained weight. However, these assumptions fail to take into account how metabolic changes that affect one person may be very different for another person. Hall and his colleagues have adopted a new mathematical model to account for such discrepancies.

(3)   The new mathematical model heralds a more individualized approach to weight loss because it acknowledges that some people actually do lose weight faster than others. That is, the model reveals how the same 500-calorie reduction per day may have more results for the relatively trim and muscular person than for the morbidly obese one. The model also takes into account the plateau effect that every person who has ever tried to lose weight knows, but which has not heretofore been scientifically acknowledged. Specifically, some measure of weight, such as those first ten pounds or so, may come off relatively easily, but then, with continued reductions, weight loss does not steadily continue.

(4)   By using a simulator, available online through NIH, individuals and their doctors can at last make reasonable and more realistic predictions about weight loss regimens and their probable effects over time. One must keep in mind that these simulators only serve as research tools for assisting in weight loss rather than weight-loss guides to be used by the public at large. Researchers intend to use the data they collect from the simulators in a more universal capacity that will help the public at large lose weight eventually. Therefore, it is imperative that the public take advantage of these online simulators to further the National Institutes of Diabetes and Digestive and Kidney Diseases' very worthy cause.

(5)   As Hall explained to the *Lancet*, "By using our model to track progress, clinicians can help people re-evaluate their goals and ability to achieve them at the pace they want... It's a good reality check for how long weight-loss takes, and what changes in eating and exercise are required to achieve and maintain goal weight." National Institutes of Diabetes and Digestive and Kidney Diseases director Griffin P. Rodgers, M.D., added, "This research illustrates how the interdisciplinary skills of NIH scientists, like a physicist doing obesity research, can help lead to innovative ways to test, understand and treat a major public health epidemic. Advancing research from the laboratory to the bedside enables us to make the discoveries that can better people's lives."

Directions: This section consists of selections from prose passages and questions on their content, form, and style. After reading each passage, choose the best answer to each question and then fill in the corresponding circle.

1. According to the second paragraph, prediction of weight loss in the past
   A. assumed universal baseline characteristics.
   B. accounted for changes in metabolism.
   C. often underestimated the amount of weight loss.
   D. was always inaccurate.

2. As used in the third paragraph, the word *plateau* means a(n)
   A. region of little or no change.
   B. extensive level land area.
   C. extensive level sea area.
   D. state of leveling off.

3. In the last sentence, the author mentions the website in order to
   A. support the contention that the model is effective.
   B. suggest how the reader can learn more about the specific model.
   C. show the reader how to individualize a weight-loss plan.
   D. raise questions about earlier conventional wisdom on the topic of weight loss.

4. Which statement from the passage best shows the author's attitude toward the new model?
   A. "In the past a kind of gross accounting of reduced calories tended to suggest unrealistic and overstated weight loss." (paragraph 2)
   B. "That is, the same 500-calorie reduction per day may have more results for the relatively trim and muscular person than for the morbidly obese one." (paragraph 3)
   C. "Specifically, some measure of weight, such as those first ten pounds or so, may come off relatively easily, but then, with continued reductions, weight loss does not steadily continue." (paragraph 3)
   D. "By using a simulator, available online through NIH, individuals and their doctors can at last make reasonable and more realistic predictions about weight loss regimens and their probable effects over time." (paragraph 4)

5. Which would be the best title for the passage?
   A. "Why One Size Does Not Fit All During Weight Loss"
   B. "New Research in Obesity"
   C. "A New Mathematical Model for Weight Loss"
   D. "How to Lose Weight"

6. Which of the following is the author's thesis statement?

- **A.** "Common knowledge once suggested that ingesting less than 3,500 calories per day was the key to shedding a pound of fat."
- **B.** "These developments are the work of brilliant physicist and obesity researcher Kevin Hall, Ph.D, and his colleagues at the National Institutes of Diabetes and Digestive and Kidney Diseases."
- **C.** "As a 2011 *Lancet* paper describes, Hall and the team have at last devised a convenient mathematical model that more realistically predicts weight loss than anything else to date."
- **D.** "In the past, a kind of gross accounting of reduced calories tended to suggest unrealistic and overstated weight loss."

7. The ideas in paragraphs 2 and 3 are mainly related by

- **A.** problem and solution.
- **B.** cause and effect.
- **C.** sequence.
- **D.** compare and contrast.

8. Which statement from the passage reflects the author's opinion?

- **A.** "Hall and his colleagues have adopted a new mathematical model to account for such discrepancies."
- **B.** "The new mathematical model heralds a more individualized approach to weight loss because it acknowledges that some people actually do lose weight faster than others."
- **C.** "By using a simulator, available online through NIH, individuals and their doctors can at last make reasonable and more realistic predictions about weight loss regimens and their probable effects over time."
- **D.** "Therefore, it is imperative that the public take advantage of these online simulators to further the National Institutes of Diabetes and Digestive and Kidney Diseases' very worthy cause."

9. Which statement from the passage leads most credibility to Kevin Hall's statement that the mathematical model for predicting weight loss is "a good reality check for… what changes in eating and exercise are required to achieve and maintain goal weight"?

- **A.** "Hall and his colleagues have adopted a new mathematical model to account for such discrepancies."
- **B.** "That is, the model reveals how the same 500-calorie reduction per day may have more results for the relatively trim and muscular person than for the morbidly obese one."
- **C.** "By using a simulator, available online through NIH, individuals and their doctors can at last make reasonable and more realistic predictions about weight loss regimens and their probable effects over time."
- **D.** "Researchers intend to use the data they collect from the simulators in a more universal capacity that will help the public at large lose weight eventually."

10. The author's tone could best be described as

A. supportive.

B. objective.

C. disapproving.

D. worried.

(1)　　As modern medical science makes rapid progress with the release and sale of new medical devices, it is often forced to take a step backward as these devices are often recalled and at great expense to Medicare. In fact, the replacement of just seven recalled medical devices has cost Medicare an astounding 1.5 billion dollars over the last ten years alone according to a recent Inspector General's report. However, another recent study indicates a solution that will no doubt take care of this ongoing problem once and for all.

(2)　　You see, researchers at Indiana University, the University of Minnesota, and the University of Wisconsin have concluded that the more regular rotation of medical inspections is a key to reducing recall of new medical devices. According to the study, the more often one particular Food and Drug Administration inspects a particular factory, the likelier it is that the devices at that plant will be released to the public prematurely and recalled. According to the study, if a particular FDA inspector inspects a medical plant for a second time, there is a 21% likelihood that devices produced at the facility will be recalled. This figure swells to a jaw-dropping 57% chance following a third visit by the same inspector. I'm sure you'll agree that such figures are completely unacceptable.

(3)　　According to the University of Wisconsin's Enno Siemsen, who helped work on the study, the increased likelihood of recall upon additional visits by the same inspector is due to the relaxation of standards that comes with increased familiarity. As a particular inspector gets to know the person in charge of the factory, that inspector is more likely to let problems slide and approve of the products made at the plant as a sort of favor to her or his new friend.

(4)　　Therefore, researchers propose regular rotation of inspectors to reduce such relaxation of standards. Inspectors are less likely to establish a personal rapport with plant managers if they only visit the factory in question once. Without question this is an excellent solution to a costly problem. There can certainly be no questioning the study considering that it involved testing that examined 4,767 FDA inspection reports and 2,863 recalls of devices produced at 2,244 factories over a six-year period. Therefore, the FDA would be wise to heed the findings of this report and implement regular rotation of inspectors to alleviate an immense and avoidable burden on Medicare.

11. According to the passage, how many FDA inspection reports were examined in the study?

A. 21

B. 57

C. 2,244

D. 4,767

12. The author's primary purpose in this passage is to

A. explain how researchers conducted a study of medical device factories.

B. prove that most medical devices are faulty and have to be recalled.

C. instruct the reader about how to perform a medical device factory inspection.

D. argue in favor of the rotation of medical device factory inspectors.

13. What can be concluded from the passage?

    A. Relaxation of medical standards leads to thousands of deaths every year.

    B. The FDA is a corrupt agency that requires close monitoring.

    C. Strangers are less likely to do each other favors than friends are.

    D. Inspections are not enough to figure out the efficacy of products.

14. As used in the fourth paragraph, the word *rapport* means

    A. report.

    B. friendly.

    C. antagonism.

    D. relationship.

15. Which word or phrase from the passage best reveals the author's bias?

    A. Ongoing problem (paragraph 1)

    B. Likelier (paragraph 2)

    C. Let problems slide (paragraph 3)

    D. Without question (paragraph 4)

16. Which word best describes the author's overall tone in the passage?

    A. Familiar

    B. Disapproving

    C. Excited

    D. Amused

17. According to the passage, the relationship between paragraph 2 and the paragraph 3 is that

    A. paragraph 2 explains a problem and paragraph 3 offers a solution to that problem.

    B. paragraph 2 describes a process and paragraph 3 details the results of that process.

    C. paragraph 2 describes the cause of a situation and paragraph 3 explains the effects of that situation.

    D. paragraph 2 explains a problem and paragraph 3 provides an explanation for the cause of that problem.

18. Which statement from the passage is an example of an opinion the author holds?

    A. "As modern medical science makes rapid progress with the release and sale of new medical devices, it is often forced to take a step backward as these devices are often recalled and at great expense to Medicare."

    B. "In fact, the replacement of just seven recalled medical devices has cost Medicare an astounding 1.5 billion dollars over the last ten years alone according to a recent Inspector General's report."

    C. "You see, researchers at Indiana University, the University of Minnesota, and the University of Wisconsin have concluded that the more regular rotation of medical inspections is a key to reducing recall of new medical devices."

    D. "This figure swells to a jaw-dropping 57% chance following a third visit by the same inspector."

19. Which of these adds the most credibility to the information presented in the passage?

    A. The fact that the author states that there "can be no questioning" the report

    B. The credentials of the researchers who created the report

    C. The number of FDA reports, devices, and factories used in the researchers' report

    D. The lack of professionalism displayed by FDA inspectors

20. At the end of the passage, what does the author conclude?
- **A.** Rotating FDA inspectors at medical device factories will reduce Medicare costs.
- **B.** 2,244 factories were studied in the researchers' report.
- **C.** The FDA should fire its most unethical medical device factory inspectors.
- **D.** Recall of medical devices cost Medicare 1.5 billion dollars over the past 10 years.

ANSWER KEY AND EXPLANATIONS

1. A	**5.** C	**9.** B	**13.** C	**17.** D
2. D	**6.** C	**10.** A	**14.** D	**18.** D
3. B	**7.** A	**11.** D	**15.** B	**19.** C
4. D	**8.** D	**12.** D	**16.** A	**20.** A

1. **The correct answer is A.** Choice A is correct because this basic comprehension question directly states in the second paragraph that, in the past, a kind of gross, or unsophisticated and inaccurate, accounting took place because of the assumption of similar baseline characteristics for all. Choice B is incorrect. The second paragraph also clearly states that former reckoning did not take into account changes in metabolism during weight gain. Choice C is incorrect; the paragraph says that the methods of the past tended to overestimate, not underestimate, weight loss. Choice D is incorrect because the second paragraph does not go quite so far as to say that the methods of the past were always inaccurate; instead, it says they "tended to suggest unrealistic and overstated weight loss."

2. **The correct answer is D.** This analysis question provides context in the last sentence of the third paragraph to suggest leveling off: it says that weight loss occurs steadily but then, even with continued reductions, stops or is not as steady. Choice A may be tempting, but it should be eliminated because of the word *region,* which does not apply, as well as the fact that the plateau effect suggests a leveling off after loss. Choice B is incorrect; the paragraph does not refer to landforms, even though the metaphor of plateauing is most certainly derived from this concept. Choice C is incorrect because there is no context to suggest landforms or the sea.

3. **The correct answer is B.** This analysis question focuses on an easily identifiable bit of information and requires only that the reader keep in mind the general passage topic of a new model for weight loss and the specific and readily inferable idea that the model itself will reveal the specific variables. Choice A must be ruled out because the entire passage is about a new and therefore unproven, model, and while the website may provide some data suggesting its effectiveness, nothing in the passage makes that idea readily inferable. Even though the reader will see the variables for an individualized plan, choice C is not the best choice because the text says only that the site is a place to use the model, not a place to understand factors affecting individual weight loss. Choice D is incorrect because the last sentence states that the site provides a place to "use" the model, not an analysis of it, or of practices and ideas of the past.

4. **The correct answer is D.** This evaluation question requires you to determine the author's overall attitude toward the model. To do so, you have to pick up on the clues that tell you that the author thinks the new model is good: for example, the author says that it *heralds* (that word is welcoming and positive) a new era in weight-loss calculation. Furthermore, the models of the past were "unrealistic"; they "overstated" weight loss. The truth according to the author is that some people "actually" do lose weight faster

than others; thus, according to the author, the old models were wrong, and the new one, which takes this fact into account, is better. In which of the statements does the author actually express this positive attitude? It is the statement that sums up the fact that "individuals and their doctors can at last make reasonable and more realistic predictions. The words *at least, reasonable,* and *realistic* all show the author's positive attitude toward the new model. Choice A is incorrect; it shows the author's attitude toward the old model. Choice B is incorrect; it is a simple statement of fact and not an opinion. Choice C is incorrect because it simply explains the concept of a "plateau effect," it does not state an opinion.

5. **The correct answer is C.** Choice C is the correct answer to this evaluation question based on the entire passage. It is not the only possible answer, but it is the best one because it includes the central topics of weight loss and a new model for predicting it. Choice A must be ruled out because, while the passage begins to explain this in the second paragraph, the bulk of the passage is about the model itself. Choice B should be eliminated because, even if the model is based on research in obesity, the topic of the passage is not obesity, and the passage is only about the new model and not about new research in general. Choice D is incorrect because the paragraph gives no advice or strategies on the topic of weight loss.

6. **The correct answer is C.** Choice C sums up the main point of the passage, so it is the thesis statement. Thesis statements may be the first sentence of a piece of writing, but this is not always the case, and since the first sentence of this passage does not clearly state the passage's point, choice A is incorrect. Choice B is too vague to be a clearly composed thesis statement—after all, what are the "developments" to which

the sentence refers? Choice D may serve as a sort of thesis statement for the second paragraph, but the question is asking you to find the thesis statement for the whole passage.

7. **The correct answer is A.** Paragraph 2 establishes a problem: the old model for predicting weight loss was highly flawed. Paragraph 3 establishes the solution to this problem as it explains that there is a new, more accurate mathematical model for predicting weight loss. Therefore, choice A is the best answer. While one might conclude that the problem described in paragraph 2 was the cause for the effect of researchers developing the solution described in paragraph 3, the problem/solution relationship is stronger than the cause/effect relationship between these two paragraphs, so choice B is not the best answer, which is what this question is asking you to find. Choice C has a similar issue—the new model described in paragraph 3 does follow the old method described in paragraph 4 sequentially, but there is always a sequential order when it comes to problem/solution relationships, so choice C is not the best answer. While there are two different methods described in the two paragraphs, the author does not really compare or contrast them in any explicit way, so choice D is not the best answer either.

8. **The correct answer is D.** Whether or not something is "a very worthy cause" is always a matter of opinion, so that phrase signals that choice D reflects the author's opinion rather than an indisputable fact. Furthermore, the author's demand that something is "imperative" is an example of extreme language that further signals an opinion rather than a fact. Choices A and B cannot be disputed, so they are facts rather than reflections of the author's personal opinions. Choice C may seem like an opinion because a word such as "reasonable" is often used to express

an opinion, but in this particular context, it is used factually; even if the mathematical model is not as perfect as the author seems to think it is, it is a fact that the model is more accurate than the old method.

9. **The correct answer is B.** Choice B is the only answer choice that provides specific information to support Hall's general statement about the efficacy of his mathematical model. Choices A and C are general statements that indicate that the model is effective, but neither statement provides specific information about what the model accomplishes as choice B does, so they provide weak support for Hall's statement. Choice D only explains how the data will be used; it does not provide any specific information indicating how the new model will help people decide what changes to make to their diets or exercise regimens.

10. **The correct answer is A.** While this passage is expository as a whole, the author makes his or her opinions about the new mathematical model known by using words such as "convenient," "at last," "imperative," and "very worthy cause," all of which reveal a supportive tone, so choice A is the best answer. Something cannot be supportive and objective, which indicates a total lack of personal opinion, so choice B is incorrect. Choice C, disapproving, is the opposite of supportive, so it is incorrect as well. The author seems confident about the efficacy of the new mathematical model and never implies any concerns about it, so the tone can hardly be described as worried. Therefore, choice D can be eliminated.

11. **The correct answer is D.** This particular supporting detail can be found in the final paragraph of the passage, which states that the study "involved testing that examined 4,767 FDA inspection reports." Choice D is the correct answer. Choice A, 21, is the percentage of the likelihood that medical devices would be recalled after the second time the same inspector inspected a particular factory. Choice B, 57, is the percentage of the likelihood that medical devices would be recalled after the third time the same inspector inspected a particular factory. Choice C, 2,244, is the number of factories involved in the study.

12. **The correct answer is D.** The author explains a study concluding that the rotation of inspectors at medical device factories is a solution to recall issues while also strongly championing those findings and concluding with a direct appeal to the FDA to heed them. Therefore, choice D is the most accurate description of the author's primary purpose. While the research method is explained in the passage, this is just a detail that supports that author's overall purpose, so choice A is not the best answer. Choice B is too extreme; the author never suggests that *most* medical devices need to be recalled. Extreme statements without direct passage support should always be eliminated. Choice C implies that the author is directly addressing FDA inspectors, but there is no real evidence of this in the passage, so it is not the best answer.

13. **The correct answer is C.** The author suggests that FDA inspectors striking up friendly relationships with medical device factory managers can result in the inspectors relaxing standards as a favor to the managers. Therefore, it is reasonable to reach the conclusion in choice C, which is the best answer. Choice A includes specific information that is not supported by any details in the passage, so it is not a reasonable conclusion. There may be issues related to a lack of professionalism among some FDA inspectors, but to conclude that the entire agency is "corrupt," as choice B does, is much too extreme. The author never implies that

inspections are not enough to figure out the efficacy of medical devices; the author only suggests that those inspections need to be performed differently. So choice D is not the best answer.

14. **The correct answer is D.** The sentence indicates FDA inspectors striking up a friendly, personal relationship with medical device factory managers, so choice D is the best answer. Choice A may sound like *report*, and the passage does discuss a report at length, but *report* makes no sense when used in place of *rapport* in the context of the fourth paragraph. A rapport may suggest friendship, but *rapport* is a noun and *friendly* is an adjective, so they cannot share the same meaning. Choice B must be eliminated. Choice C, *antagonism*, is the opposite of *rapport*, so it must be eliminated too.

15. **The correct answer is B.** Bias is revealed in the expression of personal opinion, and to suggest that something cannot be questioned often signals a personal opinion since most things can be questioned. Therefore, choice B best reveals the author's bias in favor of the rotation of FDA inspectors at medical device factories. That the regular recall of medical devices is an ongoing problem is not really a personal opinion since the author backs this assessment up with data about how much the recalls are costing Medicare, so choice A is not the best answer. That one thing is likelier than another is not an opinion either, so choice B does not really reveal bias on the part of the author. *Let problems slide* is merely an idiom that means *to neglect*, and the author does show that some FDA inspectors neglect to report problems at certain medical device factories. Therefore, the phrase is used factually in paragraph 3 and does not signal the author's bias, which makes choice D incorrect.

16. **The correct answer is A.** The author establishes a familiar tone by addressing the reader directly with phrase such as "you see" and "I'm sure you'll agree." So choice A is the best answer. While the author disapproves of unethical practices during inspections of medical device factories, the author also expresses approval of a study of such practices, so to say that the overall tone of the passage is *disapproving*, as choice B does, is inaccurate. An excited tone would be indicated by a lot of strong adjectives and exclamation marks, and this passage has neither, so choice C is not an accurate description of the passage's overall tone. The author takes the circumstances described in the passage very seriously, so to indicate that he or she establishes an *amused* tone, as choice D does, is also inaccurate.

17. **The correct answer is D.** Paragraph 2 mainly explains the problem of the likelihood of medical devices being recalled depending on the same FDA inspector inspecting the same factory multiple times. Paragraph 3 suggests that increased friendliness between inspectors and factory managers is the cause of that problem. Therefore, choice D is the best answer. Since a solution to that problem is not offered until paragraph 4, choice A is incorrect. Choice B is completely inaccurate. Choice C correctly recognizes a cause/effect relationship between the two paragraphs, but it mixes up which paragraph describes the cause and which one describes the effect.

18. **The correct answer is D.** The key word in choice D is *jaw-dropping*, which is an idiom indicating that something is surprising. Whether or not something will be surprising is a matter of personal opinion. Choice A is factual information without any indications of personal opinion. Choice B is factual as well, and it even begins with the phrase *In fact*, which introduces factual information when used correctly. Choice

C is a bit familiar, since it begins with the personal phrase *You see*, but such phrases do not necessarily signal a personal opinion, and there is no such opinion in this sentence.

19. **The correct answer is C.** Researchers examined thousands of FDA reports, medical devices, and factories in their report. That is a tremendous amount of data by any standards, and those numbers do lend credibility to the information presented in the passage. Choice C is the best answer. Choice A reveals a bit of lazy bias on the part of the author and manipulative phrases such as these do not lend reliable credibility to anything. The fact that the researchers come from a particular university may be somewhat impressive, but in terms of lending credibility to the report, the numerical data is much more significant, so choice B is not the very best answer. While FDA inspectors guilty of relaxing their standards do display a lack of professionalism, this alone does not exactly lend credibility to the findings

in the passage. This question is asking you to find concrete and convincing supporting data, and that is what choice C provides and choice D does not.

20. **The correct answer is A.** The conclusion in choice A is stated pretty explicitly in the final sentence of the passage. Choice B is just a detail in the fourth paragraph; it is not the passage's ultimate conclusion. The author never suggests that anyone should be fired, so choice C does not reflect the conclusion of this particular passage accurately. Choice D is closely related to the thesis, since it helps establish the problem explained in the passage. Its failure to indicate a solution to that problem means it does not serve as a conclusion. Also, concluding statements are never included in the first paragraph of a piece of writing, and the information in choice D is mentioned in the first paragraph of this passage.

SUMMING IT UP

- A PCAT passage will typically be four to six paragraphs long and be followed by seven to ten questions.

- Most PCAT Reading Comprehension questions require fairly sophisticated critical thinking. Questions may ask about tone and bias and may require varying levels of inference on the part of the reader.

- Passages cover historical, contemporary, cultural, ethical, political, and technical topics that relate to issues pertaining to natural sciences, social sciences, and humanities.

- Passages may be informative, persuasive, or speculative.

- Strategies for reading the passages include:

  o   Outline the passage as you read, using the erasable board and markers provided.

  o   Read between the lines to understand what is implied in the passage.

  o   Identify the terms that are important.

  o   Know when to stop reading the passage and begin answering the questions.

- Read question stems carefully. Some questions indicate the paragraph, sentence, or word in the passage that is the subject of the question.

- There are three types of questions on the Reading Comprehension subtest of the PCAT: 1. basic comprehension, 2. analysis, and 3. evaluation.

  1.   Comprehension questions include Words in Context, Main Idea, Supporting Details, and Drawing Conclusions questions.

  2.   Analysis questions include Relationship Between Ideas, Author's Purpose, Author's Tone, Facts/Opinions, and Rhetorical Strategies questions.

  3.   Evaluation questions include Bias, Support in an Argument, and Author's Conclusion/ Thesis questions.'

- Basic comprehension questions ask you to recall information or to make fairly easy, fairly obvious inferences. Usually, these questions focus on small, specific pieces of the passage. You do not have to understand the entire passage to get them right.

- Analysis questions ask you to break information down in order to figure out the correct answer. They require a deeper level of inference than needed to answer the basic comprehension questions. Analysis questions may also ask about relationships and the meaning of a given word in a specific context.

- Answering evaluation questions require judgments and applications. You will still be using information in the passage, but you will have to think beyond the specific words, word order, and the thesis and supporting phrases. Instead of focusing on small bits of information, these questions are likely to test your understanding of the passage as a whole.

- Create a study plan that involves getting familiar with the specific material on the PCAT Critical Reading subtest, taking practice tests, and keeping track of and evaluating your most common errors.

- Choose a skills based or time based study plan for yourself and stick to your schedule.

- Sharpen your Critical Reading skills for the PCAT by outlining passages, reading between the lines, deciding which terms matter the most, and knowing when to stop reading.

- Sharpen your skills every day by applying the Critical Reading skills you've learned to everything you read.

PART IV
BIOLOGICAL PROCESSES

General Biology

Chapter 5

OVERVIEW

- **Classification**
- **Cell Structure**
- **Enzymes**
- **Energy**
- **Cellular Metabolism**
- **DNA Structure and Replication**
- **Protein Synthesis**
- **The Cell Cycle and Cell Division**
- **Genetics**
- **Evolution**
- **Practice Questions**
- **Answer Key and Explanations**
- **Summing It Up**

General biology covers the basics of living organisms and the systems and processes that underlie living things. This chapter provides an overview of the most important points. Sixty percent of the PCAT Biology subtest will test your knowledge of general biology. That means approximately 29 questions. All three sections of the Biology subtest will be combined on your score report.

CLASSIFICATION

All biological organisms are classified, or organized, according to the rules of taxonomy. *Taxonomy* is the specific branch of biology that formally orders all species into a hierarchal arrangement of groupings. The highest level of organization of a species is its domain. There are three domains of life: Bacteria, Archaea, and Eukarya.

Domains

The domains Bacteria and Archaea both consist of prokaryotes, most of which are unicellular, microscopic organisms. The Bacteria domain includes almost all of the common prokaryotes such as the pathogenic species that cause strep and staph infections and other diseases, such as pneumococcal infections. There are also many types of bacteria that are beneficial for proper nutrition and metabolism. Archaea have many traits in common with bacteria, but they also have some traits in common with eukaryotes. The difference is that organisms in the Archaea domain are found in extreme environmental conditions, such as very high or very low temperatures (*thermophiles*) or areas of very high salt concentrations (*halophiles*). Other archaea, known as *methanogens*, obtain energy by using CO_2 to oxidize H_2, releasing methane gas in the process. All *eukaryotic organisms* (organisms with cells that contain a nucleus) belong to the Eukarya domain.

Kingdoms

Domains are further classified into kingdoms. There is some debate as to how many kingdoms species can be divided into. Currently, in the United States, it is acceptable to classify species into one of six kingdoms: Animalia, Plantae, Fungi, Protista, Archaea, and Bacteria. In the past, Archaea and Bacteria were classified as one kingdom known as Monera. Under the six-kingdom system of taxonomy, the kingdom Bacteria falls under the domain Bacteria; the kingdom Archaea falls under the domain Archaea; the domain Eukarya includes the kingdoms Protista, Plantae, Fungi, and Animalia.

Phyla

Kingdoms are further classified into phyla. A *phylum* is a grouping of all classes of organisms that have the same basic body plan and developmental organization. Organisms in the same phylum also have a certain degree of genetic relatedness or similarity. The kingdom Animalia is classified into about 40 different phyla. Humans belong to the phyla Chordata, which includes all vertebrates and some closely related invertebrates. Other common Animalia phyla are Anthropoda, Annelida, Cnidaria, Echinodermata, Nematoda, Mollusca, Platyhelminthes, and Porifera. Currently there are twelve phyla in the kingdom Plantae, six phyla in the kingdom Fungi, and about ten phyla in the kingdom Protista. The kingdom Bacteria has twenty-nine recognized phyla and the kingdom Archaea has five phyla.

Classes and Orders

Phyla are grouped into classes. The species included in each class have characteristics that they share with other members of the same class, but that are not found in other classes. Humans, for example, belong to the Mammalia class, which includes all mammals. Classes are further divided into orders. Humans, for example, are classified into the order Primates.

Families, Genera, Species, and Subspecies

Orders can be further classified into families (humans are in the family Hominidae), and families are classified into genera (the singular form is genus). Humans are classified into the genus *Homo*. Finally, members of each genus are divided into different species. Humans belong to the species *Homo sapiens*. There are also more specific classifications for each species. For example, modern-day humans are classified in the species *Homo sapiens* and the subspecies *sapiens*, which is why we are referred to as *Homo sapiens sapiens*.

Figure 1. Classification of a Human

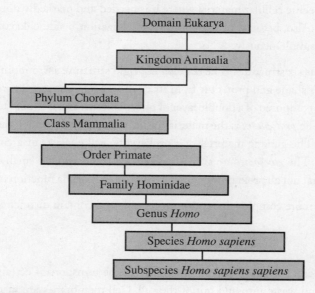

CELL STRUCTURE

Cell theory states the following:

- All living organisms are composed of at least one cell.
- The cell is the smallest biological unit that has all the characteristics of a living organism.
- All cells arise from preexisting cells.
- Cells contain hereditary information that is passed to new cells during cell division.
- Organisms of a similar species have cells with a similar chemical composition.

Complex multicellular organisms contain many types of specialized cells that work cooperatively to maintain the structure and function of the whole organism. A *cell* is a small membrane-bound structure that contains all the various chemicals and molecules that are essential for life. Therefore, an understanding of cell structure is necessary to understand the complex intercellular and intracellular interactions that take place within an organism.

Although there are many different types of cells, and they greatly differ from one another, all cells share certain characteristics and structures. Cells must remain small in order to function most efficiently in getting a sufficient amount of nutrients from outside the cell and eliminating waste from inside the cell. If a cell becomes too large, the surface area of the cell is insufficient to meet the demands inside the cell, and it will stop growing.

The basic structural unit of every organism is one of two types of cells: prokaryotic or eukaryotic. *Prokaryotic* cells are small and simple. They contain no internal membrane-bound organelles, and the only membrane is the outer cell membrane. Without internal membranes, the prokaryotic cell cannot compartmentalize its material into organelles. All cell and genetic material in prokaryotic cells exists together inside the cell. Bacteria and Archaea consist of prokaryotic cells, and all other organisms consist of eukaryotic cells. *Eukaryotic* cells are generally larger than prokaryotic cells. They are more complex and contain membrane-bound organelles and a nucleus to keep genetic material

TIP

Try this simple mnemonic device to help you learn lists. Learn one item in a list for each of your fingers—and toes, if necessary. Associate "All living organisms = at least one cell" with your thumb. Associate statement 2 with your index finger, etc.

separated from other cellular material. The compartmentalization of cellular material into organelles concentrates specific cellular material where it is needed and markedly improves the efficiency of cellular function. Also, because of the compartmentalization inside eukaryotic cells, many cell processes can occur simultaneously.

A prokaryotic cell has six structures. The *cell wall* is a rigid structure surrounding the cell that helps to maintain the cell's shape and protect it from its environment. The *plasma membrane*, which also surrounds the cell, is composed of a double layer of phospholipids and is similar to the cell membrane of eukaryotic cells. The *protoplasm* is the material inside the cell. The aqueous part of the protoplasm is called the *cytosol*. The genetic material of a prokaryotic cell consists of a circular ring of DNA known as a *nucleoid*. The *ribosomes* are sites of protein synthesis and are small complexes of RNA. Another structure that not all prokaryotic cells have is *flagella*. Flagella function to aid cell movement the.

Eukaryotic cells are more complex than prokaryotic cells and contain distinct organelles.

Cell Membrane

The cell membrane is a selective barrier that allows for the transport of certain molecules such as oxygen, nutrients, and waste into and out of the cell. Cell membranes are made of a double layer of phospholipids (fats) called the *lipid bilayer*. Only water and gases can easily pass through the lipid bilayer. So that larger molecules can pass through the bilayer, various proteins are attached or embedded within the bilayer, and these proteins allow for the transport of certain specific molecules into and out of the cell.

The structure of the lipid bilayer is also important for its function as a barrier to other molecules. Phospholipids are composed of a head that is *hydrophilic* (attracted to water), or polar, and a tail that is *hydrophobic* (repelled from water), or nonpolar. The hydrophobic tails make up the interior of the cell membrane and the proteins embedded in the membrane are also hydrophobic. The hydrophilic heads of each phospholipid make up the outer portions of the membrane that reside in an aqueous environment outside and inside the cell.

Figure 2. Lipid Bilayer

> The cell membrane is composed of a double layer of phospholipids. The hydrophilic heads of the phospholipids face outward into the aqueous regions both inside and outside the cell. The hydrophobic tail ends of the phospholipids face each other in the interior region of the cell membrane.

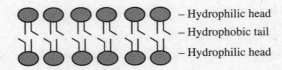

– Hydrophilic head
– Hydrophobic tail
– Hydrophilic head

Another important property of the lipid bilayer is its fluidity. The construction of the plasma membrane is often described as the *fluid-mosaic model*. The membrane is mosaic-like because the phospholipid bilayer forms a framework mixed with membrane-bound proteins. The membrane contains phospholipids, proteins, glycoproteins, and glycolipids. The fluid properties of the bilayer allow for mobility of these molecules within the lipid bilayer. There are a variety of different membrane proteins that perform various functions, but they can be divided into three different classes: integral proteins, peripheral proteins, and lipid-bound proteins. *Integral proteins* are embedded within the lipid bilayer of the cell membrane. They cannot easily be removed, but they are able to float freely within the lipid bilayer. In general, integral proteins are *transmembrane proteins*, meaning they span the entire lipid bilayer with one end in the interior of the cell and one end touching the exterior of the cell. These are the only type of membrane proteins that can perform functions both inside and outside the cell. *Peripheral proteins* are attached to the exterior of the cell membrane and can easily be separated from the lipid bilayer. Peripheral proteins tend to be less mobile than integral proteins. *Lipid-bound* proteins are positioned entirely within the lipid bilayer with no portion reaching the interior of exterior regions of the cell.

There are several ways for molecules to move across the cell membrane.

Diffusion

Diffusion is a type of passive transport. Therefore, this type of movement does not require added energy. *Diffusion* describes a gradual change in concentration of a molecule either with or along a concentration gradient. The concentration gradient describes the relative concentration of a solute within a defined area. In general, solutes move faster from areas of higher concentration to areas of lower concentration, until both areas reach an equilibrium state. Some factors that affect the rate of diffusion are the mass of the particle, temperature, the concentration gradient, and the physical state of the solute (solid, liquid, or gas). A gas will diffuse faster than a liquid, which will diffuse faster than a solid.

Osmosis

Osmosis is another form of passive transport across the cell membrane. It is defined as the diffusion of water across the membrane. There is an aqueous solution on either side of the membrane and the net movement of the water is determined by what biologists call *tonicity*. Tonicity is the osmotic pressure of the solution on either side of the semipermeable cell membrane. When a solute in the solution on either side of the cell membrane cannot cross the membrane, there is a buildup of osmotic pressure (*high tonicity*). When a solute can freely cross the membrane, there is no osmotic pressure (*low tonicity*). Water will always move from the side of the membrane with more water and less solute (*hypotonic*) toward the solution with the highest concentration of solute (*hypertonic*) in order to establish an equilibrium of solution. *Isotonic* refers to the state of equilibrium that exists when there is an equal amount of solute on both sides of the membrane.

Another way of thinking about this is the following: Water moves from a region of higher water concentration to one of lower concentration—this is just like diffusion, but with solvent moving passively, based on its concentration instead of solute.

Facilitated Transport

Facilitated transport is a third form of passive transport that relies upon the concentration gradient. Certain proteins within the cell membrane can assist in transporting molecules across the membrane. Some proteins act as channels and are, therefore, called *channel proteins*, whereas others act as transporters and are called *carrier proteins*. Facilitated transport allows specific ions or proteins to enter or exit the cell. This method relies upon natural diffusion and follows the principle that solutes will move from areas of higher concentration to areas of lower concentration. Channel and carrier proteins that are responsible for allowing solutes such as ions and small polar molecules to cross the cell membrane without the addition of energy are called *passive transport proteins*.

Active Transport

During active transport, energy in the form of ATP (adenosine triphosphate) is required to move molecules across the cell membrane and across the concentration gradient. These molecules are moved from an area of lower concentration of solute to an area of higher concentration of solute. In this type of transport, carrier or transport proteins are necessary. When these proteins interact with ATP, there is a change in the transport protein's conformation so that they bind specific ions such as Na$^+$, K$^+$, Ca^{2+}, and H$^+$ and carry them across the membrane either into or out of the cell.

Bulk Transport

The movement of large macromolecules or large quantities of molecules across the cell membrane is carried out through *bulk transport*. The process of *endocytosis* involves the ingestion of a large amount of material into the cell. In this case, the cell engulfs the aqueous solution outside the cell membrane and folds the material into the cell. The cell membrane surrounding the desired molecules fuses together and forms a vesicle known as an *endosome*. *Phagocytosis* refers to the ingestion into a cell of large molecules such as bacterial cells. Endosomes that form through phagocytosis are called *phagosomes*. Phagocytosis is common in immune cells such as neutrophils and macrophages and in amoebas, but not in all cells.

Pinocytosis refers to a process of "cell drinking." This process occurs when small droplets of liquid or dissolved matter are ingested into the cell. Pinocytosis occurs in all cell types and is a continuous process in cells, rather than a specialized function. *Exocytosis* works in the opposite direction to rid cells of material. Vesicles required for exocytosis can be *endosomes* that return to the cell membrane after depositing material or *lysosomes* that fuse with endosomes. The Golgi apparatus and the endoplasmic reticulum also create vesicles for exocytosis. These vesicles transport cell waste, such as toxins, proteins and enzymes, hormones, neurotransmitters, and antibodies, out of the cell into the extracellular fluid (ECF).

Cytoskeleton and Cytosol

Within all eukaryotic cells, the cytoskeleton and cytosol are structural elements that provide structure to the cell. The *cytoskeleton* is a network of protein filaments that organize structures and activities within the cell and allow for movement of organelles within the cell. The cytoskeleton is composed of three types of protein filaments: actin, microtubules, and intermediate filaments.

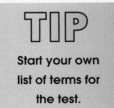

TIP

Start your own list of terms for the test.

Mixture Terminology

You should be familiar with the following terminology:

- **Solution:** a homogeneous mixture of two substances where each substance is indistinguishable from the other. The substances in a solution cannot be separated by filtration. The substance of greater amount is called the *solvent,* and the substance mixed with the solvent is called the *solute.* The solute dissolves into the solution, forming the homogeneous solution. This can pass through a solution.

- **Suspension:** a heterogeneous mixture of substances in which the substances are distinguishable from one another and can be separated by methods of filtration. Light is scattered by a suspension, and suspensions are generally opaque. In most suspensions, larger molecules of a solute in one state (solid, liquid, or gas) are mixed with smaller molecules of solvent in a liquid or gas. Therefore, the two substances are easily identified and separated.

- **Colloid:** a mixture that falls between a solution and a suspension. In general, medium-sized solute molecules are partially dissolved in a solvent. Particles in colloids are large enough to scatter light, but you cannot see through it. Therefore, it is translucent. However, particles in a colloid are small enough that they cannot be separated by filtration methods. Cream and fog are examples of a colloid.

Actin

Actin, also called microfilaments, is the thinnest fibers of the cytoskeleton. These filaments are also very flexible. In general, actin is the most abundant protein in eukaryotic cells. Actin works to provide support and structure to the cell membrane and is, therefore, found near the membrane of cells. Its main function is the maintenance of cell shape, but it is also involved in changing cell shape, muscle contraction, cell motility, and cell division.

Microtubules

Microtubules are the thickest of the three cytoskeletal protein filaments and are more rigid than actin filaments. Microtubules are long cylindrical, hollow structures composed of columns of the protein tubulin. Microtubules are located near the nucleus of the cell; in particular, they accumulate around the centrosome. Microtubules provide tracks along which organelles can travel from the center of the cell outward. They are involved in chromosome movement during cell division.

Intermediate Filaments

Intermediate filaments, as the name suggests, have a diameter in between that of actin and microtubules. They are fibrous proteins that are supercoiled into thick cable-like structures. Although they are not found in all eukaryotic cells, in those in which they are present, they form a network called the *nuclear lamina* that surrounds the nucleus of the cell. Intermediate filaments can also extend through the cell, helping it to increase the stability of the cell structure.

Cytosol

The inside of the cell is composed of a semifluid substance called *cytosol* that comprises over 50 percent of the cell's total volume. All of the organelles within a cell are arranged in the cytosol. The cytosol is also the site of protein synthesis and the location of centrosomes and centrioles, integral parts of cell division.

The Nucleus

In eukaryotic cells, the cell *nucleus* is found near the center of the cell and is one of the largest organelles in the cell. The nucleus is the site of DNA and RNA synthesis in the cell. It plays a very significant biological role in all eukaryotic organisms, as it contains almost all of the genetic material, or DNA, of the organism (some is found in the mitochondria). The nucleus is made up of two membranes that form what is known as the *porous nuclear envelope*. The nuclear envelope encloses the nucleus, separating its contents from the rest of the cell. The intermediate filaments comprising the *nuclear laminae* line the nuclear envelope, helping to maintain the shape of the nucleus. The nuclear lamina also connects the nucleus to the endoplasmic reticulum. Within the nucleus, the DNA is packaged into discrete structures called *chromosomes*. Each chromosome is made up of chromatin, a complex of protein and DNA. A prominent structure within the nucleus is the *nucleolus*, which is a nonmembraneous organelle involved in the production of ribosomes.

Ribosome

Ribosomes are organelles within the cell that carry out protein synthesis. A ribosome is made up of ribosomal RNA and proteins. Cells that have a large number of ribosomes have a high rate of protein synthesis. *Free ribosomes* are suspended in the cytosol, whereas bound ribosomes are attached to the outside of either the nuclear envelope or the endoplasmic reticulum. Most of the proteins made on free ribosomes are proteins that function within the cytosol. For example, enzymes involved in sugar metabolism are made on free ribosomes. *Bound ribosomes* are generally responsible for synthesizing proteins destined for insertion into the cell membrane, packaging within a specific organelle, or secretion out of the cell.

Endoplasmic Reticulum

The *endoplasmic reticulum (ER)* is an important structure for protein and lipid synthesis. It is the site where all transmembrane proteins are synthesized. Also, because nearly every protein secreted from the cell passes through the ER, it plays an important role in cell trafficking. The ER consists of a network of membranous tubules and sacs called *cisternae*. The membranes of the ER separate the internal compartment of the ER, called the *ER lumen*, from the cytosol. The ER membrane is joined with the nuclear envelope of the nucleus, and there are two distinct, but connected regions of the ER: *rough ER* and *smooth ER*. The rough ER is coated with ribosomes (site of protein synthesis), and the smooth ER has no ribosomes.

The smooth ER is more abundant in cells that carry out synthesis and metabolism of lipids (including oils), phospholipids, and steroids. There are also enzymes in the smooth ER that help to detoxify drugs and poisons. These are especially abundant in liver cells. Barbiturates, alcohol, and other drugs may induce the proliferation of the smooth ER and detoxifying enzymes, causing an increase in the rate of detoxification. This can increase the body's tolerance to certain drugs, and thus higher

TIP

Drawing and labeling your own diagrams of structures and organs can help you remember them. This should be especially helpful to kinesthetic learners.

doses are required to achieve the same effect. In fact, drug abuse may decrease the effectiveness of antibiotics and other useful drugs. The smooth ER also captures calcium ions from the cytosol and stores them. In muscle cells, a specialized smooth ER membrane pumps calcium ions from the cytosol into the ER lumen.

The rough ER is directly associated with the synthesis of many proteins because of the ribosomes attached to its surface. Many proteins produced by ribosomes attached to the ER are secretory proteins that contain long carbohydrate chains. The carbohydrates are attached to proteins, called *glycoproteins*, in the ER.

Golgi Apparatus

The *Golgi apparatus* is located near the nucleus of the cell and acts as the center for modifying, storing, and transporting proteins leaving the ER. The Golgi consists of a series of flattened membranous sacs, called *cisternae*. A cell can have hundreds of these Golgi stacks. A protein enters the Golgi from its *cis face* and exits the Golgi from the other side known as the *trans face*. Proteins produced in the ER always enter and exit the Golgi apparatus from the same location. In the Golgi apparatus, proteins are modified by the addition and removal of carbohydrate chains. The Golgi stacks also act to sort proteins so they are secreted to the correct location. After the Golgi sorts proteins, the membrane of the Golgi buds off, forming a small vesicle that transports the protein to a specific destination.

Lysosomes

Lysosomes are membrane sacs containing hydrolytic enzymes that digest macromolecules in the cell. These enzymes work best in an acidic environment; thus, lysosomes are acidic. Lysosomes are thought of as "cellular garbage cans" because they are responsible for ridding a cell of all debris. Proteins that have a mutation or are incorrectly folded are secreted to lysosomes to be degraded. Molecules from outside the cell are taken in through a process known as *endocytosis* and are then transported to the lysosome for degradation.

Molecules in the cell that are destined for lysosomes are secreted into membrane-bound structures called *endosomes*. Endosomes deliver the molecule to a lysosome, where they are digested. Through the help of lysosomes, a cell is able to renew itself continually. For example, a human liver cell recycles half of its macromolecules within a week. In people with rare lysosomal storage diseases such as Tay-Sachs disease, there is an accumulation of macromolecules in the cells' lysosomes. The lysosomes become engorged, which ultimately impairs other cellular functions.

Mitochondria

Mitochondria are responsible for generating ATP (adenosine triphosphate) that provides all organisms with energy. Mitochondria are often defined as the "powerhouse" of the cell. The mitochondrion is enclosed by a specialized double-membrane structure. Each membrane is a phospholipid bilayer with embedded proteins. The outer membrane layer is smooth, but the inner membrane layer is made up of a series of infoldings called *cristae*. Mitochondria are divided into two internal compartments. The first compartment exists between the smooth outer membrane and the folded inner membrane. This narrow space in known as the *intermembrane space* and contains the few proteins that are found in the mitochondria. The second compartment is the *mitochondrial matrix*, which is enclosed by the inner-folded membrane. The matrix contains many different enzymes, as well as mitochondrial DNA and ribosomes.

Peroxisome

Peroxisomes are specialized metabolic compartments within a cell that are bound by a single membrane and are found in all eukaryotic cells. The main function of peroxisomes is to break down fatty acids. Peroxisomes use oxygen molecules to oxidize organic molecules. Hydrogen peroxide is given off as a product of these oxidation reactions.

Figure 3. Diagram of a Typical Eukaryotic Cell

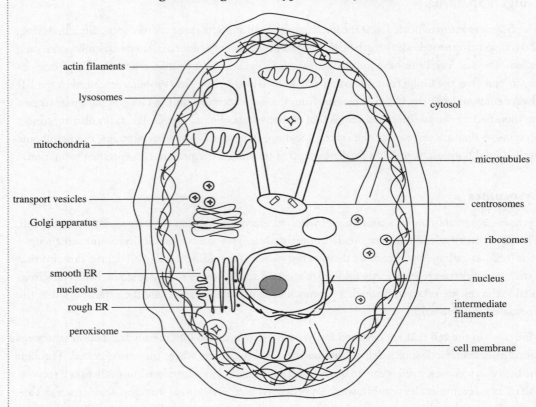

ENZYMES

In order for a chemical reaction to start, energy is required to contort the bonds of the reactant molecules so that the bonds change or break, and products form. This initial energy required to drive a reaction forward is called the *activation energy* of the reaction, and the point in the reaction at which the activation energy is achieved is known as the *transition state. Enzymes* are proteins that speed up metabolic reactions by lowering the activation energy barrier without affecting the overall free energy of the reaction. Enzymes are classified as catalysts in that they speed up a chemical reaction without being consumed by the reaction.

Enzyme activity is influenced by its cellular environment. Temperature, pH, and concentration all have an effect on enzyme activity. In general, an increase in temperature up to a maximum causes an increase in enzyme activity. Different enzymes have a different optimal temperature at which they catalyze a reaction most efficiently. Concentration of an enzyme or its substrate can also affect the performance of an enzyme. In general, an increase in the concentration of either the enzyme or its substrate will increase the reaction rate. However, as with temperature, there is an optimal concentration, and increasing the concentration above this value will not increase the reaction rate. Optimal pH levels for an enzyme reaction are dependent on the specific enzyme.

Induced Fit

The region of the enzyme that interacts with a substrate is called the *active site*. The active site is typically a groove or a pocket on the surface of the protein that is formed by a few of the enzyme's amino acids. The specificity of an enzyme for a particular substrate is attributed to the shape of the enzyme's active site and the shape of the substrate molecule. The active site does not remain a rigid shape, however. Once the substrate recognizes and binds to the active site, the enzyme changes its shape and is able to wrap around, or embrace, the substrate. This is known as an *induced fit* and allows the enzyme to be in the best position to catalyze a given reaction.

In an enzymatic reaction, the substrate is generally bound to the enzyme's active site by weak interactions such as hydrogen bonding. Once bound together, the active site of the enzyme catalyzes the conversion of reactant into product, and the product is then released from the enzyme, leaving it free to bind another substrate molecule. This cycle occurs so quickly that a single enzyme molecule can bind at least a thousand substrate molecules per second. Therefore, a small amount of enzyme can have a huge metabolic impact. It is also important to note that enzymes can catalyze both forward and reverse metabolic reactions, but they will always catalyze a reaction in the direction of equilibrium.

Figure 4. Mechanism of Enzyme Catalysis

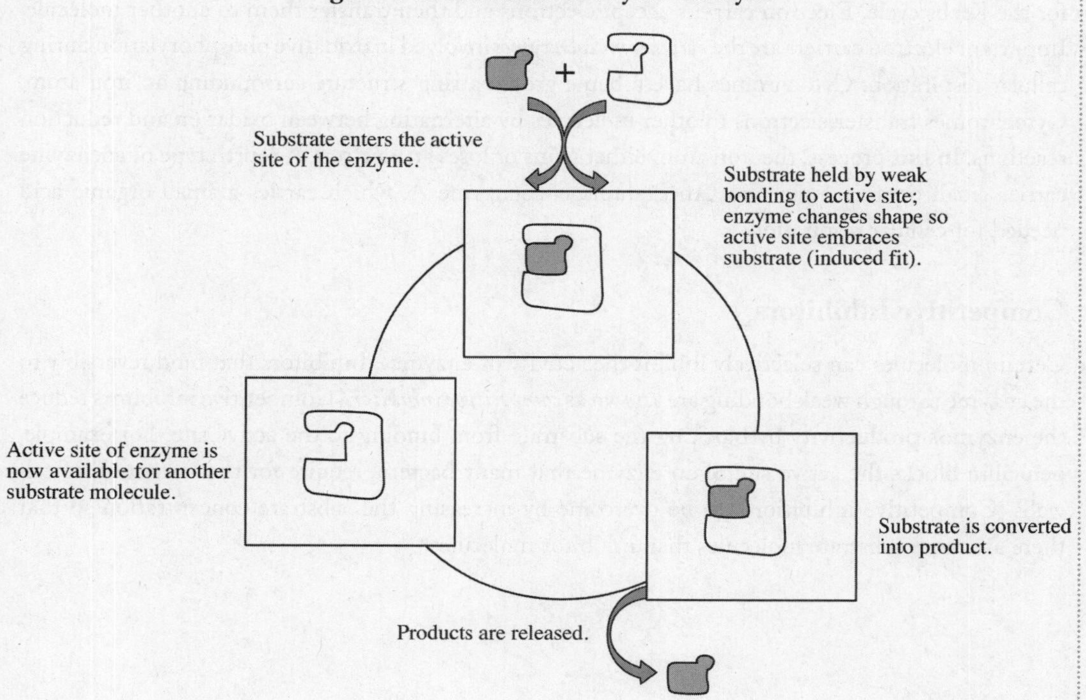

Substrate enters the active site of the enzyme.

Substrate held by weak bonding to active site; enzyme changes shape so active site embraces substrate (induced fit).

Active site of enzyme is now available for another substrate molecule.

Substrate is converted into product.

Products are released.

Enzymes lower the activation energy by interacting with one or more substrates in a reaction using a variety of mechanism. In reactions involving two or more reactants, the active site of the enzyme becomes a template on which the substrates can come together in the correct orientation for a reaction to occur. As the active site holds a substrate, the enzyme may change the substrate into its transition state confirmation. The active site of the enzyme may provide an environment more conducive to initiating a particular reaction. For example, if a reaction is more favorable in a low pH environment and the active site of an enzyme contains a cluster of acidic amino acid side chains, this localized acidic environment may catalyze the reaction. An enzyme may actively participate in a chemical reaction, but during subsequent steps of the reaction, the enzyme is restored to its original state.

Cofactors

Some enzymes require a molecule called a *cofactor* to lower the activation energy of a reaction. Cofactors can be either inorganic molecules or organic molecules. Cofactors may be tightly bound to an enzyme, or they may bind loosely and reversibly to an enzyme. Examples of inorganic cofactors are metal atoms such as zinc, iron, and copper in ionic form.

Organic cofactors are called *coenzymes*. Most vitamins are either coenzymes or the starting material from which coenzymes are made. Coenzymes function to transfer the product from one reaction to another. In this way, they can link together two unrelated molecules. There are four types of coenzymes. *Hydrogen carriers* link together two different redox (oxidation-reduction) reactions. They deliver protons (H^+) to many different enzymes. One of the most important hydrogen carriers is nicotinamide adenine dinucleotide (NAD^+), which is a key component in glycolysis and the Krebs cycle. NAD^+ is the oxidized form of the coenzyme, and NADH is its reduced form. *Flavin vitamins* are another type of coenzyme. Flavin adenine dinucleotide (FAD) is a coenzyme also important for the Krebs cycle. Electron carriers accept electrons and then transfer them to another molecule. Important electron carriers are the *cytochrome coenzymes* involved in oxidative phosphorylation during cellular respiration. Cytochromes have a heme group, a ring structure surrounding an iron atom. Cytochromes transfer electrons to other molecules by alternating between oxidation and reduction reactions. In this process, the iron atom either gains or loses an electron. A fourth type of coenzyme carries small organic molecules. An example is coenzyme A, which carries a small organic acid needed for cellular respiration.

Competitive Inhibitors

Certain molecules can selectively inhibit the activity of enzymes. Inhibitors that bind reversibly to the enzyme through weak bonding are known as *competitive inhibitors*. Competitive inhibitors reduce the enzyme's productivity by blocking the substrate from binding to the active site. For example, penicillin blocks the active site of an enzyme that many bacteria require for the formation of cell walls. Competitive inhibition can be overcome by increasing the substrate concentration so that there are more substrate molecules than inhibitor molecules.

Noncompetitive Inhibitors

Noncompetitive inhibitors do not compete with the substrate for binding to the active site. Instead, they bind to a different site on the enzyme known as an *allosteric site* and act to change the enzyme's shape so that the substrate can no longer fit into the active site.

Allosteric Regulation

Allosteric regulation is the term used to describe any case in which the function of a protein at one site is affected by the binding of a regulatory molecule at a different site. This regulatory molecule may serve to either activate or inhibit an enzyme's activity.

In the simplest examples of allosteric regulation, an activating or inhibiting molecule binds to an allosteric site on the enzyme. The binding of an activator molecule stabilizes the enzyme in a conformation that is favorable to binding substrate to the active site. Conversely, the binding of an inhibitory molecule to an allosteric site will stabilize an inactive conformation of the enzyme so that the active site of the enzyme is not accessible to its substrate.

Feedback Inhibition

In a metabolic pathway, several enzymes work together to produce the final product. In each case, the product released from an enzyme-substrate complex binds to the next enzyme in the pathway until the final product is obtained. In *feedback inhibition*, a metabolic pathway is switched off by the binding of a product of that pathway to an enzyme that is required in the initial step of the pathway. The product binds to the enzyme in an inhibitory manner, thus blocking interaction of the enzyme with its substrate. In this way, the amount of end product is regulated by itself.

ENERGY

Energy is the ability to do work or cause change. Energy exists in various forms, and cells have the ability to transform energy from one form to another.

Forms of Energy

Energy associated with the relative motion of objects is called *kinetic energy*. *Potential energy*, or stored energy, is energy that matter possesses because of its position or structure.

Within a cell, there are four basic forms of energy that are required for proper cell function. *Mechanical energy*—the sum of an object's kinetic and potential energy—is required for motion. Mechanical energy is required for muscle movement and within the cell for movement of molecules around the cytoplasm. *Chemical energy* is a term used by biologists to refer to the potential energy available in a chemical reaction. This is the amount of energy released as a reaction moves forward. *Electrical energy*, a type of potential energy, is utilized when electrons move from one orbital to another, or from one molecule to another. *Light energy*, which comes from the radiant energy of the sun and is a form of kinetic energy, is essential for photosynthesis in plant cells.

Thermodynamics

The study of energy transformations in matter is called *thermodynamics*.

- The *first law of thermodynamics* states that energy cannot be created or destroyed. Thus, energy can either be transformed into another form or be transferred from one type of matter or molecule to another.

- The *second law of thermodynamics* states that during every energy conversion or transfer, some energy becomes unavailable to do work. This energy is lost to the surrounding environment as heat. Heat is thermal energy, but it is unusable in that it cannot perform work on a system. According to this law of thermodynamics, an organism is not able to continually recycle energy within itself because, over time, the amount of usable energy in a closed system decreases. Therefore, a continuous input of energy is required for an organism to maintain organization and function. *Entropy* is a measure of disorder and randomness in the environment, and according to the second law of thermodynamics, all living systems increase the entropy of their surroundings.

Free Energy Change, ΔG

Gibbs free energy, ΔG, is most often referred to as free energy. Free energy measures the portion of energy in a system that is available to perform work at a given temperature and pressure. The free energy of a system such as a living cell can be determined from the total energy of a system, known as enthalpy, *H*, and entropy, *S*, of the system. The overall change in free energy of a system at a given temperature is determined by subtracting the change in entropy, ΔS, from the change in enthalpy, ΔH, and is represented by the following equation, where *T* is the absolute temperature of the system in degrees Kelvin:

$$\Delta G = \Delta H - T\Delta S$$

Once the value of ΔG for a reaction is known, it is possible to determine whether the reaction occurs *spontaneously* (without the input of energy from outside the closed system). Processes that have a negative ΔG value will occur spontaneously. Because of the way ΔG is dependent on entropy in the above equation, it can be determined that every spontaneous reaction decreases a system's free energy. In biological systems, spontaneous reactions can be harnessed to do work. All processes that have a ΔG value that is zero, or greater than zero, are *nonspontaneous reactions*.

Another way to think of ΔG is that it represents the difference between the free energy of a system in its initial state and the free energy of its final state:

$$\Delta G = G_{final} - G_{initial}$$

Therefore, ΔG can only be negative (spontaneous reaction) when the process involves a loss of free energy from its initial to final state. In this case, the final state has less free energy and is more stable than the initial state. Nonspontaneous reactions are more stable in their initial state than their final state (positive ΔG value). In this way, we can also think of free energy values as a measure of a system's stability. In nature, all systems tend to move toward a state of greater stability. A term used for the state of maximum stability of a system is *equilibrium*. As a reaction proceeds toward a state of equilibrium, the free energy of the reactants and products decreases. Therefore, at equilibrium, ΔG is at its lowest possible value for a system under a given set of conditions. Free energy increases as a reaction is pushed away from a state of equilibrium, for example, by additional energy added to the reaction, or due to a change in the concentration of the final products.

Based on their free energy changes, biochemical reactions can be classified in one of two ways: *Exergonic (energy outward) reactions* are those that proceed with a net release of energy. ΔG is a negative value for exergonic reactions, and these reactions occur spontaneously. *Endergonic (energy inward) reactions* are those that absorb free energy from their surroundings. Endergonic reactions have a positive ΔG value and are nonspontaneous.

ATP

Adenosine triphosphate, or ATP, is the molecule that is responsible for providing cellular energy in most cases. It acts as an immediate source of energy that powers one of three types of cellular work: mechanical, transport, or chemical. ATP is a nucleotide that is a building block of nucleic acids (DNA and RNA). ATP and all other nucleotides are composed of three different parts. A *pentose molecule* is a sugar configured in a five-carbon ring structure. The pentose molecule in an ATP molecule is ribose. The nitrogen-containing base in ATP is *adenine*. This base combines with the ribose to create a nucleoside molecule. In an ATP molecule, this nucleoside is adenosine. A *phosphate group*, PO_4, is a salt or ester of phosphoric acid. It can be denoted by the symbol, P_i, which stands for inorganic phosphate. A nucleoside molecule can be joined to one (monophosphate), two (diphosphate), or three (triphosphate) phosphate groups. ATP has three phosphate groups, hence the name "adenosine triphosphate."

Figure 5. ATP Structure

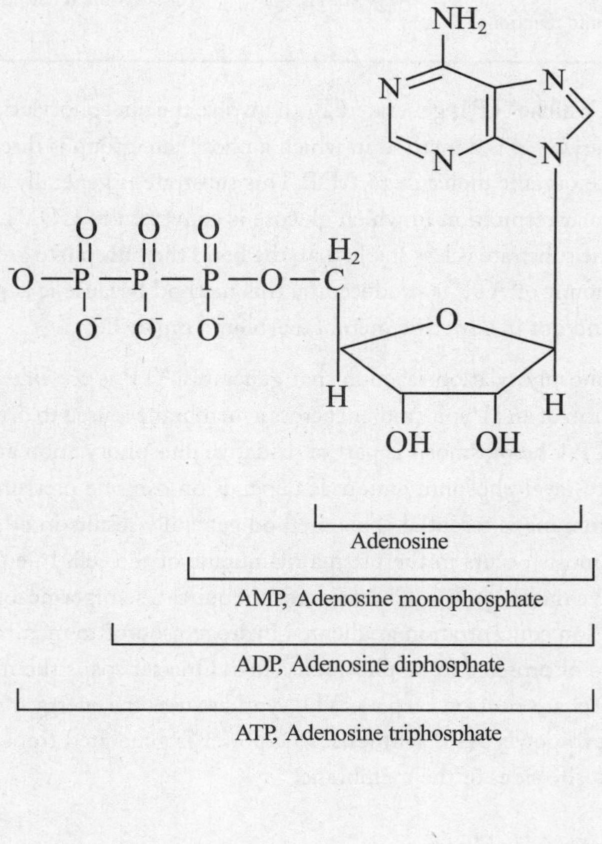

ATP provides energy for the cell because of its phosphate bonds. These are highly unstable covalent bonds that are easily broken by *hydrolysis*. The hydrolysis of ATP is an exergonic process that yields ADP and P_i. ATP releases a large amount of energy as these phosphate bonds are broken, which provides energy to cells for many metabolic processes. In fact, an endergonic reaction can be coupled to an ATP hydrolysis reaction through the transfer of a phosphate group to a molecule in the endergonic reaction, so that the overall reaction is exergonic. The recipient of the phosphate group is said to be *phosphorylated*. The key to coupling reactions is this phosphorylated intermediate that is more reactive (less stable) than its unphosphorylated form.

Each cell produces its own supply of ATP as it is needed. As a cell becomes more active, ATP production increases, and as a cell becomes less active, ATP production decreases. ATP is not transferred from one area of the body to another; therefore, its production depends upon the recycling of its components within a given cell. ATP is used continuously by cells in all organisms, but it is also a renewable resource within cells. ATP is synthesized from ADP and P_i, and this process requires an input of energy. ATP is hydrolyzed to yield ADP and P_i in a reaction that releases energy.

Figure 6. The ATP Cycle

ATP is formed from ADP and P_i and then broken down into these same molecules.

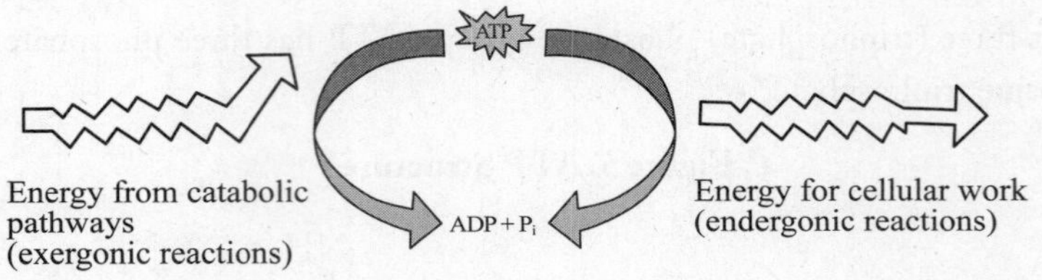

Energy from catabolic pathways (exergonic reactions)

ADP + P_i

Energy for cellular work (endergonic reactions)

There are two ways in which ATP is generated. Both involve the phosphorylation of ADP into ATP. *Substrate-level phosphorylation* is a method in which a phosphate group is directly transferred from a reactive intermediate organic molecule to ADP. This substrate is generally a substance produced by the process of cellular respiration in which glucose is converted to CO_2. The bond holding the phosphate group to the substrate is less stable than the bond the phosphate group forms with ADP. Only a very small amount of ATP is produced by this method because it is performed by cells in the aqueous cytosol and not in a specific membrane-bound organelle.

The second type of phosphorylation reaction that generates ATP is *chemiosmosis*. In this method, energy stored in the form of an H^+ ion gradient across a membrane is used to drive cellular work, such as the synthesis of ATP. Chemiosmosis is part of oxidative phosphorylation and is a more complex method than substrate-level phosphorylation. It depends on osmotic pressure, so a concentration gradient across a membrane is essential. This method generally results in a high yield of ATP. In prokaryotes, chemiosmosis occurs in the plasma membrane of the cell. In eukaryotes, it occurs in the cristae (folds) of the mitochondria. Chemiosmosis requires a semipermeable membrane to serve as a barrier for an H^+ ion concentration gradient, a hydrogen source to maintain the concentration gradient, and two sets of proteins to be phosphorylated. One set spans the membrane (ATP synthases) and the other set are electron carriers. ATP synthase uses the energy of an existing hydrogen ion (proton) gradient to power ATP synthesis. The power is generated from the difference in H^+ concentration on opposite sides of the membrane.

CELLULAR METABOLISM

In a broad sense, *metabolism* manages the material and energy resources inside a cell. A cell's metabolism is similar to a complex roadmap of many intersecting roads. In the cell, there are thousands of intersecting chemical pathways known as *metabolic pathways*. A metabolic pathway begins with a specific molecule, and this molecule is altered through a series of defined steps that ultimately lead to a specific product. Each step in a metabolic pathway is catalyzed by a specific enzyme.

Figure 7. Example of a Metabolic Pathway

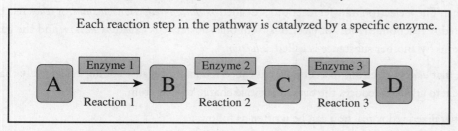

Some metabolic pathways release energy by breaking down complex molecules into more simple molecules. These are called *catabolic pathways*. Cellular respiration is a major catabolic pathway in cells. During *cellular respiration*, the sugar molecule glucose, along with other organic molecules, is broken down into carbon dioxide and water. This pathway is driven by the presence of oxygen. Energy is released from the glucose and other organic molecules, and then becomes available to do work in the cell.

Other metabolic pathways require an input of energy to build complicated molecules from simpler simple ones. These are called *anabolic*, or *biosynthetic*, pathways. Protein synthesis from simple amino acids is an example of an anabolic pathway. Energy released from a catabolic pathway can, in turn, be used as an energy source to drive an anabolic reaction.

The slowest reaction in any process is called the *rate-limiting step*. The metabolic process can never proceed faster than the rate-limiting step.

Cellular Respiration

Living cells require energy from outside sources to perform thousands of tasks. For example, animals obtain energy from the foods they eat. Some animals eat smaller animals and derive energy from them. These smaller animals may eat plant material and derive energy from the plants. In turn, the plants derive energy from sunlight. In this way, energy for all life on Earth originates from the sun. The process of *cellular respiration* involves the harvesting of chemical energy stored in organic molecules to generate ATP as a fuel source for cells. Cellular respiration that takes place in the presence of oxygen is called *aerobic respiration*. In contrast, the waste products of cellular respiration in animals, CO_2 and H_2O, become materials necessary for photosynthesis in plants. The overall process of aerobic cellular respiration can be summarized as follows:

organic compound (glucose) + oxygen → carbon dioxide + water + energy

Even though carbohydrates, fats, and proteins can all be used as a fuel source to provide energy to cells, the fuel that is most often used is glucose. The breakdown of glucose is an exergonic reaction, which means it can occur spontaneously. It is represented by the following overall equation:

$C_6H_{12}O_6$ (glucose) $+ 6O_2 \rightarrow 6CO_2 + 6H_2O +$ Energy (ATP + thermal energy)

The function of this reaction is to release the energy stored in the glucose (or other fuel source). Glucose is oxidized and releases an H^+ ion; and oxygen is reduced, so it gains an H^+ ion.

Aerobic cellular respiration can be divided into three steps: glycolysis, the Krebs cycle (citric acid cycle), and oxidative phosphorylation.

Redox Reactions

In many chemical reactions, there is a transfer of one or more electrons from one molecule to another. These electron transfer reactions are called *oxidation-reduction reactions*, or *redox* reactions. In a redox reaction, the loss of electrons from one substance is called *oxidation*, and the gain of electrons by another substance is called *reduction*.

Note that *adding* electrons to a substance is called reduction because adding a negatively charged particle to an atom reduces the overall positive charge of that atom.

A generalized redox reaction can be written as follows:

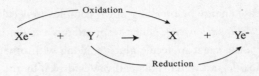

Where the substance X is the electron donor (reducing agent), and substance Y is the electron acceptor (oxidizing reagent). Y oxidizes X by removing an electron from it. Because an electron transfer requires both a donor and an acceptor, oxidation and reduction reactions are always coupled together.

A second type of cellular respiration that does not require the presence of oxygen is anaerobic respiration. Anaerobic respiration yields much less ATP per mole of starting material. Only certain prokaryotic bacteria are capable of anaerobic respiration. The general reaction requires a fuel source such as glucose and proceeds as follows:

$$C_6H_{12}O_6 \rightarrow C_3H_6O_3 \text{ (lactic acid)} + \text{Energy (ATP + thermal energy)}$$

During anaerobic respiration, glucose is oxidized and ADP is phosphorylated.

If energy is released from a fuel source all at once, it cannot be used efficiently to carry out work in the cell. Therefore, glucose and other organic fuels are broken down in a stepped metabolic pathway. Each step of the pathway is catalyzed by a different enzyme. At key steps in the pathway, electrons are removed from the glucose molecule. As is often the case in oxidation reactions, each of these electrons is transferred with a proton (H^+). The hydrogen ions that are removed from glucose do not transfer directly to the oxygen molecules to form water (one of the final products). Instead, during cellular respiration, they are passed down an electron transport chain. They are first passed to the coenzyme NAD^+. NAD^+ accepts an electron from glucose, and thus it is an oxidizing agent in cellular respiration. Enzymes known as *dehydrogenases* remove a pair of hydrogen atoms (a total of two protons and two electrons) from glucose or another substrate. The substrate is oxidized, and the enzyme then delivers two electrons and one of the H^+ protons to the coenzyme NAD^+. The other H^+ ion is released into the surroundings. Because the positively charged NAD^+ ion receives two electrons and one proton, it becomes neutrally charged as it is released as NADH. Each NADH molecule formed during cellular respiration represents stored energy (because it has accepted two electrons) that can eventually be used to make ATP once the electrons complete their transfer to oxygen in the reaction.

There are several energy-releasing steps in an electron transport chain that move the electrons stored by NADH to the oxygen molecules to make water, one of the end products of cellular respiration. The transport chain consists of several molecules, mostly proteins that are embedded in the inner membrane of mitochondrion. Electrons are transferred from glucose or another fuel source to NAD^+. Then NADH carries the electrons to the "top" of the electron transport chain. This is considered the "high-energy" end of the chain. At the bottom, or "low-energy" end of the transport chain, oxygen captures these electrons and H^+ protons to form water. Small amounts of energy are released in each step of the transport chain. Cells use the energy released to regenerate ATP.

Glycolysis

Glycolysis occurs in the cytoplasm of cells and is the breaking of glucose molecules from a six-carbon sugar into two three-carbon sugars. These smaller sugars are oxidized and their atoms are rearranged to form two pyruvate molecules. *Pyruvate* is the ionized form of pyruvic acid. The process of glycolysis consists of ten steps, which can be divided into two phases. In the *energy investment phase*, the cell actually expends ATP molecules. During the *energy-producing phase*, more ATP molecules are produced than were used in the investment phase. The initial step of glycolysis requires the input of two ATP molecules; therefore, it is an endergonic step in the pathway. The net energy yield in glycolysis is two ATP molecules and two NADH molecules. No CO_2 is released during glycolysis and all of the carbon atoms from the original glucose sugar are accounted for in the two pyruvate molecules. The steps of glycolysis are outlined below. Note that the sixth and tenth steps occur twice for each glucose molecule, so that the final yield is two pyruvate molecules, two ATP, and two NADH.

Figure 8. Glycolytic Pathway

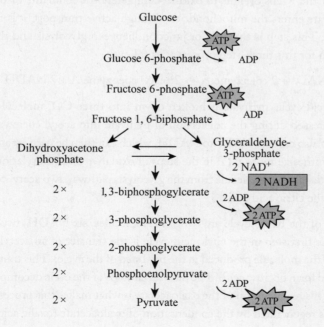

The overall glycolysis reaction can be summarized as follows:

$$C_6H_{12}O_6 + 2\ NAD^+ + 2\ ADP + 2\ P_i \rightarrow 2\ NADH + 2\ pyruvate + 2\ ATP + 2H_2O + 2H^+$$

Glycolysis may occur in both the presence and absence of oxygen. If oxygen is present during glycolysis however, the chemical energy stored in the pyruvate and NADH molecules can be extracted by the citric acid cycle and oxidative phosphorylation, respectively. In the absence of oxygen (*anaerobic*), the products of glycolysis can be used in the process of fermentation.

FERMENTATION

As long as there is a sufficient supply of NAD^+ to accept electrons during the oxidation step of glycolysis, fermentation can generate ATP in the absence of oxygen. Therefore, the fermentation process consists of glycolysis reactions and NAD^+ regenerating reactions.

In alcohol fermentation, pyruvate is converted to ethanol in a two-step process. The first step releases CO_2 from the pyruvate, and pyruvate is converted to acetaldehyde. In the second step, acetaldehyde is reduced by NADH to ethanol (ethyl alcohol). This step also regenerates the supply of NAD^+ needed for glycolysis.

In lactic acid fermentation, pyruvate is reduced by NADH to form lactate. In this process, no CO_2 is released. *Lactate* is the ionized form of lactic acid. Human muscle cells produce ATP through the process of lactic acid fermentation.

The Krebs Cycle

Glycolysis only releases a small portion of the energy stored in glucose molecules. The remainder of it remains stored in the two pyruvate molecules that are the end product of glycolysis. If there is oxygen present in the cell, the pyruvate molecules enter the mitochondrion, and the enzymes involved in the *Krebs cycle*, or *citric acid cycle*, complete the oxidation process and release the stored energy. The goal of the Krebs cycle is to oxidize completely the remnants of the original glucose molecule. As pyruvate enters the mitochondrion through active transport, it is first converted into acetyl coenzyme A. This step is the link, or junction, between glycolysis and the citric acid cycle. The overall reaction for this three-step process is as follows:

$$2\ pyruvate + 2\ NAD^+ + 2\ coenzyme\ A \rightarrow 2\ acetyl\ coenzyme\ A + 2\ NADH + 2\ H^+ + 2CO_2$$

During the citric acid cycle, pyruvate is broken down into three CO_2 molecules, and all but one CO_2 molecule is released during the conversion of pyruvate into acetyl coenzyme A (acetyl coA). This initial reaction also reduces NAD^+ to NADH, which can then be used by an electron transport system (ETS) to synthesize more ATP in the steps of oxidative phosphorylation. Also, in order to fully oxidize the initial glucose molecule from the glycolysis pathway, two acetyl coA molecules must be metabolized by the citric acid cycle.

The final products of the Krebs cycle are two ATP molecules, six NADH, two $FADH_2$, and four CO_2 molecules. The first step in the citric acid cycle is the transfer of an acetyl group from acetyl coA to *oxaloacetate* (the molecule produced in the final step of the cycle). This transfer creates a *citrate molecule* (the ionized form of citric acid). The next seven steps of the cycle decompose the citrate back into oxaloacetate. This regeneration of the oxaloacetate is what makes this process a cycle. The cycle ends when citrate is regenerated by the condensation of oxaloacetate (oxalic acid) and acetyl coA.

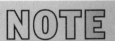

NOTE

Remember that points are not deducted for wrong answers, but don't guess indiscriminately. Use the process of elimination to discard answers that you know are wrong.

Two carbon atoms are oxidized to CO_2, which is released during the cycle. The energy from these reactions is stored in molecules of GTP, NADH, and $FADH_2$. GTP is another nucleotide triphosphate (guanosine 5′-triphosphate), which plays a role in the synthesis of DNA and RNA, and it is also involved in signal transduction. In the Krebs cycle, GTP can easily be converted into ATP. NADH and $FADH_2$ are both coenzymes that store energy and are also used in the process of oxidative phosphorylation. The overall reaction taking place in the Krebs cycle is:

$$acetyl\ CoA + 3\ NAD^+ + FAD + GDP + P_i + 3H_2O \rightarrow$$

$$CoA\text{-}SH + 3\ NADH + H^+ + FADH_2 + GTP + CO_2 + 3H^+$$

Figure 9. The Krebs Cycle (Citric Acid Cycle)

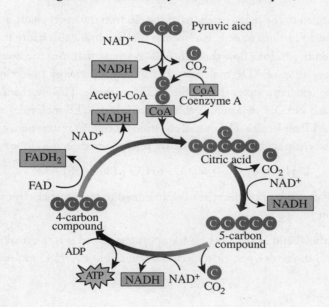

Oxidative Phosphorylation

During *oxidative phosphorylation*, chemiosmosis couples an electron transport system (ETS) to ATP synthesis. In the first two segments of cellular respiration, glycolysis, and the citric acid (Krebs) cycle, only four molecules of ATP are produced. At this point in cellular respiration, molecules of NADH (10) and $FADH_2$ account for a large bulk of the energy extracted from food. However, only ATP is a readily usable energy source in cells. These two types of electron transporters link glycolysis and the citric acid cycle to the oxidative phosphorylation pathway. The *electron transport chain*, or ETS, that is essential for oxidative phosphorylation, is a collection of membrane-bound molecules in the inner membrane of the mitochondrion. The job of the electron transport system is to oxidize molecules of NADH and $FADH_2$, so that more ATP can be produced. Electrons are removed and shuttled through a series of electron acceptors in the chain. Energy is removed from the electrons each time they are transferred to the next "link" in the chain. The electron carriers alternate between a reduced and an oxidized form as they accept and donate electrons. NADH transfers electrons to the first molecule of the electron transport chain. This first molecule is a flavoprotein. The flavoprotein is thus reduced as it accepts the electron from NADH. This flavoprotein then returns to its oxidized form as it passes electrons to the next molecule, which is an iron-sulfur protein complex. In this manner, electrons are moved through the entire transport chain through a series of redox reactions.

Figure 10. Overview of the Electron Transport Chain Essential for Oxidative Phosphorylation

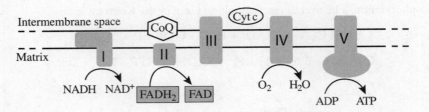

ATP synthesis is coupled to the redox reactions of the electron transport chain, and ATP synthesis is powered by the flow of H^+ ions moving back across the membrane (back into the intermembrane space of the mitochondrion). Ions flow through ATP synthase that uses the exergonic flow of H^+ to drive the phosphorylation of ADP molecules. In this way, the energy stored in the H^+ gradient across the membrane is what couples the ETS to ATP synthesis. This mechanism is an example of chemiosmosis. Each NADH molecule is able to yield three ATP molecules and each $FADH_2$ molecule yields two ATP molecules. The overall equation for cellular respiration, including all of the steps in glycolysis, the citric acid cycle, and oxidative phosphorylation is as follows:

$$C_6H_{12}O_6 + 6O_2 \rightarrow 6CO_2 + 6H_2O + (36 \text{ or } 38) \text{ ATP}$$

The number of ATP depends upon the type of shuttle used to transport electrons from the cytosol to the mitochondrion.

Oxygen is at the terminal end of the electron transport chain, and it is the final electron acceptor. For every two NADH molecules, one O_2 molecule is reduced to two H_2O molecules:

$$\frac{1}{2} O_2 + 2H^+ + 2e^- \rightarrow H_2O$$

Photosynthesis

Sunlight is the energy source that drives the *photosynthesis* reaction. The reaction converts the light energy from the sun into chemical energy in green plants. This chemical energy in plants is then passed on to animals that rely on green plants as a food source. There are three accomplishments of photosynthesis that are essential to life:

1. All stored energy in organisms stems from photosynthesis.

2. Oxygen, the waste product of photosynthesis, is required for cellular respiration. Without oxygen, cells cannot produce ATP.

3. Photosynthesis is the source of most of our fuels on Earth, including those for heating, transportation, and cooking.

The major reactants in photosynthesis are carbon dioxide, CO_2, and water, H_2O. Carbon dioxide acts as an inorganic carbon source, and water acts as a hydrogen source. Chlorophyll, a chemical inside plants, is also necessary and acts as a *photoreceptor* (captures light energy). The major products of the photosynthesis reaction are glucose, $C_6H_{12}O_6$, and oxygen gas, O_2, which is a waste product of the reaction, so:

$$6CO_2 + 12H_2O + \text{light energy} \rightarrow C_6H_{12}O_6 + 6O_2 + 6H_2O$$

Water appears on both sides of the equation because during the reaction, twelve water molecules are consumed and six molecules of water are newly formed. Glucose molecules store energy that can then be converted into ATP in animal cells. Plants convert glucose to sucrose, or they store chemical energy as starch in amyloplasts or lipids.

Like cellular respiration, photosynthesis is a redox process. During the process, water is split and electrons are transferred with hydrogen ions to carbon dioxide. Thus, carbon dioxide is reduced to a sugar. Because the electron increases in potential energy as it moves from a water to a sugar molecule, this process requires energy. The energy is provided in the form of sunlight.

Photosynthesis takes place in the *chloroplast*. The chloroplast is a green organelle with a double membrane and its own unique DNA that is separate from the nucleus of the cell. Chloroplasts are found in plant cells but not in animal cells. Each chloroplast consists of stacks of discs called *thylakoids*, where the light-dependent reactions of photosynthesis take place. Chlorophyll can be found in the thylakoids, so the thylakoids are the site of light collection. A stack of thylakoids is called a *granum*, and links between grana are called *stroma lamellae*. The light-independent reactions, or the Calvin cycle, take place in the internal cavity of the chloroplast called the *stroma*.

Photosynthesis is actually two processes, each with multiple steps. The first process is known as the *light reactions*, and the second process is known as the *Calvin cycle*. Light reactions involve the steps that convert light energy into chemical energy. Light absorbed by chlorophyll in the chloroplast drives the transfer of electrons and hydrogen from water to an acceptor called $NADP^+$ (nicotinamide adenine dinucleotide phosphate). $NADP^+$ temporarily stores the electrons. Water is split in this process; therefore, light reactions result in the release of the byproduct O_2. Light reactions reduce $NADP^+$ to NADPH, and they also generate ATP using chemiosmosis to drive the addition of a phosphate group to ADP. This process in plants is called *photophosphorylation*. The light reactions result in the production of chemical energy in the form of NADPH and ATP, but no sugar molecules are formed in these processes:

$$\text{Light (photon)} + H_2O + ADP + P_i + NADP \rightarrow O_2 + ATP + NADPH$$

Glucose is formed in the second stage of photosynthesis: the Calvin cycle. The Calvin cycle begins by incorporating CO_2 from the atmosphere into organic molecules present in the chloroplast. This process is known as *carbon fixation*. CO_2 attaches to the five carbon molecule, ribulose-1, 5-bisphosphate carboxylase oxygenase (RuBP). The fixed carbon is then reduced to a carbohydrate through the addition of electrons. The power to drive this reduction reaction comes from NADPH (which has high-energy electrons from the light reactions). ATP (also produced by the light reactions) is also required to convert CO_2 into a carbohydrate. The end result of the Calvin cycle is the production of sugar molecules. The metabolic steps of the Calvin cycle are often referred to as the *dark reactions*, or light-independent reactions. The three stages of the Calvin cycle are:

1. **CO_2 fixation:** The RuBPCO enzyme catalyzes the reaction to form a very unstable 6-carbon sugar that breaks down into two molecules of 3-phosphoglyceric acid (PGA). CO_2 is taken from the atmosphere into the plant's stroma and it attaches to RuBP.

2. **CO_2 reduction:** NADPH is the reducing agent and ATP is required to provide energy for the reaction. PGA is reduced to 3-phosphoglyceraldehyde, PGAL, as a P_i group is transferred from ATP and an H^+ ion is transferred from NADPH. The ultimate goal of the reaction is the formation of glucose.

3. **Regeneration RuBP:** The starting material of the cycle is regenerated so that the cycle can begin again when more CO_2 enters. Most of the PGAL is converted back into RuBP and this goes back into the Calvin cycle. One out of every six PGAL molecules is used to make a glucose molecule.

Overall, it takes six CO_2 molecules to produce one glucose molecule. Therefore, six cycles through the Calvin cycle are required to make one glucose molecule:

$$6 \text{ RuBP} + 6CO_2 + 18 \text{ ATP} + 12\text{NADPH} + 12H^+ + 12H_2O \rightarrow$$
$$6 \text{ RuBP} + 1 \text{ glucose } (C_6H_{12}O_6) + 18P_i + 18 \text{ ADP} + 12\text{NADP}^+$$

DNA STRUCTURE AND REPLICATION

Deoxyribonucleic acid, or DNA, is the genetic material that organisms inherit from their parents. It is a molecule necessary for all living organisms to reproduce their complex structures and components. DNA is able to provide the directions for its own replication and the synthesis of RNA. It is found in the nucleus of all eukaryotic cells.

Structure

DNA is a macromolecular structure that exists as a *polynucleotide*. This simply means that it is composed of many monomer subunits called *nucleotides*.

Nucleotide Structure

A nucleotide is composed of three parts: nitrogenous base, pentose (five-carbon sugar ring), and one, two, or three phosphate groups.

The portion without the phosphate group is called a *nucleoside*.

Figure 11. Nucleotide Structure and Four Nucleotide Bases in DNA Molecules

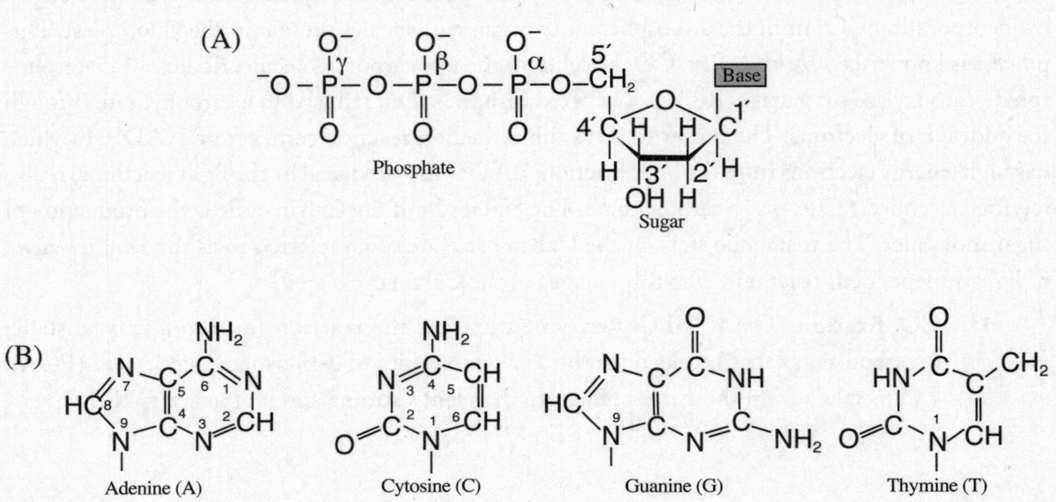

Deoxyribonucleotides can have one of four different nitrogenous bases: adenine (A), guanine (G), cytosine (C), or thymine (T). These four bases are classified as either purines or pyrimidines. Cytosine and thymine are pyrimidines and have a six-membered ring of carbon and nitrogen. Adenine and guanine are purine bases and consist of a six-membered ring fused to a five-membered ring. Each base differs in the functional groups attached to the rings.

In DNA, the five-carbon pentose is *deoxyribose*. Deoxyribose lacks an oxygen atom on its second carbon. Since all the carbons in both the base and the sugar are numbered, the carbons in the sugar are referred to as "prime" with the symbol (′) after the carbon number. Therefore, the second carbon in the deoxyribose ring is referred to as the 2′ carbon. Also, the carbon that sticks up from the ring is the 5′ carbon. The phosphate groups are attached to the nucleoside at the 5′ carbon of the sugar. A nucleotide monophosphate (one phosphate group) is called a *nucleotide*.

Nucleotides are linked together to form a *polynucleotide molecule*. In a polynucleotide, adjacent nucleotides are joined together by a phosphodiester linkage between the −OH group on the 3′ carbon of one nucleotide and the phosphate on the 5′ carbon on another nucleotide. This specific bonding creates what is called a *sugar–phosphate backbone* of DNA. The ends of each strand of DNA are referred to as either the 5′ end with a phosphate group attached, or a 3′ end with a hydroxyl group attached. DNA molecules are assembled from the 5′ end to the 3′ end. Along the sugar–phosphate backbone are appendages consisting of nitrogenous bases.

DNA Double Helix

DNA molecules have two polynucleotide chains that run in opposite directions. A polynucleotide oriented in the 5′ to 3′ direction is joined to a polynucleotide in the 3′ to 5′ antiparallel direction. These polynucleotides are joined together in a double helix structure. The structure looks like a ladder spiraled around an imaginary axis.

The sugar-phosphate backbone runs along the outside of the helical structure and the nitrogenous bases are paired together in the interior portion of the helix. The two polynucleotide chains are held together by hydrogen bonds between the paired bases and van der Waals interactions between the stacked bases. Even though hydrogen bonds are generally weak bonds, the huge number of hydrogen bonds in a DNA double helix makes the molecule very stable. Hydrogen bonds within a structure cause folding and bending, thus the double helical structure is due to the position of the hydrogen bonds between the base pairs.

Only certain nitrogenous bases can pair with one another. *Adenine* bases always pair with thymine bases, and *cytosine* bases always pair with guanine bases. Each base pair consists of one purine and one pyrimidine base. Most DNA molecules are very long, consisting of thousands of nucleotide base pairs, and one long DNA strand can include many genes in its sequence.

If the sequence of one strand of a DNA helix is known, the sequence of the other strand can be determined by following the base-pairing rules. For example, if the sequence on one strand reads 5′-GCATGCGG-3′, the sequence on the opposite strand must be 3′-CGTACGCC-5′. The two strands of the DNA are said to be complementary to each other:

5′-GCATGCGG-3

3′-CGTACGCC-5′

This feature makes it possible for genes to be copied exactly and passed on to offspring. In preparation for cell division, each strand of a double helix can serve as a template for the synthesis of a new complementary strand. This results in two exact copies of the original double-stranded DNA helix. These two copies can be passed onto each of the two daughter cells during cell division.

DNA Replication

Replication of a DNA molecule begins at a special site called the *origin of replication*. Proteins that aid in the synthesis of a new DNA strand recognize the origin sequence and what is known as a *replication bubble*, separating the two strands of the DNA helix. This prepares the DNA for replication of its sequence in both directions from the bubble.

There are six steps in the process of DNA replication:

1. The double helix unwinds. The enzyme responsible for catalyzing this reaction is called *DNA helicase*. The hydrogen bonds between the complementary bases are broken, leading to the formation of the Y-shaped replication fork. This makes each parent strand available for replication.

2. Single-strand DNA binding proteins bind to each strand of the unwound DNA and prevent the two strands from rejoining. The single-strand DNA binding proteins are also called helix destabilizing proteins.

3. Free-floating deoxyribonucleotides hydrogen bond with the exposed nucleotides on each of the two parent DNA strands. The two new strands are synthesized in the 5' to 3' direction only.

4. The enzyme *topoisomerase* helps to relieve the strain caused by untwisting the DNA. This enzyme catalyzes a reaction that causes gaps in the DNA to alleviate the strain that the unwinding causes on the helical DNA structure. Topoisomerase breaks the DNA and then joins it back together.

5. The separated strands unwind in opposite directions.

6. Enzymes called *DNA polymerases* help to add nucleotides to the free 3' end of a growing DNA daughter strand.

Ultimately, each parent DNA strand synthesizes a copy of itself, and the result is two identical double-stranded DNA molecules. The enzyme DNA polymerase III can continuously synthesize a new complementary strand in the mandatory 5' to 3' direction. This is possible on the strand running in the 3' to 5' direction, which is called the *leading strand*. The antiparallel strand that runs 5' to 3' is referred to as the *lagging strand*. DNA polymerase III still synthesizes DNA in the 5' to 3' direction, but the synthesis is not continuous on the lagging strand. Instead, short segments of DNA (about 100 to 1,000 nucleotides long) called *Okazaki fragments* are synthesized and then joined.

DNA polymerase III cannot start the synthesis of a new DNA strand without the assistance of a *primer molecule*. The primer is a short segment of RNA that has complementary bases to the unwound DNA strand. The enzyme *primase*, which is an RNA polymerase enzyme, catalyzes the reaction that synthesizes the primer on the DNA strand. DNA polymerase III then elongates the primer using DNA nucleotides. A primer is needed for the leading strand and for each of the Okazaki fragments on the lagging strand. DNA polymerase I aids in removing the RNA primers from the DNA and replacing them with the correct nucleotides. Finally, DNA ligase joins together each of the Okazaki fragments along the lagging strand.

DNA synthesis occurs at a very rapid rate of about 1,000 nucleotides per second. On average, it takes about ten minutes to replicate an entire DNA molecule.

Figure 12. Diagram of DNA Replication

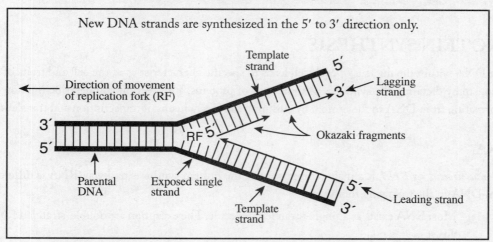

Summary of DNA Replication Proteins and Their Functions

Protein	Function on Leading Strand	Function on Lagging Strand
Helicase	Unwinds parental double helix at replication forks	Unwinds parental double helix at replication forks
Single-stranded DNA binding protein (SSB)	Binds to unwound DNA so that the strands do not base pair to each other	Binds to unwound DNA so that the strands do not base pair to each other
Topoisomerase	Corrects overwinding of DNA ahead of replication fork; breaks and rejoins DNA strands	Corrects overwinding of DNA ahead of replication fork; breaks and rejoins DNA strands
Primase	Synthesizes single RNA primer at the 5′ end of the leading strand	Synthesizes an RNA primer at the end of each Okazaki fragment
DNA Polymerase III	Continuously synthesizes new DNA strand, adding on to primer	Elongates each Okazaki fragment, adding on to its primer

DNA Polymerase I	Removes the primer from the DNA strand and replaces it with DNA	Removes the primer from the DNA strand and replaces it with DNA
DNA Ligase	Joins the 3′ end of the DNA that replaces the primer with the rest of the new strand.	Joins together the Okazaki fragments

PROTEIN SYNTHESIS

The DNA within the nucleus of each cell leads to specific characteristics of the cell and traits of an organism by dictating the synthesis of thousands of proteins. This section will describe the flow of information from DNA to the protein by outlining the mechanisms of transcription and translation.

RNA

Ribonucleic acid, or *RNA*, is a major component of the protein synthesis pathway. RNA is different from DNA in the following four ways:

1. Most RNA exists as a single-stranded molecule. The exception are double-stranded RNA viruses.

2. The pentose sugar on RNA is ribose, not deoxyribose.

3. The nitrogenous bases in RNA are guanine (G) , adenine (A), cytosine (C), and uracil (U). Like thymine, uracil can bond to adenine. Please note that uracil (U) is used only in RNA protein synthesis.

Uracil

4. RNA polymerase enzymes can join RNA nucleotides together without a preexisting RNA strand. RNA is synthesized from a DNA strand.

In eukaryotic cells, there are three main types of RNA: messenger, ribosomal, and transfer. *Messenger RNA (mRNA)* is a complimentary copy of a DNA strand. The mRNA molecule is called messenger RNA because it carries the genetic message of the DNA to the ribosomes and the protein-synthesizing machinery of the cell.

Transfer RNA (tRNA) attaches to amino acids in the cytoplasm and transports them to the ribosomes for protein synthesis. Strands of tRNA are folded into a cloverleaf structure and are then twisted into an L-shape. It is the nitrogenous base pairs that form the genetic code in DNA. The sequence of the DNA codes for specific amino acids, and the DNA is segmented into three base pair "codes," or *codons*, each of which specifies a particular amino acid. The tRNA recognizes a three-base code of mRNA that is specific for one type of amino acid, and it can only transport that one type of amino acid to the ribosome. In this way, the correct amino acid sequence is linked together so that the correct protein is synthesized. Ribosomes facilitate the specific coupling of mRNA and tRNA during protein synthesis.

Ribosomes consist of two subunits. The subunits are constructed of proteins and RNA. The RNA in ribosomes is called *ribosomal RNA (rRNA)*. About two thirds of the mass of a ribosome comes from the rRNA. rRNA is the most abundant form of RNA in cells because cells contain such a large volume of ribosomes.

Transcription

The process of synthesizing mRNA from a DNA strand is called *transcription*. mRNA is transcribed from the template strand of DNA inside the nucleus of eukaryotic cells and in the cytoplasm of prokaryotic cells. The template strand runs in the 3′ to 5′ direction, and mRNA can only be transcribed in the 5′ to 3′ direction. An enzyme called RNA polymerase II pries apart the two strands of DNA and also acts to link together the RNA nucleotides as the base pair with the complementary DNA.

The stretch of DNA that is transcribed into mRNA is called a *transcription unit*. Specific sequences along the DNA called *promoter regions* mark where transcription should begin. The promoter regions of each gene are about 40 base pairs long. RNA polymerase attaches to the promoter region directly in prokaryotic cells. However, in eukaryotic cells, a collection of proteins called *basal transcription factors* bind to the promoter region of DNA and mediate the binding of RNA polymerase II. This assembly of proteins and RNA polymerase II is called a *transcription initiation complex*. In eukaryotes, there is a crucial promoter sequence on DNA called a *TATA box*, located about 25 base pairs upstream (closer to the 3′ end of the template) from the transcription initiation site. The name TATA is given because of the sequence of DNA in this region: TATAAAA. The TATA box is significant because the first protein of the transcription initiation complex, TFIID, recognizes the TATA sequence and binds to DNA. This triggers the formation of the initiation complex and the start of transcription. Activator proteins can also bind to certain promoter regions in order to initiate the start of transcription. Once the RNA polymerase is firmly attached to the promoter region of DNA, the two strands of DNA unwind and the enzyme begins the process of transcribing mRNA. Other proteins called repressor proteins can bind and slow down the transcription process.

Once unwound, the 3′ to 5′ DNA strand acts as a template for synthesizing RNA. The promoter sequence is not transcribed, and the first region of DNA after the promoter is transcribed. This is called the *leader region* and is the portion of mRNA that will become the ribosome binding site for each mRNA.

After the leader sequence, the coding sequence is transcribed. The *coding sequence* is the region of RNA that will have the amino acid codons and will be translated into an amino acid sequence. Transcribing the coding region involves the complementary base pairing of ribonucleotide triphosphates to deoxynucleotides on the DNA strand. The RNA is bonded to the DNA through hydrogen bonding. Note that adenine on the DNA strand bonds to uracil on the RNA strand instead of thymine. Thymine is only a DNA base. Phosphodiester bonds form between the 5′C phosphate group of the nucleotide that is being inserted and the 3′C of the last nucleotide to be added to the mRNA strand. As covalent bonds form, two of the phosphate groups on the end of the triphosphates are removed, and energy

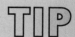

TIP

Remember to answer the question that is asked, not what you think the question is asking. Read the question quickly, but carefully.

is provided to fuel the reaction. RNA polymerase is responsible for catalyzing the reaction that joins the ribonucleotides together. It is also responsible for terminating transcription.

In higher-order eukaryotic organisms, there are some regions of DNA that do not code for genes as they are transcribed into mRNA. These regions are called *introns*. In humans, they comprise 98 percent of our chromosomal DNA. Interspersed between these intron regions are regions called *exons* that do contain genetic information. The initial piece of mRNA transcribed from DNA contains both the intron and exon sequences. This RNA is called *precursor mRNA*. Precursor mRNA has a modified guanine nucleotide at its 5′ end, which is called a *5′ cap*. The 3′ end of the mRNA is also modified by the addition of a string of A bases. This is called a *poly(A) tail*. The modified ends may better promote the export of mRNA from the nucleus to the ribosomes and also help protect mRNA from degradation. These modified ends do not translate into an amino acid during protein synthesis. RNA processing occurs in order to transform the precursor RNA into a mature mRNA strand. Introns are spliced out of the RNA sequence, and exons are joined together. These actions are performed by a protein complex called a *spliceosome*. The mature mRNA strand, therefore, has a continuous coding sequence. This process of preparing a mature mRNA molecule is called RNA splicing. This mRNA molecule is now ready to be translated into a protein.

Translation

The mature mRNA leaves the nucleus through the pores in the nuclear membrane and is transported to the ribosomes in the cytoplasm of the cell. In the process of translation at the ribosomes, the genetic message in the mRNA is interpreted and translated into a polypeptide sequence. The translated message is a series of codons along the mRNA, and the "interpreter" is tRNA. Each nucleotide codon is three bases long. A specific codon only codes for one amino acid, although several codes may be specific for the same amino acid. Because there are four nucleotides in mRNA, there are 64 (4^3) possible codons. There are 20 amino acids, so that means that there are multiple codons for each amino acid. There are also two special codons needed: a *start codon* (AUG) that indicates where translation is to begin, and a *stop codon* (UAG, UAA, and UGA) that indicates where translation is to end. The ability to extract the correct information from mRNA depends upon the nucleotides being read in the correct groupings, or reading frame. The correct polypeptide sequence can only be made if the reading frame is correct.

As mentioned earlier, eukaryotic ribosomes consist of two subunits: the 40S and 60S subunits. Each is composed of ribosomal RNA, rRNA, and proteins. The small subunit of rRNA attaches to mRNA, and two RNA binding sites are formed: the peptidyl, or P, site and the aminoacyl, or A, site.

tRNA is required for translation. On all tRNA molecules, there is a triplet of nucleotides called the *anticodon*. The anticodon sequence on tRNA base pairs with the complementary codon sequence on the mRNA molecule. On the 3′ end of tRNA, there is an amino acid attachment site containing a triplet codon specific for one amino acid. The enzyme aminoacyl tRNA synthetase catalyzes the reaction, which adds a specific amino acid to the tRNA. This reaction is called *aminoacylation*. Each amino acid has a corresponding aminoacyl tRNA synthetase enzyme. The tRNA amino acid complex is called aminoacyl tRNA. In this way, specific amino acids are bound to a specific tRNA molecule. Then the anticodon sequence on the tRNA binds specifically to the mRNA attached to the ribosome. This brings the required amino acids to the ribosome in the correct sequence.

The three steps of the translation process are as follows:

1. **Initiation:** Translation is initiated when the ribosome is attached to the mRNA. The start codon (AUG) on the mRNA indicates the point at which the mRNA attaches to the ribosome. This is called the *ribosomal binding site*, and the small 40S subunit of the ribosome binds to the mRNA first. The first tRNA then comes in at the P site on the ribosome. The initial tRNA must have the anticodon for the start codon (UAC). The anticodon binds to the start codon. The start codon codes for the amino acid methionine, so all amino acid chains have methionine as the first amino acid. Once the initiator tRNA (met-tRNA) occupies the P site, the large 60S ribosomal subunit attaches and this makes a complete initiation complex. Proteins called *initiation factors* are required to bring all the components of the subunit together.

2. **Elongation:** In the elongation stage of translation, amino acids are added one by one to the preceding amino acids, thus forming a chain. Several proteins called *elongation factors* are required for this process. Because the initiator met-tRNA is on the P site, the A site is available to bind the next tRNA and amino acid. The methionine in the P site must be attached by a peptide bond to the next amino acid. The enzyme peptidyl transferase is responsible for catalyzing this reaction. The two amino acids become joined together on the A site, and the tRNA molecule dissociates from the P site. The ribosome then moves down to the next codon on the mRNA, and the tRNA-amino acid complex moves from the A site to the P site, leaving the A site free to receive the next tRNA and amino acid. The polypeptide continues to elongate in this way, adding each amino acid that is coded for in the mRNA.

3. **Termination:** When the ribosome complex reaches a stop codon on the mRNA, no more aminoacyl-tRNAs are added to the polypeptide chain. The polypeptide chain is then released from the tRNA, and the tRNA is released from the ribosome. The large and small ribosomal subunits then dissociate from the mRNA molecule.

Figure 13. Elongation Cycle of Transcription

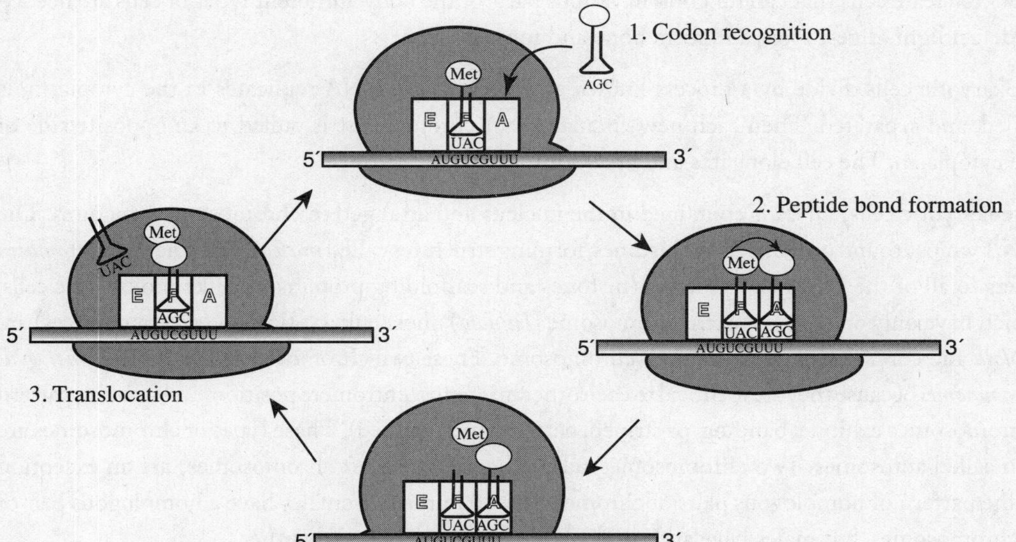

THE CELL CYCLE AND CELL DIVISION

The *cell cycle* is the series of events that takes place in eukaryotic cells in-between and during cell division. *Cell division* allows for the development of offspring from a parent organism. It enables sexually reproducing organisms to develop from a single cell into a multicellular organism. The three phases of the cell cycle can be described as follows:

1. **Interphase:** Interphase encompasses about 90 percent of the cell cycle timeline. During interphase, a cell grows and copies its chromosomes in order to prepare for cell division. This phase can be divided into three subphases: the G_1 phase (first gap), the S phase (synthesis), and the G_2 phase (second gap). The G_1 phase generally lasts about five to six hours, but the actual length of this phase is dependent on the type of cell. Cell growth begins during G_1. In the S phase, which lasts about ten to twelve hours, chromosomes are duplicated (DNA replication). The final portion of interphase, G_2, lasts four to six hours and during this time the cell grows more to prepare for mitosis.

2. **M phase:** During the M phase, the process of mitosis divides the cell nucleus, and the process of cytokinesis divides the cytoplasm. The M phase is relatively short, lasting only about one hour. In the M phase, chromosomes are divided into two daughter nuclei, and two daughter cells are produced.

3. **G_0 phase:** The G_0 phase of the cell cycle is the period in which cells are in a resting, or *quiescent*, state. There is no cell growth during this phase, and cells switch into G_0 if they do not receive a signal to move from G_1 into S. Most cells in the human body are actually in the G_0 phase at any given time.

Cell Division

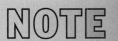

NOTE

You will have about 30 seconds to answer each question, so you need to move quickly through the items. If you are stuck on a question, mark it to return to later.

The function of cell division in multicellular organisms is growth, repair and replacement of damaged cells, and the production of gametes. The purpose of cell division in a single-celled organism is reproduction. Multicellular organisms can transform some cells into other types (*cellular differentiation*) in order to create cells that can function in various parts of the body. Different types of cells are needed to detect light, digest food, and form bone and muscle tissue.

Prokaryotic cells divide by a process known as *binary fission*. DNA replicates in the cytoplasm, is coiled, and separated. Then each new circular DNA chromosome is pulled to an opposite side of the cytoplasm. The cell elongates and breaks into two cells.

In eukaryotic cells, DNA is contained in the nucleus and arranged in chromosome structures. The DNA wraps around proteins called histones, forming structures called *nucleosomes*. The term *chromatin* refers to all of the DNA and proteins (histones and scaffolding proteins). Unlike prokaryotic cells, which have only one copy of each chromosome (*haploid*), most eukaryotic cells (except gametes) are *diploid* and contain two copies of each chromosome. These two chromosomes are called *homologous chromosomes* because they are identical to each other in length, centromere position, and staining pattern (chromosomes exhibit a banding, or striped, pattern when stained). These types of chromosomes are also called autosomes. Two chromosomes called X and Y (the sex chromosomes) are an exception to the pattern of homologous pairs of chromosomes in humans. Females have a homologous pair of X chromosomes, but males have an X and a Y chromosome paired together.

Cell division of diploid cells occurs through the process of mitosis, and the result is two diploid daughter cells.

Mitosis

Mitosis is the division of the cell nucleus and all the genetic information (DNA chromosomes) into two new nuclei. Although mitosis takes place in a short time span, it is a dynamic and essential process. Many of the events depend on the *mitotic spindle*, a structure that consists of microtubule fibers and associated proteins. The assembly of the mitotic spindle starts at the centrosome, a non-membraneous organelle in the cytosol.

There are five essential phases of mitosis, which are summarized here:

1. **Prophase:** The nucleolus disappears during this phase. The chromatin in the nucleus becomes more tightly coiled and condenses into discrete chromosomes. Each chromosome, which has been duplicated during the S phase, joins together with its sister chromatid and attaches to the center of the centromere. As the microtubule spindle begins to form, a radial array of shorter microtubules extends from the centrosomes. These arrays are called *asters*. The centrosomes move away from each other towards opposite sides of the cell as they are propelled in opposite directions by the lengthening microtubules between them. The chromosomes double from forty-six to ninety-two.

2. **Prometaphase:** The nuclear envelope disintegrates, and now the microtubules of the spindle can extend into the nuclear area of the cell and interact with the condensed chromosomes. The long microtubules extend from the centrosomes (still moving to opposite sides of the cell) towards the middle of the cell. Each of the two chromatids (or copies) of each chromosome now has a kinetochore. A *kinetochore* is a specialized protein structure that associates with specific sections of chromosomal DNA at the centromere (center point of the chromatid). Some of the microtubules attach to the kinetochore and are known as *kinetochore microtubules*. These microtubules can move the chromosomes back and forth. In this way, chromosomes can be correctly positioned by the microtubules.

3. **Metaphase:** This is the longest stage of the M phase, and it lasts approximately twenty minutes. The centrosomes are now at opposite sides of the cell, and the chromosomes are lined up across the center of the cell, in an area called the *metaphase plate*. This plate is an imaginary plane equidistant between each of the centrosomes (spindle poles). The centromere of each chromosome lies on the metaphase plate. The kinetochore of each chromatid in a chromosomal pair is attached to microtubules extending from opposite poles. Other microtubules that are not attached to chromatid (nonkinetochore microtubules) are able to extend across the metaphase plane.

4. **Anaphase:** Anaphase is the shortest stage of mitosis, and it lasts only a few minutes. Anaphase begins when the sister chromatids in each pair separate. In order for this to happen, the spindle fibers that are attached to the kinetochore of each chromatid begin to shorten. Each chromatid thus becomes a chromosome, and the two liberated chromosomes move towards opposite poles (ends) of the cell. Because the microtubules are attached to the centromeres, the chromosomes move centromere first in a "V" shape toward opposite sides. The cell begins to elongate as nonkinetochore microtubules lengthen. At the end of this phase, the opposite sides of the cell each have a complete set of chromosomes.

5. **Telophase:** During the final phase of mitosis, the daughter chromosomes reach the centrosomes at opposite poles of the cell, and two daughter nuclei begin to form. Nuclear envelopes arise from fragments of the parent nuclear envelope that remain in the cell's cytoplasm. The chromosomes become less condensed during this phase, and the process of mitosis (the formation of two genetically identical nuclei from one parent) is complete.

As mitosis is taking place in the cell, *cytokinesis*, or division of the cytoplasm, is occurring simultaneously. Cytokinesis is usually well underway by late telophase. Therefore, two daughter cells are formed shortly after the end of mitosis. In most animal cells, the cell begins to compress inward in the center, forming what is called a *cleavage furrow*. Soon, the cell splits into two identical daughter cells with all the necessary organelles and an exact copy of the original genetic material. In plant cells, a new cell wall forms between the two sets of sister chromosomes.

The result of mitosis and cytokinesis is the formation of two diploid daughter cells that are identical in all respects to the parent cell.

Meiosis

In humans, *gametes* (sperm and egg cells) contain only a single copy of each chromosome. These cells are called *haploid cells*. For humans, the haploid number of chromosomes is twenty-three (forty-six total in diploid cells). There are twenty-two autosomes and one sex chromosome (X or Y).

Meiosis is the process of division that takes place in gametes (sperm and ova cells). It avoids the problem of continually increasing the number of chromosomes in sexually reproducing organisms by reducing the number of sets of chromosomes in gamete, or sex cells, from two to one. Fertilization restores the diploid condition to the developing zygote (fertilized egg) by combining the chromosomes from a sperm cell and an ova (egg) cell.

The process of meiosis is similar to mitosis, except that a single replication of chromosomes is followed by two consecutive cell divisions (meiosis I and meiosis II). These two divisions result in the formation of four haploid daughter cells (rather than the two diploid cells that are the result of mitosis).

The nine steps of meiosis are as follows:

1. **Prophase I:** Similar to mitosis prophase, the chromatids condense, the mitotic spindle forms, and the centromeres move toward opposite sides of the cell. Homologous chromosomes loosely pair and are aligned lengthwise. Homologous chromosomes pair to form bivalents or tetrads. *Bivalent* refers to a pair of homologous chromosomes with two homologous non-sister chromatids. *Tetrad* refers to four sister chromatids.

   Unlike mitosis, where chromosomes line up individually, in meiosis, chromosomes line up in pairs. *Synapsis* is the process through which homologous chromosomes line up to form a tetrad. Between each homologous pair is a protein structure called the *synaptonemal complex*, which holds the pair tightly together. This complex is thought to facilitate pairing, synapsis, and recombination of chromosomes. Points along bivalents (non-sister chromatids) called *chiasmata* are where an exchange of genetic material (DNA) takes place. The exchange is called a *cross-over* or *recombination event*, and DNA is exchanged between the homologous, non-sister chromatids. This recombination event allows for genetic variation in offspring. The synaptonemal complex disassembles in late prophase, and each chromosome pair becomes distinct and visible under a microscope as a tetrad (four chromatids). On each tetrad, the chiasmata regions hold the homologous pairs together until anaphase I. Also during prophase I, there is a breakdown of the nuclear envelope and a dispersal of nucleoli. In late prophase I, the kinetochores of each of the homologous chromatids attaches to microtubules from one pole of the cell.

2. **Metaphase I:** At this phase, the mitotic spindle apparatus is complete, the centromeres are at opposite poles, and the tetrads line up along the metaphase plate of the cell. One chromosome of each pair faces each pole. Both chromatids of a homologous pair are attached to kinetochore microtubules from one pole. The kinetochore of the other homologue is attached to spindles from the opposite pole.

3. **Anaphase I:** The homologous chromosomes (each composed of two sister chromatids) separate and move to opposite poles, guided by the shortening on the microtubules in the spindle apparatus. Sister chromatids remain attached at the centromere and move as a single unit toward the same pole.

4. **Telophase I and Cytokinesis:** At this point, each half of the cell has a complete haploid set of chromosomes, but each chromosome is still composed of two sister chromatids. Cytokinesis occurs simultaneously with telophase I. The result is the formation of two haploid daughter cells.

5. **Interkinesis (Interphase II):** This is the period between the two cell divisions during which partial elongation of DNA takes place. The DNA does not replicate again during interkinesis.

6. **Prophase II:** The DNA condenses again in the two new daughter cells, and the nuclear membranes disintegrate. The mitotic spindle apparatus forms. In late prophase, the chromosomes (still made up of two chromatids) move toward the metaphase II plate.

7. **Metaphase II:** Chromosomes are positioned on the metaphase plate. Because of recombination of DNA during metaphase I, the two sister chromatids of each chromosome are not identical. The centrosomes move toward the poles, and the kinetochores of sister chromatids are attached to microtubules extending from opposite poles.

8. **Anaphase II:** The centromeres of each chromosome separate, and the nonhomologous sister chromatids come apart. The sister chromatids of each chromosome now move to opposite poles.

9. **Telophase II and Cytokinesis:** Two new nuclei form in each cell, and the chromosomes begin decondensing. Cytokinesis occurs at this time, and at the end of this phase, there are four new daughter cells that are genetically distinct from one another. Each unique cell has a haploid set of chromosomes.

Meiosis begins with a diploid mother cell and ends with four unique haploid gametes. The events of meiosis that contribute to genetic diversity in a species, or the mixing of the gene pool between generations, are independent assortment, random fertilization, and DNA recombination. *Independent assortment* is the random way in which homologous chromosomes are oriented on the metaphase plate during metaphase I. The number of possible orientations is 2^n, where n is the number of haploid chromosomes. In humans, the forty-six chromosome pairs have 2^{23}, or 8.4 million, possible orientations. Random fertilization refers to the fact that any of a male's 8.4 million possible genetic combinations may be contained in the sperm that fertilizes the female's ovum, which may also be in any of 8.4 million possible genetic combinations. That results in 70 trillion possible combinations. When crossover events (recombination) are considered along with independent and random assortment, the possible genetic combinations are infinite.

Spermatogenesis and Oogenesis

In males, the process of spermatogenesis occurs in the testes in adult males. *Spermatogenesis* is the production of mature sperm cells. During meiosis, one diploid spermatocyte (cell) creates four haploid spermatids. The first step occurs when a diploid male germ cell increases in size and becomes a primary spermatocyte. The spermatocyte goes through the phases of meiosis and cytokinesis to form four haploid spermatids. Finally, these haploid spermatids differentiate into mature sperm cells (haploids). Cytoplasmic material from the cell becomes the sperm head and around the anterior of the nucleus is an acrosome that contains an enzyme specific for digesting the covering of a female ovum. The tail is a single flagellum, and mitochondria are present to provide energy to the sperm. The primary function of the sperm is to deliver genetic material to the female egg.

Oogenesis, the production of a mature female ovum, occurs in the ovaries of females. At the onset of puberty, one cell is released every month. In the first step of oogenesis, a diploid female germ cell increases in size to become a primary oocyte. This cell undergoes meiosis and proceeds to prophase I. There is an unequal cytoplasmic division during meiosis of an oocyte, and the result is one haploid ovum and three polar bodies (which disintegrate over time). The potential egg gets most of the cytoplasmic material because, if fertilized, it must supply its own nutrients until it is implanted in the uterus about one week after fertilization. Only one functional gamete is produced in each round of oogenesis. Egg fertilization results in the completion of meiosis, where more polar bodies are produced along with the one fertilized egg.

Karyotypes

A *karyotype* is an organized display of the pairs of condensed chromosomes. Knowing an individual's karyotype can help to screen for genetic abnormalities. Somatic cells are isolated from an individual and treated with a drug that stimulates mitosis. The cells are arrested in metaphase when the chromosomes have condensed. Then the chromosomes are stained and viewed in a microscope. A digital picture is taken of the chromosomes, and they are arranged in pairs according to size. Patterns of stained bands help to identify specifics such as defective chromosomes, number of chromosomes, and certain congenital disorders.

Genetic Disorders

Genetic disorders can be detected during pregnancy through amniocentesis or chronic villus sampling. *Amniocentesis* involves extracting amniotic fluid and checking fetal cells for enzyme or protein abnormalities. *Chronic villus sampling* is a process in which the cells that will develop into the placenta are collected and karyotyping and biological testing are performed.

Some genetic disorders are:

- **Aneuploidy:** If there is only one copy of a particular chromosome or there are three copies, the resulting disorder is called *aneuploidy*. Monosomy (one copy of a particular chromosome) and trisomy (three copies) are the two most common types of aneuploidy.

- **Translocation:** DNA from one chromosome breaks away and attaches to a nonhomologous chromosome.

- **Reciprocal translocation:** An exchange of DNA between nonhomologous chromosomes occurs. A reciprocal switch is made between the chromosomes.

- **Nondisjunction:** One cell receives two copies of the same chromosome during meiosis and the other cell receives none. When gametes are formed, two will have two copies of the same chromosome and two will have no copies. Ultimately, after fertilization, the egg will have either one or three copies of a particular chromosome.

- **Duplication error:** One section of a particular chromosome is duplicated. The individual will have three copies of this particular gene segment instead of two.

- **Deletions:** A deletion results in a missing section of a chromosome.

The following is a list of some well-understood genetic disorders:

- **Turner syndrome:** Turner syndrome is an example of monosomy in that there is only one copy of the X chromosome in individuals. In almost 80 percent of cases of Turner Syndrome, it is the sperm that is missing the X chromosome. Individuals are infertile due to lack of ovarian development.

- **Triple X:** Individuals with this syndrome have three X chromosomes in all somatic cells.

- **Klinefelter's syndrome:** This is a trisomy disorder in which the individual has one Y chromosome and two X chromosomes. These individuals are males and tend to develop normally until puberty when they fail to develop secondary sex characteristics. They are infertile.

- **Jacob's syndrome:** This is a trisomy disorder where individuals have two Y and one X chromosome. Most individuals appear normal.

- **Down syndrome:** Down syndrome is also called trisomy 21, and individuals have three copies of chromosome 21. Some symptoms of this disorder are almond-shaped eyes, a thickening of digits, heart defects, and mental retardation.

- **Cri-du-chat syndrome:** This disorder causes an abnormal formation of the larynx and causes a newborn's cry to sound cat-like. This is a very rare syndrome.

- **Fragile X:** Fragile X syndrome is the second most common cause of mental retardation. It is due to a duplication error in the X chromosome.

GENETICS

Our modern understanding of genetics is due to the experiments of Gregor Mendel, a monk living in the nineteenth century. Mendel used a scientific approach to identify two laws of inheritance.

The Law of Segregation

Mendel developed a model to explain the inheritance pattern that he consistently observed in his experiments involving pea plants and their observable traits. There are four concepts that describe his model, one of which is called his *law of segregation*. His first observation was that variations in inherited traits are due to different versions of each type of gene. For example, the gene for flower color in pea plants exists in at least two versions; one for the color purple and one for white. Scientists call these alternative versions of genes *alleles*. Another concept that Mendel described was that for each trait, an organism inherits two alleles; one from each parent. Each somatic cell in an organism has two sets of chromosomes; one from each parent. His third idea was that if two alleles for one trait differ, the dominant allele determines the organism's appearance. The other, recessive, allele has no noticeable effect on the organism's appearance in this case. His fourth observation is known as the law of segregation. It states that two alleles for a specific inheritable character, or trait, separate (segregate) during gamete formation and end up in two different gametes (during meiosis).

The Law of Independent Assortment

The *law of independent assortment* states that each pair of alleles for a specific gene during gamete formation segregates independently of the alleles for another gene. Gene pair segregation is an independent event and occurs in an ordered fashion so that each gamete contains an allele for every gene. An exception to this law is *linked genes*. These are genes that are located close to one another on the same chromosome. These linked genes transfer together as if they were one gene.

The Role of Environment in Gene Expression

The *phenotype*, or set of physical traits, of an organism is determined by both environmental and genetic (genotype) factors. For example, a specific phenotype may be evident only under certain environmental conditions; under other conditions, it may be suppressed. Sometimes, an exact environment is required for the full expression of a gene. For example, without proper nutrition a person may not reach his/her full height potential. The expressivity of a gene is a measure of how fully that gene's traits are expressed. Environmental factors can act to switch a gene on or off.

Genetics Terms to Know

- **Allele:** Alternative forms of a gene; one member of a pair of genes for a particular trait.

- **Autosomal dominant trait:** Trait expressed because there is a dominant allele of an autosomal gene present on one homologous chromosome in a pair. Autosomal dominant genes are always expressed.

- **Codominance:** Heterozygous state in which both alleles of a specific gene are expressed phenotypically.

- **Dominant:** A gene that is favorably expressed phenotypically in heterozygous or homozygous individuals.

- **Frameshift mutation:** A deletion or insertion of a DNA nucleotide that changes the codons in the mRNA. The result is that a different polypeptide chain is translated from the mRNA strand.

- **Gene:** Sequence of DNA that codes for a specific hereditary trait. Each gene is located at a specific point on a specific chromosome.

- **Genotype:** Genetic make-up of an organism.

- **Heterozygous:** Condition in which there are two different alleles for the same gene on homologous chromosomes.

- **Homozygous:** Condition in which there are two identical alleles for a gene on each of the homologous chromosomes.

- **Incomplete dominance:** Heterozygous state in which both alleles of a particular gene are partially expressed, or are blended together. This characteristic can result in an intermediate phenotype.

- **Loci:** Location of a gene on a chromosome. Determining the loci helps locate the chromosome on which a gene is located, whether the gene is on a long or short arm of the chromosome, and the location on the arm. The specific location on the arm can be determined by staining the chromosome and determining its banding pattern.

- **Multiple alleles:** More than two possible contrasting alleles for a particular gene; for example, blood types are determined by three different alleles, A, B, and O.

- **Mutagen:** Agents that can alter genetic material, causing an increase in the number of mutations a DNA sequence has.

- **Mutation:** Changes in the DNA base sequence of a gene. Mutations can be caused by errors during cell division, exposure to radiation, chemical mutagens, and viruses. Mutations can be either harmful or beneficial to an organism.

- **Phenotype:** Observable physical traits of an organism.

- **Point mutation:** One nucleotide on the DNA strand is changed to another, which causes a different amino acid to be synthesized in that position (only one mRNA codon is changed). A point mutation can result in a *silent mutation* (the change still results in an alternate codon for the same amino acid), in a *missense mutation* in which the mutation changes the amino acid codon and that changes the resulting protein structure, and in a *nonsense mutation* in which the mutation causes a stop codon to be put in the wrong place, which results in a shortened polypeptide chain that produces an incomplete protein.

- **Recessive:** Describes a gene that is not expressed phenotypically unless there are two copies of the same allele.

- **X-linked dominant trait:** Trait caused by the presence of a dominant mutant gene on an X chromosome. Both males and females will acquire the trait with only one copy of the mutant allele.

- **X-linked recessive trait:** Trait caused by a recessive mutant gene located on the X chromosome. For females, two copies of alleles specific for the recessive trait must be present, but in males only one copy is possible (because there is only one X chromosome).

The Laws of Probability and Genetics

Mendel's laws of segregation and independent assortment reflect the rules of probability. Thus, the laws of probability are used to determine the distribution of hereditary traits. One tool that biologists use to determine the probability of inheriting a specific combination of alleles of a gene is the *Punnett square*. The Punnett square shows all of the possible combinations of alleles in offspring that result in the cross of genetic material from two individuals (parents). The percentage, or probability, of each combination can also be determined. The most common combination of alleles in a population of a given organism is called the *wild type allele*. Some alleles of a gene are dominant and are represented in a Punnett square by a single capital letter. Other alleles are recessive (only expressed if two copies are present in offspring), and they are represented by a single lower case letter. If only one trait is being analyzed, then the Punnett Square only needs to include alleles for that one trait. This is called a *monohybrid cross*. The parent generation in a cross is referred to as P, and the offspring are referred to as F_1 (first generation). Subsequent generations are labeled F_2, F_3, and so on.

In order to construct a Punnett square, it is necessary to know all the possible female gametes and all the possible male gametes. The genotypes of the parents must be known. Mendel referred to individuals that were homozygous for either the dominant or the recessive trait as *true breeding varieties*. If a parent who was homozygous for the dominant allele of a gene was bred with a parent who was homozygous for a recessive allele, 100 percent of all the offspring would be heterozygous and express the dominant trait as shown by the genotypes represented in the Punnett square below. The term *monohybrid* describes individuals who are heterozygous for one trait.

Figure 14. Punnett Square Representing a Cross Between a Homozygous Dominant Individual and a Homozygous Recessive Individual

	B	B
b	Bb	Bb
b	Bb	Bb

The mating of two heterozygous individuals is called a *monohybrid cross*. In this type of cross, 75 percent of the offspring would show the dominant trait, and 25 percent would be homozygous for the recessive trait and would show that trait. Note also that 25 percent of the offspring would be homozygous dominant, and 50 percent would be heterozygous dominant.

Figure 15. Punnett Square Representing a Cross Between Two Heterozygous Individuals

	B	b
B	BB	Bb
b	Bb	bb

The phenotypic ratio of the above cross is 3:1, and the genotypic ratio is 1:2:1 (homozygous dominant:heterozygous:homozygous recessive).

A Punnett square can also be used to predict the genotypes and phenotypes of two different traits. This type of cross was done by Mendel to identify the law of independent assortment. The traits that Mendel tested in pea plants were seed color (yellow, Y, or green, y) and shape (round, R, or wrinkled, r). In this cross, the two traits are independent of one another.

Figure 16. Punnett Square Showing a Cross Monitoring Two Different Traits in Each Parent

	YR	Yr	yR	yr
YR	YYRR	YYRr	YyRR	YyRr
Yr	YYRr	YYrr	YyRr	Yyrr
yR	YyRR	YyRr	yyRR	yyRr
yr	YyRr	Yyrr	yyRr	yyrr

The phenotypic ratio of the offspring from this cross is 9:3:3:1 (yellow and round:green and round:yellow and wrinkled:green and wrinkled).

The examples above show complete dominance of one allele over another. In cases of incomplete dominance, an alternate phenotype is created by the blending of alleles. For example, if a cross is made between two flowers of the same species, but which have different colors, a blended phenotype is the result. If a white flower, W, is crossed with a red flower, R, the result is that 100 percent of the offspring will be a blend, WR, and will have a pink phenotype. When two of the F_1 offspring (WR) are crossed, the result is a 1:2:1 phenotypic ratio (white:pink:red).

In the case of codominance, two different alleles of a gene are expressed phenotypically. A good example of codominance is blood type in humans. In the cross below, a capital I represents the dominant alleles for types A and B blood, and a lower-case i represents the recessive allele for type O blood. The codominant blood type is AB, and if a heterozygous type A female (I^Ai) is crossed with a heterozygous type B male (I^Bi), the result is 25 percent codominant phenotype type AB:25 percent heterozygous type A:25 percent heterozygous type B:25 percent homozygous recessive type O.

Figure 17. Punnett Square Showing an Example of Codominance

	I^A	i
I^B	I^AI^B	I^Bi
i	I^Ai	ii

In the case of characteristics of disease, traits can be described as being *autosomal dominant* or *autosomal recessive*. In the case of autosomal dominant traits, an individual needs only one copy of the dominant allele for a disease to show the phenotype of that allele. An example of an autosomal dominant disorder is caused by the Rh factor. RH+ is dominant, and Rh– is recessive. Both a homozygous individual (RH+, RH+) and a heterozygous individual (RH+, Rh–) express the RH+ dominant phenotype, and only individuals that are homozygous recessive (Rh–, Rh–) express the recessive Rh– phenotype.

Tay-Sachs disease is an example of an autosomal recessive trait. This is a fatal inherited disease that affects infants at about six months. In these individuals, a crucial enzyme in the brain cannot function to break down lipids, and the result is seizures, blindness, and degeneration of motor and mental performance. Only children who inherit two copies of the Tay-Sachs allele will express the disease. However, individuals with only one copy of the allele will express an intermediate phenotype.

An individual who has only one allele for a particular trait and, therefore, does not express the phenotype of that allele is said to be a *carrier* of that trait. There are many tests in place to detect carriers of certain genetic disorders.

Inheritance Patterns

Inheritance patterns are often much more complex than those dictated by simple Mendelian genetics. Often, a single gene can affect more than one trait.

Pleiotropy

Pleiotropy is the property of a gene in which it affects multiple phenotypes. Pleiotropic alleles of a gene are responsible for the multiple symptoms associated with certain hereditary disease such as cystic fibrosis and sickle cell disease. In individuals with cystic fibrosis, a mutation in the CTFR gene causes multiple symptoms because CTFR codes for a channel protein required for chloride ion channels in cell membranes. A defect in these channels causes an imbalance of water in tissue and organs and creates a problem of too much thick mucus. Cystic fibrosis is an autosomal recessive trait, so both parents need to contribute a mutant allele for the disease to be expressed.

Epistasis

In inheritance patterns involving *epistasis*, a gene at one locus on the chromosome alters the phenotypic expression of a gene at a different locus. Even though the genes are on different loci, they may be tightly linked. An example of epistasis that can be studied in mice is albinism. In mice, the allele for a black coat color is dominant and for a brown coat is recessive. However, there is another gene that determines whether or not the coat color pigment is deposited in the hair. The dominant allele is for deposition of color into the hair, and the recessive allele is for no coat color. Thus, individuals that are homozygous recessive for the deposition gene will have no coat color in their hair. These mice will be white (albino) mice. The gene for pigment deposition is said to be *epistatic* to the gene for pigment. The gene whose phenotype is masked is said to be *hypostatic*.

Polygenic Inheritance

Some traits such as human skin color vary in a population in a gradient fashion. There are many variations of the color of human skin, and this is characterized as a quantitative character. This type of variation indicates what is known as *polygenic inheritance*, which is an effect of multiple genes acting to express one phenotypic trait. Skin color, height, weight, and body shape are all traits that are controlled by multiple genes, and are common examples of polygenic inheritance.

Pedigree Analysis

Because it is unethical for geneticists to manipulate the mating patterns of humans, they study mating patterns that have already occurred. They can do this by collecting a family's genetic history with respect to a particular trait of interest. The information is assembled into a family tree, so that scientists can look for inheritance patterns. This compilation of a family's genetic history is called a *pedigree*. Pedigrees are useful in families with a history of a genetic disorder. The pedigree can help predict the outcome of future generations with respect to disease.

EVOLUTION

Evolution can be described as a change over a time in the genetic makeup of an individual population. Eventually, a population may change significantly enough that a new species is formed. On a grand scale, evolution has come to mean the gradual appearance of biological diversity from early microbial species to the vast diversity of organisms on Earth today.

Throughout evolution, mutations in genes are a method of change and modification in a species. *Microevolution* refers to a change in gene frequency within the population of a given organism in a given location. It can take only one generation for microevolution to occur, or it may take several generations. For example, fungi and insects can develop a resistance to pesticides in only one generation, but changes in higher organisms such as mammals and birds may take several generations. *Macroevolution* occurs over a much longer time frame, but the same principles of microevolution apply to macroevolution. However, macroevolution refers to the accumulation of small population-wide changes over the period of millions of years. This causes changes in a species on a more extensive scale. Macroevolution focuses on changes that occur in the family, order, and class of an organism. Fossil records can be used to study the history of macroevolution.

Stasis refers to the lack of change in a species over a long period of time. Some lineages of a species exhibit stasis for such a long period that they are referred to as "living fossils." They give evolutionary biologists a look into the past. *Character change* refers to a change in a species that happens in one direction. For example, the addition of a body segment in trilobites is a character change. *Speciation*, or lineage splitting, refers to the appearance of a new species after many generations of change. *Extinction* is the disappearance of an individual species or an entire lineage of an organism. Extinction is often due to changes in environmental factors. *Gene flow* refers to the migration of the individuals of one population to another population.

Natural Selection

Changes in a species are due to natural selection. *Natural selection* refers to Charles Darwin's theory of evolution that states that a population can change over generations if individuals with heritable traits that are better adapted to their environment survive and reproduce more frequently than other individuals of the same population. A particular gene or set of genes is passed on to offspring because the parent is able to survive its environment. Individuals who do not possess a desired trait may not survive or reproduce, and, therefore, their genes will not be passed on to offspring. Allele frequencies can fluctuate from one generation to the next. This is called *genetic drift* and can also be a factor in natural selection. Natural selection can enhance or diminish only heritable traits from one generation to the next. Thus, natural selection is a form of biological editing.

Darwin published his theory in *The Origin of the Species*, which expresses two main ideas: evolution explains the diversity and unity seen throughout the natural world, and natural selection is the cause of adaptive evolution.

Adaptation

Adaptations that organism may make to their environment are not necessarily inheritable traits and are not attributed to natural selection. However, those that are inheritable increase the fitness (survivability) of an individual so that it will survive and reproduce. An organism with a greater degree of fitness will pass on its genes more frequently. Certain adaptations of a species are specific for their environment, and, therefore, there are different phenotypic traits of similar organisms depending on where they live. For example, hares that live in the desert have longer ears than those that live in the Arctic. In the desert, the greater ear surface area helps to keep the animal cooler because more body heat can be released through the ear. In the Arctic, it is beneficial for the hare to have shorter ears so that less body heat escapes. Therefore, hares with shorter ears survived better and reproduced in the Arctic, and hares with longer ears survived better and reproduced in the desert.

Fitness of an individual is also dependent upon that individual's ability to outcompete others of the same organisms for food, water, shelter, and other natural resources. Individuals with the best reproduction rate and outcome will perpetuate their phenotypic traits. These individuals make a genetic contribution to the existing gene pool of a population when they reproduce. Emigration away from a population can diminish the gene flow and genetic variation, and immigration into a population can increase it.

The Hardy-Weinberg Theorem

The *Hardy-Weinberg theorem* is named for the two scientists who independently described the same principle in 1908. The theorem states: The frequency of alleles and genotypes within a population remains relatively constant from one generation to the next, unless the factors of evolution interfere. It describes how Mendelian genetics preserves genetic variation in species that are not evolving, but it also lays the foundation for understanding how long-term evolutionary changes occur.

If a population has individuals that donate alleles to the next generation at random and also mate at random, the population will have the same allele frequency from one generation to the next. The genotype frequencies of a generation can be predicted from allele frequencies. A population in this state is said to be in a state of *Hardy-Weinberg equilibrium*.

The Hardy-Weinberg theorem describes a hypothetical population that is not evolving. In nature, there are always intervening evolutionary factors, and allele frequencies and genotypes of a population do change over time. Other factors include nonrandom mating, restricted population size, and meiotic drive. *Meiotic drive* refers to the over-expression of certain alleles in gametes during meiosis. Because the rate of evolution is so slow, it is possible to use the Hardy-Weinberg theorem to approximate allele and genotype frequencies.

Two other effects that invalidate the Hardy-Weinberg theorem with respect to evolution are the *bottleneck effect* and the *founder effect*. Both of these effects are variations on the idea of genetic drift. The bottleneck effect is due to a drastic change in environment that greatly reduces the size of a population (forest fire, flood, human activity). After a drastic reduction in populations, there are a few survivors, and the gene pool is no longer representative of the original population. These few survivors are said to have passed through a hypothetical "bottleneck." According to chance, some alleles may be underrepresented in the gene pool, and others may be overrepresented. Others still may be completely eliminated. This can result in a large loss of variation within a species for several generations.

The founder effect is seen when a few individuals become isolated from a larger population. This smaller population may develop a gene pool that is less variable than that of the larger population. When a new population is formed with few individuals, the allele frequency is lower than its parent population. A small population size also causes a higher frequency of inbreeding, which leads to less genetic variation. The founder effect is what accounts for the high level of genetic disorders among isolated populations where inbreeding is likely to occur.

Adaptive Evolution and Natural Selection

Of all the possible factors that influence a gene pool, natural selection is likely the only one that will help a population adapt to its environment. Within any population, there are a variety of traits and reproduction rates. Therefore, not all individuals in a population reproduce to the extent they are capable. Advantageous traits that allow certain individuals to reproduce with a higher frequency than others will be passed to future generations. Trait variety, differential reproduction, and heredity are components of evolution attributed to natural selection.

Having two phenotypes for a particular trait is referred to as *dimorphism. Phenotypic polymorphism* refers to having two or more high-frequency morphs (or characteristics). A characteristic like height is due to genetic polymorphisms for alleles at several loci. The number of polymorphisms within a population is measured by determining the heterozygosity at the genetic and molecular level of an organism. Nucleotide variability is measured by determining the percent difference in the nucleotide sequence from one individual in a population to another. In general, the average heterozygosity of a population tends to be greater than the nucleotide variability because a gene consists of thousands of nucleotides. A difference of only one nucleotide is sometimes sufficient to create two different alleles of a gene.

The contribution an individual makes to a gene pool is described as *fitness*. In order to quantify this value, population geneticists define relative fitness as the contribution of a specific genotype to the

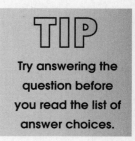

TIP

Try answering the question before you read the list of answer choices.

next generation compared to the contribution of alternate genotypes at the same chromosomal loci. However, because natural selection acts on phenotype and not genotype, the relative fitness of a particular allele depends on the entire genetic and environmental context in which it is expressed.

Natural selection can favor the extremes of a dominant or recessive phenotype, or it can favor the intermediate phenotype. When a beneficial allele is passed on at a higher-than-expected ratio, this is called *directional selection*. *Stabilizing selection* favors an intermediate phenotype. This will diminish genetic variation in an attempt to promote stability. *Disruptive selection* favors the extreme phenotypes rather than the intermediate. This method of selection increases genetic variation and may cause the division of a species into two species. Directional selection is most common when there is an environmental change or when there is a migration of a population to a new environment. This type of selection shifts the phenotypic character in a population by favoring individuals that deviate from the average.

Genetic Variation

The tendency of directional and stabilizing selection to reduce genetic variability is countered by other mechanisms that aim to preserve it. Because most eukaryotes are diploid (two copies of each chromosome), there is variability due to recessive alleles. Recessive alleles can persist because they are propagated in heterozygous individuals. This latent variation is only exposed to natural selection when an individual is homozygous for a recessive trait. A homozygous recessive individual occurs less frequently in a population than a heterozygous individual.

In some cases, selection itself can preserve genetic variability. *Balancing selection* occurs when natural selection maintains stable frequencies of two or more phenotypic traits in a population. This type of selection includes the advantage of heterozygotes and frequency-dependent selection. Heterozygote advantage refers to the fact that individuals that are heterozygous for a certain allele display a greater relative fitness than those who are homozygous for the same allele. *Frequency-dependent selection* refers to the fact that the fitness of any one morph (characteristic) tends to decline if it becomes too common within a population. Variation within a population that has little or no effect on reproductive success and natural selection is considered *neutral selection*. Another type of selection, *sexual selection*, is a natural selection for mating success. *Intrasexual selection* is a direct competition for survival and reproduction between individuals of the same sex. This occurs more frequently in males than in females. *Intersexual selection* refers to the fact that an individual of one sex (usually female) is choosy about selecting a mate.

Biological Support of Evolution

The following provide supporting evidence for the existence of evolution in nature:

- **Biogeography:** The distribution of species throughout history and geographical areas gives evidence supporting evolution. Fossil history and molecular biology are used to map evolution and the migration of species after the continents split apart.

- **Fossils:** Fossils are traces of previously existing organisms that provide evidence that changes have occurred within a particular type of organism or species. Differences have emerged over long time periods and have been documented. Fossils also reveal similarities in species.

- **Homologies:** These are structures that are anatomically alike but differ functionally. These species have shared ancestry. DNA sequence homology can indicate common ancestry and function.

- **Homoplasies:** These are structures that are similar but have a different origin. Homoplasies give evidence of convergent evolution.

- **Molecular biology:** This field of biology is used to compare nucleotide sequences in DNA and RNA and amino acid sequences in proteins of different organisms. The more similar nucleic acids and proteins are among different species, the more evidence that they are related. Examining the differences can help tell how much time has elapsed since the two species diverged.

- **Vestigial traits:** These are rudimentary structures that no longer exhibit any functionality. They may be closely related to similar yet functional structures in another species.

PRACTICE QUESTIONS

Directions: Choose the best answer for each question.

Refer to the following passage for Questions 1–5.

Tay-Sachs disease is an inherited disorder in humans affecting 1 in 3600 births in Ashkenazic Jews, about 100 times greater than the incidence in non-Jews. Affected individuals have a single faulty enzyme, gangliosidase, that is found in the brain cells of Tay-Sachs patients. As a result, the brain cells of an affected baby are unable to break down gangliosides, a type of lipid. Ganglioside buildup causes a gradual decrease in brain cell function that ultimately results in death within a few years. Symptoms are seen within a few months of birth and include seizures, blindness, and degeneration of motor and mental performance. There is no known cure.

1. Which of the following eukaryotic organelles is responsible for producing gangliosidase?
   A. Golgi apparatus
   B. Mitochondria
   C. Ribosomes
   D. Peroxisomes

2. Which of the following eukaryotic organelles is responsible for producing gangliosides?
   A. Smooth ER
   B. Rough ER
   C. Vacuoles
   D. Lysosomes

3. Gangliosidase catalyzes its reaction by
   A. increasing the substrate concentration.
   B. changing the reactants in the reaction.
   C. lowering the activation energy barrier of the reaction.
   D. increasing the activation energy of the reaction.

4. Which eukaryotic cellular organelle is the cause of the ganglioside buildup that is characteristic of Tay-Sachs disease patients?
   A. Centrioles
   B. Lysosomes
   C. Nucleolus
   D. Smooth ER

5. The substrate of gangliosidase bind to the active site of the enzyme through
   A. strong covalent bonds.
   B. weak bonding interactions.
   C. ionic bonding.
   D. double bonds.

Refer to the following passage for Questions 6–10.

Mitosis and meiosis are both processes that begin in humans with diploid cells, but the daughter cells produced in each process are quite different from one another. Meiosis also has nearly twice as many steps as mitosis, and while many of these steps mirror steps of mitosis, the increased complexity leads to more variable daughter cells with regard to chromosomes.

6. During which phase of mitosis do new nuclear membranes form around the two new sets of chromosomes?
   A. Metaphase
   B. Prophase
   C. Telophase
   D. Anaphase

7. The process of meiosis in which homologous chromosomes line up and form a tetrad is
   A. anaphase.
   B. synapsis.
   C. chiasmata.
   D. interkinesis.

8. Crossing over may occur during
   A. prophase of mitosis.
   B. prophase I of meiosis.
   C. metaphase of mitosis.
   D. metaphase I of meiosis.

9. Nondisjunction can occur during
   A. mitosis only.
   B. meiosis only.
   C. either mitosis or meiosis.
   D. neither mitosis nor meiosis.

10. Mendel's law of segregation states that
    A. the dominant allele determines an organism's appearance.
    B. the two alleles for a specific inheritable trait separate during meiosis.
    C. variations in inheritable traits are due to different alleles for each gene.
    D. alleles for one gene segregate independently from alleles for another gene.

Refer to the following passage for Questions 11–14.

Based on their chemical equations, cellular respiration and photosynthesis simply look like opposite processes, but with regard to cellular processes, the processes are much more complex. The inputs of cellular respiration are essentially the outputs of respiration, and vice versa, but the processes occur in completely different organelles within cells, and involve dramatically different steps.

11. In which stage of photosynthesis is glucose formed?
    A. Light reactions
    B. Citric acid cycle
    C. Calvin cycle
    D. Photophosphorylation

12. Which of the following eukaryotic organelles is responsible for the production of ATP in cells?
    A. Golgi apparatus
    B. Mitochondria
    C. Ribosomes
    D. Peroxisomes

13. The final products of glycolysis are
    A. two pyruvate, two ATP, and two NADH.
    B. six carbon dioxide, six water , and thirty-six ATP.
    C. two ATP, six NADH, two $FADH_2$, and four CO_2.
    D. glucose, six oxygen, and six water.

14. The light-dependent reactions of photosynthesis occur in the _____, while the Calvin cycle occurs in the _____.
    A. stroma; thylakoid membrane
    B. thylakoid membrane; stroma
    C. stomata; thylakoid membrane
    D. thylakoid membrane; stomata

Refer to the following passage for Questions 15–17.

The three domains of life are Eukarya, Eubacteria, and Archaebacteria. Eukarya consists of all eukaryotic organisms, both unicellular and multicellular. Eubacteria consist of non-extremophile bacteria, while Archaebacteria primarily include extremophile bacteria. Traditionally, there are six taxonomic kingdoms, of which Eubacteria and Archaebacteria are two. The other four kingdoms all fall under the Eukarya header.

15. The order of taxonomic ranks in the classification of species is
    A. kingdom, domain, phylum, class, order, family, genus, species.
    B. kingdom, domain, order, phylum, class, family, genus, species.
    C. phylum, order, domain, kingdom, class, family genus, species.
    D. domain, kingdom, phylum, class, order, family, genus, species.

16. Which of the following kingdoms consist of only prokaryotic organisms?

   A. Bacteria and Archaea

   B. Anamalia and Fungi

   C. Protista and Anamalia

   D. Plantae and Archaea

17. Under which domain does the protist *Euglena* fall?

   A. Eukarya

   B. Eubacteria

   C. Archaebacteria

   D. none of these

Refer to the following passage for Questions 18–20.

Polymerases are enzymes involved in several different functions, specifically replication and transcription. The suffix "-*ase*" designates polymerases as enzymes, while the rest of the name indicates that its role in each process is to generate a polymer. While translation also produces an amino acid polymer, polymerase is not involved in this particular process.

18. Which enzyme is required to unwind a DNA double helix during replication?

   A. DNA polymerase

   B. DNA topoisomerase

   C. DNA single-strand binding protein

   D. DNA helicase

19. During RNA transcription, RNA is always synthesized in which direction?

   A. Reverse

   B. 3′ to 5′

   C. 5′ to 3′

   D. Top to bottom

20. During which phase of protein synthesis does the large 60S ribosomal subunit attach to mRNA?

   A. Elongation

   B. Termination

   C. Initiation

   D. Translation

ANSWER KEY AND EXPLANATIONS

1. C	**5.** B	**9.** C	**13.** A	**17.** B
2. A	**6.** C	**10.** B	**14.** B	**18.** D
3. C	**7.** B	**11.** C	**15.** D	**19.** C
4. B	**8.** B	**12.** B	**16.** A	**20.** C

1. **The correct answer is C.** Gangliodase is an enzyme, and ribosomes are responsible for creating protein and enzyme synthesis. Choice A is incorrect because the Golgi apparatus acts as the center for modifying, storing, and transporting proteins leaving the ER. Choice B is incorrect because the mitochondria is the organelle that regulates cell metabolism. Choice D is incorrect because the main function of peroxisomes is to break down fatty acids.

2. **The correct answer is A.** The smooth ER synthesizes lipids. Choice B is incorrect because the rough ER houses ribosomes and modifies proteins. Choice C is incorrect because vacuoles store water, nutrients, or wastes, primarily in plant cells. Choice D is incorrect because lysosomes break down unneeded materials in the cell.

3. **The correct answer is C.** Enzymes lower the activation energy by interacting with one or more substrates in a reaction using a variety of mechanism. Choice A is incorrect because enzymes do not affect the substrate concentration. Choice B is incorrect because enzymes bind to a substrate in a reaction, but they do not alter the reactants. Choice D is incorrect because enzymes lower the activation energy of a reaction.

4. **The correct answer is B.** Lysosomes break down unneeded waste products like lipids. Choice A is incorrect because centrioles are involved in animal cell division. Choice C is incorrect because the nucleolus synthesizes

RNA and helps make ribosomes. Choice D is incorrect because the smooth ER produces lipids.

5. **The correct answer is B.** In an enzymatic reaction, the substrate is generally bound to the enzyme's active site by weak interactions such as hydrogen bonding. Choice A is incorrect because a substrate generally binds to an enzyme's active site through a weak bonding interaction, not a strong covalent bond. Choice C is incorrect because a substrate generally binds to an enzyme's active site through a weak bonding interaction, not an ionic bond. Choice D is incorrect because a substrate generally binds to an enzyme's active site through a weak bonding interaction, not a strong double bond.

6. **The correct answer is C.** During the final phase of mitosis, the telophase, the daughter chromosomes reach the centrosomes at opposite poles of the cell, and two daughter nuclei begin to form. Choice A is incorrect because during metaphase, the centrosomes are at opposite sides of the cell and the chromosomes are lined up along the metaphase plate. Choice B is incorrect because the nucleolus disappears during prophase and the chromatin becomes more condensed. Choice D is incorrect because during anaphase, the sister chromatid in each pair separates.

7. **The correct answer is B.** Synapsis is the process through which homologous chromosomes line up to form a tetrad. Choice

A is incorrect because during anaphase, homologous chromosomes separate and move to opposite poles in the cell. Choice C is incorrect because chiasmata are points along chromatids where an exchange of genetic material takes place. Choice D is incorrect because interkinesis is the period between the two cell divisions during which partial elongation of DNA takes place.

8. **The correct answer is B.** Prophase I is the only point during meiosis at which crossing over, the exchange of genetic material between homologous chromosomes, may occur. Choice A and choice C are incorrect because crossing over does not occur during mitosis. Choice D is incorrect because it is prophase, not metaphase, during which crossing over takes place.

9. **The correct answer is C.** Nondisjunction occurs in cell division when chromosomes fail to properly divide. Since chromosomal separations occur in both mitosis and meiosis, nondisjunction can potentially happen in either, resulting in daughter cells with improper numbers of chromosomes. Choices A, B, and D are incorrect for the same reason.

10. **The correct answer is B.** The law of segregation states that two alleles for a specific inheritable character, or trait, separate (segregate) during gamete formation and end up in two different gametes (during meiosis). Choice A is incorrect because the observation that Mendel made about the dominant allele determining an organism's traits is not part of the law of segregation. Choice C is incorrect because Mendel's first observation was that variations in inherited traits are due to different versions of each type of gene, but that is not the law of segregation. Choice D is incorrect because the law of independent assortment, not segregation, states that each pair of alleles for a specific gene segregates independently of the alleles for another gene during gamete formation.

11. **The correct answer is C.** Glucose is formed in the second stage of photosynthesis, which is the Calvin cycle. Choice A is incorrect because light reactions involve the steps that convert light energy into chemical energy. Choice B is incorrect because the citric acid cycle, or Krebs cycle, is part of cellular respiration, not photosynthesis. Choice D is incorrect because photophosphorylation involves the reduction of $NADP^+$ to NADPH and the generation of ATP using chemiosmosis to drive the addition of a phosphate group to ADP.

12. **The correct answer is B.** Mitochondria are responsible for generating ATP in eukaryotic cells and are often called the "powerhouse" of the cell. Choice A is incorrect because the Golgi acts as the center for modifying, storing, and transporting proteins leaving the ER. Choice C is incorrect because ribosomes are the organelles in which protein synthesis takes place. Choice D is incorrect because the main function of peroxisomes is to break down fatty acids.

13. **The correct answer is A.** In the process of glycolysis, steps 6 to 10 occur twice for each glucose molecule so that the final yield is two pyruvate molecules, two ATP, and two NADH. Choice B is incorrect because those products represent the overall equation for cellular respiration, including all of the steps in glycolysis, the citric acid cycle, and oxidative phosphorylation. Choice C is incorrect because the final products of the Krebs cycle are two ATP molecules, six NADH, two $FADH_2$, and four CO_2 molecules. Choice D is incorrect because glucose, oxygen, and water are the major products of photosynthesis.

14. **The correct answer is B.** The thylakoids contain the chlorophyll excited by light

during the light-dependent reactions of photosynthesis. The light-dependent reactions produced NADPH and ATP that are used in the stroma of the chloroplasts by the Calvin cycle. Choice A is incorrect because the locations are swapped. Choices C and D confuse the word "stomata" with the word "stroma"; while they look alike, stomata are the plant leaf pores that allow gases in and out of the plant leaf cells.

15. **The correct answer is D.** The taxonomic classification system organizes organisms into domain, kingdom, phylum, class, order, family, genus, species, and sometimes subspecies. Choices A, B, and C are incorrect because they list an incorrect order of classifications.

16. **The correct answer is A.** Bacteria and Archaea both consist of prokaryotes, most of which are unicellular, microscopic organisms. Choice B is incorrect because Animalia and Fungi consist of eukaryotic organisms. Choice C is incorrect because Protista and Anamalia consist of eukaryotic organisms. Choice D is incorrect because the kingdom Plantae consists of eukaryotic organisms.

17. **The correct answer is B.** Protists are eukaryotes, not prokaryotes, so they are categorized as Eukarya. Because Euglena, as protists, are eukaryotes, Choices B and C are incorrect because they categorize prokaryotes. Choice D is incorrect because Euglena are indeed eukaryotes and are categorized as Eukarya.

18. **The correct answer is D.** The enzyme responsible for catalyzing the reaction involved in unwinding double-stranded DNA during replication is called DNA helicase. Choice A is incorrect because DNA polymerases are responsible for synthesizing a complementary DNA strand during replication. Choice B is incorrect because topoisomerase catalyzes a reaction that causes gaps in the DNA to alleviate the strain the unwinding causes on the helical DNA structure. Topoisomerase breaks the DNA and then joins it back together. Choice C is incorrect because the single-strand DNA binding proteins are not enzymes, but small proteins that bind to DNA and prevent the two complementary strands from rejoining.

19. **The correct answer is C.** mRNA can only be transcribed from a DNA template in the 5′ to 3′ direction, so choices A, B, and D are incorrect.

20. **The correct answer is C.** Both the 40S and 60S ribosomal subunits attach to mRNA during the initiation phase of protein synthesis. Once the initiator tRNA (met-tRNA) occupies the P site, the large 60S ribosomal subunit attaches, which makes a complete initiation complex. Choices A and B are incorrect because the ribosomal subunits bind to mRNA during initiation. Choice D is incorrect because *translation* refers to the overall process of protein synthesis, not an individual phase of it.

SUMMING IT UP

- All biological organisms are classified, or organized, according to the rules of taxonomy.

- The hierarchical order of taxonomy is domain, kingdom, phylum, class, order, family, genus, species, and sometimes subspecies.

- Cell theory states: all living organisms are composed of at least one cell, the cell is the smallest biological unit that has the characteristics of a living organism, cells contain hereditary information, and organisms of similar species have similar cell types.

- There are two general types of cells: *prokaryotic* cells (bacteria and archaea) and *eukaryotic* cells. Prokaryotic cells have six structures and no nucleus. Eukaryotic cells have a nucleus and distinct organelles.

- The *cell membrane* is a selective barrier that allows for the transport of certain molecules into and out of the cell. It is composed of a lipid bilayer.

- The *cytoskeleton* and *cytosol* are elements that provide structure to the cell.

- The *nucleus* contains all the genetic material of the cell.

- The *ribosomes* are organelles that carry out protein synthesis.

- The *endoplasmic reticulum* (ER) is important for protein and lipid synthesis.

- The *Golgi apparatus* is important for modifying, storing, and transporting proteins that have left the ER.

- *Lysosomes* are membrane sacs containing hydrolytic enzymes that digest macromolecules in the cell.

- *Mitochondria* are responsible for generating ATP (adenosine triphosphate) that provides all organisms with energy.

- *Peroxisomes* are specialized metabolic compartments within a cell that are bound by a single membrane. The main function of peroxisomes is to break down fatty acids.

- *Enzymes* are proteins that speed up metabolic reactions by lowering the activation energy barrier without affecting the overall free energy of the reaction.

- Enzyme activity is influenced by its cellular environment.

- Once the substrate recognizes and binds to the active site, the enzyme changes its shape and is able to wrap around, or embrace, the substrate. This is known as an *induced fit*.

- Some enzymes require a molecule called a *cofactor* to lower the activation energy of a reaction. Organic cofactors are called *coenzymes*, and inorganic cofactors are often metal atoms.

- Inhibitors that bind reversibly to the enzyme through weak bonding are known as *competitive inhibitors*.

- *Noncompetitive inhibitors* bind to a different site on the enzyme known as an *allosteric site* and act to change the enzyme's shape so that the substrate can no longer fit into the active site.

- In *feedback inhibition*, a metabolic pathway is switched off by the binding of a product of that pathway to an enzyme that is required in the initial step of the pathway.

- There are two general types of energy: kinetic and potential.

- The *first law of thermodynamics* states that energy cannot be created or destroyed.

- The *second law of thermodynamics* states that during every energy conversion or transfer, some energy becomes unavailable to do work.

- *Free energy* measures the portion of energy in a system that is available to perform work at a given temperature and pressure.

- The overall change in free energy of a system at a given temperature is determined by the equation: $\Delta G = \Delta H - T\Delta S$.

- Processes that have a negative ΔG value will occur spontaneously.

- Adenosine triphosphate, or ATP, is the molecule that is responsible for providing cellular energy in most cases.

- Each step in a metabolic pathway is catalyzed by a specific enzyme.

- *Catabolic pathways* release energy by breaking down complex molecules into more simple molecules.

- *Anabolic* or *biosynthetic pathways* require an input of energy to build complicated molecules from more simple ones.

- The overall process of aerobic cellular respiration can be summarized as follows: $C_6H_{12}O_6 + 6\ O_2 \rightarrow 6\ CO_2 + 6\ H_2O + (36\ \text{or}\ 38)\ ATP$. The function of this reaction is to release the energy stored in the glucose.

- Aerobic cellular respiration can be divided into three steps: glycolysis, the Krebs cycle (citric acid cycle), and oxidative phosphorylation.

- The final yield of glycolysis is two pyruvate molecules, two ATP, and two NADH.

- The overall reaction of the Krebs cycle is acetyl CoA + 3 NAD^+ + FAD + GDP + P_i + 3 H_2O → CoA-SH + 3 NADH + H^+ + $FADH_2$ + GTP + 2 CO_2 + 3 H^+.

- The electron transport chain, or ETS, essential for oxidative phosphorylation is a collection of membrane-bound molecules in the inner membrane of the mitochondrion.

- The major products of the photosynthesis reaction are glucose, $C_6H_{12}O_6$, and oxygen gas, O_2, which is a waste product of the reaction.

- *Photosynthesis* is actually two processes, each with multiple steps. The first process is known as *light reactions* and the second process is known as the *Calvin cycle*.

- A *nucleotide* is composed of three parts: nitrogenous base, pentose (five-carbon sugar ring), and phosphate groups.

- In the process of DNA replication, the DNA double helix unwinds, single-stranded DNA binding proteins prevent the double strands from rebinding, two new DNA strands are synthesized on each of the parent strands, topoisomerase relieves the strain caused by DNA twisting as it unwinds, and the DNA polymerase enzymes help add nucleotides to the free 3′ end of a growing DNA daughter strand.

- In eukaryotic cells there are three main types of RNA: mRNA, tRNA, and rRNA.

- The process of synthesizing mRNA from a DNA strand is called *transcription*. mRNA is transcribed from the template strand of DNA inside the nucleus of eukaryotic cells and in the cytoplasm of prokaryotic cells.

- Proteins are synthesized from mature mRNA on ribosomes in the cytoplasm.

- Eukaryotic ribosomes consist of two subunits, 40S and 60S subunits. Each is composed of ribosomal RNA, rRNA, and proteins.

- The three steps of translation are initiation, elongation, and termination.

- There are three phases of the cell cycle: interphase, M phase, and G_0 phase.

- *Mitosis*, which occurs in all diploid cells, is the division of the cell nucleus and all the genetic information (DNA chromosomes) into two new nuclei. *Cytokinesis* allows for the formation of two new daughter cells.

- There are five essential phases of mitosis: prophase, prometaphase, metaphase, anaphase, and telophase.

- *Meiosis* is the process of division that takes place in gametes (sperm and ova cells). The process of meiosis is similar to mitosis, except that a single replication of chromosomes is followed by two consecutive cell divisions (meiosis I and meiosis II).

- Mendel developed a model to explain the inheritance pattern that he consistently observed in his experiments involving pea plants and their observable traits.

- Mendel's *law of segregation* states that two alleles for a specific inheritable character, or trait, separate (segregate) during gamete formation and end up in two different gametes (during meiosis).

- The *law of independent assortment* states that each pair of alleles for a specific gene segregates independently of the alleles for another gene during gamete formation.

- Mendel's laws of segregation and independent assortment reflect the rules of probability.

- One tool that biologists use to determine the probability of inheriting a specific combination of alleles of a gene is the *Punnett square*.

- Inheritance patterns are often much more complex that those dictated by simple Mendelian genetics. Often, a single gene can affect more than one trait.

- Evolution can be described as a change over time in the genetic makeup of an individual population.

- *Natural selection* refers to Charles Darwin's theory of evolution, that states that a population can change over generations if individuals with heritable traits that are better adapted to their environment survive and reproduce more frequently than other individuals of the same population.

- Adaptations that organisms may make to their environment are not necessarily inheritable traits and are not attributed to natural selection.

- The *Hardy-Weinberg theorem* states that the frequency of alleles and genotypes within a population remains relatively constant from one generation to the next, unless the factors of evolution interfere.

- Two other effects that invalidate the Hardy-Weinberg theorem with respect to evolution are the bottleneck effect and the founder effect.

- The contribution an individual makes to a gene pool is described as *fitness*.

- The tendency of directional and stabilizing selection to reduce genetic variability is countered by other mechanisms that aim to preserve it.

Microbiology

OVERVIEW

- **Microorganisms**
- **Bacteria**
- **Viruses**
- **Fungi**
- **Practice Questions**
- **Answer Key and Explanations**
- **Summing It Up**

The three types of microorganisms that will be discussed in this chapter are bacteria, viruses, and fungi. The two most widely understood infectious microorganisms are bacteria and viruses. Bacteria and fungi are classified taxonomically as distinct kingdoms, but viruses are not. Viruses are not classified as living or cellular entities and cannot survive without a host. Approximately ten questions on the PCAT will test your knowledge of microbiology.

MICROORGANISMS

Microorganisms, in general, have the following characteristics:

- They are extremely small. These microscopic organisms are measured in terms of micrometers (or microns) and nanometers.

- Most microorganisms are unicellular (bacteria) or acellular (viruses). However, fungi, with the exception of yeast, are multicellular microorganisms.

- Microorganisms are simple organisms. In general, with the exception of viruses, microorganisms can survive independent of any other cells. Therefore, if one surviving cell is left, a whole new colony of cells will arise.

- Microorganisms are difficult to destroy. Because they are simple and in most cases independent of other cells, it is difficult to kill them.

Chapter 6

Microorganisms can be classified into three basic types:

1. **Pathogens:** Pathogens are microorganisms that cause harm to host organisms. The amount of harm or damage a pathogen can cause to humans depends on the ability of the immune system to respond to and attack the pathogen.

2. **Opportunistic pathogens:** These are microorganisms that cause harm to a host under ideal conditions. In cases of a host that has a suppressed immune system, opportunistic pathogens thrive. They can also thrive in certain areas of the body where they can exist in ideal conditions or in a symbiotic relationship with another organism.

3. **Nonpathogens:** These are microorganisms that almost never cause harm to a host. However, under the correct conditions, even these microorganisms can harm their host.

Almost 99 percent of all known microorganisms are nonpathogenic. For example, *E. coli* is a bacterial microorganism that lives in the gut of humans and most mammals. It is very beneficial to its host and helps maintain the correct conditions in the gut. However, under the right conditions, *E. coli* can become an opportunistic pathogen that causes harm to its host.

BACTERIA

Bacteria are prokaryotic organisms, and they are thus simple and easy to study. The main component of the genome of most bacteria is a circular double-stranded DNA molecule. Bacteria can be classified by:

1. shape
2. optimal oxygen and temperature requirements
3. optimal pH conditions
4. nutritional requirements

Bacterial Shapes

There are three main bacterial shapes. Most bacteria fall into one of these three categories; however, there are exceptions in which bacteria takes on a different shape.

1. **Cocci:** These are spherical-shaped bacteria. They do not have flagella to aid in movement, and they are about 1 micrometer (μm) in size. Cocci are named according to how many cells are linked together:

   a. **Coccus:** single cocci

   b. **Diplococcus:** two bacterial cells

   c. **Streptococcus:** chain of cocci

   d. **Staphylococcus:** irregular bunches of cocci

   e. **Tetrad:** groups of four cocci

   f. **Sarcine:** cubes of eight cocci (2μm in diameter)

2. **Bacilli:** These are rod-shaped bacteria that have flagella. The average size of bacilli is 0.5 μm wide and 1 to 5 μm long. Bacilli are also named according to how many cells are linked together:

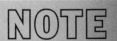

    a. **Bacillus:** single bacilli cell

    b. **Diplobacillus:** pairs of cells

    c. **Streptobacillus:** chains of cells

3. **Spirilla:** These are spiral-shaped bacteria that have flagella. Spirilla are further classified as follows:

    a. **Vibrio:** incomplete spiral; half-moon shape

    b. **Spirillum:** multi-bending spiral; thick with an average width of 1 μm; 5 to 50 μm long

    c. **Spirochete:** thin, flexible spirilla with a width of about 5 μm and a length between 5 and 25 μm

Oxygen Requirements

Different strains of bacteria require different levels of oxygen for optimal survival.

- **Obligate aerobe:** These bacteria grow only in the presence of oxygen. Energy for these bacterial cells comes from aerobic respiration.

- **Microaerophile:** These bacteria require only a low concentration of oxygen. Energy comes from aerobic respiration.

- **Obligate anaerobe:** These bacteria grow only in the absence of oxygen. Their growth is inhibited, and often they will die in the presence of oxygen. Energy for growth of these bacteria comes from anaerobic respiration or fermentation.

- **Aerotolerant anaerobe:** These bacteria do not require oxygen for growth, but they can tolerate the presence of oxygen. Energy for these bacteria cells comes from anaerobic respiration.

- **Facultative anaerobe:** These bacteria can grow either with or without the presence of oxygen, but they grow best in oxygenated environments. Energy for growth comes from aerobic respiration, anaerobic respiration, or fermentation. Most bacteria are classified as facultative anaerobes.

Temperature Requirements

Different strains of bacteria require different temperatures for optimal growth.

- **Thermophile:** These bacteria are heat-loving. Their optimal temperature for growth is between 45°C and 70°C. These bacteria typically grow in hot springs and compost heaps.

- **Psychrophile/cryophile:** These bacteria are cold-loving. Their optimal temperature for growth is between –5°C and –15°C. These bacteria typically grow in the Arctic and Antarctic regions. They are also found in cold streams that are fed by glaciers.

- **Mesophile:** These bacteria thrive in moderate temperatures. The optimal temperature range for their growth is between 25°C and 45°C. Most bacteria are mesophiles. This includes bacteria found in the human body and bacteria that grow in soil.

- **Hyperthermophiles:** These types of bacteria grow in extremely high temperatures. The optimal temperature for growth is between 70°C and 110°C. These organisms are usually classified as archaea. They grow near hydrothermal vents on the ocean floor, hot springs, and solfataric fields of boiling mud near volcanoes.

pH Requirements

Bacteria generally prefer to grow in a pH environment of 6.8 to 7.2. Because the pH of our blood is between 7.35 and 7.45, bacteria will not grow effectively in blood. Salt, brine, and vinegars are used to lower the pH of foods, so that bacteria cannot grow. The pH of human skin is generally around 5 to 6, but skin infections do occur, especially on children's skin, which tends to be about pH 7.

Nutritional Requirements

The basic nutritional requirements of bacteria include a source of:

1. carbon
2. nitrogen
3. hydrogen
4. sulfur
5. phosphorus
6. oxygen

Bacteria also need:

7. minerals such as iron, zinc, potassium, and calcium
8. vitamins, including niacin, riboflavin, and vitamin B_6
9. water.

In order to obtain all of these nutritional requirements, it is usually beneficial for bacteria to live on a host. Bacteria have the ability to compete with their host for nutrients.

Basic nutrients for bacterial cell growth can be in the form of light or chemicals. Cells that get energy from light are called *phototrophs*, and cells that get energy from chemicals are called *chemotrophs*. Photosynthetic bacteria that use light as an energy source and depend upon carbon dioxide to produce their own food are called *photoautotrophs*. Photosynthetic bacteria that use light as an energy source and produce their own nutrients from a carbon source other than carbon dioxide are called *photoheterotrophs*. Likewise, chemotrophs that get energy from inorganic molecules and produce their own nutrients using carbon dioxide from their environment are called *chemoautotrophs*. Chemotrophs that get energy from an inorganic source and obtain carbon from organic sources other than carbon dioxide are called chemoheterotrophs. Chemotrophs that require whole blood or tissue to get energy are called *fastidious chemoheterotrophs*.

Bacteria that require living cells and tissue as a source of nutrition are called *obligate parasites*. Those that require nonliving material as an energy source are called *obligate saprophytes*. Those that can get nutrients from both living and nonliving materials are referred to as *facultative*. Facultative saprophytes are normally parasitic in nature, but can survive for at least part of their lifecycle as a saprophyte. Facultative parasites do not rely on living tissue to complete their life cycle, but may resort to parasitic activity.

Extremophiles

In addition to hyperthermophiles that live under conditions of extremely hot temperatures, there are other types of bacteria that thrive under extreme conditions. These organisms are all classified as extremophiles. Extreme halophiles live in highly saline environments such as the Dead Sea. Some species of bacteria tolerate moderate salinity, whereas others require an environment that is several times saltier than seawater. *Methanogens* are another type of extremophile. These bacteria use carbon dioxide to oxidize hydrogen molecules. This process releases methane gas as a waste product, hence the name "methanogens." Methanogens are poisoned by oxygen, and most types of methanogens live in swamp areas and marshes where other microorganisms have consumed all the available oxygen.

Major Bacteria Groups

Several major groups of bacteria are:

- **Proteobacteria:** This is a large and diverse group of gram-negative bacteria (they become decolorized when exposed to Gram staining) that includes photoautotrophs, chemotrophs, and heterotrophs. Some proteobacteria are aerobic, and others are anaerobic. There are five subgroups of proteobacteria:

    1. **Alpha-proteobacteria:** These bacteria are closely associated with eukaryotic hosts. Genetic engineers use these bacteria to transfer select DNA into the DNA of plants.

    2. **Beta-proteobacteria:** This is a nutritionally diverse group and includes many soil bacteria.

    3. **Gamma-proteobacteria:** Some heterotrophic gamma proteobacteria are pathogens. For example, *Salmonella* is responsible for food poisoning and *Vibrio cholera* causes cholera. *E. coli* is a strain that is inside the gut of most animals and is not usually harmful.

    4. **Delta-proteobacteria:** This subgroup includes the slime-secreting myxobacteria that form elaborate colonies.

    5. **Epsilon-proteobacteria:** Most of the species of bacteria in this subgroup are pathogens. For example, *Campylobacter* causes blood poisoning and intestinal irritation, and *Heliobacter pylori* causes stomach ulcers.

- **Chlamydias:** These parasitic bacteria can only survive within an animal cell. These types of bacteria depend on their host for resources such as ATP. *Chlamydia trachomatis* is the leading cause of blindness and is the most common sexually transmitted disease in the United States.

- **Spirochetes:** These helical heterotrophs spiral through their environment by rotating internal flagellum-like filaments. Many are able to live independently, but some strains are parasitic. The parasitic strains are pathogenic to their host. *Treponema palladium* causes syphilis, and *Borrelia burgdorferi* causes Lyme disease.

- **Gram-positive bacteria:** These bacteria are another very diverse group of bacteria (become a dark blue or violet when treated with Gram stain). Soil-dwelling gram-positive *Streptomyces* are cultured by pharmaceutical companies as a source of antibiotics, including streptomycin. Other gram-positive bacteria include *Bacillus anthracis* (anthrax), *Streptococus*, and *Staphylococus*.

- **Cyanobacteria:** These bacteria are photoautotrophs with the plant-like ability to carry out oxygen-generating photosynthesis.

TIP

One way to remember a list like the major bacteria groups is to assign each one to a finger and memorize them in that order. The thumb is the alpha-protobacteria, the index finger is the beta-proteobacteria, etc.

Bacterial Growth Cycle

Bacteria reproduce asexually through the process of binary fission. During binary fission, bacteria will split in two, thus doubling the population. In general, it takes about 20 to 30 minutes for a bacteria population to double. This is called the generation time (GT). Bacteria experiences logarithmic growth: every generation is double that of the preceding one. The growth cycle occurs in the following four stages:

1. **Lag time:** 20 to 30 minutes. This is equivalent to the generation time (GT) and is the time when a new colony is establishing itself and getting ready to reproduce.

2. **Logarithmic growth period:** 12 to 24 hours. During this time, there is active doubling of bacteria through binary fission.

3. **Stationary period:** 24 to 48 hours. There is an equal rate of growth and death during this time so that the number of bacteria in a population remains constant.

4. **Decline or death period:** 48 to 96 hours. Rapid cell death by cell lysis occurs. The colony reaches its maximum capacity for the given environmental conditions. Cell lysis is occurring faster than binary fission at this point.

Figure 1. Gram Negative Bacterial Structure

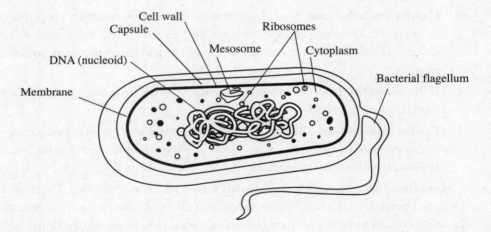

Bacterial Cell Wall and Capsule

The function of the bacterial cell wall is to maintain the correct size and shape of the bacteria and to help prevent cell lysis. Peptidoglycan is an important chemical component of bacterial cell walls. Gram-positive bacteria have a thick layer of peptidoglycan (PG) and therefore are more resistant to cell lysis than other bacteria strains. Certain antibiotics, such as penicillin and cephalosporins, target the cell wall of gram-positive bacteria by stopping the formation of PG.

Gram-negative bacteria have only a thin layer of PG; therefore, their cell walls are weaker and are easier to lyse. However, when the cell wall of gram-negative bacteria is lysed, lipopolysaccharides (LPS) are released. LPS are poison and are referred to as *endotoxin*. Endotoxins stimulate inflammation of infected tissue in the host. An infection will cause damage to host cells and cell death (necrosis). Most *E. coli* strains are harmless, but some virulent strains cause serious infections that lead to inflammation, diarrhea, bloody stool, and scar tissue. Endotoxins in the bloodstream can cause hemorrhaging and septic shock.

The cell wall of many bacteria, especially those that are pathogenic, are covered with a capsule. A capsule is a sticky layer of polysaccharides or proteins. The capsule allows bacteria to adhere to a host (substrate) or to other bacteria cells in a colony. Capsules can also shield pathogenic bacteria from an attack by a host's immune system. Because of the slimy capsule surrounding the bacteria, neutrophils cannot attach and ingest the bacteria.

Bacterial Cell Membrane

The cell membrane of prokaryotes is composed of a phospholipid bilayer, just as in eukaryotic cells. The main function of the cell membrane is to act as a semipermeable barrier for the cell. As a barrier, it can regulate the chemicals going into and out of the cell. The membrane is also capable of making cell wall repairs by filling in damaged areas with new PG or LPS. Furthermore, the cell membrane is the site of ATP production in bacterial cells. Glycolysis, the Krebs cycle, and electron transport all take place at the cell membrane.

During binary fission, or division, of a single bacteria cell into two cells, the cell membrane forms a septum caused by invagination of the membrane so that two cells form from one. After the DNA is duplicated, the cell membrane attaches to the two copies of the genome and pulls them apart. This separates the two copies of DNA on opposite sides of the cell. Then the cell begins to split in two. The cell membrane forms the septum dividing the cell into two parts. Once the cell is divided by the invagination of the membrane, the membrane facilitates the formation of a new cell wall. Between the cell wall and the cell membrane is the periplasmic space.

Some antibiotics are used to dissolve the cell membrane of bacteria by binding to the phospholipids. Polymixins, typically found in topical antibiotics, are useful for dissolving the membrane of gram-positive and gram-negative bacteria. Other membrane-damaging agents include some disinfectants (soaps and detergents) and some antiseptics (bleach).

Bacterial Flagella

Flagella are found on both bacilli (rod-shaped) and spirilla (spiral-shaped) bacteria. They function to add motility (movement) to the bacterial cell. Flagella are composed of a single strand of the protein flagellin. A bacteria with one flagellum at one end is called *polar monotrichous*, and a bacteria cell with two or more flagella at one end is called a *polar lophotrichous*. If flagella are positioned all around the cell, it is called *peritrichus*. Spirochete bacteria have flagella inside the cell that wrap around the spirochete from each end toward the middle of the cell. These are called *endoflagella*. Destroying flagella does not destroy a cell. Furthermore, cells can regrow flagella, so antibiotics are not aimed at destroying the flagella.

Flagella attach to bacteria by four anchors called rings. The innermost L ring attaches to the lipid bilayer of the membrane. The P ring attaches to PG in the cell wall. The S ring attaches to the periplasmic space. The M ring attaches to the cell membrane. The M ring wobbles and passes this vibration to the other rings, resulting in motility.

Movement of the bacterial cell is governed by taxis, the movement toward or away from a stimulus. Positive taxis is the movement of the bacteria toward an environmental stimulus, and negative taxis is movement away from an environmental stimulus. Chemotaxis is movement in response to chemicals, and phototaxis is movement in response to light.

Bacterial Pili

Pili, or fimbriae, are structures that resemble cilia (small hairs). They help to hold bacteria securely to one spot. For example, in the mouth, bacteria pili hold on to plaque. In the intestine, pili help the bacteria attach to the intestinal wall, where food is readily available. Pili hold bacteria securely in place so that they are not flushed out. Fluids are an effective means of flushing out bacteria, but pili help to combat this. *Neisseria gonorrhoeae,* the bacterium that causes gonorrhea; *Neisseria meningitides,* the bacterium that causes meningitis; and *Moraxella catarrhalis,* the bacterium that causes respiratory tract infections, all use pili to fasten themselves to the mucous membrane in the genital, urinary, and respiratory tract of a host.

Specialized pili called sex pili, or F pili, serve to link two bacteria to each other. The F pilus forms a DNA bridge, and genetic material is transferred from one cell to another across it. This process is called *sexual conjugation.*

Bacterial DNA

In the cytoplasm of bacteria, there are two major components: nuclear material and ribosomes. Bacteria have one double-stranded circular DNA chromosome. The DNA is very tightly wound and packed so that it fits inside the bacterium. The length of unwound DNA is about 1,000 times longer than the bacterium itself.

Bacterial Ribosomes

The second major component of the bacterial cytoplasm is the ribosome. Ribosomes are the site of protein synthesis in the cell. Ribosomes are composed of proteins and RNA, just as in eukaryotic cells. Some bacteria produce proteins in the ribosome that are poisonous. These poisons are called *exotoxins* and are released by living bacteria. Some examples of exotoxins include botulism, tetanus, anthrax, cholera, and diphtheria.

Antibiotics can act to damage ribosomes and interfere with protein synthesis. Aminoglycosides (streptomycin, kanamycin, gentamycin), macrolides (erythromycin, clarithromycin, and azithromycin), and tetracycline all damage the ribosomes of bacteria. These are broad-spectrum antibiotics, because they work on both gram-positive and gram-negative bacteria.

Bacterial Endospores

The ability of some bacteria to withstand harsh conditions contributes to their survival. Some bacteria can form resistant cells called *endospores.* Endospores are produced mainly in bacillus and clostridium. The original bacterial cell produces a copy of its chromosome and surrounds it with a tough wall. This creates an endospore. Water is removed from inside an endospore, and metabolism ceases inside the cell. The original cell disintegrates, leaving behind the endospore. Most endospores are so durable that they can withstand boiling water. The function of the endospore is survival, not reproduction. Endospores enable bacteria to survive under harsh conditions, and they can survive either with or without O_2, depending on the bacterium that produced them. In less hostile environments, endospores can lie dormant for centuries, yet still be viable. There are no antibiotics or disinfectants that can kill endospores; however, bleach and formaldehyde can eliminate them.

There are five major diseases caused by spore-forming bacteria: *Clostridium difficile* (a major cause of wound infection and gastrointestinal infections), *Clostrdium botulinin* (botulism), *Clostridium tetani* (tetanus), *Clostridium perfrinens* (gas gangrene), and *Bacillus anthracis* (anthrax). In each case, spores germinate bacteria and the bacteria produce exotoxin.

Genetic Recombination in Bacteria

There are three methods of exchanging genetic information between bacteria in the same generation:

1. *Transformation* is the process by which DNA that is not associated with a cell or proteins is transferred from one bacterium to another.

2. *Transduction* is the process by which DNA is carried by a bacteriaphage (virus) from one bacterium to another.

3. *Conjugation* is the transfer of DNA from one bacterium to another across F pili (DNA bridge).

VIRUSES

Viruses are the simplest of all genetic systems, yet they play a major role in causing disease and infection. Basic information about viruses follows:

- Viruses are nonliving entities, yet they carry DNA.

- Viruses have none of the structures that cells have: no cell wall, membrane, cytoplasm, or ribosomes.

- Viruses are incapable of performing metabolic processes without a host.

- Viruses are the smallest infectious agents. In fact, they are about 1,000 times smaller than a typical bacterium cell.

- Viruses consist of nuclear material (either DNA or RNA), packaged inside a protein head called a *capsid*.

- Viruses cannot reproduce, mutate, or survive on their own. They require the functions of a host cell in order to survive and reproduce.

Viral Specificity

Most viruses are specific to the organism they infect. Animal viruses infect only animal cells, and plant viruses infect only plant cells. Therefore, a virus specific to animals cannot harm plants, and a plant virus does not harm animals. However, viral mutations and some crossover to other species do occur. For example, the West Nile virus was first found only in horses. The virus then mutated to a form that was capable of infecting birds. Now the virus, often carried by mosquitoes, can infect humans. Birds are often a crossover vector, meaning they can be infected by a virus specific to one species and pass it on to another species.

Viruses are also specific to a particular tissue type. On the head of the virus, there are receptor proteins that recognize a specific protein on specific cells of a host. For example, pneumotropic viruses have proteins that are recognized only by receptor proteins on lung and respiratory tissue, dermatotropic viruses have proteins that are recognized only by receptor proteins on skin, neurotropic viruses are specific to the brain and nerve tissue, and lymphotropic viruses are specific to lymphocytes. There is some evidence of crossover of viruses to another tissue type.

It is difficult to study and grow human viruses because of the specificity of most viruses to one species and the fact that viruses are nonliving entities. Thus, vaccine development is also a difficult process. Vaccines can be made from a weakened (attenuated) form of the virus. The attenuated virus is injected into humans, and because it is in a weakened form, the immune system can attack. In this way, we build up immunity to viruses through vaccines.

Virus Shapes

The shape of a virus is defined by its viral type. It is the protein shell enclosing the viral genome that takes on various shapes. As noted earlier, this shell is called a capsid. Capsids built from a large number of protein subunits are called *capsomeres*.

- **Polyhedral:** The most common viral shape is an icosahedron: twenty triangular faces, thirty edges, and twelve vertices. Most animal viruses are icosahedral, or another polyhedral shape. The viral head is made of protein and is hollow. Inside the head is DNA or RNA. The protein head, or capsid, is built from protein subunits called capsomeres. Each face of the icosahedral head is a capsomere. In some icosahedrals, there are glycoprotein structures called *spikes* protruding from each corner. The spikes function to stick the virus to cell surfaces. In general, cold viruses do not have spikes, but influenza viruses do.

- **Cylindrical or Helical:** Most plant viruses are cylindrical in shape. Tobacco mosaic virus (TMV) has a rigid rod-shaped capsid made from over 1,000 molecules of one type of protein arranged in a helix. Some animal viruses, such as lyssaviruses (rabies and other animal viruses) are helical. Rabies is a bullet-shaped, rigid helical structure.

- **Complex Viral Shapes:** The most complex capsid shapes are found among viruses that infect bacteria. These viruses are called *bacteriophages* and *mycophages*. These phages generally have a polyhedral hollow head that contains DNA and a tail apparatus. The tail is a hollow tube, and its end has a base plate on which are attached tail fibers. The remainder of the tail is covered in a contractile sheath. Phages will land on the surface of bacteria, and pins on the ends of the tail fibers plunge into the bacteria to attach the virus. The contractile sheath on the tail acts like a thread of a screw to secure the base plate of the tail to the bacterial wall. DNA is then injected from the viral head through the hollow tube of the tail into the bacterium.

Figure 2. Virus Shapes

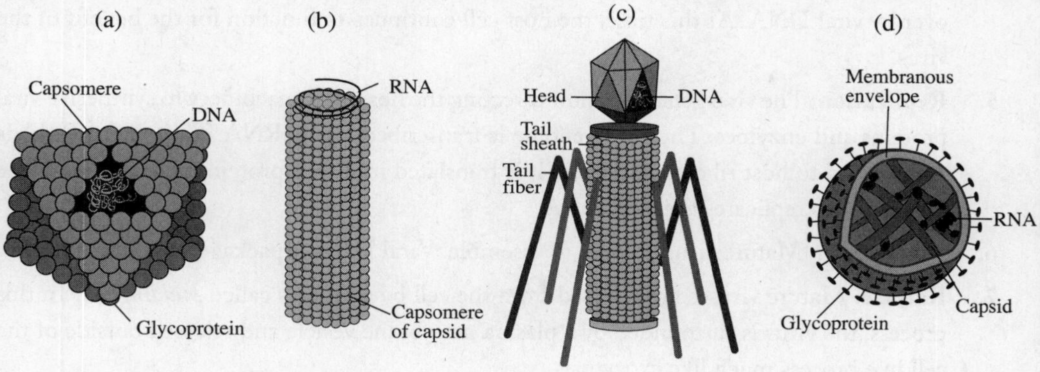

(a) Polyhedral, adenovirus. (b) Helical, tobacco mosaic virus. (c) Complex, bacteriophage T4. (d) Polyhedral, influenza virus.

Virus Life Cycle

An isolated virus is unable to reproduce or do anything except infect a host cell. Viruses are merely packages of genetic information moving from one host to another. A viral infection begins when a viral nucleic acid (DNA or RNA) makes its way into a host cell. The mechanism of nucleic acid entry varies depending on the virus and its structure. The host cell provides nucleotides for making new viral DNA or RNA, enzymes, ribosomes, amino acids, tRNA, ATP, and all other necessary components for making viral proteins and nucleic acids. Most DNA viruses use the host cell's DNA polymerase to synthesize new DNA, but viral RNA most often relies on viral encoded RNA polymerases.

Productive Life Cycle

Different types of viruses have different life cycles. An animal virus goes through the following eight steps of the productive life cycle:

1. **Attachment:** In the first step of attachment, a nonpermanent attachment of the virus to the host cell is formed. To form a more permanent attachment, the virus must have the correct proteins for the particular receptors on the host surface. If it does, it will become more tightly attached via an interaction with the receptors. If it does not have the correct protein for the host receptor sites, it will be shed from the host.

2. **Penetration:** Penetration of the virus into the host cell keeps the virus protected from the host's immune system. Penetration occurs because the host cell treats the virus like a nutrient and takes it inside the cell via endocytosis.

3. **Uncoating:** This process releases the viral genome for the capsid. The host cell digests the capsid proteins. When the viral capsid is destroyed, the viral genetic material (DNA) is released into the cell. The first genes of the viral DNA are identical to those of its host, so it is not destroyed by the cell.

4. **Transport of viral DNA to the nucleus:** The host cell identifies the foreign viral DNA as its own because some of the genes are the same. Therefore, the viral DNA is transported

into the cell nucleus. In the nucleus, it is attached to the end of a host cell chromosome. The cell then is under the control of the virus. The host cell is partially shut down and taken over by viral DNA. At this time, the host cell continues to function for the benefit of the virus.

5. **Replication:** The viral genome is now directing the host cell's machinery to synthesize viral proteins and enzymes. The viral genome is transcribed into mRNA. This viral mRNA is transported to host ribosomes, where it is translated into viral proteins and enzymes. The host cell also replicates the viral DNA.

6. **Maturation:** Mature viruses begin to assemble. Viral DNA is packaged into capsids.

7. **Release:** Mature viruses are released from the cell by a process called *budding out*. In this process, the virus is surrounded by a plasma membrane vesicle and released outside of the cell in a process much like exocytosis.

8. **Reinfection:** The process begins again with the infection of other host cells.

Viral death can only occur outside of the host cell.

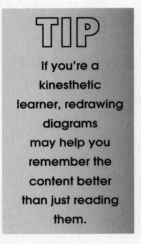

TIP

If you're a kinesthetic learner, redrawing diagrams may help you remember the content better than just reading them.

Figure 3. Simplified Diagram of a Typical Virus Life Cycle

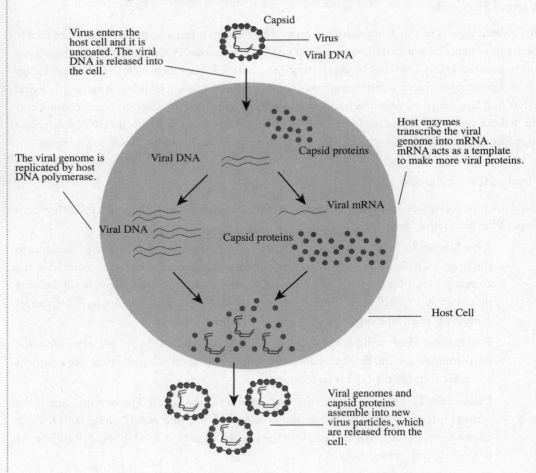

RNA Virus Life Cycle

Most RNA animal viruses have an outer membrane called a *viral envelope*. The viral envelope contains phospholipids and membrane proteins made in the host cell. The viral envelope also contains viral specific glycoproteins that protrude from the virus, forming spikes that stick to the host cell surface. The viral envelope is used by RNA viruses to enter the host cell. Viral glycoprotein spikes on the RNA virus bind to specific receptor sites on the host cell, and in this way, the virus attaches to the host. The glycoproteins on the viral envelope are produced in the ER of the host cell, and capsid proteins are synthesized in the cytosol from viral mRNA. The viral envelope is made from the host cell's plasma membrane enveloping the newly formed viral capsids. The plasma membrane envelope is studded with the newly synthesized viral glycoproteins. The enveloped viruses, once released, can infect other cells. The RNA genome of animal viruses is transcribed into complementary RNA strands in the cytoplasm of the host cell. The RNA strands serve as mRNA and as templates for the synthesis of copies of the RNA viral genome.

Provirus Life Cycle

Animal RNA viruses with the most complicated genome are the retroviruses. These viruses have an enzyme called *reverse transcriptase*, which synthesizes DNA from RNA. This is the opposite of the DNA-to-RNA information flow of normal cells. HIV (human immunodeficiency virus) is a retrovirus that causes AIDS (acquired immunodeficiency syndrome). HIV is an enveloped virus that contains two identical RNA strands and two molecules of reverse transcriptase.

After a retrovirus enters the host cell, the reverse transcriptase molecules are released into the cytoplasm and catalyze the synthesis of viral DNA. Newly made viral DNA can then enter the nucleus of the host cell and integrate into the DNA of a host chromosome. The integrated viral DNA, called a *provirus*, never leaves the host's genome, although it can go into a latency period. Viral latency is caused when the host cell does not produce the necessary viral proteins. The virus remains in the cell safe from the immune system until the host cell begins producing the necessary viral proteins.

The host cell's RNA polymerase transcribes the proviral DNA into RNA. The viral portion of the host DNA is called a *virogene*. The virogene replicates every time the host DNA is replicated. If the virogene detaches from the host DNA, it enters into a productive life cycle instead of a latent period. This RNA can then function as mRNA for the synthesis of new viral proteins and a new RNA genome for new viral particles released from the cell. An example of a virus that cycles from a productive life cycle to provirus and back to productive life cycle is the chicken pox virus. Chicken pox is productive during infection, and then enters a latent phase as a provirus. It can emerge again as shingles, which is the second productive phase of the virus.

Sometimes, a virogene detaches from its host DNA, causing a mutation to the host genome. This mutation may cause rapid cell division and the formation of a tumor. This can cause cancer to develop in the host. There are at least thirty known viruses that can stimulate tumor growth. The link between mononucleosis and Hodgkin's lymphoma is the Epstein-Barr virus. The human papilloma virus is a precursor to cervical cancer.

Lytic Life Cycle

Phages are capable of reproducing by two different mechanisms: the *lytic cycle* and the *lysogenic cycle*. The lytic cycle involves the reproduction of phage and the death of the host cell. During the last stage of viral infection, the bacterium cell lyses, or breaks open, to release the newly synthesized phages. Because the lytic cycle results in cell death, a few successive cycles can destroy a bacterial population in just a few hours. A phage that only utilizes the lytic cycle is called a *virulent phage*. The lytic cycle parallels the following same eight steps as the productive life cycle of animal viruses:

1. **Attachment:** During attachment, the bacteriophage attaches specifically to the wall of certain bacteria.

2. **Injection:** During injection, the DNA is injected through the hollow tube of the phage's tail.

3. **DNA attachment:** Next, the DNA attaches to the host cell bacterial chromosome.

4. **Shutdown:** The viral DNA partially shuts down the bacterial cell functions and the virus then takes over the cell's systems to make DNA, RNA, and proteins.

5. **Replication:** New copies of viral DNA are made (about 100 to 500 new viral heads per bacterium cell).

6. **Assembly:** New bacteriophages are assembled.

7. **Release:** The bacterial cell wall is destroyed, and the new phages are released from the cell.

8. **Reinfection:** The bacterium cell dies, and the cycle continues. The newly formed viruses can now infect new bacteria cells.

Lysogenic Life Cycle

In contrast to the lytic cycle, the lysogenic cycle replicates the phage genome without killing the host cell. Bacteriophages that use both the lytic and the lysogenic cycles are called *temperate phages*. The lysogenic life cycle parallels the four stages of the provirus life cycle:

1. **Attachment:** The virus attaches to the cell wall of specific bacterial cells.

2. **Injection:** The viral DNA is injected into the host cell.

3. **DNA attachment:** The viral DNA is incorporated into the host chromosome.

4. **No shutdown:** The virus does not take over the cell's functions. The viral DNA is copied every time the bacteria reproduce and replicate their DNA. The bacteriophage genome is integrated into the host genome. This creates what is called a *prophage*. The bacteria continue to grow and reproduce unharmed until something triggers the start of the lytic life cycle. Usually, this trigger comes from an environmental signal, such as a chemical or radiation. If the viral DNA prophage detaches from the bacterial chromosome, this will trigger the lytic cycle, and the cellular machinery will be taken over by the virus.

Combating Viral Diseases

The link between a viral infection and the symptoms it causes is not always readily known. Some viruses cause an infected cell to produce toxins, and some viruses contain their own toxic components. The damage caused by a virus is dependent on the ability of the infected tissue to regenerate

TIP

Draw the lytic life cycle and the lysogenic life cycle side by side to help you learn the differences. This should be especially helpful for kinesthetic learners.

healthy cells through cell division. Some viruses, such as cold viruses, allow for complete recovery, since epithelial cells in the respiratory tract are efficiently repaired by the production of new cells. However, the polio virus that infects nerve cells results in permanent damage because mature nerve cells do not divide and usually cannot be replaced. Many temporary symptoms that one experiences from a viral infection result from the process of the body's immune system combating the virus.

The immune system is critical to the body's defense against viral infection and is the basis for the development of vaccines. Vaccines are harmless variants, or derivatives, of pathogenic viruses that act to stimulate the immune system in defense against a pathogenic virus. Vaccines can prevent future infection, but they cannot cure a viral infection once it occurs. There are relatively few antiviral medicines available, and, thus, in most cases the symptoms of the infection are treated until the immune system fights off the virus infection. Certain antiviral drugs called protease inhibitors are used to stop the production of the viral head. However, sometimes a virus can mutate and produce different head structure proteins that are not affected by the protease inhibitor.

There are two main antiviral defense mechanisms in the body. 1. Neutralizing antibodies are proteins made by the immune system. Each virus generally needs a different specific antibody. Antibodies attach to the protein head of a virus and prevent the attachment of the virus to a host cell. Specific antibodies are not made by the immune system until the body is exposed to a particular virus. 2. B-lymphocytes in the immune system are also able to produce what are called memory B cells. These cells give us antibody protection against future infections of the same virus. This is the idea behind immunization against certain viral infections.

Interferons, or interleukins, are antiviral proteins made by cells infected with a virus. Interferons prevent viral replication in other cells. When interferons are made by an infected cell, they enter other cells, preventing viral infection over a given time period in those cells. Interferons are not specific to a particular virus, and they are only produced in cells that are undergoing active infection. Interferons are also capable of stopping the replication of tumor cells, just as they stop the replication of viruses.

FUNGI

Fungi are not only diverse and widespread eukaryotes, but they are essential components of most ecosystems. They are responsible for the breakdown of organic material and the recycling of nutrients. In fact, almost all plants depend upon a symbiotic relationship with fungi that helps their roots absorb essential minerals from the soil. However, there are some fungi that also cause disease in plants and animals.

Among the various species of fungi are those that live as decomposers (saprobes), parasites, and mutualistic symbionts. *Saprobic* fungi break down dead organic matter, such as fallen logs and animal waste, and absorb nutrients from these materials. *Parasitic* fungi absorb the nutrients from the cells of a living host. Some parasitic fungi are pathogenic and can infect animal or plant tissue. *Mutualistic* fungi absorb nutrients from a host, but are also beneficial to the host in some way.

Fungal Nutrition

Fungi, like animals, are heterotrophs, so they cannot produce their own food. However, fungi do not ingest food as animals do; instead, they digest nutrients while they are still in the environment. They

ALERT

Remember that only correct answers count. Use your time wisely, but if you get toward the end of the time limit and have a number of questions left, increase your speed, make your best guess if you have to, and answer as many questions as you can.

do this by secreting hydrolytic enzymes called *exoenzymes* into their surrounding environment. The exoenzymes break down complex molecules into simple organic molecules that fungi can absorb and use.

Body Structure

Some fungi are unicellular, such as yeasts, but most fungal species are multicellular. The morphology of multicellular fungi aids in the absorption of nutrients from the surrounding environment. The bodies of multicellular fungi typically form a network of tiny filaments called *hyphae*. Hyphae are made of tubular cell walls that are surrounded by plasma membrane. The cell walls of fungi contain *chitin*, which is a strong and flexible nitrogen-containing polysaccharide. The hyphae form an interwoven mass called a *mycelium*. Mycelia surround and infiltrate the material on which the fungus feeds. Mycelia cannot move, but they make up for a lack of mobility by extending the tips of hyphae into new spaces. In most fungi, the hyphae are divided into cells by crosswalls called *septa*. The septa have pores large enough to allow ribosomes, mitochondria, and nuclei to move from cell to cell.

Fungi that lack septa are called *coenocytic fungi*. These types of fungi contain a continuous cytoplasmic mass with thousands of nuclei. The nuclei repeatedly divide, but the cytoplasm does not. Some fungi have specialized hyphae that allow them to feed on living tissue of animals. Other fungi have specialized hyphae called *haustoria* that allow them to penetrate the tissue of their host.

Reproduction in Fungi

Fungi propagate by producing a vast number of spores. This can be carried out either through sexual or asexual reproduction.

Sexual Reproduction

Generally, sexual reproduction in fungi begins when hyphae (which have haploid nuclei), from two distinct mycelia, release sexually signaling molecules called *pheromones*. If mycelia are of different mating types, the pheromones from each bind to surface receptors on the other. Then the hyphae from each mycelia extend toward the source of the pheromones. When the hyphae eventually meet, they fuse. This contributes to genetic variability, as hyphae from the same or genetically identical mycelia will not fuse.

The joining together of the cytoplasm of the two parent mycelia is called *plasmogamy*. If the haploid nuclei from each parent mycelium do not fuse right away, the two genetically different nuclei can coexist in the mycelium. This type of mycelium is called a *heterokaryon*. In some species, heterokaryons can become mosaics. Fungi in which the haploid nuclei pair off two to a cell are called *dikaryotic*. As dikaryotic mycelia grow, the two nuclei in each cell divide in tandem without ever fusing.

The next stage of the sexual reproduction cycle after plasmogamy is karyogamy. During karyogamy, the haploid nuclei from each parent fuse together to produce a diploid cell. Karyogamy is the only stage at which diploid cells exist in most fungi. Meiosis restores the cells to the haploid state.

Meiosis occurs after karyogamy. The mycelium then produces specialized reproductive structures that disperse the fungal spores during germination. The sexual process of karyogamy and meiosis generates a great amount of genetic variation, which is important for adaptive evolution of fungi.

Asexual Reproduction

Many fungi can also reproduce asexually, and some types only reproduce asexually. During asexual reproduction, clones are produced by the mitotic production of spores. The process of asexual reproduction can vary widely among fungi. Some fungi that reproduce asexually grow as molds. Molds grow rapidly as mycelia and are able to produce spores. Spores can be spread through air or water. Another type of asexually reproducing fungi is yeast. Instead of producing spores, yeast reproduce asexually by simple cell division or by the pinching off of small buds from the parent cell.

Figure 4. Life Cycle of Fungi: Overview of Sexual and Asexual Reproduction

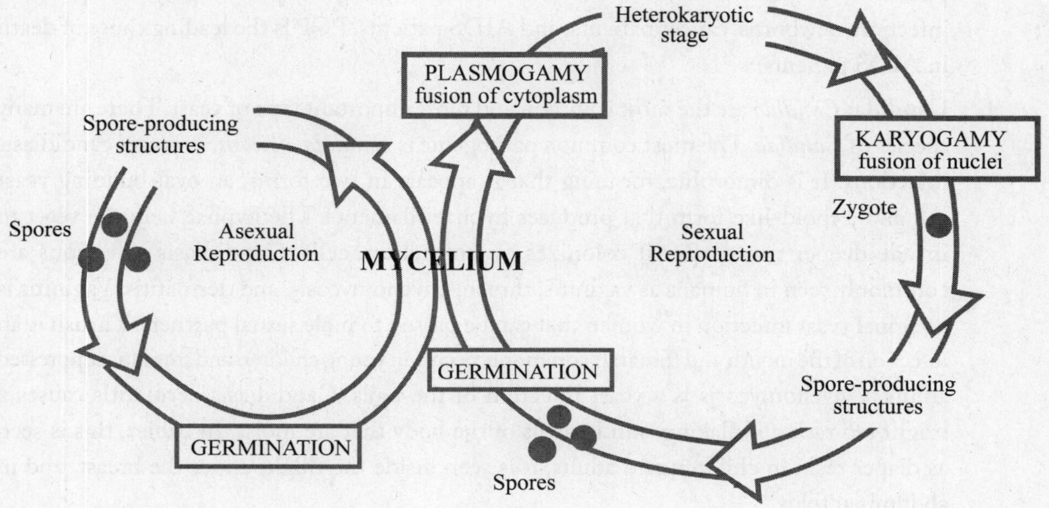

Yeasts

Yeasts inhabit liquids and moist environments, including plant sap and animal tissue. Although most often yeast reproduce asexually, they can sometimes reproduce sexually. Yeast are generally spherical or oval unicellular organisms.

During the yeast budding process (asexual reproduction), DNA is first replicated in the nucleus. The nucleus then splits and forms a daughter nucleus, which migrates to the edge of the cell. The daughter nucleus is then surrounded by cytoplasm. Cell wall material is laid between the parent and the daughter nuclei (bud). The small bud continues to grow until it separates from the parent cell. Once it separates, it is fully mature and the same size as the parent. In some strains of yeast, such as *Candida*, buds can remain attached to the parent, forming branches off the parent cell. These branches are called *pseudohyphae*.

Yeast are facultative anaerobes. They get energy from either cellular respiration or fermentation. Most yeast are nonpathogenic, and the following are four common types of yeast:

1. **Saccharomyces cervisiae:** These yeasts pose no health risk. Common examples of *Saccharomyces cervisiae* are baker's yeast and brewer's yeast. These yeasts feed on sugars such as glucose and maltose, producing CO_2 gas and alcohol as they metabolize (ferment) the sugar.

2. **Cryptococcus neoformus:** This strain of yeast is pathogenic and causes an infection called *cryptococcosis*. It is found in soil contaminated with certain types of bird droppings—for example, pigeon droppings. If humans inhale dust containing *C. neoformus*, they develop flu-like symptoms that can progress to pneumonia and lung scarring. In immune-compromised patients such as those with HIV or Hodgkin's disease, the pathogen can spread through the circulatory system to the meninges and the brain, developing into cryptococcal meningoencephalitis.

3. **Pneumocystis jirovecii:** *P. jiroveccii* affects the lungs and causes the formation of cysts. It causes pneumonia in immunosuppressed individuals. This type of pneumonia is called pneumocystis pneumonia, or PCP. There are three groups that are highly susceptible to infection: newborns, cancer patients, and AIDS patients. PCP is the leading cause of death in AIDS patients.

4. **Candida:** *Candida* are the most common and most important type of yeast. There are many species of *Candida*. The most common pathogenic is *Candida albicans*. It causes candidiasis infections. It is dimorphic, meaning that it appears in two forms: an oval-budding yeast cell and a mold-like form that produces hyphae filaments. The hyphae help the yeast to invade deeper tissue after it colonizes on epithelium cells. Candidiasis infections are commonly seen in humans as vaginitis, thrush, onychomycosis, and dermatitis. Vaginitis is a vaginal yeast infection in women that can be passed to male sexual partners. Thrush is an infection of the mouth and throat. It commonly occurs in young children and immunosuppressed adults. Onychomycosis is a yeast infection of the nails. Candidiasis dermatitis causes a bright red rash and flaking skin in areas of the body that are moist. In babies, this is seen as diaper rash; in children and adults, it is seen inside the thigh, under the breast, and in abdominal folds.

Fungal Pathogens

There are about 100,000 known species of fungi, and about 30 percent of those species are known to be parasitic. Animals are much less susceptible to parasitic fungi than plants. There are only about fifty species of fungi that are known to parasitize humans and animals. The general term for a fungal infection is *mycosis*. Skin mycoses include ringworm. The fungus that causes ringworm can infect almost any skin surface. It is commonly found to grow on the foot, causing what is known as athlete's foot. Ringworm and athlete's foot can be treated with fungicidal lotions and powders.

Systemic mycoses spread throughout the entire body and cause very serious illnesses. Systemic mycoses are typically caused by inhaled fungal spores. For example, coccidioidomycosis is a systemic mycosis that produces tuberculosis-like symptoms in the lungs.

Practical Uses of Fungi

Humans have long used yeasts to produce alcoholic beverages and breads. However, many fungi also have great medical value. For example, a compound extracted from the fungus that causes a disease in rye known as *ergot* is used to reduce high blood pressure and to stop bleeding after childbirth.

Some fungi are used to produce antibiotics that are essential in treating bacterial infections. In fact, the first antibiotic discovered, penicillin, was made from the mold *Penicillium*. Molecular biology and molecular genetics of eukaryotes are often studied in yeast.

PRACTICE QUESTIONS

Directions: Choose the best answer for each question.

Refer to the following passage for Questions 1–5.

Streptobacillus moniliformis is a non-motile, Gram-negative bacterium that lives in the respiratory tract of rats; the bacteria are provided with a habitat, but the rats are unaffected. *S. moniliformis* thrives around 37°C, a warm but average temperature. Though it grows best in an oxygenated environment, it can also grow in the absence of oxygen.

1. Based on its optimal growth conditions, which type of bacteria is *S. moniliformis*?
   A. Obligate aerobe
   B. Obligate anaerobe
   C. Aerotolerant anaerobe
   D. Facultative anaerobe

2. When *S. moniliformis* is lysed, the cell wall releases
   A. peptidoglycan.
   B. lipopolysaccharides.
   C. exotoxins.
   D. penicillin.

3. Based on its optimal growth temperature, *S. moniliformis* is a
   A. thermophile.
   B. hyperthermophile.
   C. mesophile.
   D. cryophile.

4. Which type of symbiosis is exhibited between *S. moniliformis* and rats?
   A. Commensalism
   B. Mutualism
   C. Parasitism
   D. None of these

5. In terms of shape and growth arrangement, *S. moniliformis* is
   A. circular and grows in chains.
   B. rod-shaped and grows in irregular clusters.
   C. circular and grows in irregular clusters.
   D. rod-shaped and grows in chains.

Refer to the following passage for Questions 6–8.

Fungi represent a kingdom within the eukaryotic domain. Fungi do not possess chlorophyll and must grow in the presence of organic matter in order to derive their nutrients and energy. There are a wide array of types of fungi, which can be unicellular or very complex multicellular organisms.

6. Fungi that lack septa in the hyphae have a continuous cytoplasmic mass and are called
   A. coenocytic fungi.
   B. mycelia.
   C. hyphae.
   D. cytoplasmic fungi.

7. During sexual reproduction of fungi, the haploid nuclei fuse to form a diploid cell during which process?
   A. Plasmogamy
   B. Karyogamy
   C. Meiosis
   D. Germination

8. The general term for a fungal infection is
   A. thrush.
   B. systemic mycoses.
   C. mycosis.
   D. candidiasis.

The following questions are standalone and not tied to a passage.

9. The first step of the productive viral life cycle is
   A. uncoating.
   B. attachment.
   C. transport.
   D. penetration.

10. During which viral life cycles does the host cell partially shut down as the virus takes over the cell's systems?
   A. Productive life cycle and lysogenic life cycle
   B. Lytic life cycle and lysogenic life cycle
   C. Productive life cycle and lytic life cycle
   D. Lysogenic life cycle and provirus life cycle

11. Which bacterial structure is responsible for holding the bacteria securely in place?
   A. Ribosomes
   B. Flagella
   C. Endospores
   D. Pili

12. In humans, the two main defense mechanisms against viral infection are antibodies and
   A. B-lymphocytes.
   B. vaccines.
   C. interferons.
   D. antibiotics.

13. Viruses use reverse transcriptase to
   A. produce DNA from RNA.
   B. produce RNA from DNA.
   C. produce proteins from RNA.
   D. produce RNA from proteins.

14. The shape of the influenza virus is
   A. polyhedral.
   B. helical.
   C. complex.
   D. filamentous.

15. The stage of bacterial growth during which bacteria are growing in size as they adapt to the environment, but are not undergoing binary fission, is the
   A. death phase.
   B. lag phase.
   C. log phase.
   D. stationary phase.

16. Transfer of genetic material via the pilus occurs during
   A. conjugation.
   B. transduction.
   C. transformation.
   D. all of these.

17. Bacteria that only require a low concentration of oxygen are described as
   A. facultative anaerobes.
   B. microaerophiles.
   C. obligate aerobes.
   D. obligate anaerobes.

18. A group of eight cocci is known as a
   A. sarcine.
   B. spirochete.
   C. tetrad.
   D. vibrio.

19. Athlete's foot and ringworm are caused by the same:
   A. bacterium.
   B. fungus.
   C. prion.
   D. virus.

20. Yeast reproduce asexually through
    A. hyphae.
    B. spore production.
    C. budding.
    D. karyogamy.

ANSWER KEY AND EXPLANATIONS

1. D	**5.** D	**9.** B	**13.** A	**17.** B
2. B	**6.** A	**10.** C	**14.** A	**18.** A
3. C	**7.** B	**11.** D	**15.** B	**19.** B
4. A	**8.** C	**12.** C	**16.** A	**20.** C

1. **The correct answer is D.** Facultative anaerobe bacteria can grow either with or without the presence of oxygen, but they grow best in oxygenated environments. Choice A is incorrect because obligate aerobe bacteria grow only in the presence of oxygen. Choice B is incorrect because obligate anaerobe bacteria grow only in the absence of oxygen. Choice C is incorrect because aerotolerant anaerobe bacteria do not require oxygen for growth, but can tolerate the presence of oxygen.

2. **The correct answer is B.** When the cell wall of a gram-negative bacteria is lysed, lipopolysaccharides (LPS) are released. LPS are poison and are referred to as endotoxin. Choice A is incorrect because peptidoglycan (PG) are an important chemical component of cell walls, which helps protect them from being lysed. Choice C is incorrect because LPS is an endotoxin; exotoxins are poisons that are released by living bacteria. Choice D is incorrect because penicillin is derived from a mold and is used as an antibiotic.

3. **The correct answer is C.** *S. moniliformis* grows best at an average, mild temperature, so it is a mesophile. Choices A and B are incorrect because the optimal growth temperature is not higher, and Choice D is incorrect because the optimal growth temperature is not cold.

4. **The correct answer is A.** Because the bacterium is provided with a habitat but has no effect on the rat, it is a commensal relationship. Choice B is incorrect because both organisms would benefit from a mutual relationship. Choice C is incorrect because one organism would be harmed in a parasitic relationship. Choice D is incorrect because commensalism is an accurate description of the described relationship.

5. **The correct answer is D.** The name *Streptobacillus* provides all the necessary information to deduce the shape and growth arrangement of the bacterium. *Strepto-* indicates a chain of bacteria, while *bacillus* refers to a rod shape. Choice A is incorrect because the shape has the incorrect designation. Choice B is incorrect in both shape and growth arrangement. Choice C is incorrect because the growth arrangement is incorrectly indicated.

6. **The correct answer is A.** Fungi that lack septa are called coenocytic fungi. These types of fungi contain a continuous cytoplasmic mass with thousands of nuclei. Choice B is incorrect because mycelia are interwoven masses of hyphae that surround the material on which fungi feed. Choice C is incorrect because hyphae are the filaments of fungi that form the network of the mycelia. Hyphae are made of tubular cell walls that are surrounded by plasma membrane. Choice D is incorrect because fungi with a continuous cytoplasm are called coenocytic fungi.

7. **The correct answer is B.** During karyogamy, the haploid nuclei from each parent fuse together to produce a diploid

cell. Karyogamy is the only stage at which diploid cells exist in most fungi. Choice A is incorrect because plasmogamy is the joining together of the cytoplasm of two parent mycelia. Choice C is incorrect because meiosis occurs after karyogamy and restores the fungal cell to its haploid state. Choice D is incorrect because germination is the step in fungal sexual reproduction when new fungal spores are dispersed.

8. **The correct answer is C.** The general term for a fungal infection is *mycosis*. Choice A is incorrect because thrush is a yeast infection of the mouth and throat. Choice B is incorrect because systemic mycoses refers to serious fungal infections that spread throughout the entire body. Choice D is incorrect because candidiasis infections are those caused by the yeast *Candida albicans*.

9. **The correct answer is B.** In the first step of the productive viral life cycle, the virus attaches to the host cell via an interaction with receptor proteins on the host. Choice A is incorrect because the process of uncoating capsid proteins from the virus occurs after the virus attaches to the host and penetrates into the host cell. Choice C is incorrect because transport of viral DNA to the nucleus occurs after the uncoating process. Choice D is incorrect because replication of viral DNA cannot occur until the viral DNA is transported to the nucleus.

10. **The correct answer is C.** During the transport phase of the productive life cycle, the host cell is partially shut down and taken over by viral DNA. At this time, the host cell continues to function for the benefit of the virus. Also, during the shutdown phase of the lytic life cycle, the phage (viral) DNA partially shuts down the bacterial cell functions, and the virus takes over the cell's systems to make DNA, RNA, and protein.

Choices A, B, and D are incorrect because none of these have a shutdown phase.

11. **The correct answer is D.** Pili, or fimbriae, are structures that resemble cilia (small hairs). They help to hold bacteria securely to one spot. Choice A is incorrect because ribosomes are internal structures of bacterial cells and the sites of protein synthesis. Choice B is incorrect because flagella are structures of bacteria that help with motility. Choice C is incorrect because endospores are bacterial cells that form so that the bacteria can survive, even in harsh conditions.

12. **The correct answer is C.** Antibodies produced by B-lymphocytes in the immune system can attach to the protein head of a virus and prevent it from attaching to a host cell. Interferons are a second type of defense against viruses in the human body; they prevent viral replication in cells. Choice A is incorrect because antibodies are produced by B-lymphocytes, so they are not two distinct defense mechanisms. Choice B is incorrect because vaccines are not produced in the body. Choice D is incorrect because antibiotics are used as a defense against bacterial infections, and they are not produced in the human body.

13. **The correct answer is A.** Transcription is the production of RNA from DNA, so reverse transcription, performed by reverse transcriptase, makes DNA (cDNA) from RNA. Choice B is incorrect because it describes typical transcription. Choice C is incorrect because it describes typical translation. Choice D is incorrect because it describes the reverse of translation.

14. **The correct answer is A.** The flu virus is polyhedral and enveloped. Choices B and C represent other virus shapes, including the helical tobacco mosaic virus and the complex bacteriophage. Choice D often

refers to viruses that take on the helical conformation.

15. **The correct answer is B.** Bacteria are growing in size but not number during the lag phase. Choice A is incorrect because this is the stage during which the number of living bacteria declines. Choice C is incorrect because this is the main stage during which the bacterium undergoes binary fission. Choice D is incorrect because this is the stage during which bacterial growth plateaus due to competition for resources.

16. **The correct answer is A.** During conjugation, a donor bacterium transfers genetic material to another bacterium. Choice B is incorrect because transduction involves the transfer of genetic material among bacteria via bacteriophage. Choice C is incorrect because transformation describes the uptake of environmental genetic material by competent cells. Choice D is incorrect because only Choice A is correct.

17. **The correct answer is B.** Microaerophiles require only low oxygen concentrations. Choice A describes bacteria that grow best in oxygenated environments but can grow in the presence or absence of oxygen. Choice C describes bacteria that grow only in the presence of oxygen. Choice D describes bacteria that grow only in the absence of oxygen.

18. **The correct answer is A.** A sarcine is a cluster of eight cocci. Choice B is incorrect because a spirochete is a spiral-shaped bacterium. Choice C is incorrect because a tetrad is a cluster of four cocci. Choice D is incorrect because a vibrio is a half moon-shaped bacterium.

19. **The correct answer is B.** Athlete's foot and ringworm are both caused by the same fungus skin mycosis. Choices A, C, and D are incorrect because these are not caused by bacteria, prions, or viruses.

20. **The correct answer is C.** Yeast are able to pinch off as small buds from the parent cell to form a new cell. Choice A is incorrect because hyphae are the structures that release pheromones and initiate sexual reproduction. Choice B is incorrect because some fungi indeed release spores, but yeast are not among those fungi. Choice D is incorrect because karyogamy refers to the product of a diploid cell from haploid nuclei in sexual reproduction.

SUMMING IT UP

- Microorganisms are classified as 1) pathogenic, 2) opportunistic pathogenic, and 3) nonpathogenic.

- There are three main bacterial shapes: 1) cocci, 2) bacilli, and 3) spirilla.

- Different strains of bacteria require different levels of oxygen for optimal survival. They can grow in the presence or absence of oxygen, depending on the strain of bacteria.

- Different strains of bacteria require different temperatures for optimal growth. Most bacteria found in humans require a moderate temperature.

- Bacteria generally prefer a pH of 6.8 to 7.2 for optimal growth.

- The basic nutritional requirements of bacteria include a source of 1) carbon, 2) nitrogen, 3) hydrogen, 4) sulfur, 5) phosphorus, and 6) oxygen. Bacteria also need 7) minerals, such as iron, zinc, potassium, and calcium; 8) vitamins, including niacin, riboflavin, and B_6; and 9) water.

- Photosynthetic bacteria use light as a source of energy, and chemotrophs get energy from inorganic molecules and produce their own nutrients.

- Some bacteria require living cells and tissue as a source of nutrition. These are obligate parasites. Those that require nonliving material as an energy source are called obligate saprophytes. Those that can get nutrients from both living and nonliving materials are referred to as facultative.

- Major bacterial groups include proteobacteria (gram-negative bacteria), chlamydias, spirochetes, gram-positive bacteria, and cyanobacteria.

- Bacteria reproduce through the asexual process of binary fission, in which bacteria split in two. Bacteria experiences logarithmic growth (every generation doubles the preceding one).

- The function of the bacterial cell wall is to maintain the correct size and shape of the bacteria and to help prevent cell lysis. Peptidoglycan is an important chemical component of bacterial cell walls.

- Gram-positive bacteria have a thick layer of peptidoglycan (PG); therefore, they are more resistant to cell lysis than other bacteria strains. Gram-negative bacteria have only a thin layer of PG; therefore, their cell walls are weaker and easier to lyse.

- The main function of the cell membrane is to act as a semipermeable barrier for the cell.

- *Flagella* are found on both bacilli and spirilla bacteria. They function to add motility to the bacterial cell.

- *Pili*, or fimbriae, are structures that resemble cilia. They help to hold bacteria securely to one spot.

- In the cytoplasm of bacteria, there are two major components: nuclear material and ribosomes. Bacteria have one double-stranded circular DNA chromosome.

- Some bacteria can form resistant cells called *endospores*, which allow the bacteria to survive under harsh conditions.

- There are three methods of exchanging genetic information between bacteria in the same generation: transformation, transduction, and conjugation.

- Viruses are specific to an organism and most often a specific tissue type within that organism.

- The protein shell, or capsid, enclosing the viral genome takes on various shapes. These shapes include 1) polyhedrals, in particular icosahedrals; 2) cylindrical; 3) helical; and 4) complex viral shapes such as that of the bacteriophage.

- Different virus types can undergo one of the five following life cycles: 1) productive, 2) provirus, 3) RNA virus, 4) lytic, or 5) lysogenic. Some bacteriophage viruses can alternate between the lytic and lysogenic life cycles.

- The immune system is critical to the body's defense against viral infection and is the basis for the development of vaccines.

- There are two main antiviral defense mechanisms in the body: antibodies and interferons.

- Among the various species of fungi are those that live as decomposers (saprobes), parasites, and mutualistic symbionts.

- Fungi do not ingest food as animals do; instead, they digest nutrients while they are still in the environment.

- Some fungi are unicellular such as yeasts, but most fungal species are multicellular. The bodies of multicellular fungi typically form a network of tiny filaments called *hyphae*.

- *Hyphae* are made of tubular cell walls that are surrounded by plasma membrane. The hyphae form an interwoven mass called a *mycelium*. In most fungi, the hyphae are divided into cells by crosswalls called *septa*.

- Generally, sexual reproduction in fungi begins when hyphae (which have haploid nuclei), from two distinct mycelia, release sexually signaling molecules called pheromones.

- Sexual reproduction occurs in four stages: plasmogamy, karyogamy, meiosis, and germination.

- Many fungi can also reproduce asexually, and some types only reproduce asexually. During asexual reproduction, clones are produced by the mitotic production of spores.

- Yeast are fungi that live in moist environments. In general, they reproduce asexually through the process of budding.

- There are only about 50 species of fungi that are known to parasitize humans and animals.

- The general term for a fungal infection is *mycosis*. Systemic mycoses spread throughout the entire body and cause very serious illnesses.

- Fungi have useful medical applications and are often used in the fields of molecular biology and molecular genetics to study eukaryotic systems.

Anatomy and Physiology

OVERVIEW

- **The Nervous System**
- **The Skeletal and Muscular Systems**
- **The Cardiovascular System**
- **The Lymphatic and Immune Systems**
- **The Endocrine System**
- **The Respiratory System**
- **The Digestive System**
- **The Urinary System**
- **The Reproductive System**
- **Practice Questions**
- **Answer Key and Explanations**
- **Summing It Up**

Chapter 8 describes the anatomy and physiology of the human body. Anatomy is the study of the shape and structure of organisms and their parts. Physiology is the study of the biological functions of living organisms and their parts. Questions related to these topics constitute 20 percent of the PCAT, or about ten questions.

THE NERVOUS SYSTEM

The nervous system consists of

- the brain
- the spinal cord
- circuits of neurons (nerve cells) and supporting cells
- sensory receptors

The brain and the spinal cord constitute the central nervous system. Nerve cells that connect the central nervous system (CNS) with the rest of the body constitute the peripheral nervous system (PNS). In general, there are three stages of processing in the nervous system:

- sensory input of an internal or external stimulus
- integration of the signal
- a motor output

Each stage of the process is controlled by a specialized set of neurons. Sensory neurons transmit information from the sensors that detect the external stimuli (light, sound, taste, smell, or touch), or internal stimuli (blood pressure, blood oxygen level, muscle tension, etc.). This information is then sent from the PNS to the CNS, where interneurons integrate the sensory input by analyzing and interpreting the signal. The connection between interneurons is the most complex part of the nervous system. Motor output leaves the CNS through motor neurons.

Neurons

Nerve tissue mostly consists of cells, and a single cell of the nervous system is called a *neuron*. A neuron's main function is to communicate a signal from a stimulus to the CNS. Support cells, called *glial cells*, provide nutrition and the correct pH level for neurons to function properly. The following are the three main components of neurons:

1. **Cell body:** Most of the neuron's organelles, including its nucleus, are located in the cell body. The cell body is the main hub through which ingoing and outgoing nerve impulses must travel. Clusters of neuron cell bodies are called *ganglia*.

2. **Axon:** The axon is a long, slender, branched structure that extends from the cell body. The axons carry messages from one neuron to another or from the neuron to an effector cell. The end of the axon, called the *synaptic terminal*, is where the secretory component of the neuron is located. The site of communication between the synaptic terminal and another cell is called the *synapse*. At most synapses, the information is passed from a transmitting neuron (*presynaptic cell*) to a receiving neuron (*postsynaptic cell*). This transmission is carried out through the use of *neurotransmitters*, which are specialized chemical messengers. The *axon hillocks* are sites where a signal, or action potential, is generated before traveling along the axon.

3. **Dendrites:** The dendrites are highly branched extensions of the neuron that receive signals from other neurons. There is only one very long axon per neuron, but a single neuron may have numerous dendrites.

The complexity of a neuron and its shape is reflected in the number of synapses it has with other neurons. There are three categories of neurons that can be distinguished by the number of axons and dendrites:

1. **Unipolar neurons:** Unipolar neurons are generally sensory neurons that send signals directly to the CNS. Unipolar neurons are generally found in embryos and invertebrates. They have one extension, or process, that extends from the cell body to form one axon.

2. **Bipolar neurons:** Bipolar neurons are rare in humans and are found in the retina of the eye, in olfactory tissue, and in the vestibulocochlear nerve in the ear. Thus, they are specialized sensory neurons involved in the sensory pathways for sight, smell, taste and hearing. A bipolar cell has two extensions: an axon at one end and a dendrite at the other end.

3. **Multipolar neurons:** Almost all neurons are multipolar. These neurons have many extensions (processes): one axon and numerous dendrites.

Use the margins of this book to rewrite the main points of lists like this. Rewriting information can help you remember it.

Myelin Sheath

Many axons are enclosed by a layer called the *myelin sheath*. Myelin is made of lipids and lipoproteins. The speed of the signal transmitted through the neuron is determined by the diameter of the axon and the degree of myelination. The greater the axon diameter, the faster the impulse signal travels through the neuron. Along a myelinated axon, there are spaces called the *nodes of Ranvier*. The impulse signal travels by jumping from node to node along the axon. This will increase the speed of propagation in a myelinated axon compared to a nonmyelinated axon.

Neurons can also be classified according to their three functions:

1. **Sensory or afferent neurons:** Sensory neurons are unipolar neurons that conduct nerve impulses to the CNS. The cell body of sensory neurons lies outside of the CNS (they are not found in the brain or the spinal cord). Cell bodies of unipolar sensory neurons are most often clumped together in structures called *dorsal root ganglia*.

2. **Motor or efferent neurons:** Motor neurons are multipolar neurons that conduct nerve impulses away from the CNS. The cell bodies of motor neurons are found within the CNS, and they conduct impulses from the CNS to effector cells such as muscle and gland cells. Motor neurons have a myelin sheath. There are two further divisions of the motor neurons:

   a. **Somatic:** The somatic motor neurons make up the voluntary nervous system. The somatic nervous system, which is a part of the PNS, carries nerve signals to and from the skeletal muscles. This system is called voluntary because it is subject to conscious control.

   b. **Autonomic:** The autonomic nervous system is controlled by reflexes mediated by the spinal cord to the brainstem. It conducts impulses from the CNS to the cardiac muscles, smooth muscles, and glands, as well as to the organs of the digestive, cardiovascular, excretory, and endocrine systems.

      • The sympathetic division of the automatic nervous system corresponds to arousal and energy generation, or what is called the "fight-or-flight" response.

      • The parasympathetic division is often referred to as the digestive or resting division. It promotes responses that restore the body to a resting and normal functioning state.

      • The enteric division of the autonomic nervous system consists of a network of neurons in the digestive tract, the pancreas, and the gallbladder. This division controls secretion and smooth muscle activity in these organs. The enteric division is normally regulated by both the sympathetic and parasympathetic divisions.

3. **Interneurons:** Interneurons, or associated neurons, are multipolar neurons that function in signal integration. They are neurons that lie between the sensory neurons and the motor neurons. They have a role in evaluating the sensory input and sending the correct output to the motor neurons. These neurons lie entirely within the CNS and are unmyelinated. About 99 percent of all neurons in the human body are interneurons.

Figure 1. Neurons and Myelinated Axons

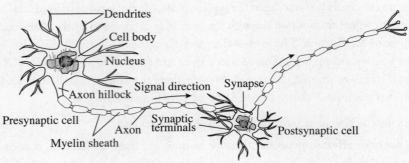

Glial Cells

Glial cells are support cells that are necessary to maintain the structural integrity of the nervous system and the normal functioning of neurons. There are several types of glial cells in the CNS and PNS. Depending on the type, glia may nourish neurons, insulate their axons, or help maintain homeostasis of the extracellular fluid surrounding the neuron. There are four types of glial cells:

1. **Astrocytes:** In the CNS, the astrocytes provide structural support for neurons, regulate the extracellular concentration of ions (Na^+ and K^+), and recycle neurotransmitters. They have many projections that attach to the dendrites of neurons. During embryonic development, astrocytes induce the formation of tight junctions between cells that line the capillaries of the brain and cells in the spinal cord. This results in the formation of the blood-brain barrier, which restricts the passage of most substances into the CNS.

2. **Radial Glia:** In a developing embryo, radial glia form tracts along which newly formed neurons can migrate from the neural tube (pre-CNS in a developing embryo) to other positions in the body.

3. **Oligodendrocytes:** These are glial cells that form a myelin sheath around the axon of neurons in the CNS.

4. **Schwann cells:** Schwann cells myelinate the axons of motor neurons in the PNS. Both Schwann cells and oligodendrocytes grow around axons, wrapping them in many layers similar to a jellyroll. Because the layers are mostly composed of lipids, the myelin sheath is also a good form of insulation for the axons. In people with the disease multiple sclerosis, the myelin sheath deteriorates, which causes a progressive loss of body function due to the disruption of nerve signal transmission.

Ion Pumps and Ion Channels

All cells have an electrical potential difference, or voltage, across their plasma membrane. This voltage is the potential energy of the cell and is called the membrane potential. The membrane potential of a typical cell is about –60 to –80 mV (millivolts), when there is no signal being transmitted by the cell. The cytoplasm inside the cell has a negative potential and the fluid outside the cell has a positive potential. The voltage across the plasma membrane of a resting cell is called the *resting potential*. The resting potential exists because of the difference in the concentration of ions in the cytoplasm compared to the fluid outside the cell.

The plasma membrane of each neuron has protein channels and pumps that allow for the passage of ions into and out of the cell. In general, the concentration of Na^+ ions is greater outside the cell and the concentration of K^+ ions is greater inside the cell. This is because sodium channels allow for very little sodium ion to diffuse into the cell. Potassium ions, however, are able to flow out of the cell more freely through potassium channels. In addition, sodium-potassium pumps actively transport Na^+ out of the cell and K^+ into the cell. The ionic gradient (high K^+/low Na^+ inside and low K^+/high Na^+ outside) produces an electrical potential difference across the plasma membrane.

Neurons also have different types of gated ion channels that open and close in response to one of three kinds of stimuli:

1. **Stretch-gated ion channels:** Stretch-gated ion channels are found in cells that sense stretch and open when the membrane is mechanically deformed (stretched).

2. **Ligand-gated ion channel:** Ligand-gated ion channels are found at synapses. These channels open and close when a specific chemical such as a neurotransmitter is bound to the channel.

3. **Voltage-gated ion channels:** Voltage-gated ion channels are generally found in axons and open and close when there is a change in membrane potential.

Gated-ion channels are essential for generating signals that travel through the nervous system.

Action Potential

A stimulus is a factor, either internal or external, that triggers a nerve signal. An *action potential* is a nerve signal that carries information from the stimulus along the axon of a neuron. Action potential is triggered when the cell reaches its threshold potential. The *threshold potential* is reached when a stimulus is applied to the cell and most activation gates of the sodium ion channels are opened and potassium ion channels remain closed. The voltage then rises from the resting potential to a threshold voltage, thus triggering the action potential. Once the action potential is triggered, the polarity of the cell is quickly reversed, with the interior of the cell becoming positive with respect to the outside. This reverse in polarity is due to the influx of Na^+ ions into the cell. Eventually, the sodium ion channels close, blocking the influx of Na^+, and the activation gates on most potassium ion channels open causing an efflux of K^+ ions. This causes the inside of the cell to become more negative again. Eventually, the membrane returns to its resting potential.

The rapid flip-flop of the membrane potential due to the movement of Na^+ and K^+ across the membrane is what causes the electrical changes of the action potential. An action potential travels along an axon from the cell body to the synaptic terminal. It travels by regenerating itself along the axon through the opening and closing of ion channels along the axon. In this way, the nerve signals travel in one direction along the axon to the synaptic terminal.

Synapses

Neurons communicate with each other at cell synapses. When an action potential reaches the synaptic terminal of an axon, it stops. Action potentials are generally not transmitted from one neuron to another. However, there is a transmission of the stimulus signal from one neuron to another. This transmission occurs at the synapse, or the space between the synaptic terminal of a neuron and another neuron.

Most synapses are chemical synapses and involve the release of neurotransmitters from the synaptic terminal of a neuron. Neurotransmitters are in a package called a *synaptic vesicle*. Common neurotransmitters include: acetylcholine, norepinephrine, dopamine, and serotonin. When an action potential reaches the synaptic terminal and the terminal membrane is depolarized through the opening of Ca^{2+} ion channels, synaptic vesicles fuse the terminal membrane of the axon and release neurotransmitters. The neurotransmitters diffuse across the synaptic cleft (the space between the presynaptic neuron and the postsynaptic cell), transferring the information from the original stimulus. In this way, chemical synapses make it possible for cells to process complex information from stimuli.

The Central Nervous System (CNS)

In the CNS, *gray matter* refers to cell bodies and all unmyelinated axons and white matter refers to myelinated axons and all glial cells. A fully developed CNS is composed of the spinal cord with cerebrospinal fluid, the brain stem, and the brain. All information from the PNS is processed in the CNS.

The brain is protected by several layers. The skin of the scalp covers the outer periosteum of the flat bones of the skull. Inside the inner periosteum of the skull bones are the *meninges*. The first meningeal layer is the *dura mater*; the second layer is the *arachnoid mater*, followed by the *subarachnoid space*. The subarachnoid space provides a path for cerebrospinal fluid to flow. Next to the subarachnoid space is the *pia mater*. It follows all the folds of brain tissue and is tightly adhered to it. Meninges also surround the spinal cord, and cerebrospinal fluid is processed in the choroid plexus, composed of capillaries with leaky junctions and glial cells. The final protective mechanism of the brain is the *blood–brain barrier*. Most brain capillaries have tight junctions so that nothing can leak out, and there is a high level of control as to the blood components that end up going to the brain.

The Brain Stem

The brain stem is composed of three regions:

1. **Medulla oblongata:** The *medulla oblongata* is continuous with the spinal cord. The function of the inferior portion is to play a role in maintaining primitive life functions, such as heart beat, respiration, blood vessel diameter, swallowing, vomiting, sneezing, and coughing. These activities help to keep the body safe from noxious substances and foreign objects. Cranial nerves VIII through XII leave the brain through the medulla oblongata.

2. **Pons:** The middle section of the brain stem is called the *pons*. It acts as a bridge to connect the higher brain centers of the cerebral hemispheres to the lower brain center in the medulla oblongata. The pons attaches to the cerebellum. It is also involved in controlling respiratory rate and sleep patterns. The cranial nerves V through VII exit the brain through the pons.

3. **Midbrain:** The midbrain is the smallest section of the brain stem. The midbrain contains centers for the receipt of different types of sensory information. It also sends sensory information to specific regions of the forebrain. The prominent centers of the midbrain are the inferior and superior colliculi (part of the auditory and visual systems).

Sketching diagrams can help you learn and remember information. Use the margin to draw a diagram of the brain.

The Diencephalon

The midbrain of the brain stem connects to the diencephalon, which is referred to as the interbrain. It is the back section of the forebrain, and there are the following three parts to the diencephalon.

1. **Epithalamus:** One of the most important features of the epithalamus is the *pineal gland*, an endocrine gland deep inside the brain. The pineal gland produces *melatonin*, a hormone essential in regulating sleep-wake cycles. Melatonin levels increase at night causing sleepiness. Melatonin is also thought to inhibit the onset of puberty and to play a role in puberty when it does begin. The *choroid plexus* in the epithalamus produces cerebrospinal fluid from blood.

2. **Thalamus:** The thalamus is the main input center for sensory information coming from all regions of the body going into the cerebrum, and the main output center for motor information leaving the cerebrum to all regions of the body. In the thalamus, sensory information is sorted and sent to the correct region of the cerebrum, and motor information is also sorted and sent to the correct region of the body.

3. **Hypothalamus:** The hypothalamus is part of the autonomic nervous system. It is one of the most important regions of the brain for homeostatic regulation, even though it is a very small portion of the brain. It is the autonomic control center for blood pressure, heart rate regulation, respiration rate, digestive tract function, and overlaps in function with the medulla oblongata. It also contains the body's thermostat and centers for regulating hunger, thirst, and other basic survival mechanisms. The hypothalamus also plays a role in sexual and mating behaviors is part of the limbic system, which controls emotional responses.

The Cerebellum

The cerebellum is often referred to as the "little brain." It is located at the back and bottom portion of the brain. It coordinates voluntary movement of the body, and is involved in balance. It is also involved in error checking during perceptual, motor, and cognitive functions. It is most likely involved in learning and remembering motor skills such as riding a bicycle. It produces smooth muscle coordination.

The cerebellum receives sensory information about the position of joints and length of muscles as well as information from visual or auditory systems. It also receives information about motor output from the cerebrum. The cerebellum then coordinates movement and balance by integrating this sensory input and motor output. Hand-eye coordination is a good example of control by the cerebellum.

The Cerebrum

The cerebrum is divided into right and left hemispheres. It is where all of the activity of the conscious is located. Each hemisphere consists of an outer covering of gray matter, the cerebral cortex (white matter), and groups of neurons collectively called *basal nuclei*. The basal nuclei are located deep within the white matter, and they are important centers for planning and learning sequences of movement.

The cerebral cortex is the largest and most complex part of the brain. In this region of the brain, sensory information is analyzed and processed, motor commands are issued based upon the sensory input into the cerebral cortex, language is also generated in this region. The cerebral cortex is also divided into right and left sides, and each side is responsible for the opposite side of the body. A thick band of axons known as the *corpus callosum* allows for communication between the left and right cerebral cortices. Each side of the cerebral cortex has four lobes: frontal, temporal, occipital, and parietal lobes. Areas within each lobe have been identified, including primary sensory areas, which receive and process sensory information. There are also association areas in each lobe that integrate the information from various parts of the brain.

The prefrontal cortex is located in the anterior, or front-most, portion of the cerebral cortex. It is the part of the brain that gives us "human" attributes such as intellect, personality type, mood, and motivation. The frontal lobe of the brain has processing centers for speech, and it also contains the motor cortex at the location known as the *precentral gyrus*. All motor output is initiated here, and there are four motor areas.

1. **Primary motor cortex:** This is a motor output center. It does not control how an action is carried out, but only that it is performed.

2. **Premotor cortex:** This area is responsible for organizing movement. It is also the site where data about learned motor skills is stored in the brain.

3. **Brocca's area:** This is the center for motor control of speech, organization of speech, and language comprehension.

4. **Frontal eye field:** This region controls the voluntary movement of the eye.

There are six sensory areas of the cerebral cortex.

1. **Somatosensory area:** The *primary somatosensory cortex* in the parietal lobe receives data from touch receptors on the skin and muscles. The somatosensory association cortex is also in the parietal lobe and is responsible for evaluating somatosensory input and analyzing the data.

2. **Visual areas:** The areas of the cerebral cortex that process visual information are found in the occipital lobe. There is a *primary visual cortex* where visual sensory input is first received in the cerebral cortex. Next, the sensory information goes to the visual association area, which is how we recognize an object that we see.

3. **Auditory areas:** The auditory areas of the cerebral cortex are found in the temporal lobe. Auditory input first goes to the *primary auditory cortex* where actual hearing takes place. The auditory association area in the temporal lobe is where the sound that we hear is interpreted.

4. **Olfactory area:** Olfactory areas are also located in the temporal lobe. The *olfactory cortex* is responsible for receiving smell input and interpreting it.

5. **Taste area:** Taste is processed and analyzed in the *gustatory cortex* located in the parietal lobe.

6. **Wernicke's area:** This is a second area that is devoted to speech and is located in the posterior portion of the temporal lobe. It is in this area that speech is comprehended.

The Spinal Cord

The spinal cord is encased in vertebrae so that it can remain anchored in place and not be jostled about by the movement of the body. The spinal cord terminates in a cone-shaped structure called the *conus medullaris*. A fibrous connective tissue called the *filum terminale* is continuous with the pia mater from the apex of the conus medullaris and enclosed within the dura mater. Extending downward, the spinal cord clings to the dura mater and attaches to the first section of the coccyx.

The spinal cord is not uniform in diameter; instead, there are two regions that are enlarged: the *cervical enlargement* and the *lumbar enlargement*. The nerves for the upper and lower limbs arise in these enlargements.

The spinal cord is made of myelinated white matter surrounding two unmyelinated gray matter butterfly-shaped sections in the middle. The two lateral gray masses in the cross section are connected by the gray commissure, which encloses the central canal. Tracts made up of axons within the CNS run the length of the spinal cord. Tracts ascending toward the brain are *sensory (afferent) tracts*, and those descending from the brain are *motor (efferent) tracts*.

The Peripheral Nervous System (PNS)

The PNS functions to transmit information to and from the CNS. It plays a large role in regulating the movement and internal environment of an organism. The vertebrate PNS consists of right-left pairs of cranial and spinal nerves along with associated ganglia. Cranial nerves originate in the brain and terminate in organs of the head and upper body. Spinal nerves originate in the spinal cord and extend to parts of the body below the head. Mammals have twelve pairs of cranial nerves and thirty-one pairs of spinal nerves. Most cranial nerves and all of the spinal nerves contain axons of both sensory and motor neurons. Some cranial nerves, such as those involved in the olfactory system, have only sensory neurons.

The PNS is divided into two parts: the *somatic* and the *autonomic* nervous systems.

1. **The somatic nervous system:** This system carries signals to and from skeletal muscles in response to external stimuli. This system regulates voluntary movement and conscious control.

2. **The autonomic nervous system:** This system regulates the internal environment by controlling smooth and cardiac muscles and the organs of the digestive, cardiovascular, excretory, and endocrine systems. There are three divisions of the autonomic nervous system: *sympathetic*, *parasympathetic*, and *enteric*.

ALERT

Use the clock to pace yourself. You will have about half a minute to answer each question. Don't get bogged down in the first questions or get tired in the middle and fall behind your pace.

Reflexes

Reflexes are controlled by a five-part neural pathway called the *reflex arc*:

1. Receptor
2. Sensory neuron (in the spinal cord)
3. Association neuron (interneuron)
4. Motor neuron
5. Effector

This pathway does not go to the cerebral cortex of the brain. The muscular response of a reflex reaction is mediated exclusively at the level of the spinal cord. Because the sensory information does not travel all the way to the cortex, the reaction is fast and reflexive. When there is only one synapse between the sensory and motor neurons without any association neuron, the reflex is *monosynaptic*. When an association or interneuron is between the sensory and motor neuron, the reflex is *polysynaptic*.

Ipsilateral responses are responses on the same side of the body as the sensory input. *Contralateral* responses are those on the opposite side of the body as the sensory input.

THE SKELETAL AND MUSCULAR SYSTEMS

The skeletal system includes all joint and bones in the body.

Joints

Joints are sites where two bones join together and articulate. Joints serve to add mobility to the skeletal structure and to hold the skeleton together. However, not all joints are movable. Joints are classified by two different systems.

1. **Functional:** The functional classification of a joint is dependent upon how the joint works.

    a. **Synarthroses:** These are immovable joints.

    b. **Amphiarthroses:** These are slightly movable joints.

    c. **Diarthroses:** These are freely movable joints.

    d. **Synostoses:** A term used to describe fused bony joints.

2. **Structural:** The structural classification of a joint is determined by how the joint is constructed.

    a. **Fibrous joints:** Fibrous joints are joined by fibrous tissue full of collagen fibers. Most fibrous joints are immovable. There is no joint cavity in a fibrous joint. *Sutures* are fibrous joints found only in the skull. The bones have a double-zigzag holding them together. These types of joints are immovable, or synarthroses. *Syndesmoses* are fibrous joints held together by ligaments. These types of joints have minimal movement and are amphiarthroses. *Gomphoses* are specialized fibrous peg-in-socket joints between the teeth and the mandible and maxilla. These joints are secured with periodontal ligament, and they are immovable.

b. **Cartilaginous joints:** Cartilaginous joints are articulating bones united by cartilage. There is no joint cavity in a cartilaginous joint. *Synchondroses* are cartilaginous joints in which a bar or plate of hyaline cartilage unites the bones. Almost all of these types of joint are synarthroses joints. *Symphyses* are cartilaginous joints in which the articular surfaces of the bones are covered with articular (hyaline) cartilage. This cartilage is fused to a pad or plate of fibrocartilage, which forms a type of shock absorber in the joint. These types of joints are *amphiarthroses*.

c. **Synovial joints:** Synovial joints are articulating bones separated by a fluid-containing joint cavity. This type of joint is freely moving, or *diarthroses*. All joints of the limbs and most joints of the body are synovial. These types of joints include ball-and-socket, hinge, and pivot joints. These joints are continuous with hyaline cartilage and have a *synovial membran*e (a membrane formed by a layer of connective tissue). It is the synovial membrane and the cartilage that define the joint cavity. The cavity contains synovial fluid that is secreted by the synovial membrane. The hyaline, cartilage, synovial membrane, and synovial fluid act as a shock absorber. Surrounding the synovial membrane is a fibrous capsule that together with the membrane forms the *articular capsule*. Movement of these joints is carried out by surrounding muscles, and muscle attachment crosses the joint.

Joint Range of Motion

There are three basic movements allowed by synovial joints.

1. **Gliding:** Gliding occurs when two surfaces of the joint slide past each other. In the femoropatellar joint, the patella glides across the patellar surface of the femur.

2. **Angular motion:** There are various forms of angular motion in joints. *Flexion* is movement in the anterior/posterior plane that reduces the angle between the articulating elements. *Extension* occurs in the same plane and increases the angle between the two articulating elements. Extension beyond a standing anatomical position is called *hyperextension*. *Abduction* is movement away from the longitudinal axis of the body, and *adduction* is movement towards the longitudinal axis. *Circumduction* is the movement of the arm or leg in a loop, independent of actually rotating a limb in a joint.

3. **Rotational movements:** Rotational movements involve the rotation of a part of the body with respect to an axis. Head rotation is either left or right, whereas limb rotation is medial or lateral. There are also special motions of the hands and feet. *Pronation* includes a rotation of the hand so that the palm is facing downward, or the rolling inward of the foot. *Supination* is the rotation of the hand into a palm-up position, or the rolling outward of the foot.

There are six basic types of synovial joints.

1. **Hinge joint:** This type of single-axis joint can only be flexed or extended through angular motion in a single plane. Examples of hinge motion are seen in movement of the jaw or the knee.

2. **Plane joint:** Plane joints have flattened or only slightly curved faces that allow gliding motion. An example of a plane joint is the femoropatellar joint.

3. **Pivot joint:** This type of joint allows rotation around a single axis. The radius and the ulna rotate around each other at both the proximal and distal end.

4. **Condyloid joint:** In this type of joint, there is angular motion in two planes and circumduction. The radiocarpal joint of the wrist moves in a condyloid fashion.

5. **Saddle joint:** This type of joint resembles a saddle. It allows angular motion in two planes and circumduction, but not rotation. An example of this type of joint motion is seen at the base of the thumb, or carpometacarpal joint.

6. **Ball-and-socket joint:** These types of joints have the greatest range of motion. They allow for various combinations of angular and rotational movement. The shoulder and hip joints are examples of ball-and-socket joints.

Figure 2. The Human Skeletal System

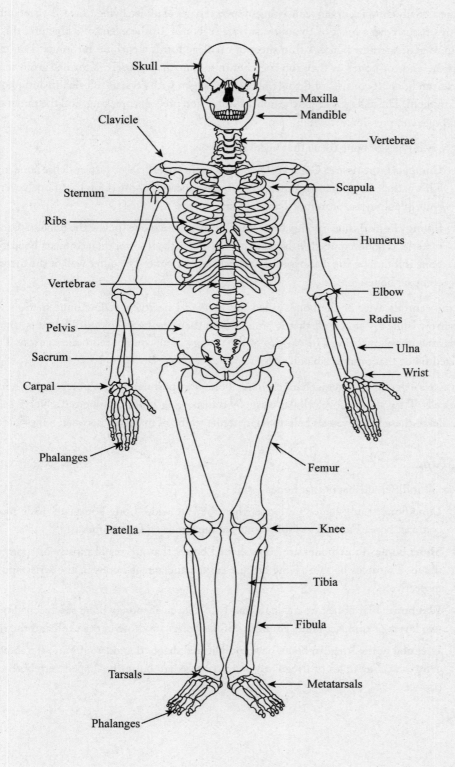

Bones

Bones are actually complex organs consisting of several types of moist, living tissue. A sheet of fibrous connective tissue covers most of the outer surface of bones. In the event of a fracture, this tissue will help to generate new bone. A thin sheet of cartilage forms a cushion for joints. This cushion protects the ends of bones as they rub together in a joint. *Bone matrix* is formed from materials secreted from bone. It consists of flexible fibers of collagen with crystals of calcium and phosphate bonded to them. The collagen keeps the bones flexible and prevents breaking, and the minerals help to resist bone compression.

There are two types of bone tissue that make up a bone.

1. **Compact bone tissue:** Compact bone tissue is the superficial or surface dense bone material. This is the reason that the outside of a bone appears smooth. Compact bone covers both ends of epiphyses, or rounded ends, of long bones.

2. **Spongy bone tissue:** Spongy bone is the deeper bone tissue (below the bone surface). This material is honeycombed with small cavities that make it softer than compact bone. Spongy bone is found on the diaphysis, or midsection, of a bone. The outer wall of the diaphysis is compact bone.

Inside the central cavity of the bone, called the *medullary cavity,* is yellow bone marrow. Yellow bone marrow is mostly stored fat that is brought into the bone by the blood. The fat is what gives bone marrow its yellow color. The cavities of the spongy bone contain red bone marrow. This is a specialized tissue that produces blood cells.

Blood vessels extending through channels in the bone transport nutrients and regulatory hormones to bone cells. They also remove cellular waste by transporting it out of bone cells. Nerve cells that run parallel to these blood vessels help to regulate the traffic of materials between bones and blood.

Bone Shape

There are four different shapes that bones form.

1. **Long bone:** Long bones are longer than they are wide. Long bones are made mostly of compact bone. Examples of long bone are the femur and the humerus.

2. **Short bone:** Short bones are cube-shaped bones that are made mostly of spongy bone tissue. Examples of short bone are the carpus and tarsus bones in the wrist and ankle, respectively.

3. **Flat bone:** Flat bones are made primarily of a layer of spongy bone sandwiched between two layers of compact bone. Examples of flat bones are those in the skull and the ribs.

4. **Irregular bone:** Irregular bones have complicated shapes that do not fit into the above three categories. Examples of irregularly shaped bones are butterfly-shaped vertebrae and the coccyx.

Bone Function

The following are the five common functions of bones:

1. **Support framework:** Bones function to support the body and protect organs.

2. **Movement:** Muscles are attached to bones with tendons that use bones as levers to help move body parts.

3. **Protection:** Fused bones of the skull protect the brain, vertebrae surround and protect the spinal cord, and ribs protect the vital organs in the thoracic region.

4. **Storage:** Long bones store fat in the form of yellow bone marrow. The minerals calcium and phosphate are stored in bone tissue. There is a constant flow of input and output of minerals in bones. If there is a deficiency of calcium in the diet, the body will remove calcium from bone tissue. Growth factors such as insulin-like growth factor, transforming growth factor, and bone morphogenic protein are also stored in bones.

5. **Blood cell formation:** Bones are the site of blood cell formation. This blood cell formation, called *hematopoiesis*, occurs in the medullary cavities, or the marrow cavities, of certain bones.

Compact Bone

A cross section of compact bone reveals highly organized patterns of concentric rings. These rings are cylindrical structures called *osteons*. Osteons are the basic structural units of compact bone. Each osteon is cylindrical and parallel to the long axis of the bone. The cylindrical structure is a conduit for blood vessels, nerves, and lymphatic vessels of the immune system. Each osteon has a series of layers called *lamellae*. Compact bone is sometimes referred to as *lamellar bone*. The network of osteons is called the *Haversian system*.

A structure called the *Haversian canal* runs along the bone axis and through the core of each osteon, and arteries run through the canal. These canals are lined with a connective tissue lining called *endosteum*. *Volkmann's canals* run at right angles perforating out from the central Haversian canals. Volkmann's canals connect the blood and nerve supply to the periosteum, to the central Haversian canals, and to the medullary cavity of the bone. The *periosteum* is the outer fibrous layer of dense irregular connective tissue on the outside of the bone. *Sharpey's fibers* are dense fibrous irregular connective tissue that connects the periosteum to the bone.

Osteocytes are mature bone cells that are found throughout the cylindrical osteons. The osteocytes are found within hollow cavities called *lacunae*. *Canaliculi* are small hairlike canals that connect lacunae to each other and to the central Haversian canal. *Medullary cavities* are located in the bone's center and contain the yellow bone marrow.

Spongy Bone

The honeycomb structure of spongy bone allows the bone to remain light. Spongy bone is composed of small needlelike or flat pieces called *trabeculae*. Trabeculae line up along stress lines of the bone to help the bone resist stress as much as possible. Trabeculae have irregularly arranged lamellae and osteocytes interconnected by canaliculi. Nutrients for spongy bone come through the canaliculi from capillaries and endosteum.

Bone Composition

Bone is composed of both organic and inorganic materials.

1. **Organic bone composition:**

   a. **Osteogenic cells:** Osteogenic cells are mitotic cells found in the periosteum and endosteum of bone. These cells originate from mesenchyme. Some osteogenic cells differentiate into *osteoblasts*, which help to build bone tissue. Some osteogenic cells become bone stem cells to provide osteoblasts at a later time. Other osteogenic cells become *osteocytes*, which are mature bone cells that secrete a matrix.

   b. **Osteoclasts:** Osteoclasts are cells that arise from hematopoietic stem cells that produce macrophages. These are large multinucleate cells that break down bone tissue. Lysosomal enzymes and HCl are used by osteoclasts to convert calcium salts to a soluble form of calcium.

   c. **Osteoid:** Osteoid is part of the organic matrix that is secreted by osteocytes. Osteoid is composed of collagen and glycoproteins, both of which provide flexibility to bones. Collagen also provides strength to bone structure.

2. **Inorganic bone composition:** Sixty-five percent of the inorganic part of the bone matrix is *hydroxyapatites*, which are mineral salts. Tightly packed calcium phosphate crystals surround the collagen fibers in the extracellular matrix of the bone. This imparts hardness to the bone, so it is able to resist compression.

Bone Development

Bone development is dependent on the type of bone. In the early stages of development, all long bones are composed of hyaline cartilage. Hyaline cartilage is a slimy mass with firm consistency and large amounts of collagen. It is a flexible semitransparent substance of pearly blue color. Hyaline cartilage undergoes a four-stage process called *endochondral ossification*:

1. Hyaline structure is supported by a bone collar. A primary ossification center forms in the middle of the diaphysis.

2. Secondary ossification centers form at the two epiphyses at the ends.

3. The medullary cavity forms at the primary ossification center. As ossification of the shaft continues, the bone hollows out.

4. A cartilaginous wedge forms between the epiphyses and the diaphysis. These are known as the *epiphyseal plates*. Ossification of the epiphyses continues. When ossification is complete, the only hyaline that is left is in the epiphyseal plates.

Bone is a dynamic and constantly changing structure in the body. Osteoclasts play an important role in the buildup and breakdown of bone tissue. There is a dynamic relationship between osteoblasts and osteoclasts. Normal aging of the body will alter the proportion of bone cell breakdown to buildup. Healthy bones maintain a balance of osteoblasts and osteoclasts, which determines the relative bone deposition and reabsorption. The entire process of bone maintenance is under the direction of growth hormones.

Flat bone forms from the intermembraneous ossification of connective tissue. Flat bones are formed from fibrous connective tissue in the following four-step process:

1. A single ossification center is formed in the middle of a mesenchyme cell cluster that becomes an osteoblast.

2. Osteoblasts produce the organic bone matter called *osteoid*. Osteoid is mineralized, which creates spongy bone called *diploë*.

3. Compact bone is laid down on either side of the diploë. The periosteum forms.

4. Diploë vascular tissue becomes red bone marrow.

Common Bone Fractures

1. **Compression:** In a compression fracture, the bone is crushed. Compression fractures are most common in porous or osteoporotic bones.

2. **Comminuted:** In a comminuted fracture, the bone is broken into three or more pieces. This type of fracture is common in old or brittle bones.

3. **Spiral:** A spiral fracture is due to excessive twisting that causes a ragged break. This type of fracture is a common sports injury.

4. **Depressed:** In a depressed fracture, the bone is pushed inward and makes a dent. Skull fractures are the most common type of depressed fracture.

5. **Greenstick:** A greenstick fracture is an incomplete break in which the bone cracks, but does not break all the way through. This type of fracture occurs in the softer, more flexible bones of children.

6. **Torus fracture:** This is also called a "buckle" fracture. The topmost layer of bone on one side of the bone is compressed, causing the other side to bend away from the growth plate. The bone does not separate. This is another common fracture in children, especially in the wrist.

7. **Growth plate fracture:** This is also called a physeal fracture and occurs at or across the growth plate. Usually, the fractures are common in the wrists of children and affect the growth plate of the radius.

The Muscular System

The skeleton and muscles interact to provide movement of the body. The bones act as a lever to produce movement, which is controlled by muscles. Muscles are connected to bones by tendons. The action of the muscle is always to contract, which shortens the length of the muscle. The relaxation of the muscle back to its extended position is a passive process. All animals have antagonistic pairs of muscles that apply force in opposite directions in order to move parts of the skeletal structure and body.

Muscle Tissue

There are three types of muscle tissue:

1. **Skeletal muscle:** Each skeletal muscle fiber is wrapped by a delicate layer of connective tissue. This layer is called the *endomysium*, and it interconnects adjacent muscle fibers. Endomysium-wrapped fibers bundle together in a parallel arrangement to form a *fascicle*. Each fascicle is covered by *perimysium*, a layer of collagen fibers. The entire muscle is surrounded by the *epimysium*, which is a dense layer of collagen fibers. The volume of skeletal muscles is mostly made up of discrete protein bundles consisting of contractile proteins such as actin and myosin. *Myofibrils* are the bundle structures formed by the myofilaments of myosin and actin. Skeletal muscle is also called *striated muscle* because the arrangement of these proteins creates a striped pattern along the length of the myofibril. The pattern of horizontal stripes is caused by alternating bands of thin actin filaments (along with troponin and tropomysin) and thick myosin filaments. The following are the five distinct bands and zones of filaments:

   a. **I-band:** An I-band is a light-colored section of myofibril in which only thin myosin filaments are present.

   b. **A-band:** An A-band is a dark band of myofibril that has both thick and thin overlapping filaments.

   c. **Z-disc:** A Z-band is the midline of an I-band that acts to anchor the filaments.

   d. **H-zone:** An H-zone is the midsection of an A-band. It is composed of thick filaments only.

   e. **M-line:** An M-line is a dark line that vertically bisects the H-zone.

   One unit of the repeated striated pattern is called a *sarcomere*. A sarcomere is defined as the distance from one Z-disc to another. It is an A-band with half of an I-band on either side.

   The *epimysium* separates the muscle from surrounding tissue and organs. The collagen fibers of the endomysium and perimysium are interwoven and blend into one another. At the end of each muscle, the collagen fibers of the epimysium, perimysium, and endomysium form a bundle known as a *tendon*, or a broad sheet called an *aponeurosis*. These structures attach the muscle to bone. Tendons are firmly attached to bone by extending into the bone matrix.

2. **Smooth muscle:** Smooth muscle tissue occurs within almost every organ. It forms sheets, bundles, or sheaths around other tissues. In contrast to skeletal muscles, smooth muscle cells have a single nucleus. Smooth muscle has no myofibrils or sarcomeres, and no striations like skeletal muscle. Therefore, it is called *nonstriated muscle*. Smooth muscle contractions are innervated by the autonomic nervous system. Both sympathetic and parasympathetic signals cause involuntary contractions in smooth muscles.

   Smooth muscles organized in bundles, layers, or sheets play a role in many biological systems. In the digestive and urinary systems, smooth muscle regulates the movement of materials. Rings of smooth muscle called *sphincters* regulate the movement of material. In the intergumentary system, smooth muscles that surround blood vessels regulate the flow of blood to the skin and act to elevate hairs on the skin surface. In the cardiovascular system, muscle surrounding blood vessels controls blood flow and regulates blood pressure. In the respiratory system, muscle contraction or relaxation changes the resistance to air flow. In the urinary system, smooth muscle tissue in the walls of small blood vessels alters the rate of filtration in the kidneys. Smooth muscle contractions in the bladder help force urine out of the bladder. In the reproductive system, layers of smooth muscle help move sperm along the reproductive tract in males and help move oocytes along the reproductive tract in females.

3. **Cardiac muscle:** A cardiac muscle cell is relatively small compared to other muscle cells, and it is sometimes called a *cardiocyte* or *cardiac myocyte*. In general, it contains a centrally located nucleus (some cells have two nuclei). This type of muscle tissue is striated and contains intercalated discs connecting the ends of adjacent cells. It is organized into sarcomeres. This type of muscle tissue is only found in the heart, and contractions of this type of muscle, called *myocardial contractions*, are controlled by the autonomic nervous system. Cardiac muscle contractions require more calcium than other types of muscle contractions.

Sliding Filament Theory

According to the sliding filament model of muscle contraction, a sarcomere contracts, or shortens, when the thin filaments slide across the thick filaments. When the muscle is fully contracted, the thin actin filaments overlap in the middle of the sarcomere. Thus, the contraction shortens the sarcomere, but does not change the length of the microfilaments. A muscle can shorten in length up to 35 percent when all of its sarcomeres contract.

The structure of myosin is important for the movement of thin filaments. The head portions of the myosin (thick) filaments move by pivoting back and forth in an arc pattern. The heads are clustered at the ends of the sarcomere (tails are found in the middle). As the head swings toward the thin actin filament, it binds to an actin molecule, thus dragging the thin filament through the arc pattern. The action of hundreds of myosin heads acting on a thin filament causes it to slide toward the center of the sarcomere. The details of this interaction are as follows:

- The myosin head binds an ATP molecule. Myosin bound to ATP is in a low-energy position. Note that prior to the binding of myosin to actin, actin is bound to troponin I (TnI). TnI is bound to troponin C (TnC), which is bound to a calcium ion ($Ca2^+$). TnC is also bound to troponin T (TnT), which is bound to tropomyosin. Tropomyosin blocks the myosin head binding site on the actin. As more $Ca2^+$ binds TnC, there is a calcium-activated conformational change, and tropomyosin comes off the myosin head binding site. The myosin head can now bind to the site on actin.

- Myosin hydrolyzes the ATP to ADP and inorganic phosphate. This hydrolysis reaction releases energy, which acts to move the myosin closer to the actin filament.

- Both the actin and the myosin have complementary binding sites. The myosin head and the actin filament bind together and form a cross-bridge.

- ADP and phosphate are released, and the myosin goes back to its low energy state. This action is called the *power stroke* and pulls the thin filament toward the center of the sarcomere.

- The cross-bridge remains intact until another ATP molecule binds the myosin head.

At each subsequent power stroke, the myosin head binds to an actin filament, ahead of the previous one. The sequence of detach, extend, attach, and pull occurs over and over during muscle contraction. In the presence of ATP, the contraction continues until the signal to contract stops.

Figure 3. The Sliding Filament Model of Muscle Contraction

The thick filaments are shown in dark gray and the thin filaments are shown in light gray.

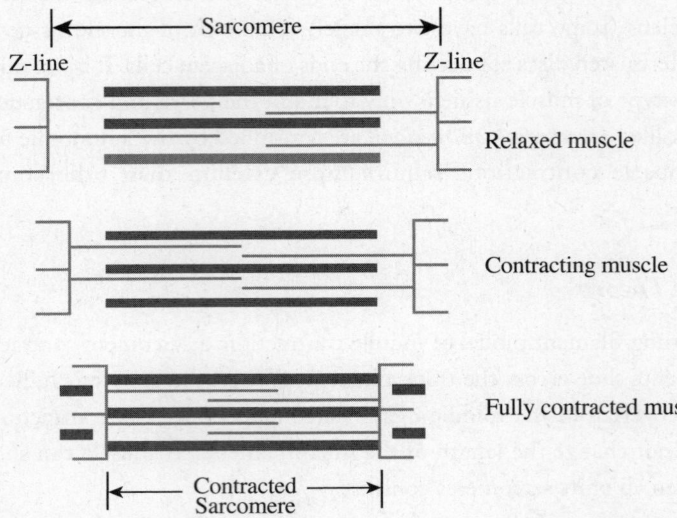

THE CARDIOVASCULAR SYSTEM

The human cardiovascular system is made up of three components: heart, blood, and blood vessels. All three components work together to pump blood through the body.

The Heart

The four-chambered heart is central to the cardiovascular system. It simultaneously pumps oxygen-poor blood to the lungs and oxygen-rich blood to the rest of the body. The pumping mechanism of the heart is a rhythmic cycle of contraction and relaxation. When the heart contracts, it pumps blood out toward different parts of the body. When the heart relaxes, its chambers are filled with blood. The continuous pumping and filling is known as the *cardiac cycle*.

The heart is located inside the medial cavity of the thorax. This cavity is called the *mediastinum*. It is partially covered by the lungs and off to the left side of the center of the body. The point of maximal intensity (PMI) is the apex of the heart located between the fifth and sixth ribs. The heart is enclosed in a double-layered sac called the *pericardium*. The outermost covering is called the *fibrous pericardium*. The fibrous pericardium has the following three functions:

1. **Protection:** The fibrous outer layer protects the heart from injury.
2. **Anchoring:** The fibrous pericardium anchors the heart in place.

3. **Prevention of overfilling:** The fibrous pericardium prevents the heart from filling with an excess amount of blood.

The inner layer of the pericardium is called the *serous pericardium*. The serous (moist membrane tissue) pericardium is further divided into two layers:

1. **Parietal layer:** The parietal layer is the more superficial of the two layers. It acts to contract the inner surface of the fibrous pericardium.

2. **Visceral layer:** The visceral layer of the serous pericardium is the deep layer. It is part of the outer portion of the heart wall and is also called the *epicardium*.

The space between the parietal layer and the visceral layer is called the *pericardial cavity*. It helps to decrease friction between the layers because it is filled with fluid. However, this region can become infected and inflamed. Also, if there is too much fluid in the pericardial cavity, it constricts the beating of the heart, a condition known as *cardiac tamponade*. Cardiac tamponade can be relieved by draining the excess fluid through the insertion of a needle.

The heart itself is made up of two layers:

1. **Myocardium:** The myocardium is the bulk of the heart. It is the contractile muscle tissue of the organ. The left ventricle of the heart pumps blood out of the heart to the body. It is thicker than the right ventricle because it must withstand higher pressure. The thickness of the walls keeps it from collapsing. Blood is pumped from the left ventricle to farther regions of the body than blood from the right ventricle, which pumps blood to the lungs. However, there are always equal amounts of blood in the left and right ventricles. When arteries become blocked and oxygenated blood cannot return to the heart, the heart muscle dies, and scar tissue develops. This is the primary cause of heart attacks, or myocardial infarctions.

2. **Endocardium:** The endocardium is the innermost layer of the heart. It lines the chambers of the heart, covers the valves, and is continuous with the blood vessels. The endocardium is made up of epithelial cells and connective tissue.

There are three main structures of the heart:

1. **The heart chambers:** The heart is divided into four chambers that are connected by valves. The two lower chambers of the heart are the *left* and *right ventricles*. The two upper chambers of the heart are the left and right atrium. Ventricles are responsible for pumping blood from the heart to other areas of the body, and *atria* receive blood returning to the heart from the body. Because more force is required to pump blood out of the heart than to receive blood back into the heart, the walls of the ventricle chambers are thicker than those of the atria.

   a. **The right ventricle:** The right ventricle receives blood from the right atrium and pumps it to the main pulmonary artery. The main pulmonary artery branches into the left and right pulmonary arteries, which both extend into the lungs. In this way, the oxygen-poor blood in the heart travels to the lungs where it picks up oxygen and is sent back to the heart via pulmonary veins. The right atrium receives oxygen-poor blood from the upper body through a vein called the *superior vena cava*, and the blood from the lower part of the body empties into the right atrium through the vein called the *inferior vena cava*. Blood from the heart is collected by the coronary sinus. All of this oxygen-poor blood is emptied into the right ventricle.

    b. **The left ventricle:** The left ventricle receives oxygen-rich blood from the left atrium of the heart. The left atrium receives the blood through the four pulmonary veins extending from the lungs. The left ventricle pumps the blood to the aorta. The aorta is the largest blood vessel of the body. The aorta carries and distributes oxygen-rich blood to the rest of the body.

2. **Septum:** The septum divides the chambers of the heart. The *interventricular septum* divides the left and right ventricles. The *interventricular sulci* are grooves located on the outside of the heart that mark the location of the interventricular septum. The *interarterial septum* divides the atria of the heart. On the anterior portion of the right atrium, the wall separating it from the left atrium contains bundles of muscles called the *pectinate muscles*. These muscles form ridges that look like the teeth of a comb. The interarterial septum has a shallow depression called the *fossa ovalis*, which is a residual from a structure called the *foramen ovale*. The latter serves as an opening for fetal circulation, but is not used after birth.

3. **Valves:** Heart valves are flap-like structures that allow blood to flow in one direction only. The heart valves prevent the back flow of blood as it is pumped from the atrium to the ventricle. The heart has two kinds of valves:

    a. **Atrioventricular valves:** *Atrioventricular valves* (AV valves) are composed of endocardium and connective tissue. They are located in the atria and the ventricles. The *mitral valve* is located between the left atrium and the left ventricle. The *tricuspid valve* is located between the right atrium and the right ventricle.

    b. **Semilunar valves:** The semilunar valves are flaps of endocardium and connective tissue reinforced by fibrous material. The fibers help prevent the valve from turning inside out. These valves have a half-moon shape. The *aortic valve* is located between the left ventricle and the aorta and prevents the backflow of blood into the ventricle as it is being pumped into the aorta. The *pulmonary valve* is located between the right ventricle and the pulmonary artery. It prevents the back flow of blood as it is pumped out of the right ventricle into the pulmonary artery.

Figure 4. The Human Heart

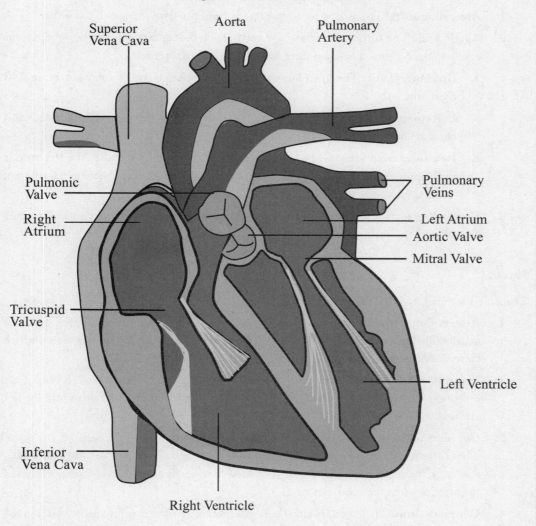

The Aorta

The aorta is the largest artery in the human body, and it functions to carry blood away from the heart. The aorta branches out of the left ventricle of the heart, forms an arch, and then extends down into the abdomen. Once in the abdomen, it branches out into smaller arteries. The walls of the aorta consist of three layers composed of connective tissue and elastic fibers.

- The *tunica adventitia* is the strong outer covering of arteries and veins. The collagen and elastic fibers of the tunica adventitia allow it to stretch and prevent overexpansion due to pressure exerted from the flow of blood from the heart.

- The *tunica media* is the middle layer of the walls of arteries and veins. It is composed of smooth muscle and elastic fibers. Arteries such as the aorta have a thicker tunica media layer than veins.

- The *tunica intima* is the inner layer of arteries and veins. In arteries, it is composed of an elastic membrane lining and smooth endothelium covered by elastic tissue.

The aorta has three basic branches:

1. **Ascending aorta:** The ascending aorta extends from the left ventricle of the heart.

2. **Aortic Arch:** The aortic arch arches over and to the left. It curves downward, right in front of the spinal column. There are three branches off the aortic arch:

   a. **Brachiocephalic:** The brachiocephalic artery supplies blood to the head, brain, and right arm.

   b. **Left common carotid:** The left common carotid artery supplies blood to the neck and chest areas.

   c. **Left subclavian artery:** The left subclavian artery supplies blood to the left arm. It runs below the clavicle, and the branches from this artery serve the vertebral column, spinal cord, and brain.

3. **Descending aorta:** The descending aorta travels through the chest to the abdomen. Branches extend from the aorta through this region.

Vessels

There are four main types of vessels in the body.

1. **Artery:** Blood vessels that carry blood away from the heart are called arteries. They are usually filled with oxygen-rich blood. One exception is the main pulmonary artery, which carries oxygen-poor blood to the lungs.

2. **Veins:** Blood vessels that carry oxygen-poor blood back to the heart are called veins. One exception is the pulmonary veins that carry oxygen-rich blood from the lungs into the left atrium.

3. **Coronary arteries:** There are left and right coronary arteries that branch off the aorta. These arteries deliver oxygenated blood to the heart muscle. When the heart (ventricle) contracts, the arteries are constricted and blood flow nearly stops. Blood is pumped out of the arteries when the ventricles relax.

4. **Coronary sinus:** The coronary sinus is a collection of veins that form a large vessel in the heart and collect the blood from the myocardium. The coronary sinus then delivers the oxygen-poor blood to the right atrium of the heart.

Blood Flow Through the Heart

The flow of blood through the heart follows a closed circuit. The following eight steps outline the flow of blood through this circulatory system, starting at the right ventricle:

1. The right ventricle pumps oxygen-poor blood to the lungs through the pulmonary arteries.

2. Blood flows through capillaries in the lungs, picks up oxygen, and gets rid of carbon dioxide.

3. Oxygen-rich blood flows back to the heart through the pulmonary veins that lead to the left atrium.

4. Oxygen-rich blood flows from the left atrium to the left ventricle.

5. The left ventricle pumps oxygen-rich blood out of the heart and through the body (systemic circuit). Blood leaves the left ventricle through the aorta.

6. Branches of arteries off the aorta lead to the heart muscles, the head, chest, and arms. The aorta descends through the abdomen and supplies blood to the lower body.

7. Oxygen-poor blood from the upper body returns to the heart via the superior vena cava, and oxygen-poor blood from the lower body returns to the heart via the inferior vena cava. The venae cavae empty blood into the right atrium of the heart.

8. Blood flows from the right atrium into the right ventricle.

Cardiovascular Circuits

There are three distinct pathways through which blood flows through the body.

1. **Pulmonary circuit:** The pulmonary circuit of blood flows from the heart to the lungs and then back to the heart.

2. **Systemic circuit:** The systemic circuit flows from the heart to the upper and lower regions of the body and then back to the heart.

3. **Coronary circuit:** The coronary circuit delivers blood to the myocardium.

Contraction of Cardiac Cells

There are two types of cells in the heart. *Autorhythmic cells* do not contract. They act by depolarizing spontaneously and keeping the heart moving at the same pace. These cells are part of what is called the *intrinsic conduction system*. In this way, the heart controls itself. *Contractile cells* are the second type of cells in the heart. They work together to contract the heart. All cells work in unison so that either all contractile cells contract, or none do.

An average heart rate of about 72 beats per minute corresponds to a cardiac cycle of rhythmic contractions that takes about 0.8 seconds. When the entire heart is relaxed, it is in the *diastolic phase*. In this phase, blood flows into all four of its chambers. The valves between the atria and the ventricles are open in this phase. The diastole lasts about 0.4 seconds, and during this time the ventricles nearly fill with blood.

The contraction phase of a heart beat is called the *systolic phase*. Systole begins with brief (0.1 second) contractions of the atria that completely fill the ventricles with blood. The ventricles contract for about 0.3 seconds, and the force of their contraction closes the AV valves and opens the semilunar valves located at the exit from each ventricle. Heart sounds that are heard through a stethoscope are caused by the closing of heart valves. (A heart murmur, which produces a hissing sound, may indicate a defect in one or more heart valves.)

Blood is then pumped into the large arteries leading out of the heart. Blood flows back into the atria during the second part of systole. The volume of blood that each ventricle pumps per minute is called the *cardiac output*, and this volume is equal to the amount of blood pumped by a ventricle each time it contracts multiplied by the heart rate (beats per minute). In an average human, a drop of blood can travel through the entire systemic circuit in about one minute. Because the left ventricle pumps blood to the entire body through the systemic circuit, the left ventricle contracts with a greater force than the right ventricle. This is the reason that the walls of the left ventricle are thicker than those of the right ventricle.

Heartbeat Tempo

Cardiac muscles contract and relax independently of any signals from the nervous system. A specialized region of the heart called a *pacemaker*, or *sinoatrial node* (SA node), sets the pace, or rate, at which all heart muscles contract. The pacemaker is located in the upper wall of the right atrium in the heart. It generates an electric signal similar to the signal produced by nerve cells. Cardiac muscle cells are electrically connected by specialized regions called *gap junctions*. Therefore, the signal spreads quickly and allows both atria to contract together. The signal also passes through what is called the *atrioventricular node* (AV node) that is located in the wall between the right atrium and the right ventricle. There is about a 0.1 second delay in the signal at this stage to ensure that the atrium contracts and is empty before the ventricle contracts. Cardiac muscle fibers then relay the signal to the apex of the heart and up through the walls of the ventricles. This signal triggers the strong contraction of the ventricles that pumps blood out of the heart. This entire process regulates the tempo at which the heart beats.

Heart Defects

Defects in the heart and its contractions can often be detected using an electrocardiogram (ECG or EKG). Electric signals generated by the heart generate electrical changes in the skin, which can be detected by electrodes attached to the skin. EKGs can provide useful data about the health of a heart. Some defects of the heart include:

- **Arrhythmia:** An arrhythmia is an irregular heartbeat caused by the depolarization of cardiac cells at an irregular rate.

- **Fibrillation:** Fibrillation is caused by irregular muscle contractions in the heart. These irregular contractions render the heart useless for pumping blood through the different circuits. Defibrillation is the process of administering a shock to the heart to "reset" the contractions.

- **Ectopic focus:** Ectopic focus occurs when there is an abnormal pacemaker in the heart. This can often be caused by nicotine and caffeine. The premature contractions caused by ectopic focus generally dissipate easily and are usually temporary.

Blood

Blood is composed of connective tissue, and is the only fluid tissue in the body. The function of blood is three-fold:

1. **Distribution:** Blood distributes oxygen (O_2) to all cells in the body, and returns CO_2 to the lungs so that it can be expelled from the body. Blood also provides essential nutrients to cells and deposits waste in the kidneys.

2. **Regulation:** Blood aids in the regulation of body temperature. Blood flow is constricted to extremities when the external temperature is relatively cold. This is done to keep the blood around vital organs in order to keep them warm and functioning. Blood also regulates the proper pH in the body.

3. **Protection:** Components in the blood that cause it to clot help to prevent excess blood loss. Also, as part of the immune system, blood carries white blood cells and antibodies that help to fight infection.

Blood is composed of the following:

- **Red blood cells:** Red blood cells (RBCS) or *erythrocytes* are not actually true cells because they lack a nucleus. Whole blood is approximately 45 percent RBCs. RBCs are the densest component of blood and settle to the bottom when blood is separated through centrifugation. The function of RBCs is to transport O_2 and CO_2. They carry *hemoglobin*, which is a protein that binds O_2 and CO_2. Erythrocytes are formed in the red bone marrow, and there are three precursor cells that form before mature RBCs. 1. *Hemocytoblasts* are the RBC stem cells. 2. *Proerythroblasts* are cells that have committed to becoming RBCs. Then the cells make ribosomes, accumulate hemoglobin, eject their nucleus, and become reticulocytes. 3. *Reticulocytes* are released by red bone marrow. Reticulocytes persist for two days in the bloodstream and then form *erythrocytes* (mature RBCs). The entire process takes about 15 days.

- **White blood cells:** White blood cells (WBCs), or *leukocytes*, are bigger than RBCs and contain a nucleus. They comprise about 1 percent of whole blood. There are five types of WBCs and can be classified as granulocytes or agranulocytes. Those that are defined as *granulocytes* have visible cytoplasmic granules and include neutrophils, eosinophils, and basophils. *Agranulocytes* have no visible cytoplasmic granulocytes and include monocytes and lymphocytes.

    a. **Neutrophils:** Neutrophils are the most abundant type of WBCs and are part of the immune system. Neutrophils are recruited to sites of injury, and are the hallmark of inflammation at the site of a wound or injury such as a bruise. When neutrophils encounter bacteria, they phagocytize the bacterial cell to fight off infection in the body.

    b. **Eosinophils:** These WBCs contain digestive enzymes and are part of the immune system that combats multicellular parasites and certain other infections. Eosinophils also respond to allergic reactions by destroying some of the chemicals released during an allergy attack.

    c. **Basophils:** Basophils are the least abundant of all WBCs. They are involved in the inflammatory response to an allergic reaction. Basophils also attract more WBCs to infected areas to help reduce infection. They also contain the anticoagulant heparin that prevents blood from clotting too quickly.

    d. **Monocytes:** Monocytes are very large and easily identifiable WBCs. When they leave the bloodstream, they become macrophages and attack virus-infected cells and some types of bacteria. An elevated monocyte count is usually an indicator of a chronic, long-term infection.

    e. **Lymphocytes:** Lymphocytes are generally not found in the bloodstream, but rather reside in lymphatic tissue. One type of granular lymphocyte called a *natural killer (NK) cell* destroys cells that do not carry self markers. Agranulocytic lymphocytes include T-lymphocytes (T cells), phagocytic cells that respond to virus-infected cells and tumor cells, and B-lymphocytes (B cells), which are not phagocytic, but instead produce antibodies.

- All WBCs start from hemocytoblasts and differentiate into either myeloid stem cells or lymphoid stem cells. Myeloid stem cells become myeloblasts, which are the precursor for all granulocytes and monocytes. Lymphoid stem cells become lymphoblasts and are the precursor for lymphocytes.

- **Platelets:** The function of platelets is to play a role in clotting. All platelets are formed from hemocytoblasts. Through a series of mitotic division, megakaryocytes are formed that have multiple nuclei. Once mature, they extend cytoplasmic extensions into the bloodstream. The extensions break off, the megakaryocyte seals itself up, and platelets are formed.

- **Plasma:** Plasma is the liquid component of blood. It is about 90 percent water with many dissolved solutes. The most important protein in plasma is albumin, which acts as a carrier, shuttling substances from one place to another. Plasma also contains many ions and gases.

Blood Types

Blood groups in humans are A, B, and O. They are named for the antigens found on the surface of red blood cells. There are four different blood types: A, B, AB, and O. Blood types A and B have those specific antigens on their surface, and type AB has both antigens on the surface of RBCs. Individuals who have blood type O have no antigens present on the surface of their RBCs.

Type O blood types are universal donors: they can donate blood to anyone. Type AB blood types are universal receivers: they can receive any blood type. Blood type can easily be determined with a sample of blood and the addition of anti-A or anti-B antibodies. For example, if anti-A antibodies are added to a blood sample and clumps of dead cells form, this indicates the presence of A antigens. This individual has blood type A.

Individuals with a specific type of antigen on their RBCs will not produce specific antibodies. For example, those with type A blood will have the A antigen on the surface of their RBCs, and they will not produce anti-A antibodies because this would cause the destruction of their own blood cells. These individuals will however produce anti-B antibodies. Individuals with type AB blood will not produce any antibodies against A or B.

Another factor in blood type is the Rh factor, or D antigen. Individuals are either Rh$^+$ or Rh$^-$. If they are negative, they do not have the D antigen, and if they are positive, they do. Rh$^-$ individuals are able to form D antibodies if they are exposed.

THE LYMPHATIC AND IMMUNE SYSTEMS

The lymphatic system returns excess body fluid back into the circulatory system. It functions as part of the immune system in fighting infection. The immune system defends the body against infection and cancers.

The Lymphatic System

The lymphatic system consists of a network of branching vessels: lymph nodes, which are rounded organs packed with macrophages and lymphocytes; the tonsils and adenoids; the spleen; and the appendix. It also includes yellow bone marrow and the thymus, sites at which WBCs develop.

Lymphatic vessels carry a fluid called *lymph*. This fluid is similar to interstitial fluid except that it contains less oxygen and fewer nutrients. Lymph flows toward the heart. Lymphatic capillaries are the smallest lymphatic vessels. They are found throughout the body except in bone, teeth, and the central nervous system. Lymphatic capillaries are permeable so that fluids can pass in and out of them, and the capillaries can pick up interstitial fluids.

Figure 5. The Human Lymphatic System

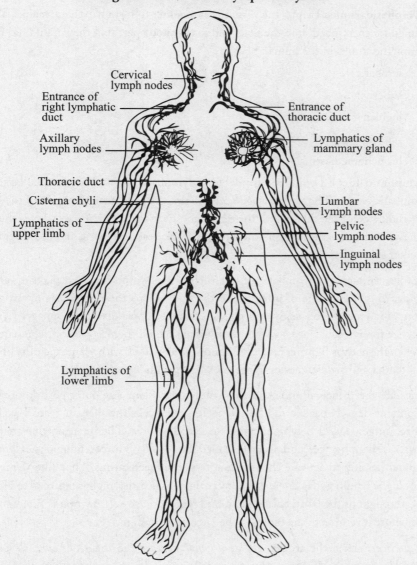

Minivalves are made up of endothelial cells that are not tightly joined. The cells form flaps that become the minivalves.

Collagen fibers secure the capillaries to surrounding tissue. Collagen fibers also keep the lymphatic capillary from collapsing under the pressure exerted by interstitial fluids. Once the fluid gets inside the capillary, it is called the lymph.

Lymph drains from lymphatic capillaries into larger lymphatic vessels. The *thoracic duct* and the *right lymphatic* duct are vessels through which lymph reenters the circulatory system. Lymphatic vessels resemble veins in that they have valves that prevent the backflow of fluids toward the capillaries.

Lymph fluid is squeezed through the lymphatic vessels in much the same way that blood moves through veins. There are three types of vessels through which lymph travels:

1. **Lymphatic vessels:** Lymphatic capillaries join together to form lymphatic vessels.

2. **Lymphatic trunks:** Lymphatic vessels join together to form lymphatic trunks. Trunks are named for their location in the body and for the body part that they drain fluid from. The lymphatic trunks in the human body are

    - lumbar,

    - subclavian,

    - jugular,

    - intestinal, and

    - bronchomediastinal.

3. **Lymphatic ducts:** Lymphatic trunks form lymphatic ducts. They are the largest of the lymphatic vessels. The *right lymphatic duct* drains the right arm, right side of the head, and the right side of the thorax into the right subclavian vein. The *thoracic duct* is the larger of the two and drains the left arm, the left side of the head, and neck, and the lower body into the left subclavian vein.

As lymph cycles through the lymphatic organs such as the lymph nodes, it picks up and carries microbes and toxins from a site of infection in the body. Once these microbes or toxins enter a lymphatic organ (adenoids, tonsils, lymph nodes, spleen, or appendix), macrophages (lymph cells that phagocytize foreign substances) within these organs engulf them as part of the innate immune response. When the body is fighting infection, lymph nodes will fill with a large quantity of defensive cells causing tender and swollen nodes in the neck, armpit, and groin regions.

Lymph nodes are the principal organs in the lymphatic system. The outer portion of the lymph node that contains densely packed follicles, dendritic cells (cells that help activate T cells and act to immobilize antigens), and B-lymphocytes is called the *cortex*. The inner portion that contains B-lymphocytes, T-lymphocytes, and plasma is called the *medulla*. The two functions of lymph nodes are filtering and helping to activate the immune response mechanisms. They filter lymph so that macrophages in the lymph nodes can remove any pathogens before lymph is returned to blood. They are scattered throughout the body, clustered around lymphatic vessels. Lymph is filtered through a lymph node before it returns to the blood in the circulatory system.

Axillary lymph nodes are in the armpit. *Inguinal lymph nodes* are in the groin area. *Cervical lymph nodes* are found in the neck. Within the lymph nodes, sinuses are open spaces through which lymph flows. There is a capsule that surrounds each lymph node and dense fibrous tissue called *trabeculae* extends into the node from the capsules dividing it into compartments. Lymph capsules can pick up proteins, cells, bacteria and cancer cells. This results in swollen glands because the debris gets stuck in the node. One way that cancer metastasizes is by traveling through the lymphatic system.

Another organ of the lymphatic system is the spleen, which is surrounded by a thin fibrous capsule. The spleen has the following functions: lymphocyte proliferation, immune surveillance, processing old red blood cells, red blood cell production in the fetus, and storing blood platelets. The spleen is composed of *white pulp*, which is the location of lymphocytes on reticular fibers, and *red pulp*, which contains macrophages, lymphocytes, dendritic cells, and reticular cells. Red blood cells are processed in the red pulp.

The thymus is an organ of the lymphatic system that secretes hormones (thymopoietin and thymosin) that target T cell maturation. The thymus becomes progressively smaller with age, as it atrophies. The thymus is composed of mostly T cells.

The tonsils and adenoids are also organs of the lymphatic system. They are found in certain areas of the throat and upper respiratory systems. The palantine tonsils are located in the posterior end of the oral cavity. There is one tonsil on each side. The lingual tonsils are located at the base of the tongue. The adenoids, or pharyngeal tonsils, are located on the posterior wall of the nasopharynx. Bacteria and other materials that can cause illness get caught in the crypts of tonsils, and macrophages destroy them.

The Immune System

There are two branches of the immune system:

1. **Innate immune system:** Also called the *nonspecific immune system*, the innate immune system consists of surface barriers and internal defenses. Surface barriers are the first lines of immune defense and include skin and mucous membranes. Skin is the first point of contact for many bacteria and pathogens. Slightly acidic secretions on the skin are a chemical barrier that inhibits bacterial growth. Mucosa is also another first line of immune defense. Mucous membranes are found in many cavities of the body, including in the respiratory, digestive, and genitourinary tracts.

   In the respiratory system, mucosa has *cilia*, or small hairs, that trap dust and other particles and move these particles toward the throat to be swallowed. Mucosa of the stomach has glands that secrete hydrochloric acid (HCl) that helps to kill bacteria. Salivary and lacrimal glands have mucosa that has the enzyme lysozyme, which lyses bacteria. Body fluids such as tears, saliva, urine, and vaginal secretions, all work to flush out irritants, bacteria, and pathogens.

   Internal defense mechanisms in the innate immune system include the following:

   a. **Macrophages** are large phagocytes (neutrophils) that move around interstitial fluid, consuming bacteria and virus-infected cells. There are also fixed phagocytes that reside in specific organs. Phagocytes must bind to a bacterium of microbe. The phagocyte forms cytoplasmic extensions around the microbe. The bacteria are now engulfed, and are called *phagosomes*. The phagosomes fuse with lysosomes (phagolysosome). Hydrolytic enzymes in the phagolysosome digest the microbe, and unused particles are removed through exocytosis.

   b. **NK cells** are another type of white blood cell that attacks cancer cells and virus-infected cells by releasing chemicals that initiate cell death. NK cells target all cells that are missing the major histone compatibility (MHC) complex. Cells without MHC are not natural to the body.

   c. **Antimicrobial proteins** include *interferons*. Interferons are proteins released from virus-infected cells that help other cells in the body resist viral infection. Interferons are released once a viral infected cell dies, and they move to noninfected areas of the body to help stop the spread of a viral infection. Additional innate immunity is provided by the *complement system*. The complement system is a group of about 30 plasma proteins that circulate in an inactive form in the blood. These proteins act together with other defense mechanisms to fight off infection. Substances on the surface of many microbes trigger a cascade of steps that ultimately activates the complement system. The complement system then acts to lyse, or kill, the infected cell. Certain complement proteins also act to trigger an inflammation response to infection. The inflammatory response is a major component of innate immunity. Damage to tissue triggers the response. The major function of this response is to disinfect and clean injured tissue through an increase in WBCs at the site of inflammation. Inflammation can prevent the spread of damaging agents, dispose of cell debris, and promote healing.

d. **Inflammation,** or the inflammatory response, is directed by chemicals in the body. Macrophages release cytokines, mast cells, and basophils (immature mast cells) that release histamine. Other phagocytes and lymphocytes release kinins, prostaglandins, leukotrienes, and complement proteins. The release of these chemicals causes vasodilation. Vasodilation leads to an increase in blood flow to an infected or damaged area. This is called *hyperemia*. Hyperemia causes redness and heat. An increase in temperature and metabolic rate leads to an increase in O_2 and nutrients sent to the site of infection. This helps to promote healing. Chemicals also cause an increase in the permeability of lymphatic capillaries. This results in fluid from the blood, clotting factors, and proteins leaking into body tissue. This increase in fluids causes swelling (*edema*) and the increase in pressure due to swelling causes pain. An increase in clotting proteins to tissue can help to prevent the spread of bacteria.

e. **Essential microbiota** are normal bacteria that reside in the body and act as antagonists to certain pathogens.

f. **Fever** is a systemic response by the body to infection. Fever is induced by pyrogens, which are released by WBCs and cause the core body temperature to increase. A very high fever is dangerous because it can cause the denaturation of proteins and, therefore, the loss of essential body functions. Mild fevers, however, are beneficial for fighting infection. Mild fevers cause the liver and spleen to hold on to iron and zinc, two essential elements for bacterial reproduction. This action causes the slowing down of bacterial reproduction in the body.

2. **Acquired immune system:** When the innate immune system fails to ward off infection from a pathogen or bacteria, the acquired immune response provides an alternative line of defense. Acquired immunity is a set of defenses that are activated only after infection by, or exposure, to pathogens. Once activated, the acquired immune response provides a strong defense against pathogens that is highly specific to that pathogen. There are three characteristics of an acquired immune system:

a. **Specific:** A specific component is directed against specific pathogens.

b. **Systemic:** The systemic component is not limited to the infection site.

c.   **Memory:** The memory component of the acquired immune system involves the build-up of immunity to a specific pathogen so that when the same pathogen enters the body, the immune system can mount a stronger attack and prevent illness.

All lymphocytes of the acquired immune system originate in bone marrow. Some immature lymphocytes continue to develop in the bone marrow, and these cells become B cells. Others travel to the thymus and develop into mature lymphocytes called *T cells.* The function of T cells is dependent upon both *immunocompetence* and *self-tolerance.* Immunocompetence is the ability of the T cell to recognize a specific antigen. Self-tolerance is the ability of the T cell to be unresponsive to body cells, so that they do not attack essential uninfected cells. They do this by recognizing specific proteins called the *major histocompatibility complex* (MHC) present on all cells in the body. Both types of cells eventually make their way into the bloodstream.

The acquired immune system has two types of immune responses. The *humoral immune response* involves the secretion of antibodies by B cells (produced in bone marrow) into the blood and the lymph. The humoral system defends primarily against bacteria and viruses present in body fluids. The cell-mediated immune response is produced by T cells (produced in the thymus). The *defense system* involves the action of defense cells in the body. Certain T cells attack bacterial or virus-infected cells.

Other T cells promote phagocytosis by other WBCs and stimulate B cells to produce antibodies. Both B cells and T cells synthesize specific proteins that are incorporated into the plasma membrane. These proteins are antigen receptors that are capable of binding a specific type of antigen. Specific cells called *antigen-presenting cells* (APCs) take in, or engulf, antigens and present them to T cells. APCs can be dendritic cells, macrophages, or B cells.

Antigens

Any substance that immobilizes the immune system and provokes an immune response is an *antigen.* Antigens do not belong to the host species; thus, they are considered a foreign substance. Most antigens are large proteins or polysaccharides located on the surface of viruses or pathogenic cells. Other sources of antigenic molecules include bacteria, blood cells, or tissue cells implanted from another individual. Antigenic molecules are also found in body fluids. These can include bacteria and venom from a bee sting or spider bite. Antigens trigger the production of antibodies. There are two main types of antigens that enter the body.

1.   **Complete antigens:** Complete antigens have immunogenicity and reactivity. *Immunogenicity* means that they will activate an immune response and stimulate the production of specific lymphocytes and antibodies. *Reactivity* is the ability of antigens to react with lymphocytes and antibodies.

2.   **Incomplete antigens:** Incomplete antigens are smaller molecules such as short peptides, nucleotides, and hormones. These molecules are called *haptens.* They cause a reaction in the body, but do not stimulate the immune system on their own. They can, however, combine with MHC proteins or other antigens, and the immune system will recognize them as foreign substances.

Antigenic determinants, also known as *epitopes*, are the small surface-exposed regions of an antigen that are recognized by antibodies. An antigen-binding site on the antibody recognizes an antigenic determinant because the binding site on the antibody and the antigenic determinant have complementary shapes, much like an enzyme and a substrate. An antigen may have several different determinants so that different antibodies can bind to the same antigen.

Self-antigens are called *major histocompatibility complex*, or *MHC, proteins*. Cell bodies are coated with MHC, and they are a way for the body to recognize its own cells. MHC proteins are specific to an individual. Class I MHC proteins are found on every cell body except red blood cells (RBCs). Class II MHC proteins are only found on cells of the immune response system.

Lymphocytes that have not encountered an antigen are *naïve cells*. B cells and T cells usually encounter antigens in the lymph nodes or spleen. The process of antigens binding to immunocompetent T cells after they are released into the bloodstream is called *antigen activation*. Specific T cells are made before antigen exposure, and it is likely that some T cells will never be activated. Naïve B cells are released from bone marrow and exposed to antigens in the spleen or lymph nodes, which provokes the humoral immune response. Once an antigen binds to a specific B cell, it stimulates the naïve B cell to complete its differentiation to a specific B cell. The antigen-driven cloning of these lymphocytes is called *clonal selection*. Clonal selection is a key component in the humoral immune response against infection.

When an antigen enters the body for the first time, it is carried into the lymph node. The antigenic determinants on only a select few of the total B cells in the lymph nodes are specific to the presented antigen. The selected antigen-bound cell is activated, and it grows, divides, and differentiates into two identical cells. Both of these newly made cells are specific for the particular antigen. The first group of newly cloned cells is called *effector cells*. Effector cells called *plasma cells* produce antibodies to fight off the antigen. A smaller, second group of cells is produced by the activated B cells. These cells are called *memory cells*. Memory cells can last in the body for decades, whereas effector cells are short-lived. Memory cells will be available to attack the same specific antigen if a future infection occurs.

These initial steps in the immune response are called the *primary immune response*. When memory cells are activated during a second exposure, this is called a *secondary response*. The secondary response is much quicker than the primary response. The secondary response also produces cloned effector cells and memory cells.

Active immunity involves all the steps of clonal selection, whereas passive immunity does not involve the presentation of antigen or the development of memory cells. Immunity can occur naturally or artificially. Natural acquired active immunity occurs when the body is infected with a particular virus or pathogen. Artificially acquired active immunity occurs through the administering of a vaccine. Vaccines are usually dead or weakened pathogens that activate B cells. Naturally acquired passive immunity is the passing of immunity from a mother to a fetus through the placenta or to a newborn baby through breast milk. Artificially acquired passive immunity occurs when antibodies are administered to a patient. This gives only temporary immunity because no memory cells are produced.

T cells are involved in two types of immune response. These immune responses are dependent on glycoprotein surface receptors called *CD4 helper T cells* and *CD8 cytotoxic T cells*. T cells only respond to antigens that have been processed by the MHC complex; they cannot recognize free-floating antigens. Helper T cells activate cytotoxic, or killer, T cells. Cytotoxic T cells are the only type of T cells that can kill an infected cell. Helper T cells interact with other WBCs and immune cells that act as antigen presenting cells. Helper T cells can recognize self-protein (MHC complex) and foreign antigen (non-self complex). This system is called *double recognition*. Binding to self and non-self proteins helps activate T cells. Activated T cells help to promote an immune response by growing, dividing, and producing memory cells; activating B cells; and stimulating the growth of cytotoxic T cells. Cytotoxic T cells bind to an infected cell with a self-nonself complex. The binding activates the T cell. Activation of the T cell stimulates the synthesis of new proteins, including *perforin*. Perforin attaches to and makes holes in the surface of infected cells. T cell enzymes then enter the infected cells through the holes and promote cell death by apoptosis. Once the infected cell dies, it is destroyed.

Antibodies

Antibody structure is a basic Y shape that has six main components.

1. **Polypeptide chains:** The basic components of an antibody are its four polypeptide chains: two heavy and two light chains.

2. **Constant region:** Within each of the four chains of the antibody is a region that remains constant.

3. **Variable region:** Within each of the four polypeptide chains is a region that is variable. This region varies to create antigen-specific binding sites on each antibody. The variable regions form a pair at the tip of each arm of the Y-shaped antibody.

4. **Antigen binding sites:** There are two antigen binding sites at the tip of the Y on each antibody.

5. **Hinge region:** The heavy chain of an antibody has a hinge region that allows bending. This hinge region is responsible for the Y shape of an antibody.

6. **Disulfide bonds:** There are disulfide bonds between the antibody chains that hold the monomer together.

There are five classes of antibodies that determine the other proteins with which a specific antibody will interact. Another term for antibody is *immunoglobulin* (Ig).

1. **Immunoglobulin A (IgA):** IgA can exist as a monomer or a dimer. IgA prevents pathogen from entering the body and is found in mucous, saliva, urine, spinal fluid, and genital secretions.

2. **Immunoglobulin D (IgD):** IgD exists as a monomer and attaches to B cells. It is an important part of B cell activation, and acts as an antigen receptor on the surface of B cells.

3. **Immunoglobulin E (IgE):** IgE is a monomer, and together with basophils and mast cells releases histamines. IgE is involved in the body's defense against parasites and allergies.

4. **Immunoglobulin G (IgG):** IgG is the most abundant monomer antibody found in the body. IgG gives natural passive immunity to the fetus through the placenta, activates the complement system, and is the primary antibody in both the primary and secondary immune response.

5. **Immunoglobulin M (IgM):** IgM exists as a monomer, or several molecules can link together to form a pentamer. When B cells are activated and change into plasma cells, IgM is the first antibody released (followed by IgG).

Antigens bind to antibodies to form an immune complex, and there are four ways to form this complex.

1. **Active complement:** Active complement is the most common method of immune complex formation. In this case, antibodies bind to antigens and slightly change shape to expose a complement binding site. This allows the complement system to target antigens for lysis.

2. **Agglutination:** Agglutination occurs when antibodies bind to antigens that are cell-bound. The binding of antigens to cell-bound antigens causes the formation of cell clumps.

3. **Neutralization:** To neutralize an antigen, antibodies bind all around an antigen to cover up the harmful parts. Once the antigen is covered, it can be phagocytized.

4. **Precipitation:** In the precipitation method of immune complex formation, antibodies bind a soluble antigen. This causes the antigen to precipitate out of solution (in blood).

THE ENDOCRINE SYSTEM

Animals rely on numerous chemical signals to regulate systems in the body. Hormones are chemical signals carried by the circulatory system, and they act as chemical messengers in the body. Hormones are produced and secreted by endocrine glands. All of the hormone-secreting cells in the human body make up the endocrine system.

Endocrine Glands

The following are the nine major endocrine glands:

1. **Hypothalamus:** The hypothalamus exerts master control over the endocrine system. It uses the pituitary gland to send directives to other glands. The hypothalamus receives information from nerves about internal and external body conditions and responds by sending out the appropriate neural of endocrine signal.

2. **Pineal gland:** The pineal gland is a small pea-sized gland near the center of the brain that synthesizes and secretes melatonin. Melatonin links biorhythms with environmental light (daily and seasonal).

3. **Pituitary gland:** The pituitary gland has two parts: the anterior and posterior lobes. The gland lies at the base of the hypothalamus. The posterior lobe of the pituitary gland is an extension of the hypothalamus and secretes hormones that are made in the hypothalamus (oxytocin and antidiuretic hormone, ADH). The anterior lobe of the pituitary gland is made up of endocrine cells that synthesize and secrete hormones into the bloodstream. The hypothalamus exerts control over the anterior lobe by secreting the releasing and inhibiting hormones. Releasing hormones stimulate the secretion of pituitary hormones, and inhibiting hormones inhibit the release of pituitary hormones. Anterior pituitary hormones include growth hormone (GH), prolactin (PRL), follicle stimulating hormone (FSH), luteininizing hormone (LH), thyroid stimulating hormone (TSH), and adrenocorticotropic hormone (ACTH).

4. **Thyroid gland:** The thyroid gland is located under the larynx, and hormones secreted from the thyroid affect almost every tissue type in the body. The thyroid produces thyroxine (T4) and triiodothyronine (T3), which stimulate and maintain metabolic processes. An excess of T3 and T4 can cause hyperthyroidism, and a deficit of these hormones can cause hypothyroidism.

5. **Parathyroid glands:** There are four parathyroid glands, all embedded in the surface of the thyroid. The parathyroid glands secrete calcitonin, which lowers blood calcium levels, and parathyroid hormone, which raises blood calcium levels. The action of these two hormones maintains calcium homeostasis in the body.

6. **Adrenal glands:** Adrenal glands are located at the top of each kidney. Each adrenal gland is actually two glands fused together: the adrenal medulla (central portion) and the adrenal cortex (outer portion). Both the medulla and cortex secrete hormones that respond to stress in the body. The adrenal medulla secretes epinephrine and norepinephrine, which increase blood glucose and increase metabolic activity while constricting certain blood vessels. These hormones trigger a "fight-or-flight response." The adrenal cortex secretes glucocorticoids (increase blood glucose), such as cortisol, and mineralocortoids (promote reabsorption of Na^+ and excretion of K^+ in the kidneys), which provide a slower longer lasting response to stress in the body.

7. **Pancreas:** The pancreas produces two hormones that play a role in maintaining the body's energy supply. The pancreas produces insulin, which lowers blood glucose, and glucagon, which raises blood glucose.

8. **Gonads:** The ovaries and testes are gonads, or sex glands, that secrete sex hormones in addition to producing gametes. The testes produce androgens (including testosterone) that support sperm formation and promote development and maintenance of male secondary sex characteristics. The ovaries produce estrogen and progesterone. Estrogen stimulates growth of the uterine lining and promotes the development and maintenance of female secondary sex characteristics. Progesterone promotes growth of the uterine lining so that it can support an embryo.

9. **Thymus gland:** The thymus gland lies under the breastbone and secretes the hormone thymosin, which stimulates T cell production.

The hormones secreted by endocrine glands can be divided into two categories: peptide, or amino acid-based hormones, and lipid, or steroid-based hormones. Steroid-based hormones are only produced in the adrenal cortex and gonads. Each type of hormone has a different mechanism that controls its release.

Peptide Hormones

The mechanism of release of peptide, or amino acid-based, hormones relies on a secondary messenger. These messengers provide an amplification effect, that is, a large amount of product is released from a small amount of hormone. Amino acid-based hormones are recognized by receptors on the outside of cells since they do not pass through a cell's plasma membrane. The secondary messenger is generated by another molecule called an *effector enzyme*. The effector enzyme is activated by yet another molecule called a *G-protein*. G-protein is turned off when it is bound to GDP (guanosine diphosphate) and turned on when it is bound to GTP. G_S stimulates the enzyme adenylate cyclase, and G_I inhibits adenylate cyclase. There are six steps in this mechanism:

1. A hormone binds to a receptor site.

2. Binding the hormone (first messenger) causes the receptor to change shape. It now binds to a nearby active G-protein (bound to GTP).

3. The activated G-protein moves along the plasma membrane until it encounters the effector enzyme, adenylate cyclase, to which it binds. Once GTP is hydrolyzed to GDP, the G-protein becomes inactive.

4. Adenylate cyclase generates the second messenger, cyclic AMP (cAMP), from an ATP molecule.

5. cAMP diffuses through the cell, triggering a cascade of chemical reactions. The first protein activated in the cascade is protein kinase.

6. Protein kinase phosphorylates various proteins, activating some and inhibiting others. Kinase is responsible for mediating the cellular response to hormones.

Steroid Hormones

Steroid hormones and thyroid hormones (which are not activated in the same way as other peptide hormones) use a mechanism of direct gene activation. Receptors for these hormones are inside the cell, so that these molecules must pass through the plasma membrane. Because steroid hormones are lipid-based, they can pass through the phospholipid bilayer of the plasma membrane. Thus, there is no need for secondary messengers to activate these hormones. The six steps of direct gene activation are:

1. The hormone diffuses through the plasma membrane.

2. It binds to a receptor called a *chaperonin complex*, which is in the cell's nucleus.

3. The chaperonin dissociates from the receptor.

4. The hormone-receptor complex binds to a specific sequence of DNA, which initiates a transcription of a certain gene in the cell.

5. mRNA is formed during transcription and migrates to the cytoplasm. This mRNA synthesizes specific proteins.

6. A third signaling mechanism, a PIP-calcium signal mechanism, is initiated.

Several factors are responsible for how strongly cells are activated. A cell with more receptors will have a stronger hormone response. Higher hormone levels in the blood will also give a stronger a response. The greater affinity a hormone has for its receptor, the stronger the response will be. There are three categories of hormone activity in which more than one hormone is acting to produce a response.

1. **Synergism:** Synergism involves two hormones working together to produce one outcome. Two hormones may also work together to produce a combined effect that is greater than the effect of one hormone acting alone.

2. **Permissiveness:** Permissiveness involves the requirement of one hormone in order to bring about the full effect of a second hormone.

3. **Antagonism:** Antagonism is the effect observed when two hormones produce opposite effects from each other.

THE RESPIRATORY SYSTEM

The respiratory system involves the process of gas exchange, specifically the uptake of O_2 and the release of CO_2. Animals exchange gases across moist body surfaces such as the lungs. There are three phases of gas exchange in the human body:

1. **Breathing:** Breathing gases into and out of the lungs is called *respiration*. As O_2 is breathed in, it diffuses across the cell lining of the lungs into surrounding blood vessels. CO_2 diffuses out of the bloodstream into the lungs and is expelled out of the body.

2. **Transport of respiratory gases:** The cardiovascular system is involved in transporting O_2 from the lungs to specific tissue (through the bloodstream) and transporting CO_2 from tissue back to the lungs. The O_2 that is diffused into the bloodstream attaches to hemoglobin in the red blood cells. Hemoglobin also helps to transport CO_2 back out of the bloodstream.

3. **Internal respiration:** In the third phase of gas exchange in the body, cells in tissue take up O_2 from the blood and release CO_2 back into the bloodstream. Cells require a continuous supply of oxygen for cellular respiration.

Structures of the Respiratory System

The human respiratory system includes passageways for getting air into and out of the lungs. This is called the *conducting zone* and includes the nose, mouth, pharynx, larynx, trachea, and terminal bronchi. The respiratory system also includes the *respiratory zone*, which is the regions where the gas exchange actually takes place. The respiratory zone includes the bronchioles, alveolar ducts, and alveola sac.

Figure 6. The Human Respiratory System

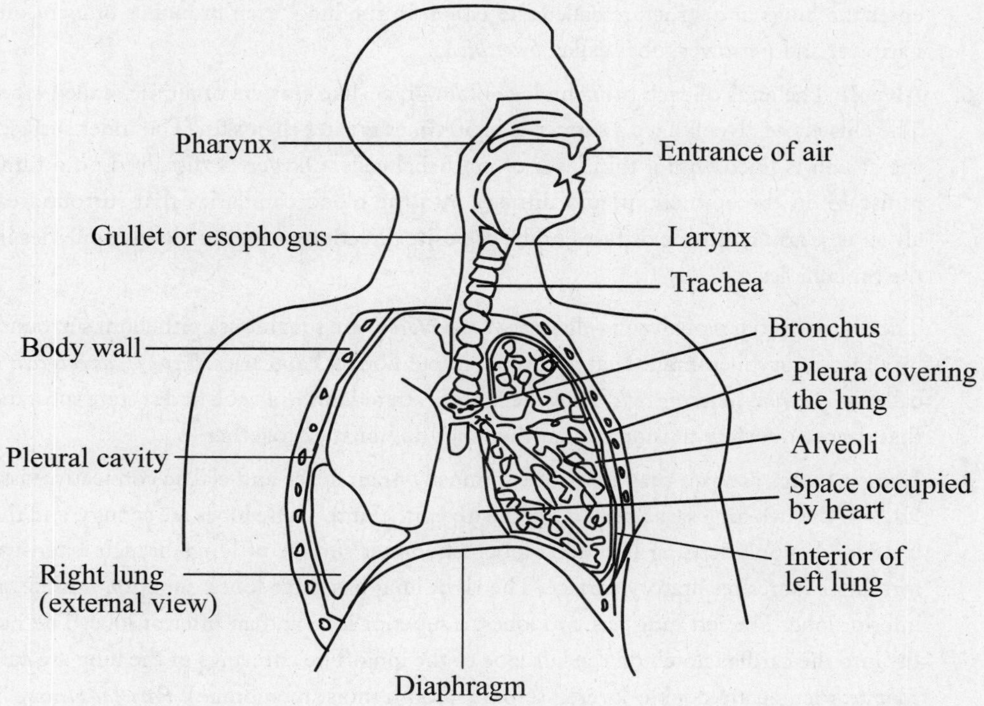

The lungs are located in the chest, or thoracic cavity, and are protected by the rib cage. The *diaphragm* is a flat sheet of muscle that separates the thoracic cavity from the abdominal cavity and helps to ventilate the lungs. The following description is the pathway that oxygen travels from outside the body into the lungs:

1. **Nose/moth:** Air is drawn into the lungs through the nose or the mouth. Both function to moisten and warm the air as it enters.

2. **Pharynx:** Air passes from the nose or mouth into the pharynx. The *nasopharynx* is located directly behind the nasal cavity. The *oropharynx* is behind the oral cavity. The *laryngopharynx* is directly posterior to the epiglottis in the back of the mouth. The laryngopharynx is the place where the paths for air and food cross one another. The upper portion of the respiratory tract moves upward as food is swallowed, and this tips the epiglottis so that it covers the trachea (windpipe), which is the pathway down which air travels. This protects the lungs from food or foreign particles. When food is not being ingested, the air passage in the pharynx remains open.

3. **Larynx:** The larynx (voice box) is the next place that air flows. The larynx contains vocal cords, and air rushing out of the larynx past the vocal cords allows the production of sound, or voice.

4. **Trachea:** The larynx leads into the trachea, or windpipe. Rings of cartilage encircle the trachea and larynx and help to reinforce the walls and keep airways open. This portion of the trachea is called the *adventitia*. The trachea is also lined with epithelium covered with cilia. A thin film of mucus coats the trachea (*mucosa layer*). The mucus acts to trap dust, pollen, and other contaminants in the air and move them up toward the pharynx where they are swallowed. The mucus in the trachea is produced by glands in the submucosa layer.

5. **Bronchi:** The trachea branches into two bronchi, one leading to each lung. The bronchi enter the lungs at a structure called the *hilum*. In the lung, each bronchus branches into narrower and narrower tubes called *bronchioles*.

6. **Alveoli:** The ends of each bronchiole contain grape-like clusters of air sacs called *alveoli*. The clusters of alveoli have a surface area 50 times greater than skin. The inner surface of the alveoli is lined with a thin layer of epithelial cells. Oxygen is dissolved on a film of moisture on the epithelium, and diffuses into the blood capillaries that surround each alveolus. Carbon dioxide diffuses in the opposite direction, from the blood capillaries into the bronchioles.

   There are two types of alveoli cells. *Type I alveoli cells* are squamous epithelium surrounded by a respiratory membrane that is covered in pulmonary capillaries. *Type II alveoli cells* are called *surfactant-secreting cells*. These cells are scattered in the alveoli and secrete substances that decrease surface tension so that the lungs do not stick together.

7. **Lungs:** Lungs are sacs that are made up mostly of air space and elastic connective tissue. Each of the two lung sacs (*lobes*) is lined with epithelium. These lobes are spongy, and there is a blood supply leading into each lobe. The inner surface of lungs branch extensively, forming a larger respiratory surface. The right lung has three lobes: superior, middle, and inferior lobe. The left lung has two lobes: a superior lobe and an inferior lobe. The heart fits into the cardiac notch on the left lobe of the lung. The coverings of the lung are called *pleurae*. Pleurae are double-layered serosa (smooth moist membrane). *Parietal pleurae* line

the thoracic cavity and the diaphragm, both of which surround the lungs. The *visceral pleurae* cover the lungs. The *pleural cavity* is the space between the two layers of serosa and is filled with liquid called *pleural fluid*. Pleural fluid allows the lungs to glide over the thorax during breathing. The pleural fluid causes adhesion between the two pleural layers, which causes the lungs to expand or contract during breathing.

Breathing

Breathing involves alternating between inhaling and exhaling air. The ventilation of lungs allows for a high concentration of O_2 and a low concentration of CO_2 on respiratory surfaces. Ventilation is dependent upon change in volume in the thoracic cavity; the pressure and volume in the thoracic cavity is dependent upon Boyle's gas law ($P_1V_1 = P_2V_2$).

During inhalation (*inspiration*), the lungs expand, and, thus, the rib cage expands in the thoracic cavity. The diaphragm contracts, moving downward and expanding the thoracic cavity. The volume of the lungs increases upon inhalation, which lowers the air pressure in the alveoli to less than that of atmospheric pressure. Air flows from a region of higher pressure (outside the body) to lower pressure (inside the expanded lungs); this is considered to be a negative breathing pressure. Pressures in the thoracic cavity are measured relative to air pressure (1 atm, or 760 mmHg). The intrapulmonary pressure, or the pressure inside the alveoli, decreases or increases during breathing, but it always equalizes to 760 mmHg. The relative intrapulmonary pressure is written as 0 mmHg because it is equal to atmospheric pressure. The intrapulmonary pressure decreases to about –1 mmHg during inhalation; then the rush of air into the lungs equalizes the pressure back to 0 mmHg. The intrapleural pressure is the pressure inside the pleural cavity. The air pressure between the visceral and parietal pleurae is always 4 mmHg less than 760 mmHg (atmospheric pressure), so it is written as –4 mmHg.

The lungs' natural tendency is to collapse due to the surface tension of the alveoli fluid. The elasticity of the chest wall exerts an opposing force on the lungs and works to keep them expanded. Thus, in a healthy individual, these forces balance out, preventing lungs from collapsing. Transpulmonary pressure is the difference between the intrapulmonary pressure and the intrapleural pressure. Transpulmonary pressure prevents the lungs from collapsing.

During exhalation (*expiration*), the rib muscles and the diaphragm relax. This causes a decrease in the volume of the rib cage and the thoracic cavity. The rib cage gets smaller, and the diaphragm moves upward into its relaxed position. The elastic lungs recoil passively and the intrapulmonary volume decreases as the intrapulmonary pressure increases to +1 mmHg. This increase in pressure causes air to be pushed back out of the lungs, and the pressure in the lungs returns to 0 mmHg.

There are two factors that may affect proper ventilation:

1. **Airway resistance:** Airway resistance is the resistance to gas flow or a friction within respiratory passages. As resistance increases, the flow of air decreases ($F = \Delta P/R$, where F is gas flow, P is pressure, and R is resistance). Airway restriction can occur when there is a restriction in the size of the diameter of the bronchi (as in the case of asthma).

2. **Alveolar surface tension:** Alveolar surface tension can also affect ventilation. Alveoli are lined with fluid, mostly water. The alveolar fluid acts to constrict alveoli, so there is less available surface area exposed to gas. Type II alveoli surfactants also decrease the surface tension in alveoli. Without surfactant, alveoli would collapse. The surfactants break up the

NOTE

The human body needs a daily supply of clean and safe water and nutrients for maintaining optimal biological and physiological functions. The body can compensate for a short-term deficiency, but long-term deficiencies can result in dangerous metabolic disruptions. A sensible and balanced diet helps to maintain overall good health.

cohesiveness of the water molecules in the alveolar fluid so that less energy is required to overcome these forces and expand the lungs.

Respiratory Volume

Respiratory volume is measured with an instrument called a spirometer. The amount of air that is breathed in and out during a resting state is called the *tidal volume*. In a healthy individual, the tidal volume is 500 mL. The volume that can be forcefully inhaled after a normal tidal volume inhalation is called the *inspiratory reserve volume*. This is equal to about 3100 mL in a healthy individual. The volume that can be forcefully exhaled from the lungs after a normal tidal exhalation is called the *expiratory reserve volume*. This volume is about 1200 mL. The volume of air remaining in the lungs after a forced exhalation is called the *residual volume*. This volume is about 1200 mL. The residual volume helps prevent the collapse of lungs.

The capacity of normal healthy lungs is as follows:

- **Vital capacity:** The vital capacity of healthy lungs is about 4800 mL, or 4.8 L. This is the maximum amount of air that can be expired after a maximum inhalation. This capacity is equal to the tidal volume (500 mL), the inspirational reserve volume (3100 mL), and the expiratory reserve volume (1200 mL).

- **Inspirational capacity:** The inspirational capacity is 3600 mL, or 3.6 L. This is the maximum volume of air that can be inspired after a normal expiration.

- **Functional residual capacity:** The functional residual capacity is 2400 mL. This is the volume of air that remains in the lungs after a normal tidal volume expiration. It is the sum of the expiratory reserve volume (1200 mL) and the residual volume (1200 mL).

- **Total lung capacity:** The total lung capacity of a healthy individual is 6000 mL, or 6 L. It is the sum of the vital capacity (4.8 L) and the residual volume (1.2 L).

THE DIGESTIVE SYSTEM

The human digestive system is involved in nutrient uptake, digestion, and absorption. It is also involved in the process of ridding the body of waste. The digestive system consists of an alimentary canal (the gastrointestinal tract) and associated glands. The function of the gastrointestinal (GI) tract is to digest food and absorb nutrients. There are several processes that occur during digestion:

1. **Ingestion:** Food is taken in through the mouth. It is chewed into small pieces in the mouth and pushed by the tongue into the pharynx.

2. **Propulsion:** The tongue pushes food into the pharynx and triggers the swallowing reflex. Once food is swallowed into the pharynx, it is propelled through the alimentary canal by the process of *peristalsis*. Peristalsis involves alternating involuntary waves of contraction and relaxation of the smooth muscles lining the GI tract.

3. **Mechanical digestion:** Mechanical digestion is a multistep process that involves chewing food in the mouth, churning or mixing of food in the stomach, and continued churning, mixing, and breaking down of food in the small intestine.

4. **Chemical digestion:** Chemical digestion takes place all along the digestive tract from the mouth to the small intestine. The breakdown of food is carried out by chemicals and enzymes specific to each location. Salivary glands in the mouth secrete saliva, which contains glyco-proteins that help to lubricate food, buffers that neutralize acidic foods, antibacterial agents that kill off some of the bacteria that enters the mouth, and digestive enzymes that break down food. Muscular, ring-like valves called *sphincters* regulate the passage of food into and out of the stomach. The sphincter leading out of the stomach closes it off so that food remains in the stomach for about 2 to 6 hours. This is long enough for gastric juices—stomach acids, mucous, and enzymes—to begin digestion. In the small intestine, digestion continues. Two large organs, the liver and the pancreas, aid in digestion in the small intestine. The liver produces bile that helps to make fats more digestible by enzymes. The pancreas produces pancreatic juice, a mixture of digestive enzymes and alkaline solution.

5. **Absorption:** Absorption of nutrients from food into the bloodstream occurs mostly in the small intestine. Some nutrients are absorbed by simple diffusion, and others are pumped against concentration gradients into epithelial cells. Epithelial cells line the inner wall of the small intestine. There are small finger-like projections called *villi*; each villus has many even smaller projections called *microvilli*. The microvilli extend into the lumen of the intestine and greatly increase the surface area available for the absorption of nutrients. Large vessels transport nutrients from the intestine directly to the liver. The liver plays a key role in body metabolism by regulating the amount of glycogen it stores and the amount of glucose that is released into the bloodstream.

6. **Defecation:** Defecation includes ridding the body of waste material in the form of feces. This occurs through the large intestine, or colon. Waste products consist mostly of indigest-ible plant fibers and bacteria. The large intestine also absorbs water from the alimentary canal and about 90 percent of this water is reabsorbed back into the blood and tissue fluids.

Figure 7. The Human Digestive System

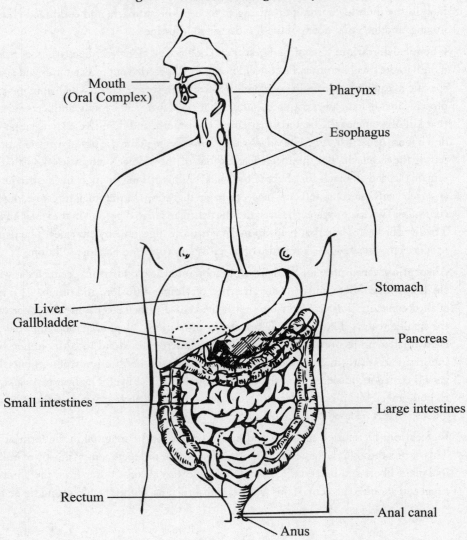

Mouth (Oral Complex)

Pharynx

Esophagus

Liver
Gallbladder

Stomach

Pancreas

Small intestines

Large intestines

Rectum

Anal canal

Anus

Within the abdominal cavity is a lining of serous membrane called the *peritoneum*. The peritoneum supports the organs in the abdominal cavity and supplies them with blood, lymph, and nerve impulses. The *visceral peritoneum* surrounds the organs, and the *parietal peritoneum* lines the abdominal and pelvic cavity. *Mesentery* consists of a double layer of peritoneum fused back-to-back from the abdominal wall to the organs. The mesentery anchors the organs in place and provides a medium for blood, lymph, and nerves and stores fat.

Layers of the Gastrointestinal (GI) Tract

The gastrointestinal tract consists of four layers.

1. **Mucosa:** The mucosa is the innermost layer of the GI tract. It secretes a mucous that contains digestive enzymes and hormones. There are three sublayers of the mucosa: the *epithelium* containing the goblet cells that produce mucous; the *lamina propria*, which is the middle layer made up of connective tissue and capillaries that play a role in absorption and immune functions; and the *muscularis mucosa*, which is the outermost sublayer of smooth muscle cells that produce local movements.

2. **Submucosa:** The submucosa is a layer of connective tissue. It allows for distension of the stomach after a large meal, and the regaining of the proper shape after digestion.

3. **Muscularis externa:** The muscularis externa is responsible for *peristalsis*, propelling food through the GI tract and churning of food as it digests. There is a circular inner layer of smooth muscle cells and a longitudinal outer layer of smooth muscle cells.

4. **Serosa:** The *serosa*, also called the *visceral peritoneum*, is the outermost layer of the GI tract. It is made up of connective tissue and is a protective layer covering all digestive organs.

Organs of the GI Tract

The components included in the GI tract are the

- mouth
- pharynx
- esophagus
- stomach
- small intestine
- large intestine

Accessory glands and components of the digestive system aid the GI tract either by providing secretions or by helping to break down food. Accessory components of the digestive system include the

- tongue
- salivary glands
- teeth
- liver
- gallbladder
- pancreas
- **Mouth:** The oral cavity is made up of stratified squamous epithelium. The mouth is formed by the lips and the cheek, which aid in keeping ingested food in place, and the palate, which is the roof of the mouth. The palate is composed of a hard palate anteriorly and a soft palate posteriorly.

- **Tongue:** The tongue forces food up against the hard palate during chewing, and in this way it is involved in the breakdown of ingested food. The tongue manipulates food during the chewing process and helps to mix it with saliva to form a food *bolus*, or ball shape. The *lingual frenulum* is a fold of mucosa that secures the tongue to the floor of the mouth. It also limits the posterior movement of the tongue so that it is not swallowed. The papillae on the tongue help to provide friction to the tongue (filiform) and to form taste buds (fungiform, circumvallate, and foliate).

- **Salivary glands:** The salivary glands produce saliva that aids in cleaning the mouth and dissolving foods. Saliva acts to moisten food and form a bolus. Saliva contains enzymes that help to digest starchy foods. The *parotid salivary gland* is located anterior to the ear and expels saliva through the parotid duct. The *submandibular gland* along the mandible empties under the tongue near the lingual frenulum. The *sublingual gland* also empties salvia into the area under the tongue. The salivary glands secrete about 1.5 liters of saliva per day. Saliva is mostly composed of water and is slightly acidic. It contains the enzyme *salivary amylase*, which aids in the digestion of starch; *mucin*, which is a precursor to mucous; *lysozymes*, which act as an antibacterial agent; and IgA antibodies.

- **Teeth:** Teeth are an accessory organ to the GI tract. They act to mash and grind food into smaller particles.

- **Pharynx:** The pharynx acts to force food into the esophagus.

- **Esophagus:** The esophagus tube remains closed until food is ingested. It runs from the pharynx to the stomach. The esophagus enters the stomach at the cardiac, or gastro-esophageal, sphincter.

- **Stomach:** The stomach stores food and breaks it down with stomach acid and enzymes. The stomach can hold up to 4 liters of food. There are four regions of the stomach: the cardiac region is the area surrounding the cardiac sphincter; the *fundus* is the dome-shaped region underneath the diaphragm; the *body* is the main part of the stomach (the midsection); and the *pylorus*, or pyloric region, is the region near the pyloric sphincter that connects to the first part of the small intestine.

Gastric pits are structures within the stomach that lead to the gastric glands. Gastric pits produce mucous and are composed mostly of goblet cells. Gastric glands produce a substance called *gastric juice*. The stomach has a thick mucous wall with tightly packed cells so that gastric juices do not leak from the stomach. There are three phases in the release of gastric juices.

1. The *cephalic reflex* occurs before food enters the stomach and is triggered by food entering the mouth or by the smell of food.

2. The *gastric phase* is stimulated by stomach digestion. This phase lasts about 4 hours and provides two-thirds of the gastric juices released. Peptides enter the stomach, causing distention, which activates the stretch receptors, and acetylcholine is released. The release of acetylcholine triggers the release of more gastric juices, which triggers

the release of gastrin. Gastrin causes parietal cells to make more HCl, and it also triggers the release of histamine.

3. During the *intestinal phase*, the final phase of gastric secretion occurs in the small intestine. During the *excitatory stage* of the intestinal phase, food enters the small intestine and more gastric juice is released. During the *inhibitory stage* of the intestinal phase, the duodenum of the small intestine gets too acidic, and the enterogastric reflex kicks in. Passage into the small intestine is blocked by inhibiting the pyloric sphincter, and gastric secretions decrease.

In the stomach, pepsin catalyzes protein digestion, and the stomach produces the churning characteristic of mechanical digestion. The actions of the stomach include *receptive relaxation*, which allows for relaxation of the stomach and expansion upon swallowing; *plasticity*, in which the stomach relaxes and stretches to hold food; *stomach contractions*, which occur through peristalsis; and *stomach emptying* in which digested food (*chime*) is forced into the small intestine with each contraction of the stomach.

- **Small Intestine:** The small intestine is the main organ for chemical digestion and nutrient absorption into the bloodstream. The small intestine is about 6 meters long, and is the longest organ in the gastrointestinal tract. There are three sections in the small intestine: The *duodenum* is the first portion of the small intestine. It receives secretions from the bile duct, liver, gallbladder, pancreatic duct, cystic duct (from the gallbladder), and hepatic duct (from the liver). The left and right hepatic ducts join together to form the common hepatic duct, which exits the liver and joins with the cystic duct to form the common bile duct. The common bile duct joins the pancreatic duct and the hepatopancreatic ampulla, which enters the duodenum. The next portion of the small intestine is called the *jejunum* (about 8 feet), and the last 12 feet is called the *ileum*. The ileum joins with the large intestine at the ileocecal valve.

Chemical digestion in the small intestine is accomplished by digestive enzymes, bile, and bicarbonate ions. Absorption in the small intestine is accomplished by the villi and microvilli. Movement through the small intestine is accomplished by segmentation. Segmentations consist of back and forth contractions. There is also peristalsis in the small intestine to aid with movement. The small intestine also releases the hormone motilin.

- **Liver:** In addition to many other functions, the liver produces bile, which aids in digestion. Bile contains salts that emulsify fats and make them more susceptible to attack from digestive enzymes. Hepatocytes make bile, and bile leaves the liver via the common hepatic duct and heads in the direction of the duodenum; this is opposite of blood flow. Another function of the liver is to process nutrient-laden blood from the intestines. It removes excess glucose form the blood and converts it to the polysaccharide glycogen. The liver converts many nutrients into new substances such as proteins, essential for normal body function. The liver is able to modify and detoxify many substances absorbed by the digestive tract before the blood carries these materials back to the heart for distribution within the body. It converts alcohol and other drugs into waste products that can be secreted in urine.

The structures of the liver include the *lower lobules*, which are the hexagonally-shaped, tiny functional units of the liver that are made up of hepatocytes (liver cells); the *central vein*, which is in the center of each lobule; the *portal triad*, which are located at each corner of the liver and contain a branch of the hepatic artery; the hepatic portal veins; the bile duct and the lymphatic vessels; *sinusoids*, which are the spaces between the hepatocytes; and the *Kupffer cells*, which are part of the sinusoid walls and remove debris and bacteria. Kupffer cells act like macrophages.

- **Gallbladder:** The gallbladder is an accessory organ in the GI tract. It is a muscular sac that functions to store bile. It concentrates the bile by removing water from it.

- **Pancreas:** The pancreas produces what is called pancreatic juice, about 1.2 to 1.5 liters per day. Pancreatic juice is a mixture of an alkaline solution rich in bicarbonate and digestive enzymes. The digestive function of pancreatic juice is to neutralize chime. Bicarbonate causes the pancreatic juice to be slightly alkaline (pH 8). Pancreatic proteases (enzymes) are activated in the duodenum. The activated enzymes include *trypsin*, which, in turn, activates carboxypeptidase and chymotrypsin. Other pancreatic enzymes include *amylase*, which breaks down starches; *lipase*, which breaks down lipids; and *nucleases*, which break down nucleic acids. There are two intestinal hormones in the small intestine that regulate the release of pancreatic juices: *secretin*, which is released in response to HCl in the intestine, and *CCK*, released in response to the entry of proteins and fats in the intestine.

- **Large intestine:** The large intestine functions to absorb water from the GI tract and compact feces. The large intestine is 1.5 meters long and 5 centimeters in diameter. It connects with the small intestine at a T-shaped junction where a sphincter controls the release of unabsorbed food materials out of the small intestine. Food can remain in the large intestine for 12 to 24 hours. The large intestine forms pocket-like sacs called *haustra* due to three longitudinal muscles in the large intestine called *teniae coli*, or ribbons of the colon.

There are five regions of the large intestine. It forms a T-shaped junction where it joins the small intestine. The *cecum* is a sac-like section of one arm of the T that makes up the first part of the large intestine. The *appendix* (vermiform appendix) is a small finger-like extension that hangs off the bottom of the cecum. The appendix contains a mass of white blood cells. The third part, the *colon*, has six regions: the *ascending colon* which runs up the right side of the abdominal cavity to the level of the kidneys where is makes a right turn; the *hepatic flexure* (right colic flexure) extends from the ascending colon and is the right turn portion of the colon (anterior to the right kidney); the *transverse colon* makes its way across the abdominal cavity; the *splenic flexure* (left colic flexure) is the left-turn portion of the colon (anterior to the spleen); the *descending colon* runs down the left side of the abdominal cavity; the *sigmoid colon* is the S-shaped end of the large intestine that enters the pelvic region. The rectum has a thick muscularis externa. There are three transverse folds in the rectum called the *rectal valves*, which separate the feces from the flatus. This prevents feces from being passed with gas. The *anal canal* is the last segment of the large intestine. It is located in the perineum and is external to the abdominopelvic cavity. There are two sphincters in the anal canal: the *internal* and *external sphincters*. The internal sphincter is smooth muscle that has involuntary control, and the external sphincter is voluntary skeletal muscle.

The large intestine is inactive most of the time. However, when food is digested and presented to the large intestine, it becomes motile. Contractions of the large intestine are short-lived and sluggish. *Haustral movements* are slow segmenting movements. *Mass movement* occurs across the entire colon three to four times a day. The presence of food in the stomach activates two propulsive reflexes: the *gastroileal reflex* in the small intestine and the *gastrocolic reflex* in the colon. The process of defecation follows the movement of food through the large intestine. Once mass movement occurs, feces are forced into an empty colon which activates the defecation reflex.

Chemical Digestion and Absorption

All four types of molecules—carbohydrates, proteins, fats, and nucleic acids—are digested by enzymes in the small intestine that are specific to each type of molecule. The digestion of carbohydrates begins in the oral cavity and is completed in the small intestine. The digestion of proteins begins in the stomach and is also completed in the small intestine. Pancreatic juice that is released into the small intestine contains nucleases (pancreatic ribonuclease and deoxyribonuclease) to hydrolyze ingested nucleic acids. Nucleotidases and phosphatases continue to break down the nucleic acids in the small intestine. Fats remain undigested until they reach the duodenum of the small intestine.

The small intestine is structurally well-suited for the absorption of nutrients. It has a huge inner surface area that has many folds and projections. The villi and microvilli increase the surface of the inside lining even more. Some nutrients are absorbed by methods of simple diffusion, and others are pumped against concentration gradients. After carbohydrates are digested, the monosaccharides (for example, glucose and galactose) are absorbed across Na^+ ion channels. They enter the capillary blood in the villi and are transported to the liver (via the hepatic portal vein). Fructose is a sugar that is absorbed by facilitated diffusion. Amino acids are also absorbed via transport across Na^+ ion channels in the same way as monosaccharides and are transported to the liver in the same way.

Nucleic acids are digested, and the breakdown products are transported by active transport with membrane carrier proteins. They are absorbed into capillary blood in the villi and are transported to the liver through the hepatic portal vein. Fatty acids and monoglycerides enter the intestinal walls by diffusion. They combine with proteins inside cells to form chylomicrons. Chylomicrons are transported to the systemic circulation system via lymph (in the thoracic duct). Glycerol and short fatty acid chains are absorbed into capillary blood and transported to the liver in the same manner as monosaccharides, amino acids, and nucleic acid breakdown products.

Figure 8. Digestion in the Small Intestine

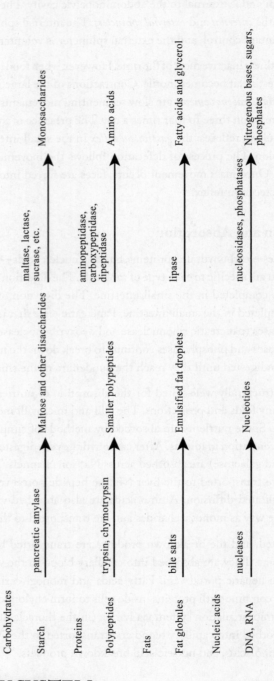

Carbohydrates	Proteins	Fats	Nucleic acids	
Starch	Polypeptides	Fat globules	DNA, RNA	

pancreatic amylase → Maltose and other disaccharides → maltase, lactase, sucrase, etc. → Monosaccharides

trypsin, chymotrypsin → Smaller polypeptides → aminopeptidase, carboxypeptidase, dipeptidase → Amino acids

bile salts → Emulsified fat droplets → lipase → Fatty acids and glycerol

nucleases → Nucleotides → nucleosidases, phosphatases → Nitrogenous bases, sugars, phosphates

THE URINARY SYSTEM

The survival of humans and other species in any environment requires a balance between the need for hydration (drinking water) and the need for waste disposal. The urinary system plays a role in homeostasis of body fluids. The key processes of the urinary system are filtration, reabsorption, secretion, and excretion. The urinary system functions to form and excrete urine, while regulating the proper levels of water and ions in body fluids. The main processing center of the urinary system is the kidneys. Each of the two kidneys in the human body is filled with about 80 km of tubules and a network of blood capillaries. The human body contains about 5 liters of blood, which circulates continuously so that about 1100 to 2000 liters of blood passes through the capillaries in the kidneys every day.

From this huge volume of blood passing through, the kidneys extract about 1.8 liters of fluid called *filtrate*. Filtrate contains water, urea, glucose, amino acids, ions, and vitamins. The human body requires many of these nutrients, and the kidneys function to concentrate the urea and return most of the water and nutrients back to the blood. Approximately 1.5 liters of urine are excreted from the body per day.

Urine gets its yellow color from urochrome. The yellow comes from the destruction of hemoglobin molecules. Urine is about 95 percent water and 5 percent solutes such as urea, creatine, and uric acid. Urine is acidic with a pH of 6 and has a higher specific gravity than water (about 1.001 to 1.035).

Figure 9. The Human Urinary System

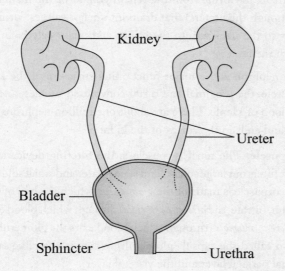

The Kidneys

The human body has two kidneys located behind the peritoneum on the right and left sides of the body. Each kidney is compact, about the size of a fist. There are several structural components to the external and internal regions of the kidneys.

The following is the external kidney anatomy:

- **Hilum:** The hilum is the region where blood vessels and lymphatic vessels enter the kidney.
- **Coverings:** There are three coverings of the kidney. The *renal fascia* is the outermost layer of the kidney, is composed of connective tissue, and serves to anchor the kidney to surrounding body structures. The *perirenal fat capsule* is a layer of fat that attaches to the posterior wall of the abdomen and serves to cushion the kidney. The *fibrous capsule* is the deepest layer of the kidney and functions to prevent infections from spreading to the kidney.

The following is the internal kidney anatomy:

- **Cortex:** The cortex is the outer most layer of the internal portion of the kidney.
- **Medulla:** The inner layer of the internal kidney is called the medulla and consists of eighteen cone-shaped subsections called *medullary*, or *renal*, *pyramids*. Renal pyramids have the following structures:
    - **Apex, or papilla:** The apex, or the papilla, is the point of the pyramid that points inward.
    - **Collecting ducts:** The collecting ducts give medullary pyramids striations. Intercalated cells help to maintain an acid–base balance. Principal cells maintain a balance of H_2O and Na^+ in the blood.
- **Renal columns:** The renal columns are cortical tissue extensions that come down between each of the 18 pyramids. The columns act to separate each pyramid from the others.
- **Renal pelvis:** The renal pelvis is a large structure that is continuous with the *ureter* (place where urine collects before it leaves the body.) The renal pelvis is composed of minor calyces (ducts that carry urine from the renal pyramid of the medulla to the renal pelvis for excretion through the ureters) that drain into major calyces. Urine travels through the collecting ducts to the papilla, into the minor and major calyces in the renal pelvis, and then on through the ureters.
- **Nephron:** The nephron is the major functioning structure of the kidneys. It consists of the renal corpuscle, the proximal and distal convoluted tubules, and the nephronic loop, also called the loop of Henle. There are about one million nephrons in each kidney. Each nephron starts and ends in the cortex of the kidney.
    - **Renal corpuscle:** The renal corpuscle is the filtering device at the opening of the nephron. It filters out large solutes and sends water and small solutes to the renal tubule. The renal corpuscle is made of the *glomerulus*, which is a ball of capillaries containing endothelium, filtrate, the *afferent arteriole* (through which blood enters the glomerulus) and the *efferent arteriole* (through which blood exits the glomerulus) and the *Bowman's capsule* (also called the capsula glomeruli), which is a cuplike sac that has two layers (the external parietal layer and the visceral layer).
    - **Renal tubule:** The renal tubule is the part of the nephron through which the filtrate passes to the collecting ducts. The renal tubule consists of the *proximal convoluted tubule* (PCT), which is a microvilli-covered tubule that leaves the Bowman's capsule and goes to the loop of Henle; the *loop of Henle* (LOH), which is made up of the descending LOH (squamous cells that are very permeable to water and impermeable to solvents) and the ascending LOH (epithelial cells that are impermeable to water, but permeable to salts); and the *distal convoluted tubule* (DCT), which is composed of cuplike epithelium that do not have microvilli and which helps to regulate the salts in the kidneys.

There are two types of nephron:

1. **Corticoid nephron:** The corticoid nephron is found mostly in the cortex of the kidney (although some are in the loop of Henle). About 85 percent of all nephrons are corticoid nephrons.

2. **Juxtamedullary nephron:** The juxtamedullary nephrons are found closer to the junction between the cortex and the medulla of the kidney.

Within the nephrons there are also three different types of capillary beds:

1. **Glomerular capillary bed:** The ball-shaped capillary bed in the glomerulus is where filtrate is formed from blood. It is the highest pressure capillary bed in the body because the diameter of the afferent arteriole is larger than that of the efferent arteriole. Thus, fluid enters faster than it can drain out.

2. **Peritubular capillary bed:** The peritubular capillary beds pick up solutes that have been filtered out in the glomerular bed and reabsorb them. The capillary beds stem from the efferent arteriole and run along the length of the renal tubules. These are low-pressure capillary beds that absorb solutes and water from the renal tubules.

3. **Juxtamedullary nephron capillary beds:** The juxtamedullary capillary beds help to concentrate urine. These capillary beds have *vasa recta*, which are straight arteries in the kidneys that are ordered and perpendicular to the loop of Helne.

The Ureter, Bladder, and Urethra

From the ureter, urine flows into the bladder. The bladder is a musculomembraneous sac in the anterior part of the pelvic cavity. It functions as a reservoir for urine flowing from the ureters. Urine is stored in the bladder until it is excreted outside the body through the urethra. The *urethra* is a canal that leads from the bladder outside the body. In females, the urethra lies between the vagina and the clitoris. In males, the urethra travels through the penis with an opening at its tip (both urine and semen are discharged through the urethra).

Overview of Processes in the Urinary System

The urinary system produces and disposes of urine using the following four major processes.

1. **Filtration:** During filtration, water and small molecules are forced through capillary walls and enter the nephron tubules from the glomerulus.

2. **Reabsorption:** Reabsorption is the first of two processes of refining the filtrate. Water and all valuable solutes (glucose, salt essential ions, and amino acids) are returned to the blood.

3. **Secretion:** During secretion, the second process to refine filtrate, substances in the blood are transported into the filtrate. For example, excess H^+ ions are secreted into filtrate to keep blood at the proper pH level. Secretion also eliminates drugs and toxic substances from the blood. In both secretion and reabsorption, water and solutes pass through interstitial fluid between tubules and capillaries.

4. **Excretion:** Excretion is the process of eliminating urine (the final product of filtration, reabsorption, and secretion). Urine passes to the external environment via the urethra.

THE REPRODUCTIVE SYSTEM

Sexual reproduction results in genetically unique offspring (except in the case of identical twins). Offspring are created by the fusion of two haploid (n) sex cells to form a diploid (2n) fertilized egg (zygote). The male gamete is the microscopic sperm that moves via its flagellum. The female gamete is the egg (ovum) that is much larger than the sperm, but not motile. The zygote carries a unique combination of genes from both the sperm and the egg.

The Female Reproductive System

The gonads (sex organ) of the female reproductive system are the *ovaries*. Ovaries produce egg cells and sex hormones. An egg is carried from the ovaries into the uterus via a series of ducts. Ovaries are suspended on each side of the uterus; there are two regions of the ovary. The *medulla* is the inner portion of the ovary and runs through the middle of the ovary. It contains blood vessels and nerves. The *cortex* is the outer region of the ovary and is involved in the formation of gametes (sex cells). The cortex is composed of *follicles* (immature eggs or oocytes). Follicle cells are those in which only one layer of cells surrounds the oocyte. Oocytes surrounded by two or more layers of cells are called *granulosa cells*.

Follicle cells specifically produce the female sex hormone estrogen. There are four types of follicles that are at different stages of maturity. *Primordial follicles* have only one layer of cells around the oocyte. These follicles mature into primary follicles. *Primary follicles* have two or more layers of cells surrounding the oocyte (granulose), and they mature into secondary follicles. A follicle becomes a *secondary follicle* when a fluid-filled space called the antrum appears. Secondary follicles become *vesicular follicles*. A *vesicular follicle* forms when the antrum becomes so large that the oocyte is pushed to one side of the follicle.

During the process of *ovulation*, an egg cell (oocyte) is ejected from a follicle. The cells and follicular tissue surrounding the egg that was ejected grow within the ovary to form a mass called the *corpus luteum*. The corpus luteum secretes additional estrogen and another hormone called progesterone, which helps to maintain the uterine lining during pregnancy. If the egg is not fertilized, then the corpus luteum degenerates and forms again when a new egg is released during the next menstrual cycle.

The ovaries are positioned next to the opening of the oviducts, or fallopian tubes. The enlarged region at the end of the oviduct closest to the ovary is called the *ampulla*. The ampulla ends in a funnel-shaped structure that is fringed with fingerlike projections covered in cilia (fimbriae). This is called the *infundibulum*. The infundibulum drapes over the ovary, but does not come in direct contact with it. The fimbriae conduct a current that is able to draw the egg into the oviduct. Fertilization typically occurs in the upper third of the oviduct. The resulting fertilized egg begins to divide as it travels along the fallopian tube.

The actual site of pregnancy and development of the embryo into a fetus is the *uterus*. The uterus, which is about 3 inches long, expands during pregnancy to accommodate the developing fetus. The uterus has a thick muscular wall and an inner lining called the *endometrium*. The endometrium contains vast amounts of blood vessels. The embryo implants in the endometrium and continues to develop into a fetus (body structures are evident). The endometrium is the innermost mucosal lining (the *startum basalis* is the deepest sublayer that newly forms after each menstrual period and the *stratum functionalis* is the surface layer that is shed during menstruation). The *myometrium* is the muscle layer that makes up most of the uterus; this muscle is used during childbirth to push the baby out. The *perimetrium* is the outermost layer of the uterus and is part of the peritoneum.

There are three regions of the uterus:

1. **Body:** The body is the main part of the uterus.
2. **Fundus:** The fundus is the rounded part of the uterus above the entrance of the oviducts.
3. **Cervix:** The cervix is the region that extends into the vagina. The cervix dilates during childbirth. A mucus plug forms a barrier in the hole between the vagina and the uterus. This plug prevents bacteria or sperm from entering. During ovulation (release of an oocyte), the mucus plug disappears so that sperm can fertilize the released egg.

The cervix exits into the vagina, which is a muscular, thin-walled chamber that acts as the birth canal through which a baby is born. Glands near the vaginal opening secrete a mucous during sexual arousal to facilitate intercourse and allow the sperm to travel through the vagina to the oviducts.

Figure 10. The Female Reproductive Organs

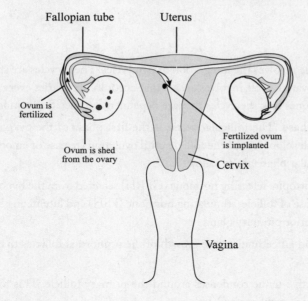

External Female Genitalia

The following four structures make up the external genitalia in females:

1. **Monis pubis:** The monis pubis is the fatty lump over the pubic bone.
2. **Labia:** The labia are the two flaps of skin and adipose tissue that extend and cover the external genitalia. There are two layers of the labia. The *labia majora* is a thick fatty ridge covered with hair, a structure parallel to the male scrotum. The *labia minora* are two soft skin folds that surround the opening of the vagina.
3. **Vestibule:** The vestibule is the region that contains the openings to the vagina and the urethra. The greater vestibular glands secrete thick mucus.

4. **Clitoris:** The female clitoris is erectile tissue, which is analogous to the penis in men. The sole function of the clitoris is sexual arousal and so has a large number of nerve endings. The clitoris consists of a short shaft that supports a rounded head, or *glans*. It is covered by a small hood of skin called the *prepuce*. The clitoris, along with the vagina and labia minora, fills with blood during arousal.

Oogenesis

Eggs form in women during the fetal period and develop into primary oocytes within primary follicles. Development of the primary oocytes freezes in prophase I of meiosis I for about ten to fourteen years. At the onset of puberty, at least one oocyte every 28 days (if a woman's cycle is "regular") completes meiosis I and produces two new cells: a secondary oocyte and a polar body, which is nonfunctional. The secondary oocyte stops in metaphase II. The secondary oocyte is released from the secondary follicle during ovulation and will complete its development only if it is fertilized by a sperm cell. Ovulation is triggered by the pituitary hormone LH (luteinizing hormone). If fertilization occurs, the oocyte completes meiosis II to yield two new cells: a polar body and an *ovum*, or mature egg. Only about 500 oocytes are released during a woman's lifetime, but there are about 250,000 oocytes in the ovaries at birth.

Ovarian Cycle

The reproductive cycle involves the integration of two cycles. These cycles are specific to the ovaries and the uterus. The ovarian cycle involves events that occur in the ovaries every 28 days (if the cycle is regular). Sex hormones link the cycles that are dependent on specific hormones.

*   **Follicular phase:** The follicular phase is the first phase of the ovarian cycle. This phase follows the development of the follicle until ovulation (release of an oocyte). The ten steps of the follicular phase are as follows:

    1. Gonadotropin-releasing hormone (GnRH) secreted from the hypothalamus stimulates the release of follicle-stimulating hormone (FSH) and luteinizing hormone (LH) from the anterior pituitary gland.

    2. FSH and LH stimulate the growth of the primordial follicles to mature into primary follicles.

    3. Connective tissue condenses around the primary follicle. This forms a theca follicle that is targeted later by LH.

    4. Primary follicles with two or more layers are targeted by FSH.

    5. Cells begin to produce estrogen. An increase in estrogen inhibits FSH and LH, which prevents the development of more follicles.

    6. Estrogen levels rise as more estrogen is produced in the ovaries. The primary follicle begins to mature into a secondary follicle.

    7. The antrum (liquid) continues to increase, and the oocyte becomes isolated on one side of the follicle. The oocyte is surrounded by a set of cells called the *corona radiate*, and the vesicular follicle forms.

8. Estrogen levels peak. FSH is no longer inhibited and activates a positive feedback loop that results in a surge of LH at the end of follicular phase.

9. The primary oocyte completes meiosis I, and the oocyte fully matures into a secondary oocyte. Ovulation occurs around day 14. The secondary oocyte is expelled from the ovaries.

10. Once ovulation occurs, estrogen levels in the ovaries decrease.

- **Luteal phase:** The second phase of the ovarian cycle starts on day 15 and continues through day 28. The four steps of the luteal phase are as follows:

   1. LH transforms the vesicular follicle into the corpus luteum. The corpus luteum begins to produce progesterone and some estrogen.

   2. When the egg is not fertilized, the corpus luteum degenerates within about 10 days. The corpus luteum leaves behind the corpus albicans (white scar tissue). The degeneration of the corpus luteum causes the levels of estrogen and progesterone to drop. A drop in these hormones causes LH and FSH levels to increase, and the cycle begins again.

   3. If fertilization occurs, the corpus luteum grows, causing an increase in progesterone production until the third month of pregnancy. After the third month, progesterone is produced in the placenta.

   4. In the first three months of pregnancy, the progesterone and estrogen produced inhibit FSH and LH, but the corpus luteum needs LH in order to grow. As LH levels drop, they are replaced by *human chorionic gonadotropin* (HCG), which is an LH-like hormone that stimulates production of estrogen and progesterone.

Uterine Cycle

The uterine, or menstrual, cycle is also about 28 days and is coordinated with the ovarian cycle so that the uterus is prepared to receive an egg. The egg is released, and it takes about six or seven days for it to travel through the oviduct to the uterus. There are three phases of the menstrual cycle:

1. **Menstrual phase:** During days 1 through 5 of the uterine cycle, the uterus sheds the stratum functionalis (endometrium). The shed lining leaves the uterus through the cervix and leaves the body through the vagina.

2. **Proliferation phase:** During days 6 through 14, the endometrium rebuilds the stratum functionalis. This action is stimulated by rising estrogen levels.

3. **Secretory phase:** During days 15 through 28, the endometrial lining prepares for implantation of an egg. If an egg implants, progesterone will maintain the corpus luteum. If the egg does not implant, the corpus luteum degrades and endometrial cells die off. The cycle returns to day 1 of the menstrual phase.

The Male Reproductive System

The male reproductive system has some similarities to the female system. Both sexes have a pair of gonads and organs that produce gametes. Both have ducts that deliver the gamete to the appropriate place. The five main structures of the male reproductive system are the following:

1. **Testes:** The testes are the male gonads. They have two coverings called tunics. The *tunica vaginalis* is the outside covering and is a continuation of the peritoneum. The *tunica albuginea* is the inside covering of the testes and is composed of mostly fibrous connective tissue. The testes are divided into two structures called *lobules*, separated by the *septula testes* (fibrous septa). Each lobule of the testes contains a series of tubules called the *seminiferous tubules* (composed of myoid and interstitial cells). Sperm are produced in these tubules.

2. **Spermatic cord:** The spermatic cord is composed of nerves, blood cells, lymphatic vessels, and the vas deferens (travels from the epididymis through the inguinal canal to each testicle).

3. **Scrotum:** The scrotum is a sac outside the abdominal cavity that holds the testes. The scrotum holds the testes at a temperature that is lower than body temperature so that the sperm-forming cells can function properly.

4. **Ducts:** The function of ducts is to deliver sperm to the epididymis (place where sperm is stored while it develops). There are four ducts in the male reproductive system.

    a. **Epididymis:** The epididymis is a tightly coiled tube that stores sperm as they develop. It is divided into three sections: the head, the body, and the tail. Microvilli function in the epididymis to absorb extra testicular fluids.

    b. **Vas deferens:** The vas deferens, also called the *ductus deferens*, is part of the spermatic cord. Muscular contractions propel sperm from the epididymis to the vas deferens. The vas deferens passes upward into the abdominal cavity and loops around the bladder. The end of the vas deferens is called the *ampulla*, and it joins to another duct called the ejaculatory duct.

    c. **Ejaculatory duct:** The ejaculatory duct is formed from the vas deferens and a short duct extending from the seminal vesicle (gland helps to provide energy to sperm). The action of peristalsis moves sperm along the ejaculatory duct.

    d. **Urethra:** The urethra receives the sperm from the ejaculatory duct. It is part of both the reproductive and urinary systems in males. The *prostatic urethra* is the portion surrounded by the prostate gland. The *membranous urethra* acts as the urogenital diaphragm. The spongy, or penil urethra, is the portion that is inside the penis. It allows urine and sperm to flow outside the body.

5. **Glands:** There are three sets of glands in the male reproductive system.

    a. **Seminal vesicles:** The seminal vesicles secrete a thick fluid that contains fructose, ascorbic acid, prostaglandins, and other substances that promote motility. The fructose provides most of the energy used by sperm to propel itself through the female reproductive tract. About 60 percent of the total volume of semen is from seminal vesicles.

    b. **Prostate gland:** The prostate gland secretes a thin fluid that further nourishes sperm. This fluid is a milky, acidic fluid that contains citrate, enzymes, and prostate-specific antigen (PSA).

c. **Bulbourethral glands:** The two small bulbourethral glands secrete a thick, clear alkaline mucus that may act to neutralize the acidity of urine. It is also known as the *Cowper's gland* and lubricates the glans penis.

Figure 11. The Male Reproductive System

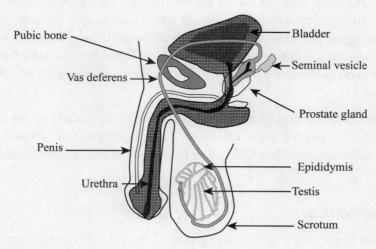

Spermatogenesis

The glandular secretions and sperm make up what is called semen. *Semen* is ejaculated from the penis through a series of rhythmic, involuntary contractions. Only about 2 to 5 teaspoons of semen are ejaculated at one time. About 95 percent of the fluid is glandular secretions, and the other 5 percent is made up of a few hundred million sperm.

Sperm is alkaline to protect it from the acidic environment in the male urethra and the female vagina. A substance called *seminal plasma* destroys any bacteria to protect sperm. Sperm are produced in the seminiferous tubules in a process called *spermatogenesis*. After a male reaches puberty, about 400 million sperm are produced each day. The process of spermatogenesis begins with diploid stem cells called *spermatogonia*, which undergo mitosis to produce two types of cells.

Type A cells stay in the basal laminae of the seminiferous tubules and maintain the germ line. Type B cells are pushed toward the lumen of the seminiferous tubule where they are transformed into *primary spermatocytes*. Primary spermatocytes undergo the process of meiosis I and become *secondary spermatocyte*s. Secondary spermatocytes undergo the process of meiosis II to become *spermatids* (haploid cells). Each original stem cell produces four spermatids. Special cells called *nurse cells*, or sustentacular cells, in the seminiferous tubules surround sperm cells and help in their maturation process.

There are three regions to a mature sperm.

1. **Head:** The head of the sperm is the portion that contains the nucleus and all the genetic information (DNA). The *acrosome* is a specialized piece on the head that has enzymes to digest the covering of an ovum. In this way, the sperm can enter the egg to fertilize it.

2. **Midpiece:** The midpiece of the sperm provides fuel. It contains many mitochondria and is the metabolic portion of the sperm.

3. **Tail:** The tail section of the sperm provides motility so that the sperm can travel to the egg.

Hormone Regulation

Within the male body, there are interactions between the hypothalamus, anterior pituitary gland, and testes. These interactions are referred to as the *brain-testicular axis*, and they regulate spermatogenesis and androgen production. The hypothalamus releases GnRH, which, in turn, regulates the release of FSH and LH in the anterior pituitary gland. The male testes release the male sex hormone, *testosterone*. FSH stimulates the nurse cells in the seminiferous tubule to release androgen-binding protein (ABP). ABP triggers the concentration of testosterone in spermatogenic cells and also allows for spermatogenic cells to be more receptive of testosterone. Concentrated testosterone then triggers spermatogenesis and inhibits any further release of GnRH from the hypothalamus. When the sperm count in the epididymis is high, the nurse cells release *inhibin*, which inhibits the release of more FSH and LH.

Testosterone is the male sex hormone that promotes the development of all male sex organs (ducts, glans, penis, testes). Testosterone is also responsible for the development of secondary sex characteristics such as facial hair, pubic hair, and axillary hair; bone and muscle growth; voice deepening; and sex drive.

External Male Genitalia

The structure that comprises the external male genitalia is the penis. The penis functions to deliver sperm to the egg inside the female oviduct. There are three regions of the penis: the root is attached to the body, the shaft (body) hangs free from the rest of the male body, and the glans penis is the expanded end, or head, of the penis. Foreskin covers the glans penis unless circumcision has been performed.

The *penile urethra* is the section of the urethra that travels through the penis. There are three bodies of cylindrical tissue that runs along the length of the penis. This tissue is spongy because it consists of connective tissue with spaces that fill with blood during an erection. *Corpus spongiosum* is the connective tissue surrounding the urethra that serves to keep the urethra open during an erection. *Corpus caverosa* are two bodies of connective tissue that form the bulk of the penis.

PRACTICE QUESTIONS

Directions: Choose the best answer for each question.

Refer to the following passage for Questions 1–4.

The respiratory and circulatory systems collaborate to oxygenate blood for use in energy production throughout the human body. The pulmonary artery carries blood from the right side of the heart to the lungs to pick up a fresh supply of oxygen, and the pulmonary vein returns oxygenated blood from the lungs to the left atrium of the heart. The aorta later initiates the distribution of the oxygen-rich blood throughout the body.

1. Which of the following are the three vessels of the right atrium of the heart?
   A. Superior vena cava, inferior vena cava, coronary sinus
   B. Superior vena cava, right pulmonary vein, coronary sinus
   C. Superior vena cava, inferior vena cava, aorta
   D. Superior vena cava, inferior vena cava, right pulmonary vein

2. Ventilation of the lungs is dependent upon the
   A. volume of pleural fluid in the lungs.
   B. concentration of CO_2 in the lungs.
   C. concentration of O_2 in the lungs.
   D. change in volume in the thoracic cavity.

3. Total capacity is the sum of which two types of lung capacity?
   A. Vital capacity and inspirational capacity
   B. Vital capacity and functional residual capacity
   C. Vital capacity and residual volume
   D. Vital capacity and airway resistance

4. Which artery supplies blood to the brain?
   A. Left common carotid artery
   B. Left subclavian artery
   C. Brachiocephalic artery
   D. Coronary arteries

Refer to the following passage for Questions 5–11.

The nervous system is responsible for direct control of both the endocrine and reproductive systems, as well as the organs that are linked with them. By sending nerve impulses, the nervous system can cause the body to secrete hormones, as well as release eggs and sperm, the female and male gametes.

5. Which part of the neuron transmits the stimulus signal from neurons to an effector cell?
   A. Cell body
   B. Dendrite
   C. Axon
   D. Myelin sheath

6. Hormones that stimulate and maintain metabolic processes are secreted from the
   A. hypothalamus.
   B. thyroid gland.
   C. anterior pituitary gland.
   D. pineal gland.

7. Which of the following types of hormone activity is best described as two hormones working together to produce one outcome?
   A. Synergism
   B. Permissiveness
   C. Antagonism
   D. Active complement

8. During the ovarian cycle, which of the following hormones are inhibited by the presence of estrogen?

  A. FSH and LH

  B. GnRH and FSH

  C. GnRH and LH

  D. Progesterone and LH

9. The division of the peripheral nervous system that conducts signals towards the CNS is the

  A. sensory or afferent division.

  B. motor or efferent division.

  C. sympathetic nervous system.

  D. parasympathetic nervous system.

10. In which portion of the sperm does cellular metabolism take place?

  A. Head

  B. Midpiece

  C. Tail

  D. Nucleus

11. Joints that are composed of articulating joints separated by a fluid-containing joint cavity are

  A. fibrous joints.

  B. cartilaginous joints.

  C. synarthroses joints.

  D. synovial joints.

The following questions are standalone and not tied to a passage.

12. The largest of all of the types of lymphatic vessels are

  A. lymphatic capillaries.

  B. lymphatic trunks.

  C. lymphatic ducts.

  D. lymphatic nodes.

13. Which of the following are examples of enzymes involved in the digestion of disaccharides?

  A. Maltase, lactase, sucrase

  B. Aminopeptidase, carboxypeptidase, dipeptidase

  C. Lipases

  D. Nucleosidases, phosphatases

14. In general where is the concentration of Na^+ greatest?

  A. Inside a neuron

  B. Outside a neuron

  C. In the plasma membrane of a neuron

  D. It is the same inside and outside of the cell.

15. Which of the following functions to prevent infection from spreading to the kidneys?

  A. Renal fascia

  B. Perineal fat capsule

  C. Fibrous capsule

  D. Hilum

16. Which of the following structures attaches muscle to bone?

  A. Joints

  B. Tendons

  C. Epimysium

  D. Ligaments

17. As primary follicles mature into secondary follicles, which of the following features appears?

  A. Oocytes

  B. Corpus luteum

  C. Antrum

  D. Ampulla

18. The structure in nephrons that filters out large solutes is the

  A. loop of Henle.

  B. distal convoluted tubule.

  C. renal tubule.

  D. renal corpuscle.

19. Kupffer cells function in the liver to
    A. produce bile.
    B. remove debris and bacteria.
    C. process nutrient-laden blood.
    D. remove excess glucose from blood.

20. With the exception of red blood cells, all cells in the body are coated with
    A. antigenic determinants.
    B. antibodies.
    C. class I MHC proteins.
    D. class II MHC proteins.

ANSWER KEY AND EXPLANATIONS

1. A	**5.** C	**9.** A	**13.** A	**17.** C
2. D	**6.** B	**10.** B	**14.** B	**18.** D
3. C	**7.** A	**11.** D	**15.** C	**19.** B
4. C	**8.** A	**12.** C	**16.** B	**20.** C

1. **The correct answer is A.** The right atrium receives blood from the upper part of the body through the superior vena cava and from the lower part of the body through the inferior vena cava. The right atrium receives blood from the heart through the coronary sinus. Choice B is incorrect because all of the pulmonary veins enter into the left atrium of the heart. Choice C is incorrect because the left ventricle pumps blood through the aorta. Choice D is incorrect because the right pulmonary vein enters the heart from the left atrium.

2. **The correct answer is D.** Ventilation is dependent upon change in volume in the thoracic cavity, and the pressure and volume in the thoracic cavity is dependent upon Boyle's gas law ($P_1V_1 = P_2V_2$). Choice A is incorrect because pleural fluid allows the lungs to glide over the thorax during breathing. The pleural fluid causes adhesion between the two pleural layers, which causes the lungs to expand or contract during breathing. Choice B is incorrect because ventilation is not dependent upon O_2 concentration. Choice C is incorrect because ventilation is not dependent upon CO_2 concentration.

3. **The correct answer is C.** The total lung capacity of a healthy individual is 6000 mL, or 6 L. It is the sum of the vital capacity (4.8 L) and the residual volume (1.2 L). Choice A is incorrect because the total lung capacity is dependent upon the vital capacity and the residual volume, not the inspirational

capacity. Choice B is incorrect because the total lung capacity is dependent upon the vital capacity and the residual volume, not the functional residual capacity (expiratory reserve volume and the residual volume). Choice D is incorrect because the total lung capacity is measured as the sum of the vital capacity and the residual volume, not airway resistance.

4. **The correct answer is C.** The brachiocephalic artery supplies blood to the head, brain, and right arm. Choice A is incorrect because the left common carotid artery supplies blood to the neck and chest areas. Choice B is incorrect because the left subclavian artery supplies blood to the left arm. Choice D is incorrect because coronary arteries deliver oxygenated blood to the heart muscle.

5. **The correct answer is C.** The axon is a long slender branched structure that carries a stimulus signal from one neuron to another or to an effector cell. Choice A is incorrect because the cell body is the main hub through which incoming and outgoing nerve impulses must travel, but it does not transmit the signal. Choice B is incorrect because dendrites are highly branched extensions of the neuron that receive signals from other neurons, but they do not transmit the signal. Choice D is incorrect because the myelin sheath is made up of lipids and lipoproteins and is a coating covering the axon.

6. **The correct answer is B.** The thyroid gland produces and secretes thyroxine (T4) and triiodothyronine (T3), which stimulate and maintain metabolic processes. Choice A is incorrect because the hypothalamus exerts master control over the endocrine system. It uses the pituitary gland to send directives to other glands. Choice C is incorrect because the anterior pituitary gland secretes hormones, including growth hormone (GH), prolactin (PRL), follicle-stimulating hormone (FSH), luteininizing hormone (LH), thyroid-stimulating hormone (TSH), and adrenocorticotopic hormone (ACTH). Choice D is incorrect because the pineal gland synthesizes and secretes melatonin.

7. **The correct answer is A.** Synergism involves two hormones working together to produce one outcome. Two hormones may also work together to produce a combined effect that is greater than the effect of one hormone acting alone. Choice B is incorrect because permissiveness involves the requirement of one hormone in order to bring about the full effect of a second hormone. Choice C is incorrect because antagonism is the effect observed when two hormones produce opposite effects from each other. Choice D is incorrect because active complement is a method of immune complex formation in which antibodies bind to antigens and slightly change shape to expose a complement binding site.

8. **The correct answer is A.** During the ovarian cycle, an increase in estrogen inhibits FSH and LH. This prevents the development of more follicles. Choice B is incorrect because estrogen does not affect the secretion of GnRH. Choice C is incorrect because estrogen does not affect the secretion of GnRH. Choice D is incorrect because estrogen does not inhibit the production of progesterone.

9. **The correct answer is A.** Sensory, or afferent, neurons are unipolar neurons that conduct nerve impulses to the CNS. Choice B is incorrect because motor, or efferent, neurons are multipolar neurons that conduct nerve impulses away from the CNS. Choice C is incorrect because the sympathetic division of the automatic nervous system corresponds to arousal and energy generation, or what is called the "fight-or-flight" response. Choice D is incorrect because the parasympathetic division is often referred to as the digestive, or resting, division. It promotes responses that restore the body to a resting and normal functioning state.

10. **The correct answer is B.** The midpiece of the sperm provides fuel, contains many mito-chondria, and is the metabolic portion of the sperm. Choice A is incorrect because the head of the sperm is the portion that contains the nucleus and all the genetic information (DNA). The acrosome is a specialized piece on the head that has enzymes to digest the covering of an ovum. In this way, the sperm can enter the egg to fertilize it. Choice C is incorrect because the tail section of the sperm provides motility so that the sperm can travel to the egg. Choice D is incorrect because the nucleus is included in the head section of the sperm, and the midpiece is the region that contains the mitochondria that are necessary for metabolism.

11. **The correct answer is D.** Synovial joints are articulating bones separated by a fluid-containing joint cavity. This type of joint is freely moving, or diarthroses. Choice A is incorrect because fibrous joints are joined by fibrous tissue full of collagen fibers; most fibrous joints are immovable. Choice B is incorrect because cartilaginous joints are articulating bones united by cartilage; there is no joint cavity in a cartilaginous joint. Choice C is incorrect because synarthroses joints are immovable joints.

12. **The correct answer is C.** Lymphatic ducts are the largest of the lymphatic vessels. The right lymphatic duct drains the right arm, right side of the head, and the right side of the thorax into the right subclavian vein. The thoracic duct is the larger of the two and drains the left arm, the left side of the head and neck, and the lower body into the left subclavian vein. Choice A is incorrect because lymphatic capillaries are the smallest of all the types of lymphatic vessels. Choice B is incorrect because lymphatic trunks join together to form the larger lymphatic ducts. Choice D is incorrect because lymph nodes are the principal organs in the lymphatic system. The two functions of lymph nodes are filtering and helping to activate the immune response mechanisms.

13. **The correct answer is A.** Carbohydrates are digested by pancreatic amylases to form disaccharides. The disaccharides are broken down further into monosaccharides by enzymes such as maltase, lactase, and sucrose. Choice B is incorrect because peptidase enzymes function to digest small polypeptides formed from ingested proteins. Choice C is incorrect because lipases are digestive enzymes that function in the breakdown of fats to fatty acids and glycerol. Choice D is incorrect because nucleosidases and phosphatases are involved in the digestion of nucleosides formed from DNA and RNA.

14. **The correct answer is B.** In general, the concentration of Na^+ ions is greater outside the cell and the concentration of K^+ ions is greater inside the cell. Choice A is incorrect because the concentration of Na^+ ions tends to be greater outside the cell than inside. Choice C is incorrect because the plasma membrane has ion channels to help Na^+ and K^+ ions pass into or out of the cell, but it does not hold these ions in the membrane. Choice D is incorrect because there is a concentration gradient of Na^+ ions, not an equilibrium of Na^+ ions.

15. **The correct answer is C.** The fibrous capsule is the deepest layer of the kidney; it functions to prevent infections from spreading to the kidney. Choice A is incorrect because the renal fascia is the outermost layer of the kidney, is composed of connective tissue, and serves to anchor the kidney to surrounding body structures. Choice B is incorrect because the perirenal fat capsule is a layer of fat that attaches to the posterior wall of the abdomen and serves to cushion the kidney. Choice D is incorrect because the hilum is the region where blood vessels and lymphatic vessels enter the kidney.

16. **The correct answer is B.** Tendons are firmly attached to bone by extending into the bone matrix, and they attach muscle to bone. Choice A is incorrect because joints join two bones together. Choice C is incorrect because the epimysium separates the muscle from surrounding tissue and organs. Choice D is incorrect because fibrous joints are held together by ligaments.

17. **The correct answer is C.** Primary follicles have two or more layers of cells surrounding the oocyte (granulose), and they mature into secondary follicles. A follicle becomes a secondary follicle when a fluid-filled space called the antrum appears. Choice A is incorrect because all follicles contain oocytes. Choice B is incorrect because the corpus luteum is a mass that forms from the cells and follicular tissue after the oocyte is ejected from a follicle. Choice D is incorrect because ampulla is the enlarged region at the end of the oviduct that is closest to the ovary.

18. **The correct answer is D.** The renal corpuscle is the filtering device at the opening of the nephron. It filters out large solutes and sends water and small solutes to the renal tubule.

Choice A is incorrect because the loop of Henle is involved in filtering salts from the kidneys. Choice B is incorrect because the distal convoluted tubule is a portion of the renal tubule and functions in the regulation of salts in the kidneys. Choice C is incorrect because the renal tubule is the portion of the nephron through which filtrate passes after the large solutes have been removed in the renal corpuscle.

19. **The correct answer is B.** Kupffer cells are part of the sinusoid walls of the liver and remove debris and bacteria; Kupffer cells act like macrophages. Choice A is incorrect because hepatocytes in the liver function to produce bile. Choice C is incorrect because although producing nutrient-laden blood from the intestines is a function of the liver,

it is not specific to Kupffer cells. Choice D is incorrect because the liver functions to remove excess glucose from blood; this is not carried out by Kupffer cells.

20. **The correct answer is C.** Cell bodies are coated with MHC, and they are a way for the body to recognize its own cells. MHC proteins are specific to an individual. Class I MHC proteins are found on every cell body except red blood cells (RBCs). Choice A is incorrect because antigenic determinants, or epitopes, are the small surface-exposed regions of an antigen that are recognized by antibodies. Choice B is incorrect because antibodies are produced in response to infection. Choice D is incorrect because class II MHC proteins are only found on cells of the immune response system.

SUMMING IT UP

- The *nervous system* consists of the 1) brain, 2) spinal cord, 3) circuits of neurons (nerve cells) and supporting cells, and 4) sensory receptors.

- In general, there are three stages of processing in the nervous system. These include 1) sensory input of an internal or external stimulus, 2) integration of the signal, and 3) a motor output.

- *Sensory neurons* transmit information from the sensors that detect either external stimuli or internal stimuli.

- *Interneurons* integrate the sensory input by analyzing and interpreting the signal. The connection between interneurons is the most complex part of the nervous system.

- Motor output leaves the CNS via motor neurons.

- There are three main components of neurons: 1) cell body, 2) axon, and 3) dendrites.

- There are three categories of neurons based on complexity: 1) unipolar neurons, 2) bipolar neurons, and 3) multipolar neurons.

- Neurons can be classified according to function as 1) sensory neurons, 2) motor neurons, and 3) interneurons.

- Neurons also have different types of gated ion channels that open and close in response to one of three kinds of stimuli: 1) stretch-gated, 2) ligand-gated, and 3) voltage-gated ion channels.

- Neurons communicate with each other at cell synapses.

- All motor output is initiated in the prefrontal cortex of the brain, and all sensory information is processed in the six sensory areas of the brain.

- The PNS is divided into two parts: 1) the somatic and 2) the autonomic nervous systems.

- Joints are sites where two bones join together and articulate. Joints serve to add mobility to the skeletal structure and to hold the skeleton together.

- The functional classification of a joint is dependent upon how the joint works.

- The structural classification of a joint is determined by how the joint is constructed.

- There are three basic movements allowed by synovial joints: 1) gliding, 2) angular motion, and 3) rotational movements.

- There are six basic synovial joints: 1) hinge, 2) plane, 3) pivot, 4) condyloid, 5) saddle, and 6) ball-and-socket.

- There are two types of bone tissue that make up a bone: 1) compact bone and 2) spongy bone.

- There are four different shapes that bones form: 1) long, 2) short, 3) flat, and 4) irregular.

- There are five common functions of bones: 1) framework support, 2) movement, 3) protection, 4) storage, and 5) blood cell formation.

- Bone is composed of both 1) organic and 2) inorganic materials.

- Bone development is dependent on the type of bone. For example, in the early stages of development, all long bones are composed of hyaline cartilage. Flat bone forms from the intermembraneous ossification of connective tissue.

- There are three types of muscle tissue: 1) skeletal muscle, 2) smooth muscle, and 3) cardiac muscle.

- According to the *sliding filament model* of muscle contraction, a sarcomere contracts, or shortens, when the thin filaments slide across the thick filaments. When the muscle is fully contracted, the thin actin filaments overlap in the middle of the sarcomere.

- The structure of myosin is important for the movement of thin filaments. The head portions of the myosin (thick) filaments move by pivoting back and forth in an arc pattern.

- The human cardiovascular system is made up of three components: 1) heart, 2) blood, and 3) blood vessels. All three components work together to pump blood through the body.

- The heart is enclosed in a double-layered sac called the *pericardium*. The fibrous pericardium has three functions: 1) protection, 2) anchoring, and 3) prevention of overfilling the heart. The serous pericardium is divided into a visceral and a parietal layer.

- The heart is made up of two layers: 1) the myocardium and 2) the endocardium. The heart has 1) four chambers (left and right atrium, left and right ventricle), 2) a septum, and 3) valves.

- The aorta is the largest artery in the human body and functions to carry blood away from the heart.

- There are four main types of vessels in the body: 1) arteries, 2) veins, 3) coronary arteries, and 4) coronary sinus.

- There are three distinct pathways through which blood flows through the body: 1) the pulmonary circuit, 2) the systemic circuit, and 3) the coronary circuit.

- *Autorhythmic cells* in the heart do not contract. They act by depolarizing spontaneously and keeping the heart moving at the same pace. These cells are part of what is called the intrinsic conduction system.

- *Contractile cells* work together to contract the heart. All cells work in unison so that either all contractile cells contract, or none do.

- A specialized region of the heart called a *pacemaker*, or sinoatrial node (SA node), sets the pace, or rate, at which all heart muscles contract.

- The function of blood is three-fold: 1) distribution of O_2 and return of CO_2 to the lungs, 2) regulation of body temperature, and 3) protection against infection.

- Blood is composed of 1) red blood cells and 2) white blood cells (neutrophils, eosinophils, basophils, monocytes, lymphocytes).

- There are four different blood types in humans: A, B, AB, and O.

- The *lymphatic system* consists of a network of branching vessels: 1) lymph nodes, which are rounded organs packed with macrophages and lymphocytes; 2) the tonsils and adenoids; 3) the spleen; and 4) the appendix. It also includes 5) yellow bone marrow and 6) the thymus, sites at which WBCs develop.

- Lymphatic capillaries are permeable so that fluids can pass in and out of them, and they can pick up interstitial fluids.

- There are several different types of vessels through which lymph travels: 1) lymphatic vessels (capillaries), 2) lymphatic trunks, and 3) lymphatic ducts.

- As lymph cycles through the lymphatic organs, such as the lymph nodes, it picks up and carries microbes or toxins picked up from a site of infection in the body.

- The outer portion of the lymph node that contains 1) densely packed follicles, 2) dendritic cells (cells that help activate T cells and act to immobilize antigens), and 3) B-lymphocytes is called the cortex. The inner portion that contains 1) B-lymphocytes, 2) T-lymphocytes, and 3) plasma is called the medulla.

- The *thymus* is an organ of the lymphatic system that secretes hormones.

- There are two branches of the immune system: 1) the nonspecific, or innate, immune system and 2) the acquired immune system.

- Internal defense mechanisms in the innate immune system include 1) phagocytes, 2) natural killer cells (NK cells), 3) antimicrobial proteins, 4) essential microbiota, 5) fever, and 6) inflammation.

- *Acquired immunity* is a set of defenses that are activated only after infection, or exposure to pathogens. There are three characteristics of the acquired immune system: 1) specific, 2) systemic, and 3) memory.

- The acquired immune system has two types of immune responses: 1) the humoral immune response and 2) the cell-mediated immune response.

- Any substance that immobilizes the immune system and provokes an immune response is an antigen. There are two main types of antigens that enter the body: 1) complete antigens and 2) incomplete antigens.

- Cell bodies are coated with MHC, and it is a way for the body to recognize its own cells. MHC proteins are specific to an individual. Class I MHC proteins are found on every cell body except red blood cells (RBCs). Class II MHC proteins are only found on cells of the immune response system.

- T cells are involved in two types of immune response. These immune responses are dependent on glycoprotein surface receptors called CD4 helper T cells and CD8 cytotoxic T cells.

- Antibody structure is a basic Y shape that has six main components: 1) polypeptide chain, 2) constant region, 3) variable region, 4) antigen binding sites, 5) hinge region, and 6) disulfide bonds.

- There are five classes of antibodies: IgA, IgD, IgE, IgG, and IgM.

- There are four ways in which to form an antigen-antibody complex: 1) active complement, 2) agglutination, 3) neutralization, and 4) precipitation.

- The major endocrine glands are: 1) the hypothalamus, 2) the pineal gland, 3) the pituitary gland (posterior and anterior), 4) the thyroid gland, 5) the parathyroid gland, 6) the adrenal glands, 7) the pancreas, 8) the gonads, and 9) the thymus gland.

- The mechanism of release of peptide, or amino acid-based, hormones relies on a secondary messenger and is a six-step process.

- There are three categories of hormone activity in which more than one hormone is acting to produce a response: 1) synergism, 2) permissiveness, and 3) antagonism.

- The *respiratory system* involves the process of gas exchange, specifically the uptake of O_2 and the release of CO_2)There are three phases of gas exchange: 1) breathing, 2) transport of respiratory gases, and 3) internal respiration.

- The *conducting zone* of the respiratory system includes the 1) nose, 2) mouth, 3) pharynx, 4) larynx, 5) trachea, and 6) terminal bronchi.

- The *respiratory zone* of the respiratory system includes the 1) bronchioles, 2) alveolar ducts, and 3) alveola sac.

- Ventilation is dependent upon change in volume in the thoracic cavity, and the pressure and volume in the thoracic cavity is dependent upon Boyle's gas law ($P_1V_1 = P_2V_2$).

- Airway resistance and alveolar surface tension affect proper ventilation.

- The capacity of lungs is measured by 1) vital capacity, 2) inspirational capacity, 3) functional residual capacity, and 4) total lung capacity.

- The *digestive system* consists of the 1) alimentary canal (the gastrointestinal tract) and 2) associated glands.

- There are several processes that occur during digestion: 1) ingestion, 2) propulsion, 3) chemical digestion, 4) absorption, and 5) defecation.

- The *gastrointestinal tract* consists of four layers: 1) mucosa, 2) submucosa, 3) muscularis externa, and 4) serosa.

- Organs of the GI tract include: 1) mouth, 2) tongue, 3) salivary glands, 4) teeth, 5) pharynx, 6) esophagus, 7) stomach, 8) small intestine, 9) liver, 10) gallbladder, 11) pancreas, and 12) large intestine.

- All four types of molecules—1) carbohydrates, 2) proteins, 3) fats, and 4) nucleic acids—are digested by enzymes in the small intestine that are specific to each type of molecule.

- The urinary system plays a role in homeostasis of body fluids. The key processes of the urinary system are 1) filtration, 2) reabsorption, 3) secretion, and 4) excretion.

- The external kidney anatomy consists of the 1) hilum and three types of coverings, 2) renal fascia, 3) fat capsule, and 4) fibrous capsule

- The internal kidney is composed of the 1) cortex, 2) medulla, 3) renal columns, 4) renal pelvis, and 5) nephrons.

- The *nephron* is the major functioning structure of the kidneys. It consists of the 1) renal corpuscle, 2) proximal and distal convoluted tubules, and 3) nephronic loop.

- Within the nephrons, there are also three types of capillary beds: 1) glomerular, 2) peritubular, and 3) juxtamedullary.

- Sexual reproduction results in genetically unique offspring created by the fusion of two haploid (n) sex cells to form a diploid (2n) fertilized egg (zygote).

- An egg is carried from the ovaries into the uterus through a series of ducts.

- Follicle cells are those in which only one layer of cells surrounds the oocyte. Oocytes surrounded by two or more layers of cells are called granulosa cells.

- Four types of follicles develop at different stages of maturity: 1) primordial, 2) primary, 3) secondary, and 4) vesicular. During the process of ovulation, an egg cell (oocyte) is ejected from a follicle.

- Fertilization typically occurs in the upper third of the oviduct. The resulting fertilized egg begins to divide as it travels along the fallopian tube.

- The *uterus* is the site of embryo implantation and fetus development. It has three regions: 1) body, 2) fundus, and 3) cervix.

- The cervix exits into the vagina, a muscular, thin-walled chamber that acts as the birth canal.

- There are four structures that make up the external female genitalia: 1) monis pubis, 2) labia, 3) vestibule, and 4) clitoris.

- *Oogenesis* involves the processes of egg maturation through meiosis I and meiosis II.

- The *female reproductive cycle* involves the integration of the ovarian and uterine cycles. There are two phases of the ovarian cycle: 1) follicular phase and 2) luteal phase. There are three phases of the uterine (menstrual) cycle: 1) menstrual, 2) proliferation, and 3) secretory.

- The main structures of the male reproductive system are 1) testes, 2) spermatic cord, 3) scrotum, 4) glands, and 5) ducts.

- *Spermatogenesis* is the production of mature sperm in the seminiferous tubules. There are three regions in a mature sperm: 1) head, 2) midpiece, and 3) tail.

- Interactions between the hypothalamus, anterior pituitary gland, and testes help to regulate male sex hormones (testosterone).

- The *penis*, composed of spongy connective tissue, is the external male genitalia.

PART V
CHEMICAL PROCESSES

General Chemistry

OVERVIEW

- **Matter**
- **Atomic Theory**
- **Detailed Atomic Structure**
- **The Periodic Table of Elements**
- **Ions, Molecules, and Compounds**
- **Chemical Bonding**
- **Chemical Equations and Reactions**
- **Gases**
- **Solids and Liquids**
- **Solutions**
- **Acid-Base Reactions**
- **Redox Reactions and Electrochemistry**
- **Thermochemistry**
- **Chemical Kinetics and Equilibrium**
- **Practice Questions**
- **Answer Key and Explanations**
- **Summing It Up**

The field of chemistry involves the study of matter and the changes it undergoes. A basic knowledge of chemistry is essential for understanding the physical world and other disciplines of science, including biology, physics, geology, and ecology. In addition, chemists in the pharmaceutical industry are researching and developing drugs that will have few or no side effects to treat cancer, viruses, diabetes, and many other diseases and illnesses.

MATTER

Matter is defined as anything that occupies space and has mass. Matter is made up of smaller units called *molecules*. Molecules are comprised of even smaller units of matter called *atoms*. Atoms are distinct elements that cannot be broken down into a more simple form.

The primary focus of chemistry is to understand the behavior of atoms and molecules. A *substance* is a form of matter that has distinct properties and a composition that is constant. All chemical substances can be described in terms of their physical and chemical properties.

- **Physical properties:** Physical properties of matter are those that can be determined by observation without changing the composition or identity of the substance. Examples of physical properties are color, taste, density, boiling point, melting point, and solubility.

- **Chemical properties:** Chemical properties of a substance are those observed when a chemical change of the substance takes place. For example, the property of hydrogen gas burning in the presence of oxygen to form water is a chemical property of hydrogen. Flammability, the heat of combustion, and the ionization energy of an element are all examples of chemical properties.

Changes in a chemical substance can also be either physical or chemical. Physical changes do not alter the chemical composition of a substance. For example, when water freezes, it still remains the chemical H_2O, so freezing produces a physical change. Chemical changes are those that alter the composition of a substance. For example, when iron rusts, the resulting iron oxide is a different chemical substance than the original iron.

States of Matter

Chemical substances can exist in one of four states, or phases, of matter, depending on the temperature and pressure of the substance.

1. **Solid:** In a solid, the molecules are held together closely in an orderly fashion. The electron interactions between neighboring atoms or molecules (intermolecular forces) keep matter in a fixed shape and volume.

2. **Liquid:** The molecules in a liquid are held close together, but are not held as rigidly as in a solid. Molecules in a liquid can move past one another, which gives liquids the property of *fluidity*. Intermolecular forces keep matter in a fixed volume, but allow liquids to take the shape of their container.

3. **Gas:** In a gas, the molecules are separated by a larger distance than in a solid or liquid, and intermolecular forces have a limited effect. A substance in the gaseous state will expand to fill its container.

4. **Plasma:** Plasma is formed when gases are exposed to very high temperature. The high temperature causes gases to ionize. This fourth state of matter is not common under normal conditions on Earth.

The four states of matter are interchangeable within a substance, without changing the chemical composition of the substance. The inverse effects of temperature and pressure on a substance and its state are depicted in a phase diagram.

Figure 1. Phase Diagram

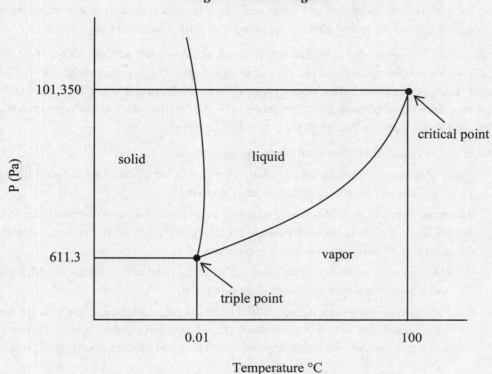

There is a unique point on the graph which is the exact temperature and pressure at which all three phases, or states, can exist simultaneously. This is called the *triple point*. Upon heating a solid, it will melt into a liquid. The temperature at which this occurs is called the *melting temperature* (also called the *freezing temperature*). Further heating of the liquid substance will cause a phase change from a liquid to a gas. The temperature at which this phase change occurs is called the *boiling point*. Lowering the temperature of a gas will cause it to condense back into a liquid, and further lowering of the temperature will convert the liquid back into a sold.

Classification of Matter

An *element* is defined as a substance that cannot be broken down into another form by chemical means. Atoms are the basic units of all elements that can enter into a chemical combination. A *molecule* is an aggregate of at least two atoms in a definite arrangement. A *compound* is formed from the combination of two or more elements in a fixed proportion.

There are several laws that were proposed by early chemists to define matter.

- **Law of conservation of mass:** The law of conservation of mass states that matter cannot be created or destroyed. Therefore, the mass of all matter on Earth remains constant, even if it changes state or chemical composition.

- **Law of definite proportions:** The law of definite proportions states that different samples of the same compound always contain its same constituent elements in the same mass proportion.
- **Law of multiple proportions:** The law of multiple proportions states that if two elements combine to form more than one compound, the mass of one element that combines with a fixed mass of the second element are in ratios of small whole numbers.

A combination of different substances that vary in composition is called a *mixture*. These types of physical (nonchemical) mixtures can be heterogeneous or homogeneous. In *heterogeneous mixtures*, the individual components of the mixture remain physically separate (sand and salt mixed together). In a *homogeneous mixture*, the composition of the mixture is such that the combined substances become indistinguishable from one another (e.g., sugar dissolved in water).

Substances can be classified as either pure substances or mixtures.

- **Pure substances:** Pure substances include elements (a list of elements is found in the Periodic Table of Elements), molecules, and compounds.
- **Mixtures:** Mixtures are combinations of two or more pure substances that physically mix, but one does not alter the chemical bonds of the other, nor do they interact with one another. Mixtures may be homogeneous or heterogeneous:
  - Homogeneous mixtures include solutions, *alloys* (e.g., a mixture of metals such as steel), and *amalgams* (alloy of mercury and another metal).
  - Heterogeneous mixtures include *colloids* (particles are small enough not to settle, but large enough not to dissolve), *emulsions* (liquid-liquid mixtures), *dispersions* (visually heterogeneous), and *suspension* (large solid particles in a liquid; particles eventually settle).

ATOMIC THEORY

In 1803, John Dalton formulated the atomic theory that gives a precise definition of the indivisible building blocks of all matter, that is, atoms. The basic atomic theory can be summarized as follows:

1. Elements are composed of very small particles called atoms.
2. All atoms of any given element are identical in size and chemical properties. They can differ slightly in their mass due to variations in the number of neutrons in their nucleus, which will be discussed later.
3. Compounds are composed of atoms of more than one type of element. The ratio of the numbers of atoms of each element is a small whole number, or a simple fraction.
4. A *chemical reaction* involves the separation, combination, or rearrangement of atoms. Atoms are not created or destroyed in a chemical reaction.

The Structure of an Atom

An atom is defined as the basic unit of an element that can be chemically combined with like or different elements. However, atoms actually possess an internal structure of even smaller particles. These particles—protons, neutrons, and electrons—are called *subatomic particles*.

Protons

A *proton* is a positively charged subatomic particle that is found in the nucleus of an atom. The nucleus is the dense central core of an atom. Each proton in an atom carries a +1 charge, and the total charge of the protons in the atom is equal and opposite to the total charge of electrons in an atom; therefore, an atom has a neutral charge. Even though the proton has an equal and opposite charge from that of an electron, a proton has a mass about 1840 times larger than the mass of an electron. An element's *atomic number*, Z, is defined as the number of protons the element has. The number of protons in an atom does not vary.

Neutrons

Neutrons are electronically neutral subatomic particles that have a mass slightly larger than that of a proton. Neutrons are also found in the nucleus of the atom. It is the mass of the protons and neutrons that gives the nucleus its dense quality. The number of neutrons in an atom can vary, which gives rise to various isotopes of an element.

Electrons

The negatively charged particles of an atom are called *electrons*. Electrons have an exceedingly small mass (about 1840 times less than that of a proton or neutron). Electrons surround the nucleus of an atom and are arranged in different orbits around the nucleus. These orbits have different energy levels, and the closer an electron is to the nucleus, the higher its energy level. Electrons can be added or removed from an atom in a process called *ionization*. Ionization leads to an overall positive (loss of electrons) or negative (gain of electrons) charge of the atom.

Atomic Number, Mass Number, and Atomic Mass

All atoms can be characterized and identified by the number of protons and neutrons they contain. The atomic number Z refers to the number of protons in the nucleus of a given atom. In a neutral atom, the number of protons is equal to the number of electrons so that the atomic number is also an indicator of the number of electrons in the atom.

The *mass number A* is the total number of neutrons and protons present in the nucleus of an atom of a given element. The mass number is generally given by the formula:

$$A = Z + \text{number of neutrons}$$

Thus, the number of neutrons in an atom is equal to the difference between the mass number and the atomic number.

Atoms of a given element do not always have the same mass. Most elements have two or more isotope forms. *Isotopes* are atoms that have the same atomic number (number of protons), but different mass numbers (different number of neutrons). An element can be written in the form $_{Z}^{A}X$, where X is any element, A is the mass number, and Z is the atomic number. Since the atomic number is the same for all isotopes of the same element, an isotope form of an element can be written as ^AX. For example, there are three isotopes for the element hydrogen:

1. Hydrogen, H, has one proton and no neutrons, ^1H.

2. The isotope deuterium contains one proton and one neutron and is represented by the symbol ^2H.

3. The isotope tritium has one proton and two neutrons, and is written as the symbol, ^3H.

Chemical properties of an element can be determined by the protons and electrons in the atom. Neutrons are not involved in chemical interactions between atoms. Therefore, different isotopes of the same element have similar chemical properties.

Atomic mass M is defined as the mass of an atom relative to the mass of one carbon-12 atom (^{12}C). An atomic mass unit, *amu*, is a mass exactly equal to one twelfth the mass of one ^{12}C atom. The mass of an individual atom depends on the number of electrons, protons, and neutrons it contains. Since atoms are so small and the mass of a single atom cannot be measured, the atomic mass of one atom is measured relative to another (^{12}C). Setting the mass of ^{12}C at a value of 12 amu provides a standard of measuring the atomic mass of other elements.

Atomic mass is a physical constant for a given atom. However, a sample of a naturally occurring element generally has a mixture of isotopes. The average atomic mass of an element is defined as the sum of the percentage of each isotope times its atomic mass. For example, the average atomic mass of natural carbon is:

Average Atomic Mass = (0.989)(12.00000 amu) + (0.011)(13.00335 amu) = 12.01 amu

where 98.90 percent of natural carbon is ^{12}C and 1.10 percent of natural carbon is ^{13}C, and the atomic mass of ^{12}C is 12.00000 amu and the atomic mass of ^{13}C is 13.00335 amu.

The International Union of Pure and Applied Chemistry (IIPAC) has published average atomic masses of each element, and the accepted average, or relative, atomic mass for each element is listed in the Periodic Table of Elements.

Avogadro's Number and Molar Mass

Atomic mass units are able to provide a relative scale for the mass of an element, but atoms have such small masses that it is nearly impossible to weigh them. In chemistry, macroscopic qualities of elements are used, and, therefore, it is convenient to have a special unit to help define these very large numbers of atoms. The special unit defined in terms of standard international (SI) units is the *mole*. A mole is the amount of a substance that contains as many atoms (or molecules, or particles) as there are atoms in exactly 12 grams (g) of ^{12}C. The actual number of atoms in 12 g of ^{12}C has been determined experimentally, and this value is known as *Avogadro's number* (N_A). The accepted value for Avogadro's number is $N_A = 6.0221367 \times 10^{23}$.

This number is generally rounded to the thousandth and is given as 6.022×10^{23}. Thus, one mole of any particular element contains 6.022×10^{23} atoms.

The molar mass (M) of a particular element is defined at the mass (in grams or kilograms) of one mole of atoms. In general, the molar mass (in grams) of an element is numerically equal to its atomic mass (in amu). For example, the molar mass of ^{12}C is 12 g. The molar mass of sodium is 22.99 g, and its atomic mass is 22.99 amu. By knowing the molar mass and Avogadro's number, the mass of a single atom of a given element can be calculated.

Molecular Mass

In a given molecule, if the atomic masses of each type of atom are known, it is possible to calculate the mass of the entire molecule. The *molecular mass* (also called the molecular weight) is the sum of all the atomic masses (or molar masses) in a molecule. Thus, the molecular mass can be calculated by multiplying the atomic mass of each element by the number of atoms of that element present in each molecule and adding all the values for each specific element. For example, the molecular mass of water, H_2O, is:

$$2(\text{atomic mass of H}) + \text{atomic mass of O}$$

$$\text{Molecular Mass of } H_2O = 2(1.008 \text{ amu}) + 16.000 \text{ amu} = 18.02 \text{ amu}$$

DETAILED ATOMIC STRUCTURE

Early physicists assumed that molecules behaved like rebounding balls. This model allowed them to understand some macroscopic phenomenon such as pressure exerted by a gas, but it did not explain the forces that hold atoms together. Physicists took a long time to realize that the physical laws that govern larger objects do not apply to atoms. The quantum theory developed in the 1900s by Max Planck explained the electronic structure of atoms.

Properties of Waves

In order to understand Planck's quantum theory, it is necessary to understand the nature of waves. A *wave* is any form of vibrating disturbance by which energy is transmitted. Waves are characterized by their height and length and by the number of waves that pass through a fixed point in one second. The *wavelength*, λ, is defined as the distance between identical points of successive waves (for example, the distance from the peak of one wave to the peak of the next wave) and is measured in units of meters, centimeters, or nanometers. The *wave frequency*, ν, is defined as the number of waves that pass through a particular point in one second, and is measured in hertz (Hz). The *amplitude* of a wave is defined as the vertical distance from the middle of a wave to its peak (highest point) or trough (lowest point).

Wave speed is another important property that depends on the nature of the wave and the medium through which it moves. The speed of a wave, u, is calculated by multiplying the wavelength by the wave frequency $u = \lambda\nu$.

NOTE

You may find some questions involving the molecular weight of some of the more common elements (O, H, etc.), so it is a good idea to be familiar with those values.

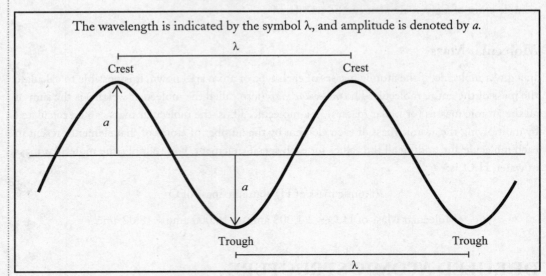

Figure 2. Wavelength and Amplitude

The wavelength is indicated by the symbol λ, and amplitude is denoted by *a*.

Electromagnetic Radiation

James Clerk Maxwell determined that visible light, ultraviolet (UV) light, and infrared (IR) light were all composed of electromagnetic (EM) waves of differing frequencies. All these different types of electromagnetic waves travel at the speed of light, which is a constant value. The wave theory of electromagnetic radiation relates the transverse wave velocity to the frequency. In a vacuum, this value is a constant known as the speed of light, *c*. The value of *c* is 2.998×10^8 m/sec, or 3×10^8 m/sec. In other media, light waves may travel more slowly, but their frequency remains the same. Thus, it is the medium that determines the extent to which radiation is slowed.

An electromagnetic wave has both an electric field component and a magnetic component. These two components of the EM wave have the same frequency and wavelength, but they travel in perpendicular planes to one another. *Electromagnetic radiation* is the emission and transmission of energy in the form of electromagnetic waves.

Planck's Quantum Theory

Classic physics assumed that atoms and molecules could emit or absorb an arbitrary amount of radiation. Planck studied the radiation emitted from heated objects and found that the frequency of the wave oscillation from these particles was not continuous. Instead, Planck found that atoms and molecules could only emit or absorb energy in discrete quantities, or bundles. Planck gave the name *quantum* to the smallest quantity of energy that can be emitted or absorbed in the form of electromagnetic radiation. The energy, *E*, of a single quantum is given by the equation:

$$E = h\nu$$

where *h* is Planck's constant and ν is the wave frequency of radiation. Planck's constant has a value of 6.63×10^{-34} J·s. Since the frequency can also be expressed in terms of wavelength using the equation $\nu = \dfrac{c}{\lambda}$, the energy of a single quantum can also be determined by the equation known as the Planck-Einstein equation:

$$E = h\,\frac{c}{\lambda}$$

Photoelectric Effect

In 1905, Albert Einstein used Planck's quantum theory to explain another problem in physics: the photoelectric effect. The *photoelectric effect* is a phenomenon in which electrons are ejected from the surface of certain materials as they are exposed to light of a given minimum frequency (threshold frequency). The number of electrons ejected from a material is proportional to the intensity of the light, but the energy of the electrons was not proportional to the intensity of the light. Einstein suggested that the beam of light shining on the material is actually a stream of particles called *photons*. Einstein deduced that each photon contains a *quanta* of energy expressed by the equation $E = h\nu$, where ν is the frequency of light.

Atomic Emission and Absorption Spectra

During the mid-1800s, studies were conducted to investigate the emission and absorptions of the visible light spectrum. Through these studies, three laws of spectroscopy were developed.

1. A continuous spectrum is produced by a hot solid object or a hot dense gas.

2. Spectral lines at discrete wavelengths are produced by hot, low-density gases. These discrete wavelengths are dependent on the energy levels of the atoms in the gas. This is called the *atomic emission spectra* and is a line spectra of radiation emitted by substances. The line spectra are light emissions at specific wavelengths.

3. A hot solid object that is viewed through a cool, low-density gas produces light with a continuous spectrum that has gaps at discrete wavelengths depending on the energy level of the atoms in the gas. This is called the *atomic absorption spectra*.

Hydrogen gas has been shown to emit a series of four distinct visible spectra emission lines. These lines are called the *Balmer series* of lines. The Balmer series was used to expand the idea of emission spectra lines to other atoms, in particular, alkaline metals. This work was done by Johannes Rydberg who used the inverse wavelength $1/\lambda$ and an empirical constant called the *Rydberg constant*, R, to develop the Rydberg formula to predict emission line spectra for other atoms. The Rydberg constant has the value $2.18 \times 10^{-18,}$ and the Rydberg formula is expressed as follows:

$$1/\lambda = R\,\frac{1}{n_f^2} - \frac{1}{n_i^2}$$

The Bohr Model

Niels Bohr's model of the atom included the idea of electrons moving in orbits around the nucleus of the atom. Bohr applied Planck's quantum theory to classical mechanics. Bohr theorized that an electron could orbit a nucleus without emitting radiation or losing energy, but the orbit would be limited to integral or quantized levels. These integrals are multiples of $h/2\varpi$, where h is Planck's constant. The quantized angular momentum of an electron can be calculated by the equation:

$$L = m_e v_n r_n = n\frac{h}{2\pi} = n\hbar$$

Where $n = 1, 2, 3, \ldots$ and is called the principle quantum number. When $n = 1$ this minimum radius is also called the *Bohr radius*. The constant $h/2\varpi$ can also be written as $\hbar$ ("h-bar") and is called the *reduced Planck constant*.

In Bohr's model, the energy of the electron orbitals is derived from photon energies given by the Planck-Einstein equation. Assuming that electrons release energy in the form of photons when they move from a higher energy orbital to a lower energy orbital, the following equation can be derived:

$$E_{photon} = \Delta E_{atom} = E_{initial} - E_{final} = hc\frac{1}{\lambda}$$

The photon energy released when an electron moves from a higher energy orbital (n_i) to a lower energy orbital (n_f) can be determined by substituting the Rydberg formula into the above equation.

$$E_{initial} - E_{final} = hcR_H\left[\frac{1}{n_f^2} - \frac{1}{n_i^2}\right] = -hcR_H\left[\frac{1}{n_f^2} - \frac{1}{n_i^2}\right]$$

By using the Rydberg constant for hydrogen (R_H in units of m^{-1}), the Planck constant (6.63×10^{-34} J·s), and the speed of light (2.998×10^8 m/sec), Bohr calculated hcR_H to be 2.179×10^{-18} J·s. Thus, Bohr was able to express the energy level of an electron orbital as follows:

$$E_n = -2.179 \times 10^{-18}\,\text{J}\,\frac{1}{n^2}$$

Therefore, when an electron moves from a higher energy orbital to a lower energy orbital, the energy drop within the atom equals the energy of an emitted photon. Photon emissions are *exothermic* in nature; ΔE for the atom is negative and the photon energy is positive. Absorptions are thus *endothermic*; ΔE for the atom is positive and is equal to the energy of the absorbed photon.

The negative sign in the above equation indicates that the energy of an electron in an atom is lower than the energy of a free electron, which is infinitely far from a nucleus. Thus, the energy of an electron in an orbital increases as the orbital increases in distance from the atomic nucleus. A free electron is arbitrarily assigned an energy value of zero. The most negative energy value is reached in the $n = 1$ orbital. This corresponds to the most stable energy state and is called the *ground state*, or ground level. The ground state refers to the lowest energy state of a system. The stability of an electron decreases as the value of n increases. Each of these levels ($n = 2, 3, 4\ldots$) is called an *excited state*, or excited level. Each of these levels is higher in energy level than the ground state.

Bohr's theory enables the explanation of the observed emission line spectra for a hydrogen atom. Radiant energy absorbed by the atom causes it to move from a lower energy state (lower n-value) to a higher energy state (higher n-value). In addition, radiant energy in the form of a photon is emitted when the electron moves from a higher energy state to a lower energy state. The amount of energy involved in the movement of the electron to either a higher or lower energy orbital is determined by the distance between the initial and final orbitals.

Figure 3. Bohr Atomic Model

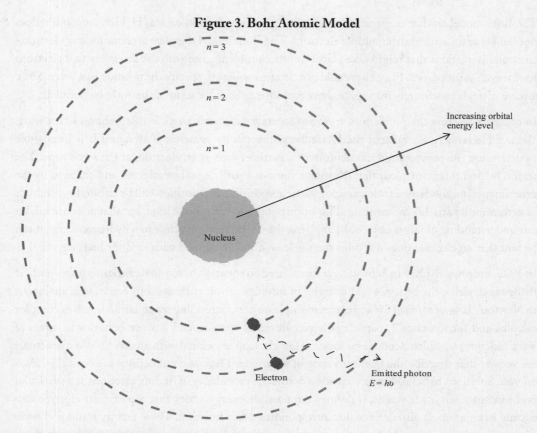

The Quantum Mechanics Atom Model

Physicists were puzzled by Bohr's theory, however. They questioned why the energies of a hydrogen electron would be quantized. For about a decade, no one could provide a reasonable explanation as to why an electron was restricted to orbiting the nucleus at fixed distances. It was Louis de Broglie who provided an explanation to this puzzling question. He reasoned that if light waves can behave like a stream of particles (photons), then perhaps particles such as electrons can behave as waves. De Broglie reasoned that an electron bound to a nucleus behaves as a standing wave (it does not travel in any direction). A standing wave possesses nodes at which there is no motion at all (the amplitude is zero at each node). If an electron bound to the nucleus behaves like a standing wave, the length of the wave must exactly fit the orbital circumference. Otherwise, it would partially cancel itself out on each orbit and eventually be reduced to zero.

De Broglie concluded that waves can behave like particles, and particles can behave like waves. Particle and wave properties can be related by the expression:

$$\lambda = \frac{h}{mu}$$

where the wavelength, λ, is related to Planck's constant (h); the mass, m, of the particle (electron); and its velocity, u. Note that the left side of the equation involves the wave property of wavelength, and the right side of the equation deals with properties attributed to particles such as mass and velocity (speed).

The Bohr model holds true for an atom containing a single electron such as H, He^+, Li^{2+}, but it does not hold true for atoms with multiple electrons. The Bohr model does not account for any electron-electron interactions that might take place. Another problem arose with the discovery that electrons have wavelike properties. Physicists could not determine how to specify the position of a wave. Since a wave extends indefinitely into space, how could the precise location of the wave be defined?

In order to describe the problem of trying to locate a subatomic particle that behaves like a wave, Werner Heisenberg formulated the Heisenberg uncertainty principle that states: It is impossible to determine the position and momentum of a particle, such as an electron, at the same time. The reason behind this principle is that the momentum of a particle will be affected and changed by the experimental methods used to determine a particle's position, and position will be affected by methods to determine a particle's momentum. This uncertainty is on an atomic level, but that does not hinder our understanding of larger objects. In applying the uncertainty principle to a hydrogen atom, it can be said that an electron does not orbit the nucleus in a well-defined path as Bohr had suggested.

In 1926, the physicist Erwin Schrödinger formulated an equation based on de Broglie's wave-particle theory to describe the behavior and energies of submicroscopic particles. His equation is analogous to Newton's laws of motion for larger macroscopic objects. Schrödinger's equation involves complex calculus and incorporates 1. particle behavior in terms of mass, and 2. wave behavior in terms of wave function, ψ, which depends on location (an electron associated with an atom). Wave functions are vectors that describe the quantum state of a particle. These wave functions are typically called *orbitals*. Solutions to Schrödinger's equation define the probability of finding electrons at a particular point in space. In other words, it defines the possible energy states that a particular electron can occupy in an atom. It also defines the corresponding wave function. These energy states and wave functions are characterized by a set of quantum numbers. Even though quantum mechanics states that the location of an electron in an atom cannot be pinpointed exactly, a particular region of the atom that the electron may occupy at any given time can be defined. The probability that an electron will be found in a particular region of the atom is described as *electron density*. The electron density in an atom is defined by the square of the wave function and is a three-dimensional space around the nucleus (an orbital). Orbitals with a high probability of containing an electron have a high electron density. Each atomic orbital has a characteristic energy and a characteristic electron density.

Heisenberg, Max Born, and Pascual Jordan formulated the basics of quantum mechanics, and their ideas helped to explain the behavior of multiple-electron atoms. The quantum mechanics model maintains that electrons move in orbitals of defined space, but that these orbitals are not necessarily circular. Within these orbitals, position and momentum, as described by classical physics, are not clearly defined.

Quantum Numbers

In quantum mechanics there are four quantum numbers that describe the distribution of electrons in an atom. These quantum numbers are all derived from the Schrödinger equation:

1. **Principle quantum number:** The principle quantum number, n, is an integer (1, 2, 3, . . .) whose value determines the energy level of the orbital. The principle quantum number also relates the average distance of the electron from the nucleus in a particular orbital. The larger the value of n, the greater the distance the orbital is from the nucleus of the atom.

2. **Angular momentum quantum number:** The angular momentum, ℓ, indicates the shape of the orbital. The values of ℓ depend on the value of the principle quantum number. For a given value of n, ℓ has possible values from 0 to $n-1$. Therefore, if $n = 1$ the only possible value of ℓ is 0. The value of ℓ is designated by the letters $s, p, d, f, \ldots$ These letters are representative of the description of the orbit. The value s is for sharp, p for principle, d for diffuse, f for fundamental. After the letter f, the orbitals are named alphabetically ($g, h, i, \ldots$). A collection of orbitals with the same n value is typically called an *electron shell*. A collection of one or more orbitals with the same n and ℓ values is called a *subshell*.

3. **Magnetic quantum number:** The magnetic quantum number, m_ℓ, describes the orientation of the electron orbital in space. For each value of ℓ, there are $(2\ell + 1)$ integral values of m_ℓ in a subshell. For example, if $\ell = 1$, then there are $[(2 \times 1) + 1]$, or three values of m_ℓ. These values are $-1, 0$, and 1. The number of m_ℓ values indicates the number of orbitals in a subshell of a particular ℓ value.

4. **Electron spin quantum number:** The electron spin quantum number, m_s, takes into account that there are two possible spinning motions (rotations) of an electron, clockwise or counterclockwise. Thus, m_s has a value of either $+1/2$ or $-1/2$. The Pauli exclusion principle and Hund's rule address restrictions on electron spin when filling orbitals. As another example, consider the situation in which $n = 2$ and $\ell = 1$. These values would indicate a $2p$ subshell with three orbitals (three values of m_ℓ: $-1, 0, 1$). The spin number of the electron can be either $+1/2$ or $-1/2$.

Atomic Orbitals

The three orbitals s, p, and d have distinct characteristics. Although it is difficult to determine the exact shape of an orbital because the wave function that characterizes the orbital extends from the nucleus to infinity, these orbitals are assigned the following three approximate shapes to help in the understanding and nature of chemical bonding:

1. *s* **orbitals:** The $1s$ orbital is represented as a sphere surrounding the nucleus of an atom. All s orbitals are spherical in shape, but differ in size. The size of the sphere increases as the principle quantum number increases. This spherical shape is represented in a boundary surface diagram which approximates the electron density of each orbital.

2. *p* **orbitals:** The smallest possible principle number for any p orbital is 2 (if $n = 1$, then there is only a $1s$ orbital). If $n = 2$ there are three p orbitals called $2p_x$, $2p_y$, and $2p_z$. The subscript indicates the axis along which the p orbital lies. The three p orbitals are identical in size, shape, and energy, and they differ only in there orientation. Boundary surface diagrams indicate that the shape of the p orbitals is that of two lobes on opposite sides of the nucleus. This gives the p orbitals a "dumbbell" shape. As in the case of s orbitals, p orbitals increase in size with increasing values of n.

3. *d* **orbitals:** d orbitals and other higher energy orbitals correspond to an ℓ value of at least 2. If $\ell = 2$, then there are five values of m_ℓ. The lowest value of n for a d orbital is three. There are five possible d orbitals ($-2, -1, 0, 1, 2$), which are labeled $3d_{xy}, 3d_{yz}, 3d_{xz}, 3d_{x^2y^2}, 3d_{z^2}$

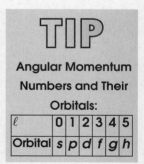

TIP

Angular Momentum Numbers and Their Orbitals:

ℓ	0	1	2	3	4	5
Orbital	s	p	d	f	g	h

Figure 4. Atomic Electron Orbitals Showing the Directional Characteristics of *s*, *p*, and *d* Orbitals

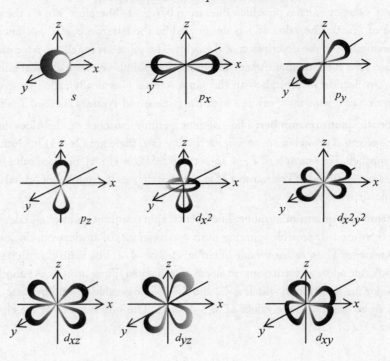

The energy level of each atomic orbital will reflect the way in which the electrons are arranged in the atom. The energies of the orbitals in the hydrogen atom (single electron) increase as follows:

$$1s < 2s = 2p < 3s = 3p = 3d < 4s = 4p = 4d = 4f < \ldots$$

The energy levels for many-electron atoms are more complex. The energy of an electron in this type of atom is dependent upon the angular momentum quantum number as well as the principle quantum number. For electrons with many atoms, the 3*d* energy level is very close to the 4*s* energy level. The total energy of the atom depends on the sum of the orbital energies and the repulsive forces between the electrons in these orbitals. Each orbital can only hold two electrons.

Figure 5. Orbital Electron Levels of an Atom with Many Electrons

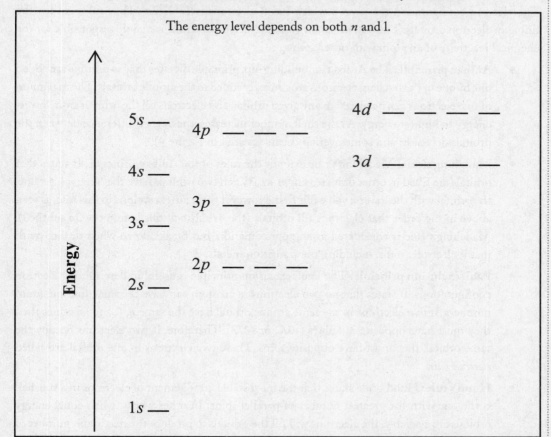

The energy level depends on both n and l.

Electron Configuration and Orbital Filling

The four quantum numbers allow for the labeling of every electron in every orbital of an atom. This labeling identifies the location of the atom. The four quantum numbers are listed in the order (n, ℓ, m_ℓ, m_s). For example, the four quantum numbers for the $2s$ orbital are (2, 0, 0, +1/2) or (2, 0, 0, –1/2). The value of m_s determines how the electron is arranged in an orbital, but not the size, shape, or energy of the orbital.

The rules of electron configuration state that electrons are added to the allowable orbitals for each atom starting with the lowest energy level, and increasing in energy levels until all the electrons occupy an orbital. Electrons fill the orbitals in the following order:

$$1s \rightarrow 2s \rightarrow 2p \rightarrow 3s \rightarrow 3p \rightarrow 4s \rightarrow 3d \rightarrow 4p \rightarrow 5s \rightarrow 4d \rightarrow 5p \rightarrow 6s \rightarrow 4f \rightarrow 5d \rightarrow 6p \rightarrow 7s \rightarrow 5f \rightarrow 6d \rightarrow 7p$$

The electron configuration of an atom is the details of how electrons are distributed among the many atomic orbitals. Knowing the electron configuration helps to understand the electronic behavior of the atom. For example, the single electron in the hydrogen atom occupies the $1s$ orbital. The electron configuration of hydrogen is $1s^1$, where 1 represents the principle quantum number, s represents the angular momentum, and the superscript 1 denotes the number of electrons in the orbital or subshell. The electron configuration for oxygen which has 8 electrons is $1s^2 2s^2 2p^4$. Four rules govern the filling of electron orbitals. The outermost, or valance, shell of electrons is mainly responsible for the chemical reactivity of an atom with other atoms.

- **Aufbau principle:** The Aufbau, or building-up, principle dictates that as protons are added one by one to the nucleus, electrons are similarly added to the atomic orbitals. The maximum of two electrons can be placed in any given orbital, and electrons fill the orbitals from lowest energy to highest energy. As the shell number increases, the energy difference between the orbitals decreases and some overlap occurs (as seen in Figure 4).

- **Madelung's rule:** Madelung's rule extends the rules of the Aufbau principle. It states that orbitals are filled in order of increasing $n + \ell$. When two orbitals have the same $n + \ell$ value, the orbital with the lower n value fills first. However there are exceptions to this rule, as seen above in the order that electrons fill orbitals (the $4s$ subshell fills before the $3d$ subshell). Madelung's rule is considered as an approximation, but breaks down when dealing with many-electron atoms, including the transition metals.

- **Pauli exclusion principle:** The Pauli exclusion principle is useful in determining electron configurations. It states that no two electrons in an atom can have the same four quantum numbers. If two electrons in the same atomic orbital have the same n, ℓ, and m_ℓ values then they must have opposite m_s values (+1/2 or –1/2). Therefore, if two electrons occupy the same orbital, they must have opposite spins. These two electrons in one orbital are called *electron pairs*.

- **Hund's rule:** Hund's rule states that the most stable arrangement of electrons in a subshell is the one with the greatest number of parallel spins. In other words, when equal energy orbitals are available, the electrons will fill the orbitals to produce the maximum number of half-filled orbitals with parallel spins (same m_s value). For example, in the p subshell, one electron will fill each of the p_x, p_y, and p_z orbitals with electrons of the same spin number, and the fourth electron will pair with the electron in the p_x orbital.

The Pauli exclusion principle and Hund's rule can be confirmed by the concepts of paramagnetism and diamagnetism. If two electrons in one orbital had the same or parallel spins, they would exhibit *paramagnetism*. Paramagnetic substances are those that contain net unpaired spins and are attracted by a magnet. Conversely, if electron spins are paired or antiparallel to each other in an orbit, they do not contain net unpaired spins and are slightly repelled by a magnet. Measurements of magnetic properties of atoms indicate that helium atoms that have two electrons do not have a magnetic field. This means that the atom is *diamagnetic*, and the electrons are paired in an antiparallel fashion.

THE PERIODIC TABLE OF ELEMENTS

Recurring patterns in the elements were observed by the Russian chemist Dmitri Mendeleev. He also noted that these patterns in their properties corresponded to their atomic weight. Mendeleev created the first known Periodic Table of Elements in 1869. Later, in 1913, Henry Moseley found a correlation between the frequency of X-rays generated by hitting an atom with high-energy electrons and the atomic number. Moseley also found that in general the atomic number increases in

TIP

For the Chemical Processes subtest, a periodic table including each element's symbol, atomic mass, and atomic number will be available by clicking on "Periodic Table" in the lower left corner of each item the same order as the atomic mass. For example, sodium is the 11th element in order of increasing atomic mass, and it has an atomic number of 11.

The Periodic Table of Elements derived by both Mendeleev and Moseley followed the same periodic law. The *periodic law* states that the chemical and physical properties of elements tend to follow certain trends when arranged and ordered by their atomic numbers. By 2011, the Periodic Table of Elements listed 118 elements, whereas Mendeleev's table listed only 66 known elements. Only 94 of the elements in the current table occur naturally on Earth, and only 80 elements have stable isotopes. The elements with atomic numbers 43, 61, and all those with atomic numbers 84 and greater do not have stable isotopes. The Periodic Table lists each element with its name, symbol, atomic number, and the average atomic mass.

Figure 6. The Hydrogen Atom as Represented in the Periodic Table of Elements

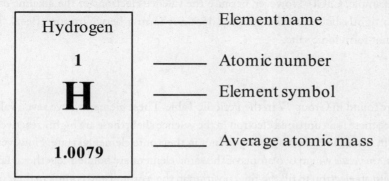

The Periodic Table provides a summary of chemical information for each element. The 18 columns of the table are called *groups*, and the seven rows are called *periods*. Elements can also be categorized based on their electron subshells.

Groups

The columns of the Periodic Table are numbered 1 through 18. All elements in each group (column) have the same valence (outer) electron configuration that plays a large role in determining the chemical reactivity of each element or group of elements. The main group elements have only *s* and *p* orbitals; the transition elements have *d* orbitals.

Hydrogen

Hydrogen is found at the top of group 1, but it does not follow the same trend as the rest of the group. Hydrogen exists in nature as a gas and has more in common with the noble gases in group 18 than the alkali metals in group 1. Hydrogen has only a single electron and readily loses this electron to become a hydrogen ion, H^+.

Alkali Metals

The rest of the first column of elements is considered Group 1, and these elements are called alkali metals. They all have one valence electron in an *s* orbital. This single valence electron can be easily removed, which makes alkali metals highly reactive elements. In fact, these metals are so highly reactive that they are never found in their pure elemental state. They can react with water to produce hydrogen gas and the corresponding metal hydroxide. Alkali metals also react with oxygen gas in the air to form metal oxides, or peroxides. Alkali metals react with halogens to form salts, for example, sodium chloride, NaCl. All alkali metals have low melting points and low densities, which makes them soft malleable metals.

Alkaline Earth Metals

The alkaline earth metals form Group 2 on the Periodic table. They all have two valence electrons in an s orbital. Because there is an electron pair filling the s orbital, these elements are much less reactive than alkali metals. Unlike alkali metals, alkaline earth metals have a high melting point. When these elements lose the outer two valence electrons, they can react with halogens to form ionic salts, for example, $CaCl_2$. However, because the valence electrons of the alkaline earth metal beryllium are so tightly bound to the atom, it does not form a beryllium ion (Be^{2+}). Therefore, beryllium does not form ionic salts.

Halogens

The halogens are found in Group 17 in the Periodic Table. These elements have seven valence electrons (s^2p^5). Since there is an unpaired electron in the valence shell, these are highly reactive elements. They are found in nature as compounds or ions, not in their pure elemental state. However, they can exist as a *diatomic molecule* where two atoms of the same element are bonded together. Halogens are able to readily gain an electron to fill the final position in the p orbital and complete their outer shell, making it s^2p^6. Fluorine, a halogen element, is the most electronegative (ready to receive an electron) and most chemically reactive of all the elements of the Periodic Table. Within the halogen group, there are elements that occur naturally as a solid, some that occur as a gas, and others that occur as a liquid. For example, fluorine and chlorine exist naturally as gases, bromine as a liquid, and iodine and astatine as solids. Astatine is the rarest naturally occurring element in the Table.

Noble Gases

The elements in Group 18 are called the noble gases. All these elements have a full outer electron shell (s^2 for helium and s^2p^6 for all the other noble gases). Since their outer shell is completely filled, noble gases have a low chemical reactivity. For the most part, they are unreactive. These gases have been called *inert gases*, and there are very few compounds with noble gases. All noble gases are colorless, odorless, tasteless, and nonflammable under standard conditions.

Transition Elements

The elements in Groups 3 through 12 make up what are known as the transition elements. These elements are also called *transition metals* and are very hard, but malleable elements. These elements all have valence electrons in the d orbitals. The five d orbitals hold their electrons very loosely, and most of these elements are characterized by high melting points, high electrical conductivity, low ionization energies, and many oxidation states. These elements are capable of forming ions in water. They are often brightly colored elements due to electron transitions in the d orbitals.

Periods

The period numbers in the Periodic Table correspond to the principle quantum number of the element. Progression across each row on the Periodic Table corresponds to the filling of a given electron shell. In the main group, elements' similarities and trends seem to be by group, whereas the transition elements seem to exhibit similarities by period.

Blocks

The blocks of the Periodic Table can be defined based on the subshell that contains the outermost electron. The *s* block includes hydrogen, helium, the alkali metals, and the alkaline earth metals. The *p* block includes Groups 13 through 17. The *s* and *p* blocks of the Table include all the main group elements. The *d* block includes Groups 3 through 12 covering all the transition elements. The *f* block includes all lanthanides and actinides (inner-transition elements).

Element Categories

There are three broad categories of the elements in the Periodic Table.

1. **Metals:** Metals include the alkali metals, the alkaline earth metals, the transition elements, inner-transition elements, and some other metals (Al, Ga, In, Tl, Sn, Pb, Bi, Zn, Cd, Hg). In general, metals are solid at room temperature. They are shiny in appearance, ductile, malleable, and thermally and electrically conductive.

2. **Nonmetals:** Nonmetals include the elements to the far right of the Periodic Table such as the noble gases, halogens, and some other nonmetals (H, C, N, O, P, S, Se). Nonmetal elements are generally dull in appearance, dry and brittle, and nonconductive either thermally or electrically as solids.

3. **Metalloids:** Metalloids are found on the right side of the Periodic Table (B, Si, Ge, As, Sb, Te, Po). There is a great variation in characteristics in this category, but in general these elements possess characteristics between that of a metal and a nonmetal.

Periodic Properties of Elements

The arrangement of elements in the Periodic Table corresponds to the order that electron shells are filled. Following the trend across a period, the number of protons in the elements increases, and electrons are added to existing valence shells. Observing the trends down a particular group of elements, it is evident that as the principle quantum number increases, this corresponds to electrons filling additional shells. These additional shells hold the electrons in a space farther from the nuclear charge (protons), and these electrons are shielded from the nuclear charge by the electrons in the inner shells. These trends alter the effective nuclear charge of the elements (Z_{eff}). The changes (Z_{eff}) have effects on elemental properties such as the atomic radius, electron affinity, ionization energy, and electronegativity.

Atomic Radius

The atomic radius is half the distance between the nuclei of two touching atoms of an element. As the nuclear charge across a period increases, the electrons are drawn closer to the nucleus. This causes a decrease in the atomic radius of elements from left to right across the period. For example, the atomic radius of lithium is nearly three times that of neon. Moving down a group adds electron shells and increases the atomic radius.

Electron Affinity

The electron affinity, E_{ea}, of an element is the energy change when an electron is added to an atom in its gaseous state to form an anion (negatively charged ion). Conversely, the electron affinity also represents the energy needed to pull an electron away from a negatively charged anion. A positive electron affinity value indicates an electron acceptor. The equation for electron affinity is:

$$X_{(g)} + e^- \rightarrow X^-_{(g)} + E_{ea}$$

Electron affinity increases across a period, and it decreases down a period. In general, nonmetals have a higher electron affinity than metals. Chlorine attracts electrons most strongly, whereas mercury attracts electrons most weakly. Since halogens need only one more electron to complete their outer shell (octet rule), they tend to have a strong electron affinity. Conversely, since the noble gases have a completely filled outer shell (stable octet), they have an electron affinity close to zero.

Ionization Energy

Ionization energy is the minimum energy required to remove an electron from an atom in its gaseous state. Energy is always required to remove an atom from an electron, but some atoms more readily give up their electrons than others. Thus, the magnitude of ionization energy is a measure of how tightly the electrons are held to an atom. The higher the ionization energy, the more difficult it is to remove an electron from the atom. The energy required to remove the first valence electron from a ground state atom is called the *first ionization energy*. As the atom becomes ionized (charged), removal becomes more difficult and ionization energy increases. The energy required to remove the second electron is called the *second ionization energy*.

Ionization energies increase going across a period because the increase in the nuclear charge and the reduced atomic radius hold the electron to the atom more tightly. Moving down a group in the Periodic Table, ionization energy decreases because the valence electrons are further from the nucleus, more shielded from the nuclear charge, and, thus, easier to remove. Alkali metals are the group with the lowest ionization energies, and, therefore, they readily give up electrons.

Electronegativity

Electronegativity is the ability of an atom to attract electrons toward itself in a chemical bond between two atoms. Since electronegativity involves the interaction of two atoms, it is a relative measurement. Linus Pauling devised a method for measuring the relative electronegativity of elements. In general, electronegativity increases across a period, and it decreases down a group on the Periodic Table. Smaller, higher nuclear-charged atoms tend to have a higher relative electronegativity.

IONS, MOLECULES, AND COMPOUNDS

Although there are 118 elements in the Periodic Table of Elements, there are only six (the noble gases) that exist in nature as single atoms. Most matter in nature exists in the form of a ion, molecule, and compound.

Ions

An ion is an atom or group of atoms that has an overall positive or negative charge. Since the number of protons in the nucleus remains constant, it is the gain or loss of electrons that determines the charge. The loss of one or more electrons from an atom results in an overall positive charge. This ion is called a *cation*. The gain of one or more electrons to an atom results in an overall negative charge. This type of ion is called an anion. In general, metals tend to form cations, and nonmetals tend to form anions. When two ions of opposite charge join together, an ionic compound forms.

An atom can gain or lose more than one electron. Examples of atoms that gain or lose more than one electron are Ca^{+2}, Mg^{2+}, Fe^{3+}, N^{3-}, S^{2-}, Cl^-. *Monoatomic ions* are those that contain a single type of atom. If two or more atoms combine to form a positive or negative ion, they form what is called a *polyatomic ion*. Examples of polyatomic ions include OH^-, CN^-, and NH^{4+}.

Molecules

A molecule is composed of at least two or more atoms in a definite arrangement and held together by chemical forces, or bonds. A molecule may consist of atoms of the same element, or it may be composed of atoms of different elements. In molecules that contain more than one type of element, the atoms are joined together in a fixed ratio in accordance with the law of definite proportions.

Diatomic molecules consist of two atoms. Hydrogen is a diatomic molecule, H_2. It contains only two atoms, and both are hydrogen. Other elements that are normally found as diatomic molecules are nitrogen (N_2), oxygen (O_2), fluorine (F_2), chlorine (Cl_2), bromine (Br_2), and iodine (I_2). Some diatomic molecules are composed of two different atoms, such as hydrogen chloride (HCl) and carbon monoxide (CO).

Polyatomic molecules are those that contain more than two atoms. These can be composed of three or more of the same type of atom in the case of ozone (O_3) or a combination of two or more elements in the case of water (H_2O).

Compounds

A compound, by definition, is made up of two or more different types of elements joined together in a fixed ratio. All compounds are molecules, but not all molecules are compounds. Water is considered a molecular compound; it contains two hydrogen atoms and one oxygen atom. Water exists in a 2:1 ratio of hydrogen to oxygen (H_2O). Compounds can form from both neutral atoms and ions.

Naming Compounds

Since there are over 20 million compounds known today, chemists have devised a way to systematically name compounds. This system is known as *nomenclature*. All organic compounds contain carbon, usually in combination with hydrogen, oxygen, nitrogen, and/or sulfur. All other compounds are considered *inorganic*. Some carbon-containing compounds such as carbon monoxide (CO), carbon dioxide (CO_2), carbon disulfide (CS_2), carbonate-containing compounds (CO_3^{2-}), and bicarbonates (HCO^{3-}) are also considered inorganic compounds. Inorganic compounds can be further categorized as

- **Ionic Compounds:** Ionic compounds are composed of cations and anions, and most cations are formed from metal ions. Many ionic compounds form from just two elements and are called *binary compounds*. The naming of binary compounds is derived by naming the metal cation, followed by the nonmetal anion. For example, NaCl is formed from a Na^+ ion and a Cl^- ion, and the ionic compound is called sodium chloride. The anion is named by taking the first part of the element name and adding the suffix *-ide* to the end.

- **Molecular compounds:** Molecular compounds contain discrete units. They are usually composed of nonmetallic elements. Many molecular compounds are binary compounds because they form from only two elements. In naming a binary molecular compound, the name of the first element is followed by the name of the second element with the suffix *-ide* added to the end. For example, the compound HCl is called hydrogen chloride. One pair of elements is capable of forming multiple compounds. For example, carbon and oxygen can combine to form carbon monoxide (CO) and carbon dioxide (CO_2).

  In naming compounds, the prefix can be added to the first or second element to indicate how many of these atoms are bound to form the compound (*mono-, di-, tri-*). In the case of the first element in the compound, the prefix *mono-* is generally not used.

  Molecular compounds containing hydrogen are given names that do not follow systemic nomenclature. For example, methane (CH_4), ammonia (NH_3), and water (H_2O) all use names that do not follow the above nomenclature. However, in general, the nomenclature of compounds is straightforward and corresponds to the elements present. For example, PCl_3 is called phosphorus trichloride, and it contains one phosphorus atom and three chlorine atoms. Some compounds are better known by common names than their systemic chemical names (e.g., baking soda, chalk, table salt).

- **Acids and Bases:** An acid is a substance that yields hydrogen (H^+) ions when dissolved in water (to form H_3O^+ ions). Acids contain one or more H atoms and an anionic group. The acid called hydrochloric acid is composed of an H^+ ion and a Cl^- ion. *Oxacids* are those that contain oxygen, hydrogen, and another element (sulfuric acid, H_2SO_4; nitric acid, HNO_3; carbonic acid H_2CO_3).

  A base is a substance that produces hydroxide, OH^-, ions when dissolved in water. Some bases are sodium hydroxide, NaOH; potassium hydroxide, KOH; and barium hydroxide, $Ba(OH)_2$. Ammonia, NH_3, is also considered a base even though it does not contain hydroxide ions. It does, however, yield hydroxide ions when dissolved in water. In fact, when ammonia dissolves in water, it reacts with the water to yield NH^{4+} and OH^-.

- **Hydrates:** Hydrates are compounds that have a specific number of water molecules attached to them. These water molecules can be removed by heating the molecule. The resulting compound after heating is referred to as an *anhydrous compound*. This simply means that the compound no longer has water molecules associated with it. For example, copper sulfate pentahydrate ($CuSO_4 \cdot 5H_2O$) is reduced to anhydrous copper sulfate ($CuSO_4$) upon heating.

> ### Naming Oxacids
>
> Often, oxacids have the same central atom with a different number of O atoms. In general, oxacids end with the suffix *-ic*. Following are six rules for naming oxacids and oxanions:
>
> 1. The addition of an O atom to an oxacid (suffix *-ic*) changes the name of the acid by the addition of the prefix *per-*. For example, adding O to $HClO_3$ changes chloric acid to perchloric acid, $HClO_4$.
>
> 2. The removal of an O atom from an oxacid (suffix *-ic*) changes the suffix to *-ous*. Nitric acid, HNO_3, becomes HNO_2, nitrous acid.
>
> 3. The removal of two atoms from an oxacid is indicated by the prefix *hypo-* and the suffix *-ous*. Bromic acid, $HBrO_3$, is converted to hypobromous acid, $HBrO$.
>
> 4. When an H is removed from an oxacid (suffix *-ic*), the new anion has the suffix *-ate*. Carbonic acid, H_2CO_3, is converted to carbonate, CO_3^{2-}.
>
> 5. When all the H ions are removed from an *-ous* acid (removal of an O atom), the name of the anion, or oxanion, takes the suffix *-ite*. Chlorous acid, $HClO_2$ (derived from chloric acid, $HClO_3$), is converted to the oxanion chlorite, ClO^{2-}.
>
> 6. The names of anions in which one or more, but not all, hydrogen atoms have been removed indicate the number of H ions present. The anions derived from phosphoric acid, H_3PO_4, are dihydrogen phosphate, H_2PO^{4-}; hydrogen phosphate, HPO_4^{2-}; and phosphate, PO_4^{3-}.

CHEMICAL BONDING

The forces that hold atoms together are called chemical bonds. The two types of bonds, *ionic* and *covalent*, stabilize molecules, ions, and compounds. In forming bonds, atoms tend to combine to achieve a more stable configuration.

Electronegativity

Electronegativity is defined as the ability of an atom to attract electrons toward itself in a chemical bond. Therefore, atoms with a higher electronegativity more strongly pull electrons toward their nucleus. A *polar covalent bond* is one in which electrons spend more time closer to one atom in the bond than the other. This unequal electron sharing can be thought of as a partial sharing of the electrons or a shift in electron density.

The Ionic Bond

Ionic bonds are electrostatic forces between two oppositely charged ions. An ionic bond usually forms when electrons are transferred from a metal ion to a nonmetal atom. In general, if the electronegativity difference between two ions is greater than or equal to two, an ionic bond can form. The electrons

TIP

Understanding and memorizing the trends in the Periodic Table will help to predict products and the bonding behavior of elements in a chemical reaction.

are not shared equally between the atoms; instead, electrons are transferred from the atom with the lower electronegativity value to the atom with the higher electronegativity.

In an ionic bond, the electron donor becomes the positively charged ion, or cation, and the electron acceptor becomes a negatively charged ion, or anion. In general, elements in Group 1 and 2 on the Periodic Table form ionic bonds with elements in Groups 16 and 17. Elements in Groups 1 and 2 are metals with a low electronegativity, and those in Groups 16 and 17 are nonmetals with high electronegativity. For example, consider the ionic compound NaCl:

$$Na\cdot + :\ddot{C}l\cdot \rightarrow Na^+ + :\ddot{C}l:^-, \text{ or NaCl}$$

In this reaction, the sodium atom donates an electron to the chlorine atom to form a sodium cation and a chloride anion. The result is the formation of an ionic bond and the ionic compound sodium chloride.

Lattice Energy

In their solid state, ionic compounds form a crystal lattice structure in an arrangement that maximizes the number of ions in a given space. The ions form alternating cations and anions. The lattice energy is the measure of bond strength of a particular ionic compound in its solid state. It is defined as the amount of energy required to completely separate one mole of solid ionic compound into individual ions in their gaseous state. The bond strength depends on two factors:

1. **Ionic radius:** Ions that have a small radius will pack closer to one another, which results in a decrease in the charge separation and an increase in bond strength.

2. **Ionic charge:** The greater the charge difference between the two ions in an ionic compound, the stronger the bond. Thus, the more electrons that are transferred to form ions, the stronger the ionic bond between them. *Divalent ions*, or those that are the result of two electrons transferring, are stronger than *monovalent ions*, where only one electron is transferred.

The lattice energy of an ionic compound cannot be measured directly, but it can be calculated based on the compound's structure and composition by using *Coulomb's law*. Coulomb's law states the potential energy, *E*, between two ions is directly proportional to the product of their charges and inversely proportional to the distance between the two ions.

Lattice energy can also be determined indirectly by assuming that the formation of an ionic compound occurs through a series of steps. The *Born–Haber cycle* relates lattice energies of ionic compounds to ionization energies, electron affinities, and other atomic and molecular properties.

Characteristics of Ionic Compounds

Ionic compounds, in general, have similar characteristics, including the following:

- **Solid at room temperature:** Ionic compounds are solids at room temperature. They have characteristically high melting and boiling points due to strong electrostatic bonds that form between ions.

- **Soluble in polar solvents:** In general, ionic compounds are highly soluble in water and other polar solvents.

- **Electrical conductivity in solution:** Ionic compounds are electrically conductive in their aqueous or molten state, but not in a solid state.

- **Low thermal conductivity:** Ionic compounds are poor thermal conductors and do not release much heat upon reacting.

The Covalent Bond

A bond in which electrons are shared between two atoms is called a covalent bond. Compounds can contain both covalent and ionic bonds within the same molecule. Atoms with a small degree of electronegativity generally combine by sharing electrons. Covalent bonds only involve the interaction of valence shell electrons. This allows for atoms to achieve a stable octet (where all valence orbitals are filled) in a fixed geometric structure of a molecule or a compound. In the case of a fluorine molecule, F_2, the electron configuration of each fluorine atom is $1s^2 2s^2 2p^5$. Therefore, each fluorine atom has seven valence electrons ($2s^2 2p^5$). Since there are eight possible positions for electrons in the $2s$ and $2p$ valence shell, each fluorine atom has one unpaired electron. Those two electrons are shared by each fluorine atom to form a covalent bond and the molecule F_2. This allows for a stable octet in the valence shell of each of the two atoms. Only two valence electrons participate in forming the covalent bond; the other electrons in the valence shell are called *lone pairs*, and they are not involved in the bond.

Covalent compounds are generally neutral and do not carry a charge. Thus, the electronegativity difference between the atoms forming the bond is zero. The strength of a covalent bond is derived from the attraction of the shared electrons to the nuclei of the atoms. Atoms that share one electron pair form what is called a *single bond*. Atoms that share two electron pairs form a *double bond*, and those that share three electron pairs form a *triple bond*. The number of individual bonds in a covalent bond is called the *bond order*. Higher bond orders (triple bonds) indicate stronger, more stable bonds. Covalent bonds are characterized by their bond length, bond dissociation energy, and bond energy.

- **Bond length:** Bond length is defined as the distance between the two nuclei of covalently bound atoms in a molecule. Multiple bonds are shorter than single bonds because the atoms are more strongly pulled toward one another. Triple bonds are shorter than double bonds, which are shorter than single bonds.

- **Bond dissociation energy:** Bond dissociation energy, D_0, is a measure of the energy required to break a covalent bond. The energy required to break a bond is related to the bond order and inversely related to bond length.

- **Bond energy:** The bond energy, E, is an aggregate measurement of the strength of the bonds in a molecule. Bond energy measures the heat required to break a molecule back into individual atoms. For diatomic molecules, this bond energy is equal to its dissociation energy.

Characteristics of Covalent Compounds

In general, covalent compounds exhibit the following characteristics and properties:

- **Various states at room temperature:** The state of a covalent compound varies with the individual elements that form the compound. Unlike an ionic compound, covalent compounds may exist as solid, liquid, or gas at room temperature.

- **Variable melting and boiling points:** The melting and boiling points of covalent compounds are generally lower than those of ionic compounds, but will vary depending on the elements and their arrangements within the compound.
- **Variable solubility:** The solubility of a covalent compound is also dependent on the elements forming the compound. However, covalent compounds usually have a lower solubility in water than ionic compounds.
- **No electrical conductivity:** Most covalent compounds do not exhibit electrical conductivity.
- **Low thermal conductivity:** In general, covalent compounds have low thermal conductivity.

Types of Covalent Compounds

The nature of a covalent bond depends on the relative electronegativity of each of the atoms sharing the electron pairs. Covalent bonds can be either polar or nonpolar in nature. This distinction depends upon the difference in electronegativity between the atoms in the bond.

1. *Polar covalent bonds* form between atoms that have different electronegativities. The bonding electron pair is not shared equally, but instead it is pulled closer to the atom with the higher electronegativity. Thus, the more electronegative atom obtains a partial negative charge, δ^-, and the less electronegative atom acquires a partial positive charge, δ^+. A dipole moment exists between the atoms of a polar bond. The dipole moment is a vector quantity, μ, that is defined as the product of the charge magnitude, q, and the distance between the partial charges, r. The equation to calculate a dipole moment is:

$$\mu = qr$$

   The dipole moment is represented by an arrow pointing from the partially positive to the partially negative charge.

2. A *nonpolar covalent bond* is formed between atoms of the same electronegativity. In this type of covalent bond, the bonding electron pair is shared equally between the two atoms. Nonpolar bonds exist in all diatomic molecules (H_2, O_2, N_2).

3. A coordinate covalent bond is a bond in which the shared electron pair comes from the lone pair of one of the atoms in the molecule. Coordinate covalent bonds are typically found in Lewis acid-base compounds. A *Lewis acid* is an acid that readily accepts an electron pair, and a *Lewis base* is a compound that readily donates an electron pair.

The Geometry and Polarity of Covalent Compounds

In general, covalent compounds (molecules) will assume a geometry that minimizes repulsion between atoms. This approach to molecular geometry is called the *valence-shell electron-pair repulsion (VSEPR) model*. The VSEPR model accounts for the geometric arrangement of electron pairs around a central atom in terms of the electrostatic repulsion between the electron pairs. There are two general rules of the VSEPR model:

1. Double and triple bonds are treated like single bonds. This generalized approximation is sufficient for qualitative purposes.

2. If a molecule has two or more resonance structures, the VSEPR model can be applied to any one of them.

The geometry of a covalent molecule can be predicted using the following three steps pertaining to the VSEPR model:

1. Draw the Lewis dot diagram of the molecule.

2. Count the total number of bonding and nonbonding electron pairs in the valence shell of the central atom.

3. Arrange the electron pairs around the central atom so that they are as far apart for each other as possible.

Molecules with a central atom that has no lone pairs adopt certain geometrical structures. Molecules with two electron pairs are linear. Those with three electron pairs form a trigonal planar structure. Molecules with four electron pairs form a tetrahedral shape. Molecules with five electron pairs in the valence shell form a trigonal bipyramid, and those with six electron pairs form an octahedral.

Figure 7. Arrangement of Atoms Around a Central Atom with No Lone Pairs

Electron pairs	Example	Molecular Geometry	Arrangement of Electron Pairs	Shape
2	$HgCl_2$	B—A—B	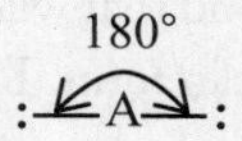 180°	Linear
3	BF_3	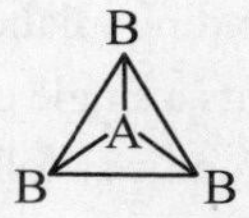	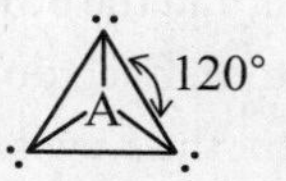 120°	Trigonal planar
4	NH_4	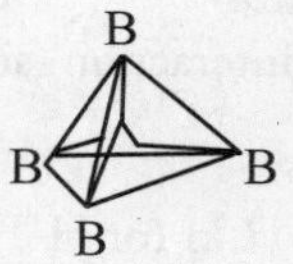	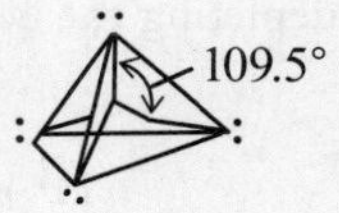 109.5°	Tetrahedral
5	PCL_5	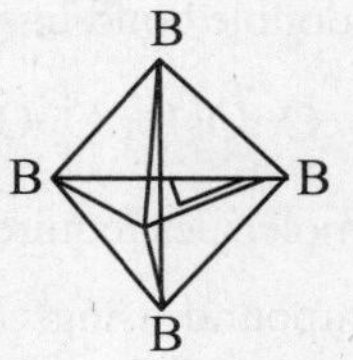	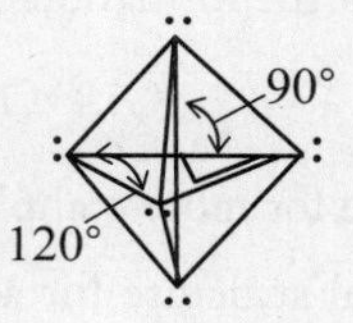 90° / 120°	Trigonal bipyramidal
6	SF_6	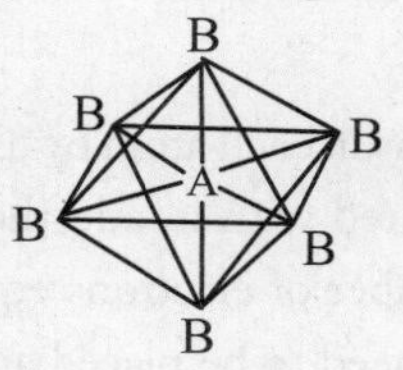	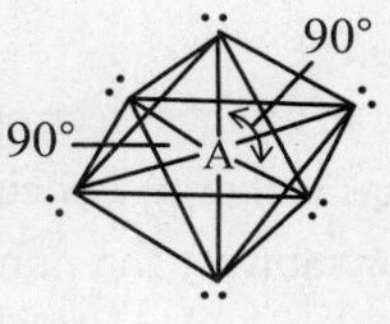 90° / 90°	Octahedral

When the central atom of a molecule has one or more lone pairs, determining the geometric shape of the molecule is more complicated. In this type of molecule, there are repulsive forces between bonding pairs, between lone pairs, and between a bonding pair and a lone pair. According to the VSEPR model, the repulsive forces decrease as follows:

lone pair vs. lone pair repulsion > lone pair vs. bonding pair repulsion >
bonding pair vs. bonding pair repulsion

The extra repulsive forces of lone pairs on the central atom cause a change in angles of the geometric shape of molecules as compared to the geometries of molecules with no lone pair on the central atom.

The geometry of molecules that contain more than one central atom is much more difficult to determine. Often, only the shape around each central atom is described.

Lewis Dot Diagrams

Lewis dot diagrams consist of the element symbol surrounded by a dot for each valence electron. Chemical bonds can be represented by this type of diagram. When atoms interact, only their outermost regions are in contact; thus, bonds are formed mainly by the interaction of valence electrons. The Lewis dot diagram helps to keep track of the electrons in each type of atom. Lewis dot diagrams are useful when dealing with Groups 1 and 2 and 13 to 18 on the Periodic Table. However, the transition metals, lanthanides, and actinides all have incomplete inner shells and, therefore cannot be easily represented by Lewis dot diagrams. Electron configuration and the Periodic Table can be used to predict the type of bond that will form between atoms and the number of bonds an atom of a particular type of element can form. The stability of the product can also be predicted.

In a Lewis structure, the shared valence electrons m, or the bonding electrons, are shown as single dots on one side of the atom, and the other nonbonding valance electrons are depicted as dots around the unbound sides of the atom. Each dot represents a single electron In the case of hydrogen, which has a single valence electron, the Lewis dot diagram is as follows:

H·

The Lewis dot diagram depicting the bonding interaction (single) of two hydrogen molecules is as follows:

H· + H· → H:H (or H-H)

The Lewis dot diagram for the formation of a double bond in an oxygen molecule, O_2 is as follows:

·Ö: + ·Ö: → :Ö::Ö: (or Ö=Ö)

Creating a Lewis structure for more complex molecules requires the following four steps:

1. Write the skeletal structure for a compound using chemical symbols. Place the bonded atoms next to one another. In general, the least electronegative atom occupies the central position.

2. Count the number of valence electrons in each atom by using the Periodic Table of Elements. If the molecule has a charge associated with it, add the number of electrons equal to the negative charge or subtract the number of electrons equal to the positive charge. The net number is the number of dots that need to be placed around the element symbol.

3. Draw a single covalent bond between the central atom and each of the surrounding atoms. Complete the octets for each atom bonded to the central atom. Electrons that are not involved in bonding are shown as lone pairs. The total number of electrons has already been established in step 2. Start with the most electronegative element and work toward the least

electronegative element (the central atom). Each bond pair counts toward the octet of each individual atom in the bond.

4. If the central atom has fewer than eight electrons after completing step 3, add double or triple bonds between the central atom and surrounding atoms, using lone pairs from surrounding atoms to complete the octet of the central atom.

Since electrons are shared in a bond, electrons in a bonding pair are divided equally among the atoms forming the bond. An atom's formal charge is the difference in the electrical charge between the valence electrons in a single atom and the number of electrons assigned to that atom in a Lewis structure of a molecule or compound. In order to assign the number of electrons on a Lewis structure of a compound or molecule, the following procedure is used:

- Assign all the nonbonding electrons to an atom.
- Break the bond between the two bonded atoms and assign half the bonding electrons to each bonded atom.

For molecules, the sum of formal charges must add up to zero, since molecules are neutral in charge. For all cations in an ionic compound, all charges must add up to a positive value. For all anions in an ionic compound, the charges must add up to a negative value. These formal charges are not necessarily the actual charge separation, but it helps to keep track of valence electrons.

Resonance

In the case of some molecules, there is more than one possible Lewis dot diagram. For example, in the case of the molecule ozone, O_3, there are two possible Lewis structures:

$$\ddot{O} = \ddot{O}^+ - \ddot{O}^{\dot{\cdot}} \leftrightarrow \ddot{O}^{\dot{\cdot}} - \ddot{O}^+ = \ddot{O}$$

Both are representative of the structure of the ozone molecule. The double bond can be between either of the two oxygen atoms. Each of these structures is called a *resonance structure*. A resonance structure is simply one of two or more Lewis dot diagrams that can represent a single molecule that cannot be accurately represented by a single diagram. The actual molecule exists as a mixture of all the possible resonance structures. This type of molecule is called a *resonance hybrid*. The molecule does not shift back and forth between the two structures, but has its own unique stable structure.

Formal Charge

The formal charge of an atom is equal to the difference of the number of electrons officially assigned to an atom in a bond and the number of valence electrons in a free atom. The formal charge, C_f, can be calculated using the following formula:

$$C_f = V - \left[\frac{1}{2} N_{bonding} + N_{nonbonding} \right]$$

where V is the number of valence electrons in a free atom, $N_{bonding}$ is the number of valence electrons in the bonded atom that bond to another atom, and $N_{nonbonding}$ is the number of lone pair valence electrons.

There are several guidelines to be considered when determining the more stable resonance structure based on a calculated formal charge of a molecule:

- For resonance structures of the same molecule, the most stable structure is that with the fewest formal charges. This structure will contribute the most to the actual resonance structure.

- Negative formal charges on more electronegative molecules are more favorable, and positive charges are more favorable on less electronegative atoms.

- The calculation of a formal charge assumes nonpolar covalent bonding in the molecule.

- The sum of formal charges of the component atoms should equal the total molecular charge.

Intermolecular Forces

The forces of attraction between two or more molecules are known as intermolecular forces and there are three types of intermolecular forces:

1. **Dipole-dipole interactions:** Dipole-dipole interactions are attractive forces between polar molecules. Polar molecules are arranged so that the partially positive end of one molecule is in close proximity to the partially negative end of another molecule. This forms a dipole-dipole interaction between the molecules, since the opposite ends of each molecule are attracted to each other. Dipole-dipole interactions occur in molecules in their solid or liquid state, but this type of interaction is negligible in the gaseous state.

2. **Dispersion forces:** Dispersion, or *London*, forces are the attractive forces that are the result of a temporary dipole induced in a nonpolar atom or molecule by a surrounding molecule. Dispersion forces are temporary forces. An induced dipole in a molecule can be caused by its proximity to an ion or polar molecule. Dispersion forces are generally weaker than other intermolecular forces. They only exist over short distances, but they tend to increase with increasing molar mass of molecules. Large molecules with electrons positioned far from the nucleus are easier to polarize than smaller molecules, and, therefore, they possess greater dispersion forces than smaller molecules. Dipole-dipole interactions and dispersion forces are also called *van der Waals forces*.

3. **Hydrogen bonding:** Hydrogen bonding is a special type of dipole-dipole intermolecular force between a partially positively charged hydrogen atom in a polar bond and a partially negatively charged electronegative atom. Molecules that utilize hydrogen bonding tend to have high boiling points because a large amount of energy is required to break the hydrogen bonds that form between molecules. Hydrogen bonding is particularly important in understanding the behavior of water molecules.

CHEMICAL EQUATIONS AND REACTIONS

A chemical reaction is a process in which a chemical substance (or substances) is changed into one or more new substances. A chemical reaction is represented by a chemical equation that uses chemical formulas and symbols to show what happens during a chemical reaction. In each chemical reaction, the law of conservation of mass is observed. This law states that matter cannot be created or destroyed, and, therefore, the quantity of matter that is present at the start of a reaction is the same amount of matter that is present at the end of the reaction. Matter can change states and can be combined with other reactants, but the end products have the same number of each type of atom as the starting reactants.

Types of Chemical Reactions

There are four general types of chemical reactions.

1. **Combination reaction:** A combination reaction is one in which two or more elements or molecules are combined to form a product. This is a very common type of reaction that is seen in all divisions of chemistry. The general formula for a combination reaction is $A + B \rightarrow AB$ in which two reactants, A and B, yield the product AB.

2. **Decomposition reaction:** A decomposition reaction involves the chemical breakdown of a substance into two or more products. These two products can usually be combined to reform the original substance. A decomposition reaction is written using the general formula $AB \rightarrow A + B$. Decomposition reactions can occur spontaneously in unstable molecules.

3. **Single or double displacement reaction:** In a single displacement reaction, an atom from one molecule is transferred to another molecule. This type of reaction is written using the following formula: $AY + BX \rightarrow AX + BY$. Displacement reactions are commonly seen in reactions involving ionic compounds. In a double displacement reaction, two different compounds displace each other to form new compounds.

4. **Neutralization reaction:** A neutralization reaction is a specialized reaction that involves acids and bases. In this type of reaction, an acid and a base combine to form a salt and water. An example of a neutralization reaction is the combination of hydrochloric acid, HCl, with the base sodium hydroxide, NaOH, to form sodium chloride (NaCl). The reaction that takes place is represented as follows:

$$HCl + NaOH \rightarrow NaCl + H_2O$$

Writing Chemical Equations

Chemical equations are always written with the reactants, or starting material, on the left side of a reaction arrow, $\rightarrow$, and the products, or ending materials, on the right side of the reaction arrow. For example, the formation of water from hydrogen gas and oxygen gas is written as:

$$H_2 + O_2 \rightarrow H_2O$$

In this chemical equation the plus sign (+) means that H_2 reacts with O_2. The reaction arrow indicates that these two reactants "yield" ($\rightarrow$) the final product, H_2O. Therefore, this equation can be read as "molecular hydrogen reacts with molecular oxygen to yield water."

The above equation, however, does not follow the law of conservation of mass because there are more oxygen molecules on the left side of the equation than on the right. According to the law of conservation of mass, there must be an equal amount of hydrogen and oxygen molecules on each side of the equation. This equation can be balanced by adding number coefficients to the reactants and products so that there is an equal number of each type of atom on the left and right sides of the reaction arrow:

$$2H_2 + O_2 \rightarrow 2H_2O$$

Additional information regarding the physical state of each of the reactants and products can also be added to a chemical equation. Each state can be represented by a letter: g = gas, ℓ = liquid, and s

= solid. In the case of the formation of water, the reaction can be written to show the physical state of each substance as follows:

$$2H_{2(g)} + O_{2(g)} \rightarrow 2H_2O_{(\ell)}$$

Balancing Chemical Equations

Once the reactants and products of an equation have been identified, they can be written into the format of a chemical equation. This chemical equation can then be balanced to make sure that the same number of each type of atom appears on both sides of the equation. An equation is balanced by following the six steps below:

1. Identify all the reactants and products and write their correct chemical formulas on the appropriate side of the reaction arrow.

2. Begin balancing the equation by adding different numerical coefficients to make the number of atoms of each element equal on both sides of the arrow. The coefficients are the numbers that precede the chemical formula. These numbers can change, but the numbers in the subscript within the chemical formula cannot.

3. Next, look for elements that appear only once on each side of the equation. The chemical formulas containing these elements must have the same coefficient.

4. Then, look for elements that appear only once on each side of the equation, but in unequal numbers of atoms. Balance these elements by adding an appropriate coefficient.

5. Balance the elements that appear in two or more chemical formulas on the same side of the equation.

6. Lastly, check the balanced equation to be sure that there is the same number of each type of atom on both sides of the reaction arrow.

Example: Balance the following equation for the combustion of ethane gas (C_2H_6):

$$C_2H_6 + O_2 \rightarrow CO_2 + H_2O$$

Because the number of each type of atom is not the same on both sides of the equation, it must be balanced. Since C and H appear only once on each side, it is best to balance these first.

$$C_2H_6 + O_2 \rightarrow 2CO_2 + 3H_2O$$

Now there are two carbons on each side of the equation and six hydrogen atoms on each side. However, the O atoms are still not balanced. Since it is common to use whole number coefficients, the coefficients for C and H will have to be adjusted to allow for the O atoms to be balanced. The equation then becomes:

$$2C_2H_6 + 7O_2 \rightarrow 4CO_2 + 6H_2O$$

TIP

It is helpful to draw up a balance sheet for the reactants and products and add up the total number of each atom for both sides of the equation. It is common practice to use the simplest possible set of whole number coefficients to balance an equation.

The tally for each element in this final equation shows that it has been balanced:

Reactants	Products
C4.	C4.
H(12)	H(12)
O(14)	O(14)

Stoichiometry

Stoichiometry is the quantitative study of reactants and products in a given chemical reaction. Balanced equations contain information that is useful in determining mass relationships, limiting reagents in a reaction, and product yields. The units for any given reaction can be in moles, grams, liters, or other units, but moles are always used to calculate the amount of product formed. This is called the *mole method* and implies further that the stoichiometric coefficients in a chemical equation can be assumed to be the number of moles of each substance. The following equation can be written for the combustion of carbon monoxide (CO):

$$2CO_{(g)} + O_{2(g)} \rightarrow 2CO_{2(g)}$$

The stoichiometric coefficients of this equation indicate that two moles of carbon monoxide combine with one mole of oxygen to form two moles of carbon dioxide. Thus, the stoichiometric molar ratio of CO to CO_2 is 2:2, or 1:1, and the ratio of CO to O_2 is 2:1.

If the number of grams of CO is known, the number of grams of CO_2 produced can be determined based on the stoichiometric molar ratio. To calculate the grams of CO_2 produced, the mass of CO needs to be converted into moles. Then the number of moles of CO_2 produced can be determined and this value can be converted into grams. For example, if the starting amount of CO is equal to 8 grams (g), it is is converted into moles by using the molar mass of CO (28.01 g/mol):

$$\text{moles of CO} = 8 \text{ g} \times \frac{1 \text{ mol CO}}{28.01 \text{ g/mol}} \text{ moles CO} = 0.285 \text{ mol}$$

Since CO and CO_2 are in a 1:1 molar ratio, the number of moles of CO_2 produced is 0.285 mol. Then the mass of CO_2 produced can be calculated by multiplying the number of moles by the molar mass of CO_2.

$$\text{grams CO}_2 = 0.285 \text{ mol} \times \frac{44.01 \text{g}}{\text{mol CO}_2} = 12.5 \text{ g CO}_2$$

The general approach to solving a stoichiometric problem is:

- Write a balanced equation for a given reaction.
- Convert a given mass (or comparable unit) of a particular reactant into moles.
- Use the molar ratio that is determined by the balanced equation to determine the number of moles of product formed.
- Convert the moles of product to grams (or other comparable units).

TIP

Most calculations in chemistry involve the number of moles of a substance. Remember to convert the mass of reactants or products into moles by using the molecular weight.

Limiting Reagents

The limiting reagent in a chemical reaction is the reactant whose quantity is used up first. When this reactant is used up, it is not possible to form any more product, thus the yield of product in the reaction is limited by that reagent. Conversely, *excess reagents* are those reactants that are present in quantities greater than necessary to react with the limiting reagent. In a stoichiometric calculation, the first step is to determine the limiting reagent in the reaction.

Reaction Yield

In a chemical reaction, the reaction yield is a theoretical yield that represents the maximum amount of product that can result if the entire limiting reagent is used up. The actual yield in a reaction is the amount of product that is actually obtained from a chemical reaction. The *actual yield* is almost always less than the theoretical yield. The reasons for the difference in yield vary. Some reactions are reversible and, therefore, do not proceed only from left to right as written. Sometimes, even if a reaction is complete in one direction, it is difficult to recover the entire yield. Some reactions are so complex that various side reactions of the reactants or products may reduce the overall yield.

The *percent yield* can be calculated to determine the proportion of actual yield to that of the theoretical yield. The percent yield is calculated by the following equation:

$$\% \text{ yield} = \frac{actual \text{ yield}}{theoretical \text{ yield}} \times 100$$

Factors that may influence the percent yield include the temperature and pressure at which the reaction takes place.

GASES

Under the correct conditions, almost all substances can exist as a solid, a liquid, or a gas. The physical properties of a substance are often dependent on its state. Gases tend to be simpler in their physical properties compared to solids and liquids. Gas molecules move about in a random fashion and the attractive forces between molecules in a gas are minimal. It is easier to predict the behavior of gases with respect to changes in temperature and pressure. There are several laws that have been established that govern the behavior of gases and that play important roles in the atomic theory of matter and the kinetic molecular theory of gases.

Gas exerts pressure on whatever surface it comes in contact with because gas molecules are constantly in motion. Atmospheric pressure is a constant pressure experienced on Earth. Atmospheric pressure is measured with an instrument called a *barometer*, which consists of a long glass tube closed at one end and filled with mercury. *Standard atmospheric pressure* is equal to the pressure that a column of mercury at exactly 760 mm high at sea level. This measurement is referred to as *atmosphere*. The pressure of gases other than atmospheric is also easily measurable with an instrument called a monometer that operates similarly to the barometer. A closed-tube manometer measures the pressures of gases below atmospheric pressure. The pressure of gases at or above atmospheric pressure are measured by an open-tube manometer.

TIP

Be sure to pay attention to the stoichiometric relationships of reactants and products.

Ideal Gases

There are four specific properties that are used to describe the behavior of gases: temperature (T in units of Kelvin), pressure (P), volume (V), and the number of moles of gas present (n). Several laws have been established to help understand the behavior of gases.

- **Boyle's law:** Boyle's law states that the pressure of a fixed amount of gas at a constant temperature is inversely proportional to the volume of the gas. The mathematical expression of Boyle's law is as follows:

$$P = k_1 \times \frac{1}{V}$$

where k_1 is a proportionality constant and the temperature and number of moles of gas remain constant. The proportionality constant k_1 is equal to the product of the number of moles (n), the temperature (T), and the gas constant (R = 8.314 J/K mol).

Boyle's law indicates that as long as the temperature and the number of moles of gas do not change, the product of P and V is a constant ($PV = k_1$). Therefore, Boyle's law can also be used to compare a sample of gas under two different sets of conditions at a constant temperature. The following equation compares two different volumes and pressure for the same type of gas:

$$P_1 V_1 = P_2 V_2$$

- **Charles's law:** Charles's law (also called Charles's and Gay-Lussac's law) states that the volume (V) of a constant amount of gas maintained at a constant pressure is directly proportional to the temperature of the gas (T in degrees Kelvin). This relationship is shown in the following equation:

$$V = k_2 T$$

where k_2 is a proportionality constant. The value of k_2 is dependent upon the number of moles of gas (n), the gas constant (R = 8.314 J/K mol) and the pressure of the gas (P). Like Boyle's law, this equation can be used to compare two sets of volume and temperature of a gas at a constant pressure:

$$\frac{V_1}{T_1} = \frac{V_2}{T_2}$$

Another form of Charles's law shows that for a constant volume and molar amount of gas, the pressure of the gas is proportional to its temperature (in degrees Kelvin):

$$\frac{P}{T} = k_3$$

where k_3 is a proportionality constant equal to nRV. This law can also be represented by the following equation:

$$\frac{P_1}{T_1} = \frac{P_2}{T_2}$$

- **Avogadro's law:** Avogadro's law states that at constant pressure (P) and temperature (T in degrees Kelvin), the volume of a gas (V) is directly proportional to the number of moles of the gas. This law can be represented by the equation:

$$V = k_4 n$$

where k_4 is the proportionality constant equal to RT/P. The following equation shows that under constant temperature and pressure, equal volumes of gases have an equal number of particles.

$$\frac{V_1}{n_1} = \frac{V_2}{n_2}$$

- **Ideal gas law:** The ideal gas law combines Boyle's, Charles's, and Avogadro's laws in order to describe the relationship among the four variable—P, V, n, and T—in one equation. The ideal gas equation is as follows:

$$PV = nRT$$

where R is the proportionality constant known as the gas constant ($8.314\,J/K\,mol$). The value of R is derived from standard conditions of temperature and pressure. Standard pressure is 1 atmosphere (atm), and standard temperature is 273.15K (0°C). One mole of an ideal gas under standard conditions occupies 22.414 L. Substituting all of these values into the ideal gas law equation and solving for R gives the value $0.082\,L\cdot atm/K\cdot mol$. This value of R can be converted to $8.314\,J/K\cdot mol$.

An ideal gas is a hypothetical gas whose pressure-volume-temperature behavior can be completely understood by the ideal gas equation. In an ideal gas, the molecules are independent of one another (no attractive or repulsive forces), and the volume of the gas molecules is negligible compared to the volume of the container. There is no such thing as an ideal gas in nature, but the ideal gas equation gives a good approximation of the behavior of most gases.

The ideal gas equation is useful when there is no change in P, V, n, or T for a sample of gas. However, when conditions of the gas undergo a change, the ideal gas equation can be modified to the following:

$$\frac{P_1V_1}{n_1T_1} = \frac{P_2V_2}{n_2T_2}$$

The ideal gas law can also be used to calculate the density of a gas. *Density* is defined as the mass per unit volume of a substance. For gases the unit of density is grams/liter (g/L). Rearranging the ideal gas law can allow for calculations of density.

$PV = nRT$ and $n = \frac{m}{M}$ where m is mass in grams and M is molar mass in g/mol; therefore, $PV = \frac{m}{M}RT$ and $V = \frac{mRT}{PM}$. Density is expressed by the equation $d = \frac{m}{V}$; therefore, $d = \frac{m}{V} = \frac{PM}{RT}$. The molar mass of a gas can also be calculated for using this equation if the density of the gas is known.

Dalton's Law of Partial Pressures

Dalton's law of partial pressures states that the total pressure of a mixture of gases is equal to the sum of the pressure that would be exerted by each individual gas if it occupied the space on its own. The atmosphere is composed of a mixture of gases, and many experimental studies also involve gaseous mixtures as opposed to pure substances. The atmosphere is a mixture of nitrogen, oxygen, carbon dioxide, and other trace gases such as carbon monoxide. Each gas exerts a part of the total pressure of the atmosphere.

Mathematically, Dalton's law of partial pressures is represented by the equation:

$$P_{total} = P_1 + P_2 + P_3 \ldots$$

where P_1, P_2, and P_3 are the pressures of the individual gases. To determine the relationship of each partial pressure to the total pressure, a ratio can be set up:

$$\frac{P_1}{P_{total}} = \frac{\frac{n_1 RT}{V}}{\frac{n_{total} RT}{V}} = \frac{n_1}{n_{total}} = X_1$$

where X_1 is called the *mole fraction* of gas 1. The mole fraction is simply a dimensionless value that expresses the ratio of the number of moles of one gas component to the total number of moles of the gas mixture. A general representation of the mole fraction is:

$$X_i = \frac{ni}{n_{total}}$$

where i represents any gas component in a mixture. The partial pressure of each gas component can be represented by the equation:

$$P_i = X_i P_{total}$$

The Kinetic Molecular Theory of Gases

Kinetic energy is the energy of motion, or the energy expended by a moving object. The kinetic molecular theory of gases, or the kinetic theory of gases, explains the motion of gas particles on a molecular level. The following assumptions are critical to the kinetic theory:

- A gas is composed of molecules separated from one another by a distance greater than the individual dimension of each particle. The molecules have mass, but they have a negligible volume.

- Gas molecules are in constant motion and move in random directions. They frequently collide with one another, and these collisions are perfectly elastic. Thus, energy can be transferred from one molecule to another as the result of a collision, but the total energy of the system remains constant.

- Gas molecules do not exert attractive or repulsive forces on one another.

- The average kinetic energy, *KE*, of gas molecules is proportional to the gas's temperature (in degrees Kelvin). Any two gases at the same temperature will have the same kinetic energy. A molecule's average kinetic energy is given by the equation:

$$\overline{KE} = \frac{\frac{1}{2}}{m\overline{u}^2}$$

where m is the mass of the molecule and u is its speed. The horizontal bar above the speed (mu) and KE denotes an average value. Since the average kinetic energy is also proportional (α) to temperature in degrees Kelvin, the equation can be altered to the following expression:

$$\overline{KE} \; \alpha \; T$$

$$\frac{1}{2} m\overline{u}^2 \; \alpha \; T$$

$$\frac{1}{2}\,m\bar{u}^2 = CT$$

where C is a proportionality constant and T is the absolute temperature. This relationship indicates that the higher the temperature of the gas, the more energetic the molecules, and the faster they move.

Deviation from Ideal Behavior

Gases can be assumed to behave like ideal gases, but not under all conditions. Thus, it is important to determine under what conditions a gas will no longer exhibit ideal behaviors. For most real gases, the ideal gas law only holds true under low-pressure conditions, and significant deviations from the law occur as the pressure of the gas increases. At high pressures, the density of the gas increases and the molecules are drawn closer together. This close proximity of gas molecules to one another causes attractive and repulsive forces between molecules. Intermolecular forces at high pressure can become significant enough to affect the motion of molecules. Nonideal behavior is also exhibited as the temperature of a gas is lowered. The decrease in temperature causes a decrease in the average kinetic energy of the molecules, so that it is harder for the molecules to repel from each other.

To study real gases accurately, the ideal gas equation needs to be modified. The van der Waals equation was derived to account for the difference in ideal gas and real gas behavior:

$$P_{ideal} = P_{real} + \frac{an^2}{V^2}$$

where a is a constant and the corrected term for pressure, $\frac{an^2}{V^2}$, based on the fact that the frequency of intermolecular interaction increases with the square of the number of molecules, n, per unit volume, V. In this correction factor, a is the proportionality constant.

Another correction in the ideal gas law is made for the volume occupied by the gas molecules. In the ideal gas equation, V represents the volume of the container. However, in order to take into account that each gas molecule takes up a small but finite space, the corrected volume becomes:

$$V_{real} = V - nb$$

where b is a constant, n is the number of moles of gas, and V is the volume of the container. The van der Waals equation accounts for these corrections in the ideal gas equation:

$$\left[P + \frac{an^2}{V^2} \right]\left[V - nb \right] = nRT$$

The van der Waals constants and b vary for each element and are based on observed behaviors of a particular gas.

Diffusion and Effusion

1. Diffusion is the gradual mixing of one gas with another due to their kinetic properties. Diffusion occurs as gas particles move through a mixture. Despite the relatively fast speed of molecules in a gas, diffusion is a relatively slow process. The kinetic molecular theory of gases predicts that heavier gases will diffuse more slowly than lighter gases. Thomas Graham showed that under the same conditions of temperature and pressure, the rates of diffusion for gases (r) are inversely proportional to the square root of their molar masses (M). Graham's law of diffusion can be expressed in an equation:

$$\frac{r_1}{r_2} \bullet \sqrt{\frac{M_2}{M_1}}$$

2. Effusion is the process by which gas under a given pressure escapes from one compartment of a container to another compartment by passing through a small opening. The rate of effusion of a gas has the same form as Graham's law of diffusion

SOLIDS AND LIQUIDS

In liquids, molecular motion is more restricted than in gases, and in solids, molecules are packed closely together in well-defined positions so that there is little movement.

The Kinetic Molecular Theory of Liquids and Solids

The molecules in a liquid are held close together so that there is very little distance between molecules. Liquids are much more difficult to compress than gases and much denser than gases under normal conditions. The molecules in a liquid are held together by attractive forces, and molecules in a liquid do not break away from these attractive forces, as they do in gases. This property gives liquids a definite volume. Molecules in a liquid can, however, move past one another, a quality that gives liquids their fluid property. Liquids assume the shape of the container into which they are poured.

In a solid, the molecules are packed into a rigid three-dimensional conformation with almost no freedom of motion. There is even less empty space between the molecules of a solid than those of a liquid. A solid can only be slightly compressed if at all, and it possesses a definite shape and volume. With the exception of water, the solid phase of a substance is denser than its liquid or gas phase.

Van der Waals Constants for Common Gases:

Gas	a (atm·L²/mol²)	b (L/mol)
He	0.034	0.0237
Ne	0.211	0.0171
Ar	1.34	0.0322
Kr	2.32	0.0398
Xe	4.19	0.0266
H_2	0.244	0.0266
N_2	1.39	0.0391
O_2	1.36	0.0318
Cl_2	6.49	0.0562
CO_2	3.59	0.0427
CH_4	2.25	0.0428
CCl_4	20.40	0.138
NH_3	4.17	0.0371
H_2O	5.46	0.0305

Characteristic Properties of Solids, Liquids, and Gases

Phase	Volume/Shape	Density	Molecular Motion	Compressibility
Solid	definite volume and shape	relatively high	vibrate in a fixed position	virtually incompressible
Liquid	definite volume; assumes the shape of its container	relatively high	freely slide past one another	slightly compressible
Gas	assumes volume and shape of its container	relatively low	free and random motion	very compressible

Intermolecular Forces

Intermolecular forces are forces of attraction between molecules. These forces are more influential on liquids and solids than they are on gases. As the temperature drops and substances condense to their liquid phase, or freeze into their solid phase, the kinetic energy of the molecules of the substance decreases. As molecules slow down, they have less ability to break away from the attraction of other molecules. The aggregation of gas molecules as the temperature is lowered forms droplets of water, called *condensation*. As the temperature is lowered even more, molecules pack together to form a solid in the process known as *freezing*.

In general, the forces that hold two molecules together are much weaker than the forces that hold atoms together within a molecule (intramolecular forces). The different types of intermolecular forces are dipole-dipole forces, dipole-induced dipole forces, dispersion forces, and hydrogen bonding. Hydrogen bonding is a particularly strong type of dipole-dipole interaction.

Properties of Liquids

Intermolecular forces are responsible for a number of structural features and properties of liquids. Two of these properties are surface tension and viscosity.

1. **Surface tension:** Surface tension is the amount of energy required to stretch or increase the surface of a liquid by a given unit of area. Molecules in a liquid are pulled in every direction by intermolecular forces. Molecules at the surface of a liquid are pulled downward and sideways by other liquid molecules. This causes the surface of liquids to tighten like an elastic film, thus creating surface tension. Liquids that have strong intermolecular forces have a high surface tension. Since water is held together by hydrogen bonds, it has a relatively high surface tension.

   An example of surface tension is capillary action. A thin film of liquid adheres to the sides of a capillary tube. Surface tension causes the liquid to contract, and the contraction pulls the liquid upward in the capillary. Two types of forces cause capillary action: *cohesion* (attraction between like molecules), and *adhesion* (attraction between unlike molecules).

2. **Viscosity:** Viscosity is the measure of a liquid's resistance to flow (fluidity). The greater the viscosity of a liquid, the more slowly it will flow. In general, the viscosity of a liquid increases with decreasing temperature. Liquids that have strong intermolecular forces have a higher viscosity than those that have weak intermolecular forces. Since water forms hydrogen bonds, which are strong intermolecular forces, it tends to have a higher viscosity than other liquids.

Properties of Solids

Solids can be categorized as either crystalline or amorphous.

Crystalline Solids

A crystalline solid possesses a rigid, long-range order. Thus, its atoms, molecules, or ions occupy specific positions in a repeating pattern. The arrangement of particles in a crystalline solid is such that the net attractive intermolecular forces are maximized. The forces responsible for the stability of a crystal structure can vary. They can be ionic forces, covalent bonds, van der Waals forces, or 4. hydrogen bonds.

Within a crystalline solid, a *unit cell* is defined as the basic repeating structural unit. The general geometric requirements of a crystalline structure can be understood by considering all the ways that a number of identical spheres can be packed together. The *coordination number* is defined as the number of atoms, or ions, that surround a single atom (ion) in a crystal lattice. The value of the coordination number is a measure of how tightly packed the atoms are. The atoms can be packed in a simple cubic cell, body-centered cubic cell, or face-centered cubic cell.

The concept of closest packing involves the most efficient arrangement of spheres in order to minimize the empty space between atoms. Every unit cell in a crystalline solid is adjacent to another unit cell, so that most of a unit cell's atoms are shared by neighboring unit cells. In addition, atoms (molecules or ions) are packed in layers. Atomic spheres (or molecular or ionic spheres) in one layer fit into the depressions between the spheres of the next layer.

The structure and properties of crystals—melting point, density, and hardness—are determined by the forces that hold the individual particles of the crystal together. There are four types of crystal structures.

1. **Ionic crystals:** Ionic crystals are composed of anions and cations, which are generally of different sizes. Knowing the radius of each type of ion helps to determine the overall stability of the crystalline structure. Most ionic crystals have high melting points, and they do not conduct electricity unless dissolved in water.

2. **Covalent crystals:** Covalent crystals are held together in a three-dimensional pattern by covalent bonds. Diamonds are an example of a covalent crystal. The strong covalent bonds in the three-dimensional crystal give diamonds their unusual degree of hardness, and their very high melting point (3350°C). Covalent crystals are poor conductors of electricity.

3. **Molecular crystals:** Molecular crystals are composed of molecules held together by van der Waals forces or hydrogen bonds. In general, the molecules in a molecular crystal are closely packed. However, since the bonding holding these crystals together is relatively weak, molecular crystals are easily broken apart and have low melting points (generally below 100°C). Molecular crystals are also poor conductors of electricity.

4. **Metallic crystals:** Metallic crystals form a lattice in which every point is occupied by a metal atom. Metallic crystals are usually composed of body-centered units, face-centered units, or hexagonally packed atoms. Metallic crystals generally have a very high density and relatively low melting points. They are good conductors of electricity and also good thermal conductors.

Amorphous Solids

An amorphous solid, such as glass, does not have a well-defined structure, or long-range molecular order. Solids are most stable in a crystalline form, but if a solid forms rapidly, its atoms or molecules will not be able to align themselves in a rigid crystalline structure. Atoms or molecules become quickly locked into a position, and the result is an amorphous solid that lacks a regular three-dimensional arrangement.

Phase Changes

A phase change is the transformation of a substance from one physical state (solid, liquid, or gas) to another. Phase changes generally occur when energy, usually in the form of thermal energy, is added to or removed from the substance. Phase changes alter the molecular order of a substance: molecules in the solid phase have the greatest amount of molecular order, and those in the gas phase have the least amount of molecular order.

Liquid to Vapor

Molecules in a liquid are in constant motion even though they lack the total freedom of gaseous molecules. Liquids tend to be denser than gases, and, therefore, there are more collisions between molecules in a liquid compared to those in a gas. When the molecules in a liquid acquire sufficient energy (usually through an increase in temperature), they change into gaseous molecules. Evaporation, or vaporization, is the process through which liquid is transformed into a gas. As the temperature of a liquid increases, the kinetic energy of the molecules in the liquid also increases. This increase in kinetic energy causes an increase in the motion and speed of the molecules, and they are able to "escape" the surface of the liquid, causing the formation of gas, or vapor.

When a liquid evaporates, the gaseous molecules given off exert a pressure known as vapor pressure. Vapor pressure is measurable only when a sufficient amount of vapor accumulates. Furthermore, evaporation is not a continuous process. At the beginning, there are molecules moving from the surface of the liquid into empty space above the liquid. This establishes both a liquid and a vapor phase. As the concentration of molecules in the vapor phase increases, some of the vapor molecules decrease in temperature and condense back to liquid. Thus, condensation is the process of changing gaseous molecules into liquid molecules. Condensation occurs because as molecules strike the surface of the liquid, they become trapped by the intermolecular forces in the liquid.

The rate of evaporation is constant in the system, but the rate of condensation increases with an increasing number of molecules in the gaseous (vapor) phase. Dynamic equilibrium is reached when the rate of condensation is equal to the rate of evaporation. The pressure of the system at this point is called the *equilibrium vapor pressure*.

The molar heat of vaporization, ΔH_{vap}, is defined as the energy required to vaporize one mole of a liquid. This value is directly related to the strength of intermolecular forces within the liquid. A liquid with strong intermolecular forces will require a great deal of energy to remove a molecule from its surface. The relationship between the vapor pressure of a liquid and the temperature (in degrees Kelvin) is expressed in the Clausius-Clapeyron equation:

$$\ln P = -\left[\frac{\Delta H_{vap}}{RT}\right] + C$$

where $\ln P$ is the natural logarithm of the vapor pressure, R is the gas constant expressed in Joules (8.314 J/K mol), and C is a constant. If the vapor pressure and molar heat of vaporization are known at one temperature, the Clausius-Clapeyron equation can be used to find the vapor pressure of the liquid at a different temperature:

$$\ln \frac{P_1}{P_2} = \left[\frac{\Delta H_{vap}}{RT}\right]\left[\frac{(T_1 - T_2)}{T_1 T_2}\right]$$

The *boiling point* of a liquid is the temperature at which the vapor pressure of the liquid is equal to the external pressure. Bubbles of gas form within a liquid as it reaches its boiling point. The pressure inside the bubble is due solely to the vapor pressure of the liquid. When the vapor pressure inside the bubble becomes equal to the external pressure, the bubble rises to the surface of the liquid and bursts. The higher the molar heat of vaporization of a liquid, the higher its boiling point.

Gases can be converted to a liquid either by cooling them, which decreases the kinetic energy of the molecules so that they aggregate and form liquid droplets, or by applying pressure to the gas. Compression reduces the distance between molecules so that they are held together and form a liquid. The molar heat of condensation, ΔH_{con} is the energy required for the process of condensation to take place. However, every substance has a critical temperature above which a gas will not be able to condense into a liquid, no matter how great the pressure applied. Thus, this critical temperature is also the highest temperature at which the liquid phase of the substance exists. At this temperature, there is no distinction between a gas and a liquid. The critical pressure is the minimum pressure that must be applied to cause liquefaction at the critical temperature.

Liquid to Solid

Freezing is the term use to describe the transformation from a liquid to a solid. The reverse process of transforming a solid into a liquid is called *melting*. The melting point of a solid, or the freezing point of a liquid, is the temperature at which the solid and liquid phases of a substance coexist.

In order to make the transition from the solid to liquid phase, thermal energy is required because the molecules in a solid are strongly held together by intermolecular forces. The temperature of a solid must reach the melting point in order for the solid-liquid phase change to take place. The added thermal energy helps the molecules to overcome the attractive forces and increases their kinetic energy. A heating curve can be drawn for a substance and can give information about its melting and boiling points.

Figure 8. A Typical Heating Curve for a Substance

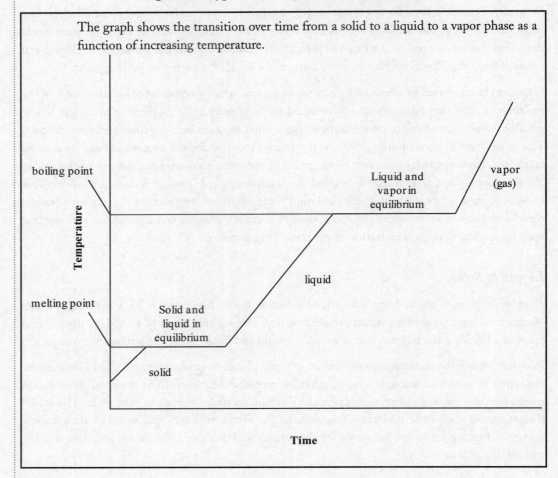

The graph shows the transition over time from a solid to a liquid to a vapor phase as a function of increasing temperature.

As heat is being absorbed by the substance so that it can overcome attractive forces, the temperature remains constant (as seen by the flat portions of the curve). During this period, an increase in kinetic energy is used to overcome the attractive forces in a solid and the cohesive forces in a liquid. Once enough molecules have transitioned to the next phase, the temperature rises again.

The *molar heat of fusion*, ΔH_{fus}, is the energy required (in kilojoules, KJ) to melt one mole of a solid. The reverse of this process is the *molar heat of crystallization*. A continued cooling of a substance leads to freezing. The phenomenon known as *supercooling* occurs when a liquid is temporarily cooled below its freezing point. Supercooling occurs when heat is so rapidly removed from a liquid that the molecules do not have the opportunity to assume the correct crystalline solid structure and remain in the liquid phase. A supercooled liquid is very unstable—so unstable that gently stirring it or adding a single solid crystal to the liquid will cause the liquid to quickly solidify.

Solid to Vapor

It is possible for a solid to undergo the process of evaporation. Thus, solids also possess a vapor pressure. *Sublimation* is the process in which molecules transition from the solid phase directly into the vapor (gas) phase. The reverse process in which a vapor transitions directly into a solid is called *deposition*. The molar heat of sublimation, ΔH_{sub}, is the energy required (in kilojoules, KJ) to sublime one mole of solid. This value is equal to the sum of the molar heats of fusion and vaporization for a substance ($\Delta H_{sub} = \Delta H_{fus} + \Delta H_{vap}$).

Phase Diagrams

A phase diagram indicates the conditions at which a substance exists as a solid, liquid, or gas (vapor). A simple diagram graphs pressure vs. temperature for a given substance.

Figure 9. A Phase Diagram for Water

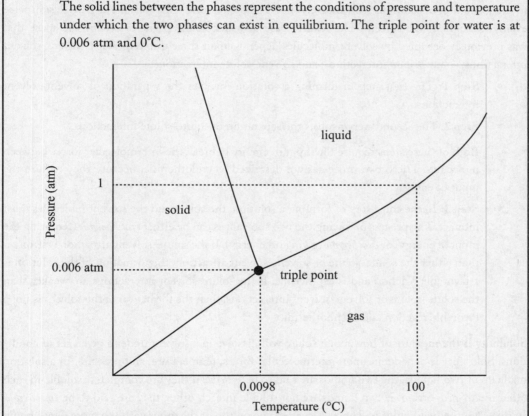

The solid lines between the phases represent the conditions of pressure and temperature under which the two phases can exist in equilibrium. The triple point for water is at 0.006 atm and 0°C.

As shown in Figure 9, a phase diagram is divided into three regions, each of which represents the substance in a pure phase. The line separating each phase represents the temperature and pressure under which the substance can exist in equilibrium in both phases. The point at which all three curves meet is the *triple point*. The triple point is the exact conditions under which all three phases (solid, liquid, and gas) exist in equilibrium. Phase diagrams are useful in predicting changes in the boiling or melting point of a substance based on external pressure.

SOLUTIONS

Many chemical reactions take place between molecules or ions that are dissolved in water or another solvent. A *solution* is a homogeneous mixture of two or more substances. Solutions can form from two liquids, two gases, a solid and a liquid, a liquid and a gas, and even from two solids. The *solute* is the substance that is present in the smaller amount, and the *solvent* is the substance present in the greater amount. The solute is completely dissolved in the solvent, and the two substances become indistinguishable once a solution is formed. The process of forming a solution is called *solvation* or *dissolution*. When water is the solvent, the reaction is called a *hydration reaction*, and the solution is referred to as an *aqueous solution*.

Intermolecular forces that hold molecules together in liquids and solids also play an important role in the formation of solutions (solvation). When a solute dissolves in a solvent, its particles disperse evenly throughout the solvent. The relative ease in which solute particles occupy the space that was previously occupied by solvent molecules depends upon three different steps: solvent-solvent interactions, solute-solute interactions, and solvent-solute interactions.

- **Step 1:** The first step in forming a solution involves the separation of solvent-solvent interactions.

- **Step 2:** The second step involves the separation of solute-solute interactions.

  Both of these steps require the input of energy to break the intermolecular forces between molecules. These two processes are described as endothermic, because they require the input of energy.

- **Step 3:** In the third step of forming a solution, the solute and the solvent molecules must interact. The process of mixing the two substances can be either *endothermic* (requiring the input of energy) or *exothermic* (giving off energy). If the solute-solvent attraction is stronger than either the solute-solute or solvent-solvent attraction, the formation of the solution is a favorable reaction and is exothermic. If the solute-solvent interactions are weaker than the solute-solute or solvent-solvent interactions, then the formation of the solvent is not a favorable reaction and is endothermic.

Solubility is the measure of how much solute will dissolve in a solvent under a given set of conditions. Solubility is dependent upon intermolecular forces, temperature, and pressure. In a solution made up of two liquids, the two liquids are said to be *miscible* if they are completely soluble in each other in any proportion. If two liquids are not soluble in each other, they are said to be *immiscible*. In this case, the two liquids will appear layered, one on top of the other with the more dense liquid below the less dense liquid.

Solutions can be characterized by the capacity to dissolve in a given solvent:

- **Saturated solution:** A saturated solution contains the maximum amount of solute that will dissolve in a given solvent at a specific temperature.

- **Unsaturated solution:** An unsaturated solution contains less solute than the maximum capacity of a given solvent at a specific temperature.

- **Supersaturated solution:** A supersaturated solution contains more solute than is present in a saturated solution. This is a very unstable solution, and the addition of a single crystal of solute will cause the solute to come out of solution and form crystals (crystallization).

Ions

Liquid solutions can contain many types of ions. Water, for example, can dissolve many ionic compounds since there is a partial negative charge on the oxygen molecule in water, and a partial positive charge of the hydrogen atoms in water. When an ionic compound is dissolved in water, the water molecules surround the cation and anion as they dissociate from one another. If electrodes are added to the water solution, the anions move toward the positive electrode and the cations move toward the negative electrode. Thus, ionic solutions are good conductors of electricity, and these ionic solutions are called *electrolytes*. Compounds that dissolve in solution, but do not ionize, are called *nonelectrolytes*.

In a net ionic equation, there are several types of ions that form, but only those that form a product in the solution are shown in the overall reaction. For example, consider the formation of silver chloride (AgCl). The total reaction involves the ionization of sodium chloride (NaCl) and silver nitrate ($AgNO_3$) and is represented by the equation:

$$Na^+_{(aq)} + Cl^-_{(aq)} + Ag^+_{(aq)} + NO^{3-}_{(aq)} \rightarrow AgCl_{(s)} + Na^+_{(aq)} + NO^{3-}$$

However, it is not necessary to include the ions that do not become part of the product. These are free ions in solution and are not involved in the reaction; this can be seen by the fact that they remain the same on both sides of the equation arrow. These are called *spectator ions*. If the spectator ions are removed, the net ionic equation becomes:

$$Cl^-_{(aq)} + Ag^+_{(aq)} \rightarrow AgCl_{(s)}$$

Solution Concentration

A quantitative understanding of solution involves determining their concentration, which is the amount of solute present in a given volume of solution. The concentration of solute in a liquid solution can be measured in terms of molarity, molality, percent mass, and the mole fraction (X).

Molarity

Molarity (M) is defined as the number of moles of solute in 1 liter (L) of solution. The equation used for determining molarity is:

$$M = \frac{\text{moles solute}}{\text{liters solution}}$$

The units of molarity are moles per liter, or mol/L. Molarity is a commonly used measurement in the laboratory. The mass of solute can be determined if the molarity, volume, and molar mass of the solute is known.

Molality

Molality (m) is defined as the number of moles of solute dissolved in 1 kilogram (kg) of solvent. Molality can be calculated using the following equation:

$$m = \frac{\text{moles solute}}{\text{mass of solvent}}$$

The units of molality are moles per kilogram, or mol/kg. From the equation for molality, the exact amounts of both solute and solvent can be determined.

Percent by Mass

The percent by mass (or percent by weight or weight percent) of a solution is the ratio of the mass of the solute to the mass of the solvent multiplied by 100. The equation for calculating the percent by mass is:

$$\text{percent by mass} = \frac{\text{mass of solute}}{\text{mass of solution}} \times 100$$

There are no units assigned to the percent by mass, because it is a ratio of two similar quantities.

Mole Fraction

The mole fraction, X, as defined earlier is a quantity that expresses the ratio of the number of moles of one component of a solution to the number of moles of all the components of the solution. The mole fraction of a solute can be expressed by the following equation:

$$X_{\text{solute}} = \frac{\text{moles of solute}}{\text{moles of solute} + \text{moles of solution}}$$

The moles of solvent can be determines in the same manner. The mole fraction has no units because it is a ratio of similar quantities.

Solution Dilution

A solution becomes dilute when a greater amount of solvent is added to a given amount of solute. The volume of the solvent increases, but the number of moles of solute remains the same. Therefore, the concentration in terms of molarity decreases. This is called a *dilution of the original solution*. The concentration in terms of molarity can be determined for the dilute solution by using the following equation:

$$M_1 V_1 = M_2 V_2$$

where M_1 and V_1 are the molarity and volume of the original solution, and M_2 and V_2 are the molarity and volume of the diluted solution.

Solution Equilibrium

There are several factors that can affect the amount of solute dissolved in a given solvent. The factor that seems to have the greatest influence is temperature. In general, there is an increase in the solubility of liquids and solids in a solution when the temperature of the solution is increased.

However, this is not always true with gases in solution. The solubility of a gas solute in a liquid follows Le Chatelier's principle: When heat is added to a gas-liquid solution, the equilibrium of the solution shifts in response to the input of thermal energy. The addition of thermal energy causes a release of gas from the solution. Therefore, in general, the solubility of a gas in a liquid decreases with increasing temperature.

The solubility of a solute is also affected by the presence of other solutes in the solvent. For example, the solubility of a salt is greatly decreased when it is dissolved in a solution that already contains ions that are also present in the salt. If the salt sodium chloride, NaCl, is dissolved in a solvent that already has Na^+ ions present, the equilibrium will shift toward the formation of solid salt (NaCl) and the sodium chloride will not dissolve in the solvent. This reduced solubility is known as the *common ion effect*, and it is another example of Le Chatelier's principle.

Colligative Properties

Colligative properties are properties of solutions and depend on the concentrations of different parts of the solution. Colligative properties include changes in vapor pressure and temperature, phase changes, and osmotic pressure.

Vapor Pressure

Raoult's law states that the vapor pressure of a solvent (P_1) over a solution is given by the vapor pressure of the pure solvent (P_1°) times the mole fraction (X_1) of the solvent in the solution. Raoult's law can be expressed mathematically in the following equation:

$$P_1 = X_1 P_1^\circ$$

When a solution contains only one solute, the mole fraction of the solute can be expressed as X_2, and the mole fraction of the solvent can be expressed by the equation $X_1 = 1 - X_2$. The expression is rewritten as:

$$P_1 = (1 - X_2)P_1^\circ$$

or

$$P_1^\circ - P_1 = X_2 P_1^\circ$$

and $P_1^\circ - P_1$ can be rewritten as ΔP, so the equation for vapor pressure becomes:

$$\Delta P = X_2 P_1^\circ$$

Thus, a change in vapor pressure of the solvent is directly proportional to the solute concentration of the solution. Furthermore, the vapor pressure of a solution is always less than the vapor pressure of a pure solvent because the solvent molecules of a solution have less of a tendency to vaporize than the molecules of a pure solvent. The result is that the vapor pressure of a solution is less than that of a pure solvent.

If both components of a solution have a measurable vapor pressure, they are said to be *volatile*. Volatile components have a measurable vapor pressure. In this case, the vapor pressure of the solution is the sum of the individual partial pressures and Raoult's law still holds true.

When two components form a solution, the boiling point and freezing point of the resulting solution may be elevated or depressed as compared to the pure solvent. The boiling point of a solution is the temperature at which the vapor pressure of the solution is equal to the external atmospheric pressure. *Boiling point elevation*, ΔT_b, is defined as the boiling point of the solution, T_b, minus the boiling point of the pure solvent, T_b°. The equation for the boiling point elevation is $\Delta T_b = T_b - T_b^\circ$. Freezing point depression, ΔT_f, is defined as the freezing point of a pure solvent, T_f°, minus the freezing point of the solution, T_f. The equation for the freezing point depression is $\Delta T_f = T_f^\circ - T_f$.

Osmotic Pressure

Osmosis is the process by which there is a selective passage of solvent molecules through a porous membrane from a dilute solution to a more concentrated solution. The porous membrane, called a *semipermeable membrane*, allows the passage of solvent molecules through it, but blocks the passage of solute molecules. The osmotic pressure is defined as the pressure required to stop the process of osmosis. The osmotic pressure pushes solvent from a more dilute area into a more concentrated area in an attempt to achieve equilibrium between the two areas. Osmotic pressure, Π, can be calculated by the equation:

$$\Pi = MRT$$

where M is the molarity of the solution (mol/L), R is the gas constant (0.0821 L atm/K mol), and T is the temperature (in degrees Kelvin). Osmotic pressure is directly proportional to the concentration of the solution. If two solutions are of equal concentration and have the same osmotic pressure, they are said to be *isotonic*. If, however, two solutions have different concentrations and osmotic pressures, the more concentrated solution is said to be *hypertonic*, and the more dilute solution is *hypotonic*.

ACID-BASE REACTIONS

Acids are those substances that ionize in water to form H^+ ions, and bases are those substances that ionize in water to produce OH^- ions. There are four major concepts that explain the behavior of acids and bases:

1. **Arrhenius concept:** The Arrhenius concept explains that acids produce H^+ cations (hydronium ions, H_3O^+) in an aqueous solution. The Arrhenius acid base reaction can be written as:

   $$\text{acid} + \text{base} \rightarrow \text{salt} + \text{water}$$

   The Arrhenius concept of acids and bases only holds true for aqueous solutions.

2. **The Brønsted-Lowry concept:** The Brønsted-Lowry concept defines acids as donors of H^+ ions and bases as acceptors of H^+ ions. This concept does not require the acid or base to be in an aqueous solution. It led to the idea of conjugate acids and bases: a strong acid has a weak conjugate base, and a weak acid has a strong conjugate base.

3. **Solvent system concept:** The solvent system concept states that ions dissociate from a solvent, and these ions can be either anions or cations. If the ions are anions, then the solution is a base, and if the ions are cations, the solution is an acid.

4. **Lewis acid-base concept:** The Lewis acid-base concept defines acids and bases in terms of electrons. A *Lewis acid* is an electron pair acceptor, and a *Lewis base* is an electron pair donor.

Properties of Acids and Bases

There are several characteristics that help to define a substance as an acid or a base.

Acids

Acids have a sour taste. They are able to react with certain metals, such as zinc, magnesium and iron. They are able to change the color of litmus from blue to red. Aqueous acidic solutions are good conductors of electricity. Acids are also able to react with carbonates and bicarbonates to produce carbon dioxide gas. A strong acid is one that completely dissociates into its components when dissolved in water. Some examples of a strong acid are hydrochloric acid (HCl), perchloric acid ($HClO_4$), nitric acid (HNO_3), and sulfuric acid (H_2SO_4). Weak acids are those that are only partially dissociated in water. An example of a weak acid is acetic acid (CH_3COOH).

Bases

Bases have a bitter taste. They are able to change the color of litmus from red to blue. Aqueous solutions that contain a base are good conductors of electricity. A strong base completely dissociates into ions in an aqueous solution. Some examples of a strong base are sodium hydroxide (NaOH), potassium hydroxide (KOH), and other soluble hydroxides. A weak base is one that only partially dissociates in an aqueous solution. Ammonia (NH_4) is an example of a weak base.

pH

The most commonly discussed property of acids and bases is their pH level. pH is defined by the equation:

$$pH = {}^-\log_{10}[H_3O^+]$$

where $[H_3O^+]$ is the concentration of hydronium ions in the solution. The range of pH values is between 0 and 14. 1. A pH of 7.00 is considered a neutral pH. 2. pH values below 7.00 are considered acidic, and 3. those above 7.00 are considered to be basic. A very low pH value indicates a strong acid, and values that approach 7.00 represent weaker acids. Similarly, a very high pH value indicates a strong base, and a pH value that approaches 7.00 from the upper end of the pH scale indicates a weak base.

Equilibrium Constant

The strengths of acids and bases can be represented by a value called the equilibrium constant, K_a. The equation used to calculate the value of the equilibrium constant for a given acidic solution is:

$$K_a = \frac{\left[H^+\right]\left[A^-\right]}{\left[HA\right]}$$

where [H+] is the concentration of hydronium ions, [A−] is the concentration of anion, and [HA] is the nondissociated acid.

The dissociation constant for a base, K_b, can be calculated in the exact same way. A high value of K_a indicates a strong acid. For example, HCl has a K_a value of 1.3×10^6. A strong acid has a low pH and a high percentage of dissociation, meaning that it readily forms hydronium ions in solution. A high K_b value correlates to a strong base and a higher pH value.

Salt Formation

A salt is an ionic compound that forms when an acid and a base react with each other. Salts contain both a cation and an anion and are electrically neutral molecules. Salts form during a *neutralization reaction* between an acid and a base, and the other product of this reaction is water. Salts release ions when dissolved in water. A salt may precipitate out or remain ionized in a solution, depending on its solubility in water. The reverse reaction in which salt ions react with water to produce an acid and a base is called a *hydrolysis reaction*.

There are four possible combinations in a neutralization reaction.

1. **Strong acid + strong base:** The products that form when a strong acid and strong base interact are a salt and water.

2. **Strong acid + weak base:** When a strong acid and a weak base interact, a salt is formed. However, very little water, if any, is formed because the cation of the salt that forms reacts with water to reform the weak acid, and the solution is going to be weakly acidic.

3. **Weak acid + strong base:** When a weak acid reacts with a strong base, the salt that forms hydrolyzes to reform the acid. Hydroxide ions form due to the hydrolysis of water and, therefore, the overall solution is basic.

4. **Weak acid + weak base:** When a weak acid and a weak base react, the resulting pH of the solution is dependent on the relative strength of each reactant.

Polyvalence and Normality

Some acids and bases are *polyvalent*, meaning that each mole of the acid or base is capable of dissociating more than one acid or base equivalent. An acid equivalent is equal to one mole of H^+ (H_3O^+) and a base equivalent is equal to one mole of OH^- ions. For example, one mole of diprotic acid (H_2SO_4) can produce two acid equivalents ($2H^+$ ions), since it contains two hydrogen atoms.

The relative acidity or basicity depends on the concentration of acid or base equivalents that can dissociate from a molecule. The degree of acidity and basicity is indicated by the normality of the solution. *Normality* is equal to the number of grams of equivalent weight of solute per liter of solution. Normality, N, is useful in dealing with salt solutions. Since salts dissolve differently in different solvents, normality takes into account the ratios of cations and anions and is dependent on the type of reaction taking place. For example, a 1 M solution of sulfuric acid (H_2SO_4) would be 2 N in an acid base reaction because it donates two H^+ ions to the reaction, but it is 1 N for a sulfate precipitation reaction because only one mole of sulfate (SO_4^{2-}) ion is dissociated from one mole of sulfuric acid.

Amphoteric Species

An *amphoteric species* can react as either an acid or a base, depending on the chemical environment. This is a common trait in biological molecules such as amino acids. Water is the most common example of an amphoteric species. When it reacts with a base (B), it behaves like an acid and donates a proton to the base:

$$H_2O + B \rightarrow \rightleftarrows HB + OH^-$$

Conversely, when water reacts with an acid (A), it behaves like a base:

$$H_2O + A \rightarrow \rightleftharpoons H_3O^+ + A^-$$

Titrations and Buffers

Titrations are a procedure used for quantifying the amount of acid or base in a solution. In a titration, a solution of an accurately measured concentration, known as a *standard solution* (acid or base), is gradually added to another solution (acid or base) of an unknown concentration. The standard solution is added to the unknown solution until the chemical reaction between the two solutions is complete. The point at which the acid has completely reacted with the base is called the *equivalence point*. The equivalence point is measured in terms of pH, and it indicates that the number of moles of H^+ ions that have reacted is equivalent to the number of moles of OH^- ions that have reacted. The equivalence point is generally signaled by a sharp change in color due to the presence of an indicator in the solution. *Indicators* are substances that have a distinctly different color in an acidic and basic environment. A titration curve is a graph showing pH on the *y*-axis and the volume of the added compound on the *x*-axis. If the concentration and volume of the standard solution is known, and the volume of the unknown solution is known, the concentration of the unknown solution can be determined using the equation:

$$M_1 V_1 = M_2 V_2$$

A *buffer* is a chemical solution of a weak acid or base and its salt. The buffer solution has the ability to resist changes in pH when small amounts of an acid or a base are added. Buffers play an important role in maintaining proper pH levels, especially in biological systems.

A buffer solution must contain a large enough concentration of both acid and base so that either can react with the appropriate ions (H^+ or OH^-) added to the solution. In addition, the acid and base components of a buffer must not undergo a neutralization reaction. This requirement is satisfied by using an acid-base conjugate pair in a buffer solution. This pair can be a weak acid and its conjugate base supplied by a salt, or a weak base and its conjugate acid. For example, a buffer for the pH range 3.8 to 5.5 can be made using acetic acid, (CH^3COOH), a weak acid, and its conjugate base in the form of the salt sodium acetate (CH^3COONa).

REDOX REACTIONS AND ELECTROCHEMISTRY

Electrochemistry is the specialized field of chemistry that studies the conversion of electrical energy into chemical energy and the conversion of chemical energy into electrical energy. Electrochemical reactions are oxidation reduction reactions in which the energy released from a spontaneous reaction is released as electrical energy, and electrical energy is used to drive a nonspontaneous reaction.

Oxidation-Reduction Reactions

Oxidation-reduction, or *redox*, reactions are reactions in which electrons are transferred from one chemical substance to another. *Oxidation* is the loss of electrons by a substance, and *reduction* is the gain of electrons by a substance. In a redox reaction, the species that oxidizes the other (removes its electrons) is called the *oxidizing agent*. The oxidizing agent is itself reduced (gains electrons), and, thus, the species that loses its electrons (oxidized) is called the *reducing agent*.

Oxidation Number

In a redox reaction, the number of electrons and the number of each type of atom must be balanced on each side of the chemical equation. The oxidation number helps to determine whether a species has been oxidized or reduced. Assigning oxidation numbers to atoms in a redox reaction helps to keep track of the redistribution of electrons during the reaction. In a sense, an oxidation number is similar to an electric charge assigned to atoms. The oxidation number is the number of charges an atom would have in a molecule if the electrons were completely transferred from one species to another. Here are some facts about oxidation numbers:

- *Pure elements* have an oxidation number of zero.

- *Monoatomic ions* have the same oxidation number as their ionic charge. For example, the oxidation number for Ca^{2+} is 2, and the oxidation number of N^{3-} is -3.

- The oxidation number in each Group 1 (IA) element is $+1$ and the oxidation number in each Group 2 (IIA) element is $+2$.

- The oxidation number in each Group 17 (VIIA) element is -1, except when the element is bound to an element of higher electronegativity.

- The oxidation number of hydrogen is $+1$, except in compounds where H is bound to an element of lower electronegativity (Groups 1 and 2). In those cases, the oxidation number of H is -1.

- In most cases, the oxidation number of oxygen is -2. If the element bound to oxygen is more electronegative, then oxygen has an oxidation number of $+2$.

- The sum of the oxidation numbers of all the elements in a neutral compound is zero.

- The sum of the oxidation numbers in a polyatomic ion compound is equal to the charge of the compound.

- Since fluorine is the element with the highest electronegativity, it always has an oxidation number of -1.

- All metallic elements always have a positive oxidation number.

Balancing Redox Equations

The most common method for balancing a redox reaction is the ion-electron method. In this method, the overall reaction is divided into two parts called *half-reactions*. One half-reaction represents the oxidation reaction, and the other half-reaction represents the reduction reaction. Each half-reaction is balanced separately. There are five steps taken to properly balance a redox reaction.

- **Step 1:** Write an unbalanced equation in ionic form. For example:

$$Fe^{2+} + Cr_2O_7^{2-} \rightarrow Fe^{3+} + Cr^{3+}$$

- **Step 2:** Separate the reaction into two half-reactions. The numbers shown in parentheses are the oxidation numbers.

$$\text{Oxidation reaction: } Fe^{2+} (+2) \rightarrow Fe^{3+} (+3)$$

$$\text{Reduction reaction: } Cr_2O_7^{2-} (+6) \rightarrow Cr^{3+} (+3)$$

- **Step 3:** Balance each half-reaction for the number and type of atom and charge. For reactions taking place in an acidic environment, add H_2O to balance the H^+ ions and O atoms. In a reaction that takes place in a basic environment, add H_2O and OH^- to balance O and H^+.

$$Fe^{2+} \rightarrow Fe^{3+} + e^-$$

$$14\ H^+ + Cr_2O_7^{2-} + 6\ e^- \rightarrow 2Cr^{3+} + 7H_2O$$

- **Step 4:** Combine the two half-reactions and balance the final equation. The electrons on both sides of the reaction arrow must cancel each other out.

$$6[Fe^{2+} \rightarrow Fe^{3+} + e^-]$$

$$14\ H^+ + Cr_2O_7^{2-} + 6\ e^- \rightarrow 2Cr^{3+} + 7H_2O$$

$$6\ Fe^{2+} + 14H^+ + Cr_2O_7^{2-} + 6e^- \rightarrow 6Fe^{3+} + 2Cr^{3+} + 7H_2O + 6e^-$$

$$6\ Fe^{2+} + 14H^+ + Cr_2O_7^{2-} \rightarrow 6Fe^{3+} + 2Cr^{3+} + 7H_2O$$

- **Step 5:** Verify that the final equation has the same number of atoms and charges on each side.

There are four major types of redox reactions that take place.

1. **Combination reaction:** A combination reaction takes place when there are one or more free elements in the reaction:

$$N_2\ (0) + 3H_2\ (0) \rightarrow 2NH_3\ (0)$$

   The oxidation number of the pure elements is 0, and the oxidation number of N is $^-3$ and of H_3 is $^+3$, so that the sum of the oxidation numbers on each side of the equation is 0.

2. **Decomposition reaction:** A decomposition reaction is the breakdown of a compound into one or more single elements:

$$2HgO\ (+2/^-2) \rightarrow 2Hg\ (0) + O_2\ (0)$$

   where the oxidation number of Hg is $^+2$ and O is $^-2$ in the compound HgO.

3. **Combustion reaction:** A combustion reaction is one in which a given substance reacts with oxygen and releases thermal and light energy in the process:

$$C_3H_{8\ (g)} + 5O_{2\ (g)} \rightarrow 3CO_{2\ (g)} + 4H_2O_{\ (\ell)}$$

4. **Displacement reaction:** In a displacement reaction, an ion or atom of a given compound is replaced by a different ion or atom. Most displacement reactions can be categorized as hydrogen displacement, halogen displacement, or metal displacement.

$$2Na\ (0) + 2H_2O\ (^+2) \rightarrow 2NaOH\ (^+2) + H_2\ (0)$$

Electrochemical Cells

The process of transferring electrons from one substance to another creates an electric current (flow of electrons). *Electrochemical cells* are contained systems in which a redox reaction takes place. If the oxidizing agent is physically separated from the reducing agent, the transfer of electrons takes place by an external electrical conductor such as a metal wire. The reaction sets up a constant flow of electrons that generates electricity. There are two types of electrochemical cells: 1. galvanic (or voltaic) cells and 2. electrolytic cells. Both types of cells contain electrodes, which are the sites of the redox reactions. 1. Oxidation occurs at the electrode called the anode, and 2. reduction occurs at the electrode called the cathode.

Galvanic Cells

The redox reaction that occurs in a galvanic cell is a spontaneous reaction. The oxidizing and reducing agents are separated into half-cells in a galvanic cell. A zinc bar is immersed in a $ZnSO_4$ solution, and a copper bar is immersed in a $CuSO_4$ solution. In this cell, the oxidation of Zn to Zn^{2+} takes place at the same time as the reduction of Cu^{2+} to Cu. A salt bridge is added and links the two half-cells together and allows for the exchange of cations and anions. The salt bridge acts to complete the circuit. The salt bridge contains an inert electrolyte solution that will not interact with other ions in the solution or with the electrodes.

Electrons transfer from the anode (Zn) to the cathode (Cu) through a metal wire that connects the two half-cells. An electric current flows from the anode to the cathode because there is a difference in electrical potential energy between the two electrodes. The difference in electrical potential energy is measured by a voltmeter, and the reading from the voltmeter is called the cell voltage. The terms *electromotive force* (*emf* or *E*) and *cell potential* are also used to denote cell voltage. The cell voltage depends on the nature of the ions as well as their concentration in the cell and the temperature of the cell.

Electrolytic Cells

A redox reaction that occurs in an electrolytic cell is a *nonspontaneous* reaction. In this case, electrical energy input is required to initiate the redox reaction. In an electrolytic cell, the two half-reactions (oxidation and reduction) are placed in one container, or cell.

Michael Faraday hypothesized that the amount of chemical charge induced by an electrolytic cell is directly proportional to the number of moles of electrons that are exchanged during a redox reaction. Faraday's constant is a value that expresses the charge carried by one mole of electrons and is measured in terms of Coulombs (C) per mole of electrons. Faraday's constant is 9.645×10^4 C/mol e^-.

In an electrolytic cell, positively charged ions (cations) migrate toward the cathode where they are reduced. Negatively charged ions (anions) migrate toward the anode where they are oxidized. This type of cell is used in industry as a major source of sodium and chlorine production, because it is effective in separating sodium chloride. The current produced in an electrolytic cell can easily be measured using a voltmeter. Each half-reaction (oxidation or reduction) has a voltage (cell potential or *emf*) measurement associated with it. The total cell potential under standard state conditions (1 *M* and 1 atm) is given by the equation:

$$E^{\circ}_{cell} = E^{\circ}_{cathode} - E^{\circ}_{anode}$$

where E is the cell potential.

Cells that function under nonstandard conditions, such as alkaline batteries, can be understood using the Nernst equation:

$$E = E^{\circ} - \left(\frac{RT}{nF}\right)\ln Q$$

where R is the gas constant, T is the temperature, n is the number of moles, F is the Faraday constant, and Q is the reaction quotient. The reaction quotient is a number equal to the ratio of the product concentrations to the reaction concentrations. In a general reaction of $aA + bB \rightarrow cC + dD$, where lowercase letters represent the stoichiometric coefficients for each species, the reaction quotient is:

$$Q = \frac{[C]^c [D]^d}{[A]^a [B]^b}$$

Reduction Potential and *emf*

Every substance has an intrinsic reduction potential. The *reduction potential* is the tendency of a substance to acquire electrons and be reduced. The substance in a reaction that will be oxidized or reduced can be determined by evaluating the reduction potential of each species. A greater value of the reduction potential indicates a greater tendency for the substance to be reduced, and a lower value indicates a greater tendency to be oxidized.

A reduction potential is measured in units of voltage and is compared to the standard hydrogen electrode (SHE), which is assigned a voltage value of 0 volts. The *standard reduction potential* is the value assigned to a reduction reaction at an electrode at 25°C, when all solutes are at a concentration of 1 M and all gases are at a pressure of 1 atm.

The *electromotive force, emf,* is the work per unit charge that is required to produce an electrical current. Standard reduction potentials can be used to calculate the standard electromotive force of a reaction. The *emf* of a reaction is determined by adding the standard reduction potential of the reduced species and the standard oxidation potential of the oxidized species:

$$emf = E^\circ_{red} + E^\circ_{ox}$$

The standard *emf* of a galvanic cell is a positive value, and the standard *emf* of an electrolytic cell is a negative value.

Thermodynamics of Redox Reactions

Thermodynamics can be used to determine the spontaneity of a reaction. *Gibbs free energy*, ΔG, is the maximum amount of useful work that can be produced by a given chemical reaction. In an electrochemical cell, the work done is related to the number of coulombs and the energy available:

$$\Delta G = -nFE_{cell}$$

In this equation, ΔG is expressed in Joules, J; n is the number of moles of electrons that are exchanged; F is Faraday's constant; and E_{cell} is the cell potential (*emf*). Under standard conditions, this equation becomes:

$$\Delta G^\circ = -nFE^\circ_{cell}$$

A negative value of ΔG° and a positive value of E°_{cell} indicate that the reaction is *spontaneous*. A positive value of ΔG° and a negative value of E°_{cell} indicate that the reaction is *nonspontaneous*. A ΔG° value of 0 and E°_{cell} value of 0 indicate that the reactants and products are equally favored in the reaction.

For reactions in a solution, ΔG° can also be determined by the equation:

$$\Delta G^\circ = -RT\ln K_{eq}$$

where R is the gas constant, T is temperature in Kelvin, and K_{eq} is the equilibrium constant for the reaction.

THERMOCHEMISTRY

Thermochemistry is the application of thermodynamics to chemical reactions. *Thermodynamics* is the study of the interconversion of thermal energy and other kinds of energy. *Thermochemistry* is the study of heat change during a chemical reaction. Heat is defined as the transfer of energy between two bodies that are at different temperatures. Energy changes in a reaction are referred to as *heat absorbed* or *heat released*. All chemical reactions obey the law of conservation of energy: Energy is neither created nor destroyed during a chemical reaction. The first law of thermodynamics is based on the law of conservation of energy and states: Energy can change forms or be transferred from one substance to another, but it cannot be created or destroyed.

Thermochemistry is useful for predicting the spontaneity of a reaction, determining the favorability of a reaction, and for calculations of heat capacity, enthalpy, and free energy. In order to analyze the energy changes that take place in a chemical reaction, the system in which the reaction takes place must be analyzed. In chemistry, the *system* usually includes the substances involved in the chemical reaction, and the *surroundings* are defined as the rest of the universe outside the system. There are three types of systems.

1. **Open system:** An open system can exchange mass and energy (usually in the form of thermal energy) with its surroundings.

2. **Closed system:** A closed system allows for the transfer of energy (heat), but not the transfer of mass.

3. **Isolated system:** An isolated system does not allow for the transfer of either energy or mass.

Heat and Work

Heat, q, is a form of energy and should not be confused with temperature. Temperature is a measure of the heat content of a substance. Heat is a form of energy that can easily transfer from or to a system. Heat added to a system from its surroundings is given a positive value, and heat lost from a system to its surroundings is given a negative value.

Heat change is the most common energy change in chemical processes. It is usually measured in units of calories (or kilocalories, Kcal) or joules (or kilojoules, kJ). An *exothermic* reaction is any process that transfers thermal energy from the reaction to its surroundings. An *endothermic* reaction is any process that requires thermal energy input from the surroundings to the system. Heat is not a property of a system. Instead, it manifests itself during a change. Therefore, the value of heat is dependent upon the reaction pathway.

Every object has a *specific heat capacity*, *C*. This value is dependent on the quantity and chemical makeup of a substance. *Specific heat capacity* is defined as the amount of thermal energy required to raise the temperature of one kilogram of a substance by 1 degree Kelvin. The units of specific heat capacity are J/kg·K and heat capacities for most substances can be found in reference books. The quantity of the amount of heat exchanged when a substance undergoes a change in temperature can be determined by the equation:

$$q = ms\Delta T$$

where s is the specific heat, m is the mass of the substance, and ΔT is the value of the temperature change. Since the specific heat capacity is defined as $C = ms$, the amount of heat exchanged can be determined by the equation:

$$q = C\Delta T$$

Work is another property that depends on the path of a chemical reaction and varies accordingly. Neither heat nor work is considered a state function (properties that are determined by the state of the system). Work is defined by force and distance in the equation:

$$w = Fd$$

where w is work, F is force, and d is distance.

State and State Functions

The states, or phases, of matter are solid, liquid, and gas. Every substance under the proper conditions can exist in any of these three states. The state of a substance or system is defined by macroscopic properties such as temperature (T), pressure (P), volume (V), the internal energy (E) of a system, enthalpy (H), entropy (S), and free energy (G). When a substance undergoes a change of state, these macroscopic properties change also. Thus, these properties are called *state functions*, because they are dependent on the state of a substance or system.

Standard reaction conditions are defined as 25°C and 1 atm. These are the conditions normally used for measuring enthalpy, entropy, and free energy of a reaction. A substance is in its most stable form under standard conditions, and it is considered to be in its standard state. Standard enthalpy changes, standard entropy changes, and standard free energy changes are all measured at 25°C and 1 atm. These measurements are represented by the symbols ΔH°, ΔS°, and ΔG°, respectively.

Enthalpy

Enthalpy is defined as the heat content of a substance at a constant pressure. The enthalpy change, ΔH, is defined by the change in heat content from the initial to the final state of a substance. The change in enthalpy is expressed by the following equation:

$$\Delta H = \Delta E + P\Delta V$$

where ΔE is the change in internal energy, P is the pressure, and ΔV is the change in volume.

Because most reactions take place under conditions of constant pressure, the change in heat of these reactions can be equated to the change in enthalpy. The enthalpy of the reaction is the difference between the enthalpies of the products and the enthalpies of the reactants ($\Delta H = H_{products} - H_{reactants}$). A negative value of ΔH indicates that energy is transferred from the system to its surroundings, and a positive ΔH value indicates that energy is transferred from the surroundings to the system.

The *standard heat of formation* is defined as the enthalpy of the formation of a compound, ΔH°_f if one mole of the compound were formed from its elements in their standard states. The value of ΔH°_f of an element in its standard state is zero. ΔH°_f values for most substances are known.

The standard heat of reaction, $\Delta H°_{rxn}$ is a hypothetical enthalpy change that would occur if the reaction were carried out under standard conditions. It is expressed as the difference between the sum of standard heats of formations of the products and the sum of the standard heats of formation of the reactants.

Hess's law states that if the overall reaction process is the sum of two or more reactions, then the overall ΔH value is the sum of all of the ΔH values of the reaction. Thus, for a multistep reaction, the overall ΔH value is the sum of the ΔH value for each step of the reaction. Hess's law also states that the change in enthalpy of a reaction is the same whether the reaction takes place in one step or in a series of steps. For example, in the formation of CO the following reactions are involved:

$$C + O2_{(g)} \rightarrow CO_{2(g)} \qquad \Delta H°_{rxn} = -393.5 \text{ kJ/mol}$$

$$CO_{2(g)} \rightarrow CO_{(g)} + \frac{1}{2} O_{2(g)} \qquad \Delta H°_{rxn} = +283.0 \text{ kJ/mol}$$

$$C + \frac{1}{2} O_{2(g)} \rightarrow CO_{(g)} \qquad \Delta H°_{rxn} = -110.5 \text{ kJ/mol}$$

Entropy

Entropy, S, is a measure of the randomness and disorder of a system. The greater the entropy value, the greater the disorder of a system. Entropy can be expressed by the equation:

$$\Delta S = \frac{q}{T}$$

where q is the heat absorbed in joules/mole. The units of entropy are J/K mol. Standard entropy values of most substances are known and can be found in a chemistry reference.

The second law of thermodynamics states that the entropy of the universe increases in a spontaneous process and remains unchanged in a process that is at equilibrium. This concept can be expressed mathematically as follows:

In a spontaneous reaction: $\Delta S_{universe} = \Delta S_{system} + \Delta S_{surroundings} > 0$

In a reaction at equilibrium: $\Delta S_{universe} = \Delta S_{system} + \Delta S_{surroundings} = 0$

The standard entropy of a reaction is given by the difference between the sum of the standard entropies of the products and the sum of the standard entropies of the reactants ($\Delta S°_{rxn} = \Sigma n S°_{products} - \Sigma n S°_{reactants}$).

The entropy of the surroundings of a system can be expressed in terms of the change in enthalpy of a system and the temperature (in Kelvin):

$$\Delta S_{surr} = \frac{-\Delta H_{sys}}{T}$$

The change in entropy of the universe is expressed as the sum of the change in energy of the system and the change in energy of the surroundings:

$$\Delta S_{univ} = \Delta S_{sys} + \Delta S_{surr}$$

TIP

In almost all mathematical calculations involving temperature, the temperature must be converted from degrees Celsius to degrees Kelvin: 0°C = 273.15K.

Gibbs Free Energy

Gibbs free energy, or free energy, is defined as the energy available to do work. In other words, it is the amount of available, or free, energy in a system. The mathematical expression that relates free energy to enthalpy and entropy is:

$$G = H - TS$$

where T is the temperature in degrees Kelvin.

The free energy value of a system can more directly express the spontaneity of a reaction as compared to enthalpy and entropy. The change in free energy, ΔG, for a system during a process of constant temperature and pressure is given by the equation:

$$\Delta G = \Delta H - T\Delta S$$

A negative ΔG value indicates the release of usable energy during a reaction. This type of reaction is spontaneous. If the value of ΔG is positive, this indicates that additional energy is required for a reaction to proceed. The reaction is nonspontaneous. A ΔG value of zero indicates that the system is at equilibrium. The spontaneity of a reaction is independent of the reaction rate. A spontaneous reaction may proceed at a very slow rate, but it is thermodynamically favored.

The standard free energy, $\Delta G°$, is defined as the ΔG of a process occurring under standard state conditions. The standard free energy of formation, $\Delta G°_f$, is the free energy change that occurs when one mole of a compound in its standard state is formed from elements in their standard state. The free energy of formation of an element in its most stable form (standard state) is zero. The standard free energy of a reaction, $\Delta G°_{rxn}$, is the free energy change when a reaction is carried out under standard conditions.

The relationship between ΔG (nonstandard state) and $\Delta G°$ (standard state) can be seen in the following mathematical expression:

$$\Delta G = \Delta G° + RT\ln Q$$

where R is the gas constant, T is temperature in degrees Kelvin, and Q is the reaction quotient. At equilibrium, this equation becomes:

$$0 = \Delta G° + RT\ln K$$

or

$$\Delta G° = - RT\ln K$$

where K is the equilibrium constant and ΔG is equal to zero.

CHEMICAL KINETICS AND EQUILIBRIUM

In order to best understand a chemical reaction, it is necessary to know the chemical components of the reaction, the conditions under which the reaction proceeds, the mechanism of the reaction, the rate at which it occurs, and 5. the equilibrium state toward which it proceeds.

Kinetics

Chemical kinetics is the study of the rates of chemical reactions, or how fast they occur. The rate of a reaction is dependent upon the mechanism of the reaction. The reaction rate is a measure of the change in the concentration of reactants and the products over time. Kinetics deals with how fast the reactants are transformed into products.

Any chemical reaction can be represented by the generic equation:

$$\text{reactants} \rightarrow \text{products}$$

This equation indicates that over the course of a chemical reaction, reactants are consumed and products are formed. Reaction rates can be expressed in terms of the change in concentration over time. The mathematical expression for the reaction rate is:

$$\text{rate} = -\frac{\Delta\left[\text{reactants}\right]}{\Delta t}$$

OR

$$\text{rate} = \frac{\Delta\left[\text{products}\right]}{\Delta t}$$

where the brackets indicate concentration, Δ indicates change, and t represents time.

Reaction Mechanisms

The mechanism of a chemical reaction is the series of steps that make up the overall reaction. In the generalized reaction below, the overall reaction can be divided into reaction steps.

$$\text{Overall reaction: } 2A + B_2 \rightarrow 2AB$$

$$\text{Step 1: } A + B_2 \rightarrow AB_2 \text{ (slow)}$$

$$\text{Step 2: } AB_2 + A \rightarrow 2AB \text{ (fast)}$$

The formation of the compound AB_2 does not fall under the category of reactant or product; therefore, it is considered an intermediate. Reaction intermediates can be difficult to detect, especially if the reaction rate is very fast. Notice that the two steps of the overall reaction occur at different rates (step 1 = slow and step 2 = fast). The slowest step in the reaction is called the *rate-determining step*. The overall rate of the reaction cannot occur faster than the rate of this step.

The stoichiometry of a chemical reaction can give an idea about the relative rates of the consumption of reactants and formation of products. For example, in the reaction:

$$2A + B \rightarrow C$$

the reactant A is used up twice as fast as the reactant B. A is also consumed twice as fast as C is formed. The rate of each component of the reaction takes into account the stoichiometric coefficient:

$$\text{rate} = \frac{-1}{2}\left(\frac{\Delta\left[A\right]}{\Delta t}\right) = -\frac{\Delta\left[B\right]}{\Delta t} = \frac{\Delta\left[C\right]}{\Delta t}$$

The value of the rate is expressed in units of moles per liter per second (mol/L s). A general equation for the rates of reaction includes the stoichiometric coefficients as a fraction ($1/x$) and the change in concentration over time.

Rate Law and Reaction Order

The rate law expresses the relationship of the reaction rate to a rate constant and the concentration of each reactant raised to a power that is determined experimentally by the order of the reaction. For the general reaction $aA + bB \rightarrow cC + dD$, the rate law is expressed by the equation:

$$\text{rate} = k[A]^x[B]^y$$

where k is the rate constant, $[A]$ and $[B]$ are the concentrations of the reactions, and the exponents correspond to the order of the reaction. The rate constant is defined as a proportionality constant between the reaction rate and the concentration of reactants. The rate constant varies for each element and can be determined experimentally if the rate and concentration of a reaction is known ($k = \text{rate}/[A][B]$).

k has the unit of 1/time in a first-order reaction, l/mol time in a second-order reaction, and mol/L time in a zero-order reaction. The order of the reaction is determined experimentally with respect to each reactant, and the overall order of the reaction is defined as the sum of each exponent (for the above reaction the order is $x + y$).

Reaction order enables one to understand how the reaction is dependent on the concentration of a given reactant. In the reaction $aA + bB \rightarrow cC + dD$, where the rate is $k[A][B]^2$, the reaction orders are $x = 1$ and $y = 2$. This reaction is first order for A ($x = 1$) and second order for B ($y = 2$). The overall reaction order is 3 ($1 + 2$), so this is a third-order equation. Thus, if the concentration of the reactant A is doubled, the reaction rate is doubled, and if the concentration of B is doubled, the reaction rate increases four-fold. An exponent of 0 (zero order) indicates that the reaction is independent of a given reactant.

In summary:

- The rate law of a reaction is determined experimentally. The reaction order can be determined by the concentration of the reactants. The rate constant is determined by the rate and the concentration of the reactants.

- Reaction order is always defined in terms of the concentration of a given reactant.

- The reaction order is independent of the stoichiometric coefficient of the reactant.

- A first-order reaction is one in which the rate depends on the reaction rate raised to the first power.

- A second-order reaction is one in which the rate depends upon 1. the concentration of the reactant raised to the second power, or 2. the concentration of two reactants raised to the first power.

- A zero-order reaction is one in which the rate is independent of a given reactant.

Collision Theory

The collision theory of chemical kinetics states that the rate of the reaction is directly proportional to the number of collisions between the molecules in a reaction. In a chemical reaction, the reaction rate almost always increases as the temperature increases. As the temperature increases, the kinetic energy of the molecules of a reaction increase, thus this tends to increase the number of collisions of the reactant molecules. An *effective collision* occurs if the molecules collide in the correct orientation and with sufficient force to break and form bonds. The *activation energy* (E_a) is the minimum energy required for the collisions to be strong enough to initiate the chemical reaction. Only a fraction of the molecules in a chemical reaction have sufficient kinetic energy to overcome the activation energy barrier. When reactants collide, they form an *activated complex*, or transition state, which is a temporary species formed by the reactant molecules as a result of the collision. The transition state complex forms before the final product is formed, and the transition state has a greater energy than either the reactants or the products.

Potential Energy Diagram

A potential energy diagram shows the relationship between the potential energy of a reaction, the activation energy, and the heats of reaction. It also shows the difference between the relative potential energy of the reactants and the products. The enthalpy change, ΔH, of the overall reaction is the difference between the potential energy of the products and the potential energy of the reactants. A negative ΔH value indicates an exothermic reaction and a positive ΔH value indicates an endothermic reaction. The transition state is found at the top of the energy barrier. The activation energy of the forward progressing reaction is the difference between the potential energy of the transition state and the reactants. The difference between the potential energy of the transition state and the products is the activation energy of the reverse reaction.

Figure 10. Diagrams of Potential Energy

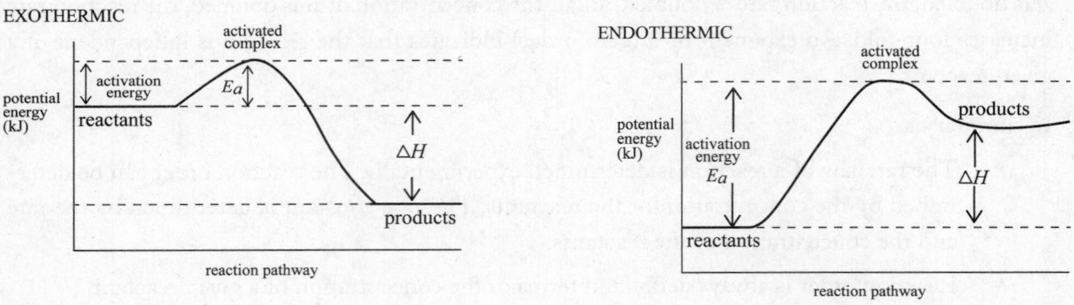

Factors That Affect Reaction Rate

The rate of a chemical reaction is dependent upon the substances that are reacting, their concentrations, and the environmental factors of the reaction:

- **Reaction concentration:** The greater the concentration of the reactants, the greater number of collisions between molecules per unit of time. Thus, an increase in concentration of reactants greater than zero order to a determined maximum level will increase the reaction rate.

- **Temperature:** In almost all reactions, an increase in temperature will increase the reaction rate. This is due to the fact that an increase in temperature causes an increase in the kinetic energy of the reactant molecules. Therefore, the proportion of the number of molecules with an energy above the activation energy barrier is greater at increasing temperatures.

- **Medium:** The rate of a reaction may be affected by the medium in which it takes place. For example, certain reactions proceed more rapidly in an aqueous (water) environment than in other solvents. The state—solid, liquid, or gas—may also have an effect on the reaction rate.

- **Catalysis:** A catalyst is a substance that increases the rate of a chemical reaction without being consumed in the reaction. A catalyst acts by lowering the activation energy barrier of a reaction. This increases the number of molecules with potential energy greater than the activation energy and, thus, increases the number of collisions, so the reaction proceeds at a faster rate.

Equilibrium

Equilibrium is a state in which no observable change occurs. When a chemical reaction reaches a state of equilibrium, there is no observable change in the concentration of the reactants and the products. However, during equilibrium, there is still activity at the molecular level. Reactant molecules continue to form products, and product molecules break down into the original reactant molecules. Chemical equilibrium is thus achieved when the rates of the forward and reverse reactions are equal, and the concentration of the reactants and the products remains constant. In the generalized equation:

$$A \rightleftarrows B$$

there is an equal concentration of both A and B and the forward and reverse reactions occur at an equal rate.

Law of Mass Action

The law of mass action maintains that for a reversible reaction at equilibrium and constant temperature, a given ratio of reactant and product concentrations has a constant value, K. This value, K, is called the *equilibrium constant*. In the generalized reaction:

$$aA + bB \rightarrow cC + dD$$

the equilibrium constant can be expressed as follows:

$$K = \frac{[C]^c [D]^d}{[A]^a [B]^b}$$

In general, the equilibrium constant for the forward and reverse reactions in a gas is not equal because the partial pressures of the reactants and products are not equal to their concentrations. The two equilibrium constants can be related in the equation:

$$K_p = K_c (RT) \Delta^n$$

where K_p represents the equilibrium constants of a gas (the p indicates that it is in terms of partial pressure) and K_c represents the equilibrium constant in terms of concentration.

The following are some basic properties that apply to the equilibrium constant:

- Pure solids and liquids do not factor into the equation for the equilibrium constant, K.

- K is characteristic of a given reaction at a specific temperature.

- The equilibrium constant helps to predict the direction in which a reaction will proceed (forward or reverse) to achieve a state of equilibrium.

- The equilibrium constant can be used to determine the equilibrium concentration of reactants and products.

- If the value of *K* is much greater than 1, the equilibrium mixture contains very little reactants as compared to products.

- If the value of *K* is more than ten-fold less than 1 (less than 0.1), the equilibrium mixture will contain very little product as compared to reactants.

- If the value of *K* is close to 1, there will be a relatively equal amount of reactants and products.

Factors That Affect Chemical Equilibrium

Changes in experimental conditions can affect the balance of a reaction and shift the equilibrium position so that either more or less of the product is formed. Variables affecting the equilibrium of a reaction are concentration, pressure, volume, and temperature. There is a general rule that helps to predict the direction in which an equilibrium reaction will move when it undergoes a change in one of these conditions. Le Chatelier's principle states: If an external stress is applied to an equilibrium reaction, or system, the system responds by adjusting the reaction in a way that offsets the stress as the system achieves a new equilibrium. *Stress* refers to a change in concentration, pressure, volume, or temperature:

- **Changes in concentration:** According to Le Chatelier's principle, increasing the concentration of a substance in a reaction will cause a shift in the reaction away from that substance in order to establish a new equilibrium. Increasing the concentration of the product will shift the equilibrium to the left (toward the reactants), and decreasing the concentration of the product will cause a shift to the right (toward the products).

- **Changes in pressure or volume:** In a system at a constant temperature, an increase in pressure causes a decrease in volume, and a decrease in pressure causes an increase in volume for gases. Changes in pressure and volume have little effect on solids and liquids, but do have an effect on equilibrium reactions involving gases. When pressure is increased (and volume decreased), the equilibrium will shift such that the side of the reaction with fewer moles of molecules will be favored. If the volume is increased (pressure decreased), the same principle applies.

- **Changes in temperature:** A change in temperature can actually alter the value of the equilibrium constant as well as shift the position of the equilibrium of a reaction. An increase in temperature favors the endothermic direction of a reaction and a decrease in temperature favors the exothermic direction of a reaction. Consequently, a temperature increase causes an increase in the equilibrium constant, and a temperature decrease causes a decrease in the value of the equilibrium constant.

PRACTICE QUESTIONS

Directions: Choose the best answer for each question.

Refer to the following passage for Questions 1–4.

Substances can exist on Earth in three states: solid, liquid, and gas. Solids are generally the densest, while gases tend to be the least dense, with liquids typically falling right in the middle. A phase diagram provides the temperatures and pressures at which a given substance exists in each of the three states.

1. The ideal gas law is expressed by the equation
   A. $P_1 V_1 = P_2 V_2$
   B. $\dfrac{P_1}{T_1} = \dfrac{P_2}{T_2}$
   C. $P_{total} = P_1 + P_2 + P_3 \ldots$
   D. $PV = nRT$

2. The temperature and pressure at which a substance can exist as a solid, liquid, and vapor is called the
   A. boiling point.
   B. melting point.
   C. critical temperature.
   D. triple point.

3. Which of the following elements exists in nature as a diatomic molecule?
   A. Oxygen
   B. Magnesium
   C. Potassium
   D. Ozone

4. Which type of connection is responsible for the low melting points of molecular crystals?
   A. Intramolecular forces
   B. Van der Waals forces
   C. Covalent bonds
   D. Ionic bonds

Refer to the following passage for Questions 5–7.

Though not a molecule of any kind, heat energy can still be an input or an output in a chemical reaction. However, the heat of a chemical reaction, the enthalpy, differs from Gibbs free energy, which determines the spontaneity of a chemical reaction.

5. Given the information below, what is the standard heat of formation of acetylene (C_2H_2)?

   Overall reaction: $2C_{graphite} + H_{2(g)} \rightarrow C_2H_{2(g)}$

   $C_{graphite} + O_{2(g)} \rightarrow CO_{2(g)} \qquad \Delta H^r rxn = $ -393.5 kJ/mol

   $H_{2(g)} + \dfrac{1}{2} O_{2(g)} \rightarrow H_2O_{(\ell)} \qquad \Delta H^r rxn = $ -285.8 kJ/mol

   $2C_2H_{2(g)} + 5O_{2(g)} \rightarrow 4CO_{2(g)} + 2H_2O_{(\ell)}$
   $\Delta H^r rxn = $ -1073.6 kJ/mol
   A. 1299.4 kJ/mol
   B. 226.6 kJ/mol
   C. -787.0 kJ/mol
   D. -1752.9 kJ/mol

6. What is the quantity of heat absorbed by a substance with a specific heat of 4.18 J/g°C and a mass of 50.0 g when the temperature changes from 15°C to 94°C?
   A. 224 J
   B. 19.6 kJ
   C. 944.9 J
   D. 16.5 kJ

7. If the potential energy of a product is greater than that of its reactants, the reaction is
   A. spontaneous.
   B. exothermic.
   C. endothermic.
   D. heat-releasing.

The following questions are standalone and not tied to a passage.

8. Which of the following is the correct order in which electrons fill the orbitals of an atom?
   A. $3s \rightarrow 2s \rightarrow 2p \rightarrow 1s$
   B. $3s \rightarrow 2p \rightarrow 2s \rightarrow 1s$
   C. $1s \rightarrow 2p \rightarrow 2s \rightarrow 3s$
   D. $1s \rightarrow 2s \rightarrow 2p \rightarrow 3s$

9. Which of the following is an example of a covalent compound?
   A. CO_2
   B. HCl
   C. NaCl
   D. $CuSO_4 \cdot 5H_2O$

10. The idea that the same type of compound always contains the same elements in the same ratio is the
    A. law of conservation of mass.
    B. law of definite proportions.
    C. law of multiple proportions.
    D. second law of thermodynamics.

11. A bond in which electrons are shared between two atoms is a(n)
    A. ionic bond.
    B. covalent bond.
    C. electronegative bond.
    D. molecular bond.

12. The angular momentum quantum number
    A. determines the energy level of an electron orbital.
    B. describes the orientation of the electron orbital.
    C. indicates the shape of an electron orbital.
    D. describes the direction of electron spin.

13. A reaction in which an atom from one molecule is transferred to another molecule is called a
    A. displacement reaction.
    B. combination reaction.
    C. decomposition reaction.
    D. neutralization reaction.

14. The particle in an element that does not vary in quantity for a given element or its ionic forms is the
    A. proton.
    B. neutron.
    C. electron.
    D. nucleus.

15. How much sodium hydroxide must be added to 250 mL of water to make a 1 M solution?
    A. 10 g
    B. 20 g
    C. 40 g
    D. 160 g

16. Which of the following elements has the smallest atomic radius?
    A. Li
    B. F
    C. O
    D. Mg

17. The oxidation number of O_2 is
    A. 0
    B. +1
    C. +2
    D. -1

18. If the rate of an equation is given as $k[A]^2[B]$, the reaction order of each reactant is
    A. A = second order, B = zero order.
    B. A = second order, B = first order.
    C. A = first order, B = zero order.
    D. A = first order, B = second order.

19. According to the VSEPR model, repulsive forces of electrons decrease as follows
    A. Bonding pair vs. bonding pair > lone pair vs. bonding pair > lone pair vs. lone pair
    B. Lone pair vs. bonding pair > lone pair vs. lone pair > bonding pair vs. bonding pair
    C. Lone pair vs. lone pair > lone pair vs. bonding pair > bonding pair vs. bonding pair
    D. Bonding pair vs. bonding pair > lone pair vs. lone pair > lone pair vs. bonding pair

20. A K_a value of 1×10^6 and a K_b value of 1×10^{-11} indicate a
    A. weak acid and a weak base.
    B. weak acid and a strong base.
    C. strong acid and a weak base.
    D. strong acid and a strong base.

ANSWER KEY AND EXPLANATIONS

1. D	**5.** B	**9.** A	**13.** A	**17.** A
2. D	**6.** D	**10.** B	**14.** A	**18.** B
3. A	**7.** C	**11.** B	**15.** A	**19.** C
4. B	**8.** D	**12.** C	**16.** B	**20.** C

1. **The correct answer is D.** The ideal gas law describes the relationship between $P, V, T,$ and n in one equation. The equation $PV = nRT$ expresses the ideal gas law mathematically. Choice A is incorrect because the equation $P_1V_1 = P_2V_2$ represents Boyle's law stating that the pressure of a fixed amount of gas at a constant temperature is inversely proportional to the volume of the gas. Choice B is incorrect because Charles's law (or Gay-Lussac's law) can be manipulated to compare two sets of volume and temperature at a constant gas pressure: $\frac{P_1}{T_1} = \frac{P_2}{T_2}$. Choice C is incorrect because the equation $P_{total} = P_1 + P_2 + P_3...$ represents Dalton's law of partial pressures, which states that a mixture of gases is equal to the sum of the pressure that would be exerted by each individual gas if it occupied the space on its own.

2. **The correct answer is D.** The triple point is the unique point on the graph that is the exact temperature and pressure at which all three phases, or states, can exist simultaneously. Choice A is incorrect because the boiling point is the temperature and pressure at which the liquid and vapor phases exist together. Choice B is incorrect because the melting point is the temperature and pressure at which a solid and a liquid exist together. Choice C is incorrect because the critical point is the temperature above which a gas will no longer change into a liquid.

3. **The correct answer is A.** Oxygen is an element that is commonly found in the form O_2, which is a diatomic molecule that is composed of two oxygen atoms. Choice B is incorrect because magnesium is commonly found as a single atom. Choice C is incorrect because potassium is commonly found as a single atom. Choice D is incorrect because ozone is a compound composed of three oxygen atoms and is considered a polyatomic molecule, not an element.

4. **The correct answer is B.** Molecular crystals are composed of molecules held together by van der Waals forces or hydrogen bonds. These very weak bonding interactions are easily broken and contribute to the low melting point of molecular crystals. Choice A is incorrect because intramolecular forces are the forces that hold individual atoms together, not molecules. Molecules are held together by intermolecular forces. Choice C is incorrect because covalent bonds are strong bonds that hold covalent crystals together. The strong covalent bonds in three-dimensional covalent crystals give them a very high melting point. Choice D is incorrect because ionic bonds are what hold ionic crystals together. These are strong interactions, and ionic crystals have high melting points.

5. **The correct answer is B.** Adding the heats of enthalpy for each stoichiometrically correct reaction step in the formation of acetylene gives a value for the overall reaction of 226.6 kJ/mol. Choice A is incorrect because 1299.4 kJ/mol is the enthalpy for the third step in the reaction where acetylene is formed from

CO_2 and H_2O. Choice C is incorrect because −787.0 kJ/mol is the heat of enthalpy for the formation of carbon dioxide from graphite and oxygen. Choice D is incorrect because −1752.9 kJ/mol is the sum of the enthalpies of reaction for each step without balancing or reversing the equations.

6. **The correct answer is D.** The heat absorbed by a reaction is determined by the equation $q = ms\Delta T$, therefore the heat absorbed by the given substance is 16.5 kJ. Choice A is incorrect because this value only takes into account the starting temperature of 15°C, not the change in temperature. Choice B is incorrect because this value only takes into account the final temperature of 94°C, not the temperature change. Choice C is incorrect because this value is calculated from rearranging the equation to $q = m\Delta T/s$, which is not the correct equation for calculating the heat absorbed by a substance.

7. **The correct answer is C.** A reaction in which the potential energy of the products is greater than the potential energy of the reactants is an endothermic reaction. This reaction requires the addition of energy, usually in the form of thermal energy, to move in the forward direction. Choice A is incorrect because a spontaneous reaction is an exothermic reaction. An exothermic reaction is one in which the potential energy of the reactants is greater than that of the products. Choice B is incorrect because an exothermic reaction is one in which the potential energy of the reactants is greater than the potential energy of the products. Choice D is incorrect because an exothermic reaction releases heat, and in an exothermic reaction the potential energy of the products is lower than that of the reactants.

8. **The correct answer is D.** The rules of electron configuration state that electrons are added to the allowable orbitals for each

atom starting with the lowest energy level, and increasing in energy levels until all the electrons occupy an orbital. Electrons fill the orbitals in the following order: $1s \rightarrow 2s \rightarrow 2p \rightarrow 3s$. Choice A is incorrect because the $3s$ orbital is the highest energy level of the four orbitals, so it would be filled last. Choice B is incorrect because the $3s$ orbital would be filled last because it has the highest energy level, and the $2s$ orbital would fill before the $2p$ orbital since the s orbitals are lower in energy than the p orbitals. Choice C is incorrect because the $2s$ orbital would fill before the $2p$ orbital because the $2s$ orbital is lower in energy.

9. **The correct answer is A.** CO_2, or carbon dioxide, is an example of a covalent compound in which each carbon atom is covalently bonded to 2 oxygen atoms (double bond in this case). Choice B is incorrect because HCl, while a gas, is considered an ionic compound because in water the hydrogen atom exists as H^+ (definition of an acid) and the chlorine atom has a negative charge as Cl^-. Choice C is incorrect because NaCl is an example of an ionic compound, formed from a Na^+ ion and a Cl^- ion. Choice D is incorrect because $CuSO_4.5H_2O$, while an example of a hydrate, is also ionic, formed by a Cu^{+2} ion and SO_4^{-2} ion.

10. **The correct answer is B.** The law of definite proportions states that different samples of the same compound always contain their same constituent elements in the same mass proportion. Choice A is incorrect because the law of conservation of mass states that matter cannot be created or destroyed. Therefore, the mass of all matter on Earth remains constant, even if it changes state or chemical composition. Choice C is incorrect because the law of multiple proportions states that if two elements combine to form more than one compound, the masses of one element that combine with a fixed mass of the second

element are in ratios of small whole numbers. Choice D is incorrect because the second law of thermodynamics states that the entropy of the universe increases in a spontaneous process.

11. **The correct answer is B.** A bond in which electrons are shared between two atoms is called a covalent bond. Choice A is incorrect because in an ionic bond electrons are transferred from one atom to another. Choice C is incorrect because there is no such thing as an electronegative bond. Electronegativity is the ability of an atom to attract electrons toward itself in a chemical bond. Choice D is incorrect because there is no such thing as a molecular bond. Molecules join together through covalent bonds.

12. **The correct answer is C.** The angular momentum, ℓ, indicates the shape of the orbital. Choice A is incorrect because the principle quantum number, n, determines the energy level of the orbital. Choice B is incorrect because the magnetic quantum number, m_ℓ, describes the orientation of the electron orbital in space. Choice D is incorrect because the electron spin quantum number, m_s, takes into account that there are two possible spinning motions (rotations) of an electron, clockwise or counterclockwise.

13. **The correct answer is A.** In a displacement reaction, an atom from one molecule is transferred to another molecule. This type of reaction is written using the following formula: $A + BX \rightarrow AX + B$. Choice B is incorrect because a combination reaction is one in which two or more elements or molecules are combined to form a product. Choice C is incorrect because a decomposition reaction involves the chemical breakdown of a substance into two or more products. Choice D is incorrect because a neutralization reaction is specialized reaction that involves acids and bases. In this type of reaction, an acid and a base combine to form a salt and water.

14. **The correct answer is A.** The number of protons in an atom does not vary, even if the element is in its ionic form. Choice B is incorrect because the number of neutrons for a given atom can vary and give rise to various isotopes of an atom. Choice C is incorrect because an atom can readily gain and lose an electron in the process of ionization. Choice D is incorrect because the nucleus of an atom is not a separate particle; it contains the protons and neutrons of the atom.

15. **The correct answer is A.** The molecular weight of NaOH is about 40 g/mol; therefore, the amount of NaOH that needs to be added to a 250 mL solution to make it 1 M is 10 g. The value of 10 g corresponds to 0.250 mol of solute, which is the amount required to make a 1 m solution. Choice B is incorrect because using the molecular weight of 40 g/mol NaOH it is determined that only 10 g of sodium hydroxide are needed to make a 1 M solution of 250 mL. Choice C is incorrect because 40 is the value of the molecular weight of NaOH (40 g/mol), not the amount of solute that must be added to make a 1 M solution. Choice D is incorrect because 160 g would be the value obtained by dividing the molecular mass of NaOH by the number of moles (0.250 mol) of solute.

16. **The correct answer is B.** As the nuclear charge increases, there is a decrease in the atomic radius. Therefore, the atomic radius decreases across the Periodic Table from left to right in a period. Within a group, the atomic radius increases down the group. Fluorine, F, is on the right side of the Periodic Table and has the smallest radius of all the elements listed. Choice A is incorrect because lithium has the largest atomic radius of all the elements listed.

Choice C is incorrect because oxygen is to the left of fluorine on the periodic table and has the larger radius of the two. Choice D is incorrect because magnesium is on the left side of the Periodic Table and has a much larger radius than F.

17. **The correct answer is A.** Pure elements have an oxidation number of zero. Therefore, pure oxygen (O_2) has an oxidation number of 0. Choice B is incorrect because pure elements have an oxidation number of 0. Choice C is incorrect because pure oxygen has an oxidation number of 0. Choice D is incorrect because pure elements have an oxidation number of 0.

18. **The correct answer is B.** The exponents of each reactant concentration in the rate equation determine the reaction order of the equation. Therefore, in the rate equation rate = $k[A]^2[B]$, the reactant A is second order and B is first order. (No exponent is necessary for a first-order equation.) Choice A is incorrect because B is first order, not zero order. Choice C is incorrect because A is second order and B is first order. Choice D is incorrect because A is second order and B is first order.

19. **The correct answer is C.** According to the VSEPR model, the repulsive forces of electrons decrease as follows: lone pair vs. lone pair > lone pair vs. bonding pair > bonding pair vs. bonding pair. Choice A is incorrect because repulsive forces decrease in the opposite direction of the order shown in this choice. Choices B and D are incorrect because repulsive electron forces decrease as follows: lone pair vs. lone pair > lone pair vs. bonding pair > bonding pair vs. bonding pair.

20. **The correct answer is C.** A high value of K_a indicates a strong acid, and a low K_b value indicates a weak base. Choice A is incorrect because the high K_a value indicates a strong acid. Choice B is incorrect because a high K_a value indicates a strong base. Choice D is incorrect because a low K_b value indicates a weak base.

SUMMING IT UP

- All matter can be described in terms of its chemical and physical properties.

- A chemical substance can exist in one of four states of matter: solid, liquid, gas, or plasma.

- The law of conservation of mass states that matter cannot be created or destroyed. Therefore, the mass of all matter on Earth remains constant, even if it changes state or chemical composition.

- Pure substances are composed of one species; they can be elements, molecules, or compounds.

- A heterogeneous mixture can be a colloid, emulsion, dispersion, or suspension.

- An *atom* is defined as the basic unit of an element that can be chemically combined with like or different elements. An atom is made up of protons, neutrons, and electrons.

- *Electrons* surround the nucleus of an atom and are arranged in different orbits around the nucleus. These orbits have different energy levels, and the closer an electron is to the nucleus, the higher its energy level.

- The *mass number, A,* is the total number of neutrons and protons present in the nucleus of an atom of a given element. The mass number is generally given by the formula $A = Z$ + number of neutrons.

- An *atomic mass unit*, amu, is a mass exactly equal to one twelfth the mass of one ^{12}C atom. The mass of an individual atom depends on the number of electron, protons, and neutrons it contains.

- A *mole* is the amount of a substance that contains as many atoms (or molecules, or particles) as there are atoms in exactly 12 grams (g) of ^{12}C. This number is defined as Avogadro's number 6.022×10^{23}.

- The molecular mass can be calculated by multiplying the atomic mass of each element by the number of atoms of that element present in each molecule and adding all the values for each specific element.

- *Electromagnetic radiation* is the emission and transmission of energy in the form of electromagnetic waves.

- Planck gave the name *quantum* to the smallest quantity of energy that can be emitted, or absorbed, in the form of electromagnetic radiation. The energy, *E,* of a single quantum is given by the equation $E = h\nu$.

- Spectral lines at discrete wavelengths are produced by hot, low-density gases. These discrete wavelengths are dependent on the energy levels of the atoms in the gas.

- *Line spectra* are light emissions at specific and discrete wavelengths.

- The atomic absorption spectra is developed from the discrete wavelengths observed when a hot solid is viewed through a cool, low-density gas. The wavelength is dependent on the energy of the atoms of the given solid.

- Bohr's model of the atom included the idea of electrons moving in orbits around the nucleus of the atom. In Bohr's model, the energy of the electron orbitals is derived from photon energies given by the Planck-Einstein equation.

- When an electron moves from a higher-energy orbital to a lower energy orbital, the energy drop within the atom equals the energy of an emitted photon.

- The amount of energy involved in the movement of the electron to either a higher- or lower-energy orbital is determined by the distance between the initial and final orbitals.

- The *Heisenberg uncertainty principle* states that it is impossible to determine the position and momentum of a particle, such as an electron, at the same time.

- De Broglie's wave-particle theory showed that waves can behave like particles, and particles can behave like waves. Particle and wave properties can be related by the expression $\lambda = h/mu$.

- Schrödinger formulated an equation based on de Broglie's wave-particle theory to describe the behavior and energies of submicroscopic particles. His equation is analogous to Newton's laws of motion for larger macroscopic objects.

- The *principle quantum number, n,* is an integer (1, 2, 3, . . .) whose value determines the energy level of the orbital.

- The *angular momentum, ℓ,* indicates the shape of the orbital. The values of ℓ depend on the value of the principle quantum number.

- The *magnetic quantum number, m_ℓ,* describes the orientation of the electron orbital in space. For each value of ℓ in a subshell, there are $(2\ell + 1)$ integral values of m_ℓ:

- The *electron spin quantum number, m_s,* takes into account that there are two possible spinning motions (rotations) of an electron, clockwise or counterclockwise. Thus, m_s has a value of either $+\frac{1}{2}$ or $-\frac{1}{2}$.

- The three orbitals—*s, p,* and *d*—have distinct characteristics. *s* orbitals approximate a spherical shape, *p* orbitals are shaped like a dumbbell, and *d* orbitals are balloon-shaped orbitals mainly in groups of four around the nucleus.

- The energies of the orbitals in the hydrogen atom (single electron) increase as follows: $1s < 2s = 2p < 3s = 3p = 3d < 4s = 4p = 4d = 4f < . . .$

- Electrons fill the orbitals in the following order: $1s \rightarrow 2s \rightarrow 2p \rightarrow 3s \rightarrow 3p \rightarrow 4s \rightarrow 3d \rightarrow 4p \rightarrow 5s \rightarrow 4d \rightarrow 5p \rightarrow 6s \rightarrow 4f \rightarrow 5d \rightarrow 6p \rightarrow 7s \rightarrow 5f \rightarrow 6d \rightarrow 7p$.

- The *Aufbau,* or *building-up, principle* dictates that as protons are added one by one to the nucleus, electrons are similarly added to the atomic orbitals. The maximum of two electrons can be placed in any given orbital, and electrons fill the orbitals from lowest energy to highest energy.

- *Madelung's rule* states that orbitals are filled in order of increasing $n + \ell$. When two orbitals have the same $n + \ell$ value, the orbital with the lower n-value fills first.

- The *Pauli exclusion principle* states that no two electrons in an atom can have the same four quantum numbers. If two electrons in the same atomic orbital have the same n, ℓ, and m_ℓ values, then they must have opposite m_s values ($+\frac{1}{2}$ or $-\frac{1}{2}$).

- *Hund's rule* states that the most stable arrangement of electrons in a subshell is the one with the greatest number of parallel spins.

- The Periodic Table lists each element with its name, symbol, atomic number, and average atomic mass.

- The eighteen columns of the Periodic Table are called *groups*, and the seven rows are called *periods*. Elements can also be categorized based on their electron subshells.

- The three broad categories of the elements in the Periodic Table are metals, metalloids, and nonmetals.

- The *atomic radius* is half the distance between the nuclei of two touching atoms of an element. As the nuclear charge across a period increases, the electrons are drawn closer to the nucleus. This causes a decrease in the atomic radius of elements from left to right across the periods on the Periodic Table of Elements.

- The *electron affinity*, E_{ea}, of an element is the energy change when an electron is added to, or removed from, an atom in its gaseous state to form an anion (negatively charged ion). On the Periodic Table, electron affinity increases across a period and decreases down a period.

- *Ionization energy* is the minimum energy required to remove an electron from an atom in its gaseous state. Ionization energies increase going across a period because the increase in the nuclear charge and the reduced atomic radius hold the electron to the atom more tightly. Moving down a group in the Periodic Table, ionization energy decreases because the valence electrons are further from the nucleus and more shielded from the nuclear charge and, thus, easier to remove.

- *Electronegativity* is the ability of an atom to attract electrons toward itself in a chemical bond between two atoms. In general, electronegativity increases across a period and decreases down a group on the Periodic Table. Smaller, higher nuclear-charged atoms tend to have a higher relative electronegativity.

- A *molecule* is composed of at least two or more atoms in a definite arrangement and held together by chemical forces, or bonds. A molecule may consist of atoms of the same element, or it may be composed of atoms of different elements.

- An *ion* is an atom or group of atoms that has an overall positive or negative charge. Since the number of protons in the nucleus remains constant, it is the gain or loss of electrons that determines the charge.

- A *compound* is made up of two or more different types of elements joined together in a fixed ratio. All compounds are molecules, but not all molecules are compounds.

- Since there are over 20 million compounds known today, chemists have devised a way to systematically name all of the compounds. This system is known as *nomenclature*.

- *Ionic bonds* are electrostatic forces between two oppositely charged ions. An ionic bond usually forms when electrons are transferred from a metal ion to a nonmetal atom.

- In their solid state, ionic compounds form a crystal lattice structure in arrangement that maximizes the amount of ions in a given space.

- Ions that have a small radius will pack closer to one another, which results in a decrease in the charge separation and an increase in bond strength.

- The greater the charge difference between the two ions in an ionic compound, the stronger the bond. Thus, the more electrons that are transferred to form ions, the stronger the ionic bond between them.

- *Coulomb's law* states the potential energy, *E*, between two ions is directly proportional to the product of their charges and inversely proportional to the distance between the two ions.

- *Ionic compounds*, in general, have similar characteristics: solid at room temperature, soluble in polar solvents, electrically conductive in solution, and 4. low thermal conductivity.

- A bond in which electrons are shared between two atoms is called a *covalent bond*. Covalent bonds only involve the interaction of valence shell electrons. This allows for atoms to achieve a stable octet in a fixed geometric structure of a molecule or a compound.

- Covalent bonds are characterized by their bond length, bond dissociation energy, and bond energy.

- In general, covalent compounds exhibit the following characteristics and properties: they exist in various states at room temperature, have variable melting and boiling points, are not electrically conductive, and have low thermal conductivity.

- In general, covalent compounds (molecules) will assume a geometry that minimizes repulsion between atoms. This approach to molecular geometry is called the *valence-shell electron-pair repulsion (VSEPR) model*.

- *Lewis dot diagrams* consist of the element symbol surrounded by a dot for each valence electron. Chemical bonds can be represented by this type of diagram.

- A *resonance structure* is simply one of two or more Lewis dot diagrams that can represent a single molecule, which cannot be accurately represented by a single diagram.

- The *formal charge* of an atom is equal to the difference of the number of electrons officially assigned to an atom in a bond and the number of valence electrons in a free atom. The formal charge, C_f, can be calculated using the following formula $C_f = V - [\frac{1}{2} N_{bonding} + N_{nonbonding}]$.

- There are several different types of intermolecular forces: 1. dipole-dipole interactions, 2. dispersion forces, and 3. hydrogen bonding.

- There are several general types of chemical reactions: combination, decomposition, displacement, and neutralization.

- Chemical equations are always written with the reactants, or starting material, on the left side of a reaction arrow ($\rightarrow$) and the products, or ending materials, on the right side of the reaction arrow.

- A chemical equation can be balanced to make sure that the same number of each type of atom appears on both sides of the equation.

- *Stoichiometry* is the quantitative study of reactants and products in a given chemical reaction. Balanced equations contain information that is useful in determining mass relationships, limiting reagents in a reaction, and product yields.

- The *limiting reagent* in a chemical reaction is the reactant whose quantity is used up first. The *reaction yield* is a theoretical yield that represents the maximum amount of product that can result if the entire limiting reagent is used up.

- The percent yield can be calculated to determine the proportion of actual yield to that of the theoretical yield. The percent yield is calculated by the following equation % yield = [actual yield/theoretical yield] × 100. Factors that may influence the percent yield include the temperature and pressure at which the reaction takes place.

- There are four specific properties that are used to describe the behavior of gases: temperature (T in units of Kelvin), pressure (P), volume (V), and the number of moles of gas present (n). Several gas laws have been established to help understand the behavior of gases.

- *Boyle's law* indicates that as long as the temperature and the number of moles of gas do not change, the product of P and V is a constant ($PV = k_1$). The following equation compares two different volumes and pressure for the same type of gas: $P_1V_1 = P_2V_2$.

- *Charles's law* (also called Charles's and Gay-Lussac's law) states that the volume, V, of a constant amount of gas maintained at a constant pressure is directly proportional to temperature of the gas, T (in degrees Kelvin). This relationship is shown in the equation $V = k_2T$. This law can also be represented by the equation $\frac{P_1}{T_1} = \frac{P_2}{T_2}$.

- *Avogadro's law* states that at constant pressure and temperature, the volume of a gas is directly proportional to the number of moles of the gas. This law can be represented by the equation $V = k_4n$.

- The *ideal gas law* combines Boyle's law, Charles's law, and Avogadro's law in order to describe the relationship among the four variables—P, V, n, and T—in one equation. The ideal gas equation is $PV = nRT$.

- *Dalton's law of partial pressures* states that the total pressure of a mixture of gases is equal to the sum of the pressure that would be exerted by each individual gas if it occupied the space on its own.

- The *kinetic molecular theory of gases*, or the kinetic theory of gases, explains the motion of gas particles on a molecular level.

- The average kinetic energy, *KE,* of gas molecules is proportional to the gas's temperature.

- For most real gases, the ideal gas law only holds true under low-pressure conditions, and significant deviations from the law occur as the pressure of the gas increases. Nonideal behavior is also exhibited as the temperature of a gas is lowered. The decrease in temperature causes a decrease in the average kinetic energy of the molecules, so that it is harder for them to repel from each other.

- *Diffusion* is the gradual mixing of one gas with another due to their kinetic properties. Diffusion occurs as gas particles move through a mixture. Despite the relatively fast speed of molecules in a gas, diffusion is a relatively slow process. Graham's law of diffusion can be expressed by this equation: $\frac{r_1}{r_2} = \sqrt{\frac{M_2}{M_1}}$.

- *Effusion* is the process by which gas under a given pressure escapes from one compartment of a container to another compartment by passing through a small opening. The rate of effusion of a gas has the same form as Graham's law of diffusion.

- Molecules in a liquid can, however, move past one another, a quality that gives liquids their fluid property. Liquids assume the shape of the container into which they are poured.

- In a solid, the molecules are packed into a rigid three-dimensional conformation with almost no freedom of motion.

- *Intermolecular forces* are forces of attraction between molecules. These forces are more influential on liquids and solids than they are on gases. The different types of intermolecular forces are dipole-dipole, dipole-induced dipole, and dispersion forces, and hydrogen bonding.

- *Surface tension* is the amount of energy required to stretch or increase the surface of a liquid by a given unit of area.

- *Viscosity* is the measure of a liquid's resistance to flow (fluidity).

- Within a crystalline solid, a *unit cell* is defined as the basic repeating structural unit. The structure and properties of crystals such as their melting point, density, and hardness are determined by the forces that hold the individual particles of the crystal together.

- Phase changes generally occur when energy, usually in the form of thermal energy, is added or removed from the substance. Phase changes alter the molecular order of a substance. Molecules in the solid phase have the greatest amount of molecular order, and those in the gas phase have the least amount of molecular order.

- Vapor pressure is measurable only when a sufficient amount of vapor accumulates. The molar heat of vaporization, ΔH_{vap}, is defined as the energy required to vaporize one mole of a liquid.

- The *boiling point* of a liquid is the temperature at which the vapor pressure of the liquid is equal to the external pressure. Bubbles of gas form within a liquid as it reaches its boiling point. The pressure inside the bubble is due solely to the vapor pressure of the liquid.

- *Freezing* describes the transformation from a liquid to a solid. The reverse process of transforming a solid into a liquid is called *melting*.

- As heat is being absorbed by the substance so that it can overcome attractive forces, the temperature remains constant. During this period, an increase in kinetic energy is used to overcome the attractive forces in a solid and the cohesive forces in a liquid. Once enough molecules have transitioned to the next phase, the temperature rises again.

- A *phase diagram* indicates the conditions at which a substance exists as a solid, liquid, or gas (vapor). A simple diagram graphs pressure vs. temperature for a given substance.

- A *solution* is a homogeneous mixture of two or more substances. Solutions can form from two liquids, two gases, a solid and a liquid, a liquid and a gas, and two solids. The *solute* is the substance that is present in the smaller amount, and the *solvent* is the substance present in the greater amount.

- *Solubility* is the measure of how much solute will dissolve in a solvent under a given set of conditions. Solubility is dependent upon intermolecular forces, temperature, and pressure.

- The concentration of solute in a liquid solution can be measured in terms of molarity, M; molality, m; percent mass; and 4. mole fraction, X.

- In general, the solubility of a gas in a liquid decreases with increasing temperature.

- *Raoult's law* states that the vapor pressure of a solvent (P_1) over a solution is given by the vapor pressure of the pure solvent (P_1°) times the mole fraction (X_1) of the solvent in the solution. A change in vapor pressure of the solvent is directly proportional to the solute concentration of the solution.

- The *osmotic pressure* is defined as the pressure required to stop the process of osmosis. The osmotic pressure pushes solvent from a more dilute area into a more concentrated area in an attempt to achieve equilibrium between the two areas. Osmotic pressure, Π, can be calculated by the equation $\Pi = MRT$.

- The *Arrhenius concept* explains that acids produce H^+ cations (hydronium ions, H_3O^+) in an aqueous solution.

- The *Brønsted-Lowry concept* defines acids as donors of H^+ ions and bases as acceptors of H^+ ions. This concept led to the idea of conjugate acids and bases. A strong acid has a weak conjugate base, and a weak acid has a strong conjugate base.

- The *solvent system concept* states that ions dissociate from a solvent, and these ions can be either anions or cations. If the ions are anions, then the solution is a base, and if the ions are cations, the solution is an acid.

- The *Lewis acid-base concept* defines acids and bases in terms of electrons. A Lewis acid is an electron pair acceptor and a Lewis base is an electron pair donor.

- pH is defined by the equation $pH = -\log_{10}[H_3O^+]$.

- The strengths of acids and bases can be represented by a value called the *equilibrium constant*, K_a:

$$K_a = \frac{[H^+][A^-]}{[HA]}$$

  The *dissociation constant* for a base, K_b, can be calculated in the same way.

- Salts form during a neutralization reaction between an acid and a base, and the other product of this reaction is water.

- Some acids and bases are *polyvalent*, meaning that each mole of the acid or base is capable of dissociating more than one acid or base equivalent.

- *Normality* is equal to the number of grams of equivalent weight of solute per liter of solution. Normality, N, is useful in dealing with acid and base titrations.

- An *amphoteric species* can react as either an acid or a base, depending on the chemical environment.

- *Titrations* are a procedure used for quantifying the amount of acid or base in a solution. In a titration, a solution of an accurately measured concentration, known as a *standard solution* (acid or base), is gradually added to another solution (acid or base) of an unknown concentration. The standard solution is added to the unknown solution until the chemical reaction between the two solutions is complete. The point at which the acid has completely reacted with the base is called the *equivalence point*.

- *Oxidation-reduction*, or *redox*, *reactions* are reactions in which electrons are transferred from one chemical substance to another. Oxidation is the loss of electrons by a substance, and reduction is the gain of electrons by a substance.

- The *oxidation number* helps to determine whether a species has been oxidized or reduced. Assigning oxidation numbers to atoms in a redox reaction helps to keep track of the redistribution of electrons during the reaction.

- The most common method for balancing a redox reaction is the *ion-electron method*. The overall reaction is divided into two parts called half-reactions. One half-reaction represents the oxidation reaction, and the other half-reaction represents the reduction reaction. Each half-reaction is balanced separately.

- There are four major types of redox reactions: combination, decomposition, combustion, and displacement.

- *Electrochemical cells* are contained systems in which a redox reaction takes place. If the oxidizing agent is physically separated from the reducing agent, the transfer of electrons takes place through an external electrical conductor such as a metal wire. The reaction sets up a constant flow of electrons that generates electricity.

- There are two types of electrochemical cells: galvanic (or voltaic) cells, and electrolytic cells. Both types of cells contain electrodes, which are the sites of the redox reactions. Oxidation occurs at the electrode called the anode, and reduction occurs at the electrode called the cathode.

- The reduction potential is the tendency of a substance to acquire electrons and be reduced. The substance in a reaction that will be oxidized or reduced can be determined by evaluating the reduction potential of each species.

- The *electromotive force, emf,* is the work per unit charge that is required to produce an electrical current. Standard reduction potentials can be used to calculate the standard electromotive force of a reaction.

- Thermochemistry is useful for predicting the spontaneity of a reaction and determining the favorability of a reaction and for calculations of heat capacity, enthalpy, and free energy.

- *Heat* is a form of energy between two bodies that are at different temperatures. Heat added to a system from its surroundings is given a positive value, and heat lost from a system to its surroundings is given a negative value.

- Heat change is the most common energy change in chemical processes. It is usually measured in units of calories (or kilocalories, Kcal) or joules (or kilojoules, kJ). An exothermic reaction is any process that transfers thermal energy from the reaction to its surroundings. An endothermic reaction is any process that requires thermal energy input from the surroundings to the system.

- The quantity of the amount of heat exchanged when a substance undergoes a change in temperature can be determined by the equation $q = ms\Delta T$.

- Work is defined by force and distance in the equation: $w = Fd$.

- *Standard reaction conditions* are defined as 25°C and 1 atm. These are the conditions normally used for measuring enthalpy, entropy, and free energy of a reaction. A substance is in its most stable form under standard conditions, and it is considered to be in its standard state.

- *Enthalpy* is defined as the heat content of a substance at a constant pressure. The *enthalpy change*, ΔH, is defined by the change in heat content from the initial to the final state of a substance. The change in enthalpy is expressed by the equation $\Delta H = \Delta E + P\Delta V$.

- The enthalpy of the reaction is the difference between the enthalpies of the products and the enthalpies of the reactants ($\Delta H = H_{products} - H_{reactants}$).

- *Hess's law* states that if the overall reaction process is the sum of two or more reactions, then the overall ΔH value is the sum of all the ΔH values of the reaction.

- *Entropy*, S, is a measure of the randomness and disorder of a system. The greater entropy value, the greater the disorder of a system. Entropy can be expressed by the equation $\Delta S = q/T$.

- The *second law of thermodynamics* states that the entropy of the universe increases in a spontaneous process and remains unchanged in a process that is at equilibrium.

- The entropy of the surroundings of a system can be expressed in terms of the change in enthalpy of a system and the temperature (in Kelvin):

$$\Delta S_{surr} = \frac{-\Delta H_{sys}}{T}$$

- *Gibbs free energy*, or free energy, is defined as the energy available to do work. In other words, it is the amount of available, or free, energy in a system.

- The change in free energy, ΔG, for system during a process of constant temperature and pressure is given by the equation $\Delta G = \Delta H - T\Delta S$.

- The relationship between ΔG (nonstandard state) and $\Delta G°$ (standard state) can be seen in the mathematical expression $\Delta G = \Delta G° + RT\ln Q$. At equilibrium, this equation becomes $\Delta G° = -RT\ln K$.

- *Chemical kinetics* is the study of the rates of chemical reactions, or how fast they occur. The rate of a reaction is dependent upon the mechanism of the reaction. The reaction rate is a measure in the change in the concentration of reactants and the products over time.

- The mathematical expression for the reaction rate is:

$$\text{rate} = -\frac{\Delta\left[\text{reactants}\right]}{\Delta t} \text{ or rate} = \frac{\Delta\left[\text{products}\right]}{\Delta t}$$

- The *mechanism* of a chemical reaction is the series of steps that make up the overall reaction. The slowest step in the reaction is called the *rate-determining step*. The overall rate of the reaction cannot occur faster than the rate of this step.

- The stoichiometry of a chemical reaction can give an idea about the relative rates of the consumption of reactants and formation of products.

- The rate law expresses the relationship of the reaction rate to a rate constant and the concentration of each reactant raised to a power that is determined experimentally by the order of the reaction. For the general reaction $aA + bB \rightarrow cC + dD$, the rate law is expressed by the equation rate $= k[A]^x[B]^y$.

- Reaction order enables one to understand how the reaction is dependent on the concentration of a given reactant.

- The *collision theory of chemical kinetics* states that the rate of the reaction is directly proportional to the number of collisions between the molecules in a reaction. In a chemical reaction, the reaction rate almost always increases as the temperature increases.

- A *potential energy diagram* shows the relationship among the potential energy of a reaction, the activation energy, and the heats of reaction. It also shows the difference between the relative potential energy of the reactants and the products.

- The *transition state* is found at the top of the energy barrier. The *activation energy* of the forward progressing reaction is the difference between the potential energy of the transition state and the reactants. The difference between the potential energy of the transition state and the products is the activation energy of the reverse reaction.

- The rate of a chemical reaction is dependent upon the substances that are reacting, their concentrations, and the environmental factors of the reaction such as temperature, the medium of the environment, and the presence or absence of a catalyst.

- When a chemical reaction reaches a state of equilibrium, there is no observable change in the concentration of the reactants and the products. However, during equilibrium, there is still activity at the molecular level.

- The *law of mass action* maintains that for a reversible reaction at equilibrium and constant temperature, a given ratio of reactant and product concentrations has a constant value, K (the equilibrium constant).

- In general, the equilibrium constant for the forward and reverse reactions in a gas are not equal because the partial pressures of the reactants and products are not equal to their concentrations. The two equilibrium constants can be related in the equation $K_p = K_c(RT)^{\Delta n}$.

- Changes in experimental conditions can affect the balance of a reaction and shift the equilibrium position so that either more or less of the product is formed. Variables affecting the equilibrium of a reaction are concentration, pressure, volume, and temperature.

- *Le Chatelier's principle* states that if an external stress is applied to an equilibrium reaction, or system, the system responds by adjusting the reaction in a way that offsets the stress as the system achieves a new equilibrium.

Organic Chemistry

Chapter 9

OVERVIEW

- **Atomic Bonding and Structure**
- **Nomenclature and Functional Groups**
- **Reaction Mechanisms**
- **Methodology**
- **Spectroscopy**
- **Practice Questions**
- **Answer Key and Explanations**
- **Summing It Up**

Organic chemistry is the study of carbon compounds. All forms of life are based on carbon. Although carbon is the principle element, almost all organic compounds also contain the element hydrogen, and many contain oxygen, nitrogen, phosphorous, sulfur, and chlorine.

ATOMIC BONDING AND STRUCTURE

In the study of organic chemistry, it is important to understand the details of *covalent bonding*. Covalent bonds are the most prevalent bonding type in organic compounds. In a covalent bond, the electrons may not be shared equally between the two atoms. The electron density may be greater for one atom than for the other.

The electron sharing that takes place in a covalent bond tightly binds the atoms because the shared electrons are pulled toward the nucleus of both atoms. The electrons are drawn to the positively charged protons of each nucleus, and at the same time, they are repelled by the electrons of each atom. At a certain distance between the atoms, there is equilibrium of the attractive and repulsive forces of the individual atoms, and the covalent bond forms. If the atoms are too close together, they will repel each other, and if they are too far apart they will not interact with each other. The optimal distance between the two atoms at which a covalent bond forms is called the *bond length*.

The Octet Rule

A single carbon atom has four valence, or outer shell, electrons that are capable of forming a bond. In order to be in its most stable, lowest energy state, the carbon atom must bind to four other valence electrons with which it can bind. This follows the *octet rule* that states:

An atom is in its most favorable, or lowest, energy configuration when it contains eight valence electrons, which is the maximum number of electrons that can fill a valence shell. Therefore, in organic compounds, carbon forms four covalent bonds.

Other organic molecules also follow the octet rule.

- Oxygen has six valence electrons and, therefore, seeks two shared electrons. It can form two covalent bonds.

- Nitrogen has five valence electrons and can form three covalent bonds as it seeks three more electrons to form a stable octet.

- Sulfur has six valence electrons and forms two covalent bonds.

- Phosphorous, like nitrogen, has five valence electrons and, therefore, can form three covalent bonds.

- Chlorine has seven valence electrons and seeks to form one covalent bond to form a stable octet. Fluorine, chlorine, bromine, and iodine all have seven valence electrons and can form single covalent bonds.

The octet rule is occasionally broken, for example, when carbon forms a carbocation (CH_3^+). However, a carbocation is very unstable and seeks to find an electron almost immediately. Nitrogen, sulfur, boron, and other elements found in organic molecules can also break the octet rule. When the octet rule is broken, a very reactive molecule is formed.

The Molecular Orbital Theory

In order to fully understand the covalent bonds formed in organic molecules, it is necessary to understand the nature of the electron orbitals involved in covalent bonding. According to the *molecular orbital theory*, when a covalent bond forms, the atomic orbital on different individual atoms combine to form molecular orbitals. These combined orbitals hold the shared electrons that make up a covalent bond. The formation of a molecular orbital can be thought of as the overlap of atomic orbitals from each individual atom to form a shared orbital between the two atoms that is a property of the whole molecule, and not the individual atoms.

In mathematical terms, a molecular orbital is the sum of the wave functions of the individual atomic orbitals. If the signs (+ or –) of the combined wave functions are the same, then a lower-energy bonding orbital is produced. If the signs of the wave functions are different, then a higher-energy antibonding orbital is produced. The higher-energy antibonding orbital does not fill with electrons, and in most chemical reactions, this antibonding orbital is not of concern to the bonds being formed.

Single Bond

In the formation of a hydrogen, H_2, molecule, each atom has a valence electron in its *ℓs* orbital. As the two spherical *ℓs* orbitals approach each other, they combine to form a new egg-shaped molecular orbital. This new molecular orbital is filled with an electron from each hydrogen orbital. This new arrangement of electrons between the two hydrogen atoms is more stable than the arrangement in each individual atom. When the atoms combine, a pair of molecular orbitals forms. One molecular orbital is lower in energy than the original atomic orbital, and the other is higher in energy than the original atomic orbitals. The two electrons from the hydrogen atoms occupy the bonding molecular orbital (lowest energy state), and the antibonding molecular orbital remains unoccupied. The bonding molecular orbital in a hydrogen molecule has an elongated egg shape formed by the combination of the two spherical orbitals of each H atom. This type of bond is formed by the head-on overlap of two orbitals, has a spherical cross-section, and is called a *sigma (σ) bond*.

A sigma bond can be formed by the combination of two *s* orbitals, two *p* orbitals, or one *s* orbital and one *p* orbital. All single bonds are σ bonds in which two electrons are shared between atoms. Sigma bonds with a shorter bond length are stronger than those with a longer bond length, since the electrons are closer to the nuclei of the atoms when the bond length is shorter.

Figure 1. Configuration of σ Bonding Orbitals

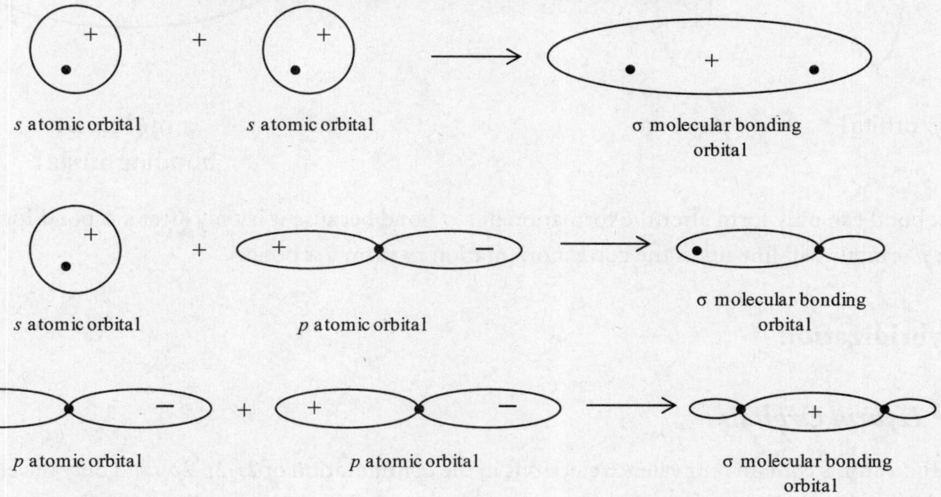

s atomic orbital   s atomic orbital   σ molecular bonding orbital

s atomic orbital   p atomic orbital   σ molecular bonding orbital

p atomic orbital   p atomic orbital   σ molecular bonding orbital

Double and Triple Bonds

The strongest covalent bond will form between two atoms when maximum overlap of the atomic orbital is achieved. In the case of two *p* orbitals, they can be oriented in a head-on fashion to form a single σ bond, or a bond can form when the two *p* orbitals overlap in a sideways fashion. This forms what is known as a *pi (π) bond*. In general, sigma bonding is more efficient than pi bonding, but it is difficult to predict which kind of bonding will lead to maximum overlap between orbitals.

When both a sigma and a pi bond exist between two atoms, a *double bond* is formed. Furthermore, when a sigma bond and two pi bonds exist, a *triple bond* forms between atoms.

Figure 2. The Formation of a π Bond from Two *p* Orbitals

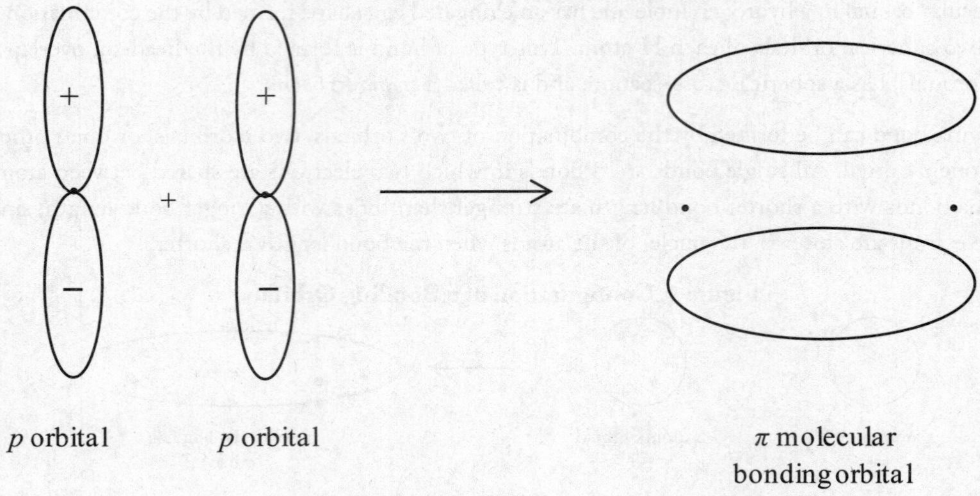

p orbital   *p* orbital   π molecular
                                                   bonding orbital

A π bond can only form after the formation of a σ bond because it is only after a σ bond forms that the *p* orbitals will line up in the correct orientation to form a π bond.

Hybridization

sp³ Hybrid Orbitals

Carbon atoms contain four valence electrons in the configuration of $2s^2 2p_x 2p_y$, and only the electrons in the *p* orbitals are unpaired. Alternatively, carbon can adopt what is called an *excited state*, where there are four unpaired valence shell electrons. In its excited state, an electron from the $2s$ orbital of a carbon atom moves into the $2p_z$ orbital, giving carbon four unpaired valence electrons.

Experimental data shows that the four sigma bonds formed in a methane molecule (CH_4) are all equal. This would not be the case if bonds were forming between both *s* and *p* orbitals of the carbon atom. Instead, it would be expected that the bonds formed between s orbitals were shorter than those formed between *p* orbitals. Linus Pauling showed that a combination of an *s* and three *p* orbitals can be mathematically hybridized, or mixed, to form four equivalent orbitals oriented towards the corners of the tetrahedral shape that a carbon molecule adopts. These new tetrahedral orbitals are called *sp³ hybrid orbitals*.

Figure 3. Formation of an sp^3 Hybrid Orbital

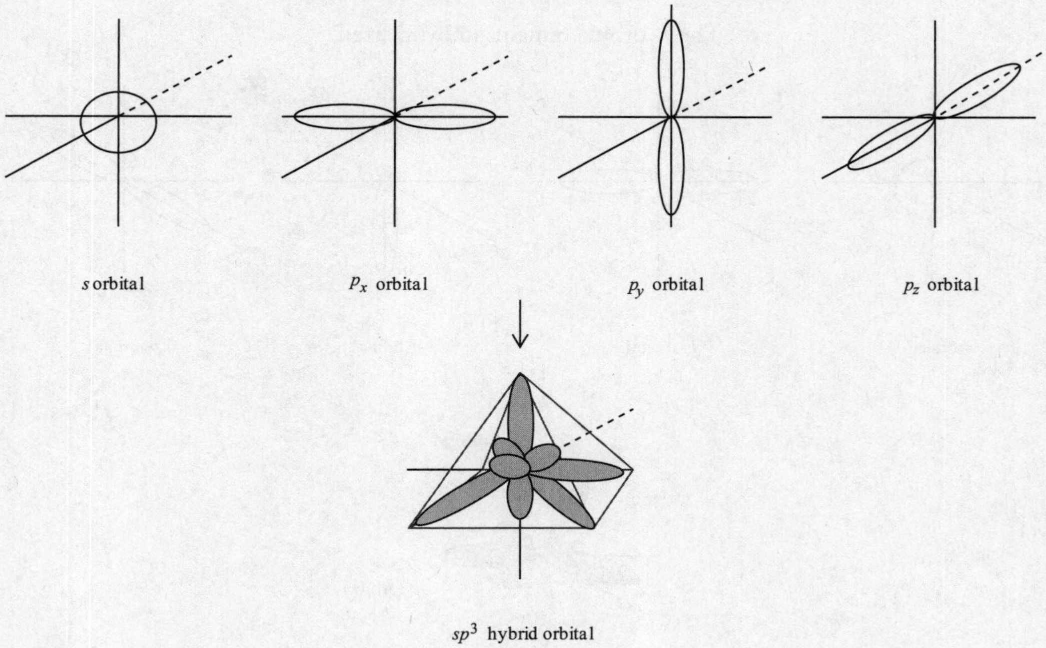

s orbital P_x orbital p_y orbital p_z orbital

sp^3 hybrid orbital

sp^2 Hybrid Orbitals

The sp^3 hybridization is the most common form of carbon's electronic state, but it is not the only type of hybridization orbital that can be formed. The combination of an s orbital with only two p orbitals (p_x and p_y) forms an *sp^2 hybrid orbital*. For example, in the molecule ethylene, C_2H_4, the two carbon atoms form a double bond between themselves. In this case, the $2s$ orbital is combined with only two of the three available p orbitals. Thus, three hybrid sp^2 orbitals are formed, and one $2p$ orbital remains unchanged. The unhybridized p orbital participates in the formation of a pi bond, such that a double bond can form between the two carbon atoms (C=C). The three sp^2 orbitals are arranged 120° apart in a triagonal planar shape. The three sp^2 orbitals participate in the double bond formation and three single C-H bonds form.

Figure 4. *sp*² Hybridization of Carbon

The p_y orbital remains unhybridized.

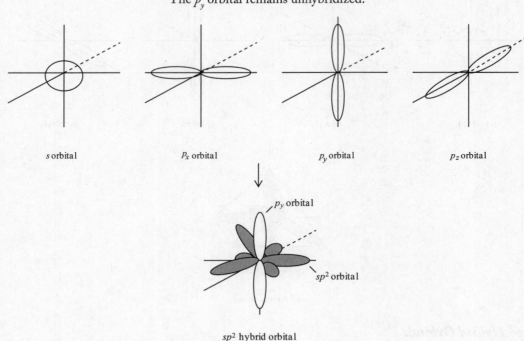

| *s* orbital | P_x orbital | p_y orbital | p_z orbital |

*sp*² hybrid orbital

sp Hybrid Orbitals

In addition to forming single and double bonds, carbon can also form *triple bonds*. In order to form a triple bond, carbon forms a third type of hybridization orbital called an *sp* hybrid. In an *sp* hybrid orbital, two of the *p* orbitals are used to form a triple bond between two carbon atoms (C≡C). The remaining *p* orbital hybridizes with the *s* orbital, forming two *sp* hybrid orbitals.

If the *sp* hybrid orbitals are close enough, they overlap head to head to form an *sp-sp* σ bond. The p_z and p_y orbitals overlap to form a p_z-p_z and p_y-p_y π bond. The σ and two π bonds form the carbon triple bond. The p_x and *s* orbitals form a hybrid orbital that has a straight 180° angle giving a linear structure to the molecule. This arrangement is found in the organic molecule acetylene, C_2H_2.

Figure 5. Formation of Overlapping *sp* Hybrid Orbitals

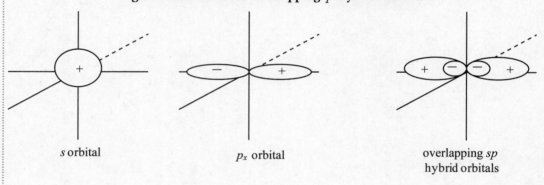

| *s* orbital | p_x orbital | overlapping *sp* hybrid orbitals |

Electronegativity

The electronegativity of an atom helps to determine the structures of organic molecules. Within a covalent bond, the electrons are not always shared equally between the two atoms. Covalent bonds can be classified as *polar* or *nonpolar* bonds. If the bonding electrons between two atoms are shared more or less equally, the covalent bond is considered to be nonpolar. If the electrons are positioned closer to the nucleus of one atom than the other, the covalent bond is considered to be a polar bond. There are different degrees of polarity, depending on the atoms forming the bond.

The relative position of the shared electrons is dependent upon the electronegativity of the atoms. *Electronegativity* is the physical property of an atom that describes its relative attraction of the shared electrons in a covalent bond. The electronegativity of an atom is related to the octet rule and the propensity of an atom to fill any unfilled orbitals in its valence shell.

The atom fluorine has the highest electronegativity of all the elements in the Periodic Table. Fluorine has seven electrons in its valence shell, and it has a strong propensity to attract electrons to fill the eighth position. A molecule such as hydrogen fluoride (HF) has a highly polar covalent bond because fluorine is highly electronegative and hydrogen has a low electronegativity. Therefore, there is a large difference in electronegativity between the two atoms, and the electrons are pulled more strongly toward the F atom (high electron density) than the H atom (low electron density). However, in a diatomic fluorine molecule, F_2, the covalent bond is nonpolar because the electronegativity and the electron density of the two bonded atoms is equal.

NOMENCLATURE AND FUNCTIONAL GROUPS

There are over 16 million known organic compounds, and new compounds are synthesized by chemists each year. Therefore, rules have been established to name organic compounds. Chemists classify compounds into groups according to structural features. In this way, instead of sorting through over 16 million compounds, there are several dozen classes of organic compounds, and the compounds in each group behave in similar ways.

Functional Groups

The structural features that allow the classification of organic compounds are called *functional groups*. A functional group is part of a larger molecule and is composed of atoms or groups of atoms with a known chemical reactivity. Therefore, a functional group will behave in much the same way in any molecule to which it is attached. So, the chemistry of a molecule is largely dependent upon its functional groups.

Functional groups such as alkenes, alkynes, and aromatic rings are only composed of carbon and hydrogen molecules. They differ in the number of carbon and hydrogen bonds they contain, and the nature of the carbon-carbon bonds. Other functional groups have different atoms such as oxygen, nitrogen, sulfur, metals, or halogens. Another important functional group in organic chemistry is the carbonyl group that consists of a carbon-oxygen double bond.

TIP

Be sure you know the relative electronegativity values of elements found in organic molecules.

Element	Relative Electro-negativity
C	2.6
H	2.2
O	3.4
N	3.0
F	4.0
P	2.2
S	2.6
Cl	3.2
Br	3.0
I	2.7

TIP

A good understanding of nomenclature helps to predict the behavior of certain compounds. Functional groups behave similarly in most chemical environments.

Hydrocarbons

Hydrocarbons, or compounds with chains of carbon and hydrogen molecules, are named by finding the highest number of carbon-carbon bonds in the molecule. If a single bond exists between two carbon atoms, the compound name ends in the suffix *-ane*. If a double bond exists between any of the carbons in the molecule, the name of the molecule ends in the suffix *-ene*. A molecule with even one carbon-carbon triple bond has a name that ends in the suffix *-yne*. Common classifications of hydrocarbons are alkanes, alkenes, alkynes, and aromatic rings. Other functional groups found in organic compounds include alcohols, ethers, carbonyl compounds, and amines.

Alkanes

Alkanes are hydrocarbons that contain only single carbon-carbon bonds. The general molecular formula for alkanes is C_nH_{2n+2}. In this formula, *n* is a positive integer. All alkanes have the suffix *-ane*. The prefixes correspond to the number of carbons in the chain. The simplest alkane molecule is methane. It has one carbon atom and $2n + 2$, or four, hydrogen atoms. Alkanes that have four or more carbon atoms may be arranged in more than one way. For example, butane, C_4H_{10}, can be arranged in each of the following structural ways:

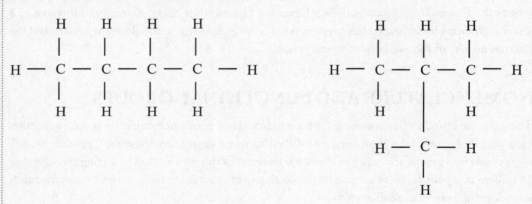

Each of the two structures has the exact same molecular formula, but they have different physical properties, for example, different melting and boiling points, which is due to the different structural orientations. These two compounds are known as isomers of butane. *Isomers* have the same molecular formula, but different structures. The structure on the left is a straight-chain butane, and the one on the right is a branched structure called isobutane. As the number of carbons in a chain increases, the number of isomers of the compound increases.

If one hydrogen group is removed from an alkane molecule, the residue is called an *alkyl group*. The *-ane* suffix is then replaced by *-yl*. For example, removing a hydrogen atom from methane (CH_4) results in a methyl group (CH_3). A branched alkyl group can be generated from hydrocarbons by removing internal hydrogen atoms. As the number of carbon atoms in a chain increases, the number of possible alkyl groups also increases. Furthermore, the prefixes *sec-* (secondary), *tert-* (tertiary) and *quat-* (quaternary) refer to the degree of alkyl substitution at a particular carbon atom. There are four possible substitution patterns for a single carbon atom: *primary*, which is one hydrogen atom substitution; *secondary*, which is two hydrogen atom substitutions; *tertiary*, which is three alkyl substituents on the carbon atom; and *quaternary*, which is four alkyl substituents on the carbon. A generalized alkyl group is represented by the symbol R.

Alkenes

Alkenes are hydrocarbons that contain at least one carbon-carbon double bond. The naming of alkenes is similar to alkanes, except that the suffix on the end of each compound name is *-ene*. The general molecular formula for alkenes is C_nH_{2n}. The simplest alkene molecule is ethane (C_2H_4):

$$H_2C=CH_2$$

Because alkenes have fewer hydrogen atoms than alkanes (due to the presence of at least one double bond), alkenes are often said to be *unsaturated*. An alkane that has the maximum number of hydrogen atoms per carbon is a saturated molecule.

Alkynes

Alkynes are hydrocarbons that contain at least one carbon-carbon triple bond. The naming convention is the same as that of alkanes and alkenes, except that the suffix used is *-yne*. Like alkenes, alkyne molecules are unsaturated because of the presence of at least one triple bond. The simplest alkyne molecule, C_2H_2, is ethyne (also known as acetylene):

$$HC{\equiv}CH$$

The general formula for alkynes is C_nH_{2n-2}. Compounds with more than one triple bond are called *diyens*, *triynes*, and so on. Compounds with both triple and double bonds are called *enyens*.

Alkanes, alkenes, and alkynes can also be cyclical molecules; the carbon atoms form a ring structure. The nomenclature for these molecules are the same as for linear molecules except that the prefix *cyclo-* is attached to the name. In a ring structure, the carbon atoms are not drawn, but occupy the positions where two bond lines meet.

Aromatics

Some unsaturated cyclic hydrocarbon molecules are known as *aromatic rings*. Benzene, C_6H_6, is the parent compound for this type of hydrocarbon. These structures have a high degree of stability because of the effects of resonance. Thus, every C-C bond in the benzene ring exists as an intermediate between a double and a single bond as shown in the following:

Aromatic compounds are formed by replacing hydrogen atoms on the benzene ring with another atom or group of atoms.

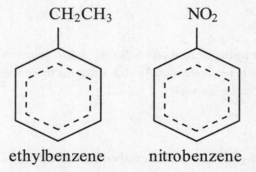

ethylbenzene   nitrobenzene

If one or more substituents are present, the compound must be labeled according to its position on the ring. The carbon atoms of benzene are numbered as follows:

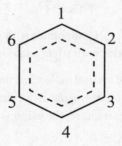

For example, the addition of a bromine molecule at position 1 and 4 forms the compound 1, 4 dibromobenzene.

Oxygen-Containing Compounds

Organic compounds often include oxygen molecules in addition to the carbon and hydrogen molecules.

Alcohols

All *alcohols* contain the functional group –OH. Alcohols are named in a similar manner to alkanes with a prefix of *-ol*. For example, the alcohol derivative of ethane is ethanol. Ethanol is similar to ethane except that one hydrogen atom is replaced with an OH group (C_2H_5OH). Oxygen atoms have a strong electronegativity, and, therefore, the hydrogen atom in the OH group can hydrogen bond to other molecules. The hydrogen bonding that alcohols can participate in typically gives an alcohol derivative a higher boiling point than its corresponding hydrocarbon.

Ethers

Ethers are organic compounds containing the general formula R-O-R' where R and R' are hydrocarbon functional groups. Ethers are formed by a reaction between an alkoxide (with an OR- ion) and an alkyl halide. An example of this reaction can be seen in the formation of dimethyl ether:

$$NaOCH_3 + CH_3Br \rightarrow CH_3OCH_3 + NaBr$$

sodium methoxide + methyl bromide → dimethyl ether + sodium bromide

Ethers do not participate in hydrogen bonding, and, therefore, they generally have low boiling points. They are often used as a solvent in chemical reactions because ethers are relatively inert chemicals.

Carbonyls

Carbonyl compounds are those that contain a carbon-oxygen double bond. A C=O bond is referred to as a *carbonyl bond*. The general structure of a carbonyl-containing compound is:

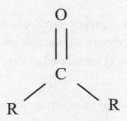

Carbonyls can be further classified depending upon the groups that attach to the carbon atom:

- **Aldehydes:** An aldehyde is formed when at least one of the R groups attached to the carbon atom is an H atom. If both R groups are H atoms, the compound formed is formaldehyde.

- **Ketones:** In a ketone, the carbon atom of the carbonyl group is bound to two hydrocarbon groups. The simplest ketone structure is the solvent acetone. Ketones are generally less reactive than aldehydes.

- **Esters:** Esters have the general formula R'COOR. R' can be either an H or a hydrocarbon, and R is a hydrocarbon group. Esters are what give many fruits their characteristic smell and flavor. For example, apples contain methyl butyrate, $CH_3CH_2CH_2COOCH_3$.

- **Carboxylic acids:** Carboxylic acid compounds contain a carboxyl group, COOH. Under the correct conditions, both aldehydes and alcohols can be oxidized to form a carboxylic acid. Carboxylic acids are weak acids that are widely distributed in the plant and animal kingdom. All amino acids have both an amino group and a carboxyl (COOH) group.

Amines

Amines are organic molecules with properties of a base. They have the general formula, R_3N, where R is an H atom or a hydrocarbon group. The simplest amine is NH_3. Like all bases, when an amine reacts with an acid, it undergoes a neutralization reaction to form salt and water.

Aromatic amines contain a benzene ring as one of the R groups. The simplest known aromatic amine is aniline, shown here:

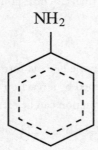

REACTION MECHANISMS

An important part of learning organic chemistry is understanding how substrates (reactants) form products. Knowing the mechanisms of chemical reactions allows for the prediction of product yield, and also the development of new compounds. Almost all of organic chemistry can be explained in terms of three generalized reaction types: polar reactions, radical reactions, and pericyclic reactions.

Polar Reactions

Polar reactions are the result of attractive forces between the positive and negative charges on molecules. Although most organic compounds are electrically neutral, specific bonds within a functional group on a given molecule may be polarized. As mentioned earlier, bond polarity is due to the intrinsic electronegativity of an atom.

In a polar reaction, bonds are formed when an electron-rich substance called a *nucleophile* donates a pair of electrons to an electron-poor substance called an *electrophile*. The bond is broken when one of the two nuclei leaves with the electron pair and separates from the other atom. This type of unsymmetrical breaking of the bond (both electrons go with one atom) is called a *heterolytic process*. In organic chemistry, this type of polar reaction is called a *nucleophilic substitution reaction*. A generalized mechanism for a nucleophilic substitution reaction is:

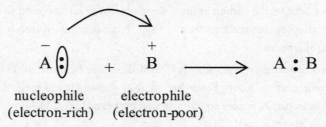

where the curved arrow shows the donation of an electron pair from the nucleophile to the electrophile. More specific types of nucleophilic substitution reactions will be discussed later on in this chapter.

Radical Reactions

In a *radical reaction*, two species called radicals donate a single electron to form a bond. All reagents in a polar reaction contain an even number of electrons distributed as electron pairs. In a radical reaction, the species contain an odd number of electrons, and the single unpaired electrons are donated to form a bond in what is called a *homogenic process*. When bonds are broken between radicals, each species leaves the bonding relationship with only one of the bonding electrons. This type of bond breakage is called a *homolytic breakage*. Most radicals are electrically neutral; however, they are highly reactive species. In most cases, this is because they aim to establish a stable octet.

The chlorination of methane is an example of a radical substitution reaction. Radical substitution reactions generally occur in three steps: the initiation step, the propagation steps, and the termination steps. The propagation and termination steps can occur multiple times in a single reaction.

1. **Initiation step:** Radical homolytic bond breakage.

$$\overset{..}{\underset{..}{:}}Cl : \overset{..}{\underset{..}{Cl}} : \quad \overset{light}{\longrightarrow} \quad 2 : \overset{..}{\underset{..}{Cl}} \cdot$$

Chlorine radicals

2. **Propagation steps:** The chlorine radicals are highly reactive and when the chlorine radicals collide with methane molecules, they abstract an H atom to form HCl and a methyl radical (CH_3). The methyl radical is also highly reactive and reacts further with the chlorine to produce chloromethane and chlorine radicals. The chlorine radical then cycles back to the first propagation step, so that the overall process is a chain reaction.

(a) $\boxed{Cl \cdot}$ + H $\overset{..}{:}$ CH_3 $\longrightarrow$ H$:$Cl   + $\cdot CH_3$

(b) $\cdot CH_3$ + Cl $\overset{..}{:}$ Cl $\longrightarrow$ Cl$:CH_3$ + $\boxed{Cl \cdot}$

(c)   Repeat steps (a) and (b) multiple times.

3. **Termination steps:** When two radicals collide and combine to form a stable product, termination of the reaction occurs. Termination steps occur infrequently because stable products between radicals form very infrequently. The concentration of radicals in a reaction is very small, and, therefore, the likelihood of two radicals colliding is also very small.

$$Cl^{\cdot} \; + \; Cl^{\cdot} \quad \longrightarrow \quad Cl{:}Cl$$

$$\text{or} \quad Cl^{\cdot} \; + \; {}^{\cdot}CH_3 \quad \longrightarrow \quad Cl{:}CH_3$$

$$\text{or} \quad {}^{\cdot}CH_3 \; + \; {}^{\cdot}CH_3 \quad \longrightarrow \quad CH_3{:}CH_3$$

There are several other types of radical reactions that all follow the same basic principle. All bonds in a radical reaction are formed and broken by the reaction of odd-electron species.

Pericyclic Reactions

Pericyclic reactions are those that involve the redistribution of bonding electrons in a cyclical manner. One type of pericyclic reaction is the *cycloaddition reaction*, which involves the addition of one reactant to another to form a cyclical product. An example is the reaction between a diene (a compound with two C=C bonds) and an alkene, which is called a *Diels-Alder reaction*. In a Diels-Alder reaction, the reactants are neither nucleophile–electrophile pairs nor radicals. A Diels-Alder reaction involves the rearrangement of electrons so that there is an overlap of p orbitals. This creates sp^3 hybrid orbitals so that new sigma bonds form, and the final product is a cyclic compound.

Consider the reaction in which 1, 3-butadiene combines with methyl propenoate to form the cyclic product methyl 3-cyclohexencarboxylate.

1, 3-butadiene   Methylpropenoate   Methyl 3-cyclohexenecarboxylate

The arrows drawn indicate the breaking of the double bonds and the placement of new sigma bonds.

Characteristics of Three Types of Organic Reaction Mechanisms

Reaction Type	Characteristics
1. Polar	Nucleophile donates a pair of electrons to an electrophile to form a new bond.
2. Radical	Bonds form when each reactant donates one electron to the new bond.
3. Pericyclic	Bonds are formed by the cyclic reorganization of electrons.

Specific Reaction Mechanisms

Although all organic chemical reactions can be classified as polar, radical, or pericyclic, they can be further categorized into specific mechanisms of reaction: substitution, elimination, condensation, dehydration, oxidation and reduction, esterification, and addition.

Substitution

The substitution reaction is one of the most common reactions in organic chemistry. As mentioned above, in a substitution reaction, a nucleophile reacts with an electrophile in a process called nucleophilic attack. There are two main categories of substitution reactions: S_N2 and S_N1.

1. **S_N2:** The term S_N2 is shorthand for substitution (S), nucleophilic (N), and bimolecular 2. In an S_N2 reaction, a nucleophile attacks an electrophile and a new covalent bond forms between the two species. During this reaction, a portion of the electrophile called the leaving group is displaced and departs from the molecule. The leaving group leaves the electrophile at the same time that the electrophile is attacked by the nucleophile. These simultaneous reactions make up a concerted reaction.

    The entering nucleophile attacks the substrate (electrophile) from a position that is 180° from the leaving group on the electrophile, and the reaction takes place all in one step without any intermediates formed. In the reaction process, as the leaving group departs from the electrophile, the remaining three groups change their orientation around the carbon atom.

    In the following example of a generalized reaction, the lone pair on the oxygen acts as the nucleophile and the electron pair is donated to the carbon on the electrophile. The nucleophile attacks on one side of the molecule, and the leaving group, Cl, leaves from the opposite side. There is a 180° angle between the attack site and the leaving group, as is the case in all S_N2 reactions.

During the transition state of this reaction, the OH forms a partial bond with the C atom, and the C-Cl bond becomes partially broken. In the case of the above example, the chlorine atom has a higher electronegativity than the carbon atom. Therefore, it draws the electron density away from the carbon atom, and the carbon becomes an electron-poor constituent (electrophile). The chlorine atom thus becomes the leaving group. Once the chlorine atom leaves with the electron it was sharing in the C-Cl bond, it has a complete and stable octet. After the S_N2 reaction, the electrophilic carbon is still in its same position, but the stereochemistry of the other groups is inverted, and the other groups flip. This occurs because the nucleophile attacks from the backside of the molecule and pushes the R groups forward.

2. **S_N1:** An S_N1 reaction obeys first-order kinetics. In this type of reaction, there is a nucleophilic attack and a leaving group departs from the electrophile. However, unlike an S_N2 reaction, the two events do not happen simultaneously. In an S_N1 reaction, the leaving group departs first, leaving a carbocation behind. This step in the S_N1 process is always a slow process and is, therefore, the rate-determining step. The nucleophile plays no kinetic role in the rate-limiting step, since it does not enter the reaction until after the leaving group has departed.

A *carbocation* (positively charged carbon atom) is extremely electrophilic, and the nucleophile can attack from any angle (front, back, above, or below). Thus, the nucleophile attacks randomly from either side, which should result in racemic products (a 50/50 mixture of both chiral enantiomers—mirror images). However, very few S_N1 reactions occur with complete racemization. Typically, there is about 80 percent racemization and 20 percent inversion.

In an S_N1 reaction, the more stable the carbocation intermediate, the faster the overall reaction. The movement of the reaction through the carbocation form is fairly quick and represents the transition state of the S_N1 reaction. An S_N1 reaction is often carried out in acidic conditions, and in these cases, water can act as a leaving group. Other excellent leaving groups include tosylates and mesylates, since they are stable in their ionic forms.

Elimination

An *elimination reaction* involves the removal of an atom or functional group from a molecule. This type of reaction usually involves an increase in the number of double or triple bonds in a final product as compared to the reactant. Elimination reactions can be divided into two types: E1 and E2 reactions.

1. **E1:** *E1 reactions* involve a leaving group that will be stable once it leaves with its newly acquired negative charge (like an S_N1 reaction). All E1 elimination reactions occur by spontaneous dissociation of the leaving group and the loss of a proton from an intermediate carbocation. As in the case of an S_N1 reaction, the loss of the proton (breaking of a C-H bond) occurs after the rate-limiting step of the dissociation of the leaving group. An example of an E1 elimination reaction is the removal of a Cl functional group from 2-chloro-2-methylpropane.

Figure 6. E1 Reaction

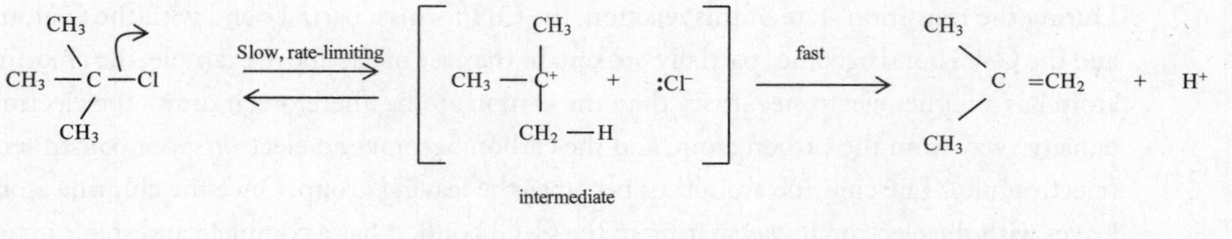

In Figure 6, the spontaneous dissociate of the tertiary chloride atom yields an intermediate carbocation (C^+) in a slow rate-limiting step. The loss of H^+ from the molecule in a fast step yields a neutral alkene product (double bond). The C-H bond electron pair goes to form the new alkene pi bond.

2. **E2:** *E2 reactions* involve two compounds in which one compound removes an atom or functional group from the other compound. The E2 reaction is the most common type of

elimination reaction. It is also analogous to the S_N2 reaction in many respects. Like the S_N2 reaction, the E2 reaction occurs in one step without any intermediates. In the generalized E2 reaction in Figure 7, a nucleophile base B attacks a neighboring C-H bond and starts to remove the H atom from the neighboring molecule. At the same time, a double bond starts to form, and the functional group X starts to leave the molecule. This brings the molecule into its transition state which is a very short-lived state. A neutral alkene (double bond) is produced after the C-H bond is fully broken, and the X group leaves the molecule with an electron pair. In the final molecule, a double bond has formed between the two central carbon atoms.

Figure 7. E2 Reaction

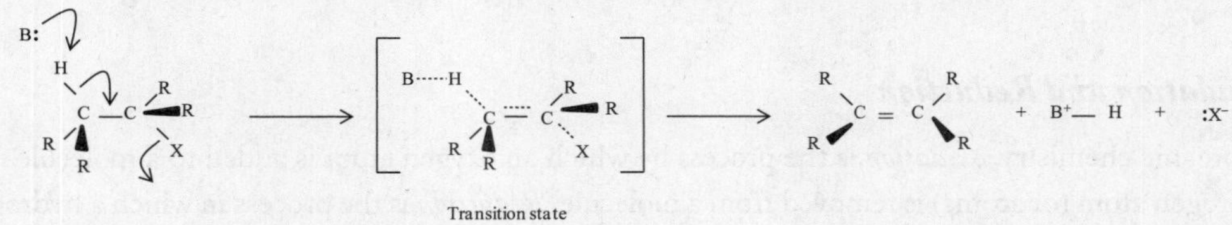

Transition state

In the above reaction, the partially formed bonds in the transition state are represented by dotted lines.

There are many similarities between substitution and elimination reactions. If the nucleophile is weak, the reaction is more likely to proceed by elimination than substitution. If the reaction takes place at a high temperature, in the presence of a strong base, or with significant steric hindrance on the electrophile, an elimination reaction is favored over a substitution reaction. Substitution reactions are favored when the reaction takes place in water, and elimination reactions are favored when the solvent in which the reaction takes place is an alcohol such as ethanol.

Condensation

An *organic condensation reaction* is one in which two molecules are united as they expel a smaller molecule such as water. Most condensation reactions take place via substitution, addition, or elimination processes. An example of a condensation reaction is the carbonyl condensation reaction. This type of condensation reaction is a combination of a nucleophilic addition reaction and a substitution reaction. The general mechanism of a carbonyl condensation reaction is shown below. In this reaction, a carbonyl with a hydrogen atom in its alpha position is converted by base (OH^-) into its anion form, called an *enolate ion*. The enolate ion acts as a nucleophile electron donor and donates an electron pair to the electrophilic carbonyl group. Protonation of the neutral intermediate yields a neutral condensation product.

Figure 8. Carbonyl Condensation Reaction

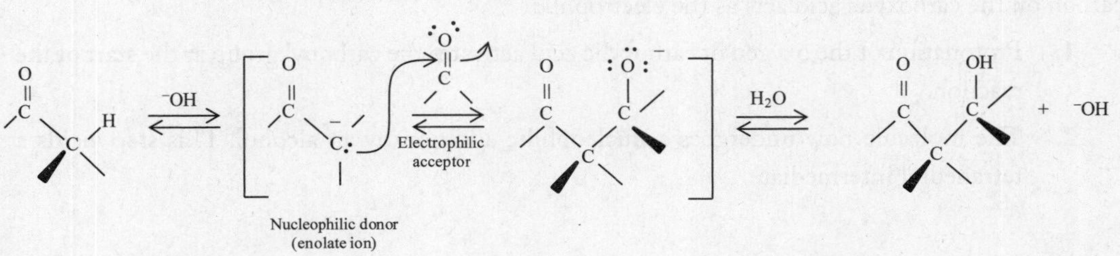

Dehydration

Dehydration reactions are special types of elimination reactions in which the leaving group is always a water molecule. Thus, a dehydration reaction is one is which water is lost. The molecule that acts as a base always contains a hydroxyl (OH) group that can leave the molecule. A reaction that involves the dehydration of an alcohol yields an alkene. During the process of dehydration, the OH group on the base must receive another H proton (H⁺), which can be donated by another reactant, the solvent, or the molecule itself.

In most cases, an acid catalyst is present to facilitate the dehydration reaction. The lone pair of electrons on the hydroxyl group attracts a proton from a strong acid. OH⁻ is a poor leaving group, but the addition of the H⁺ ion transforms it into a good leaving group by eliminating the negative charge.

Oxidation and Reduction

In organic chemistry, *oxidation* is the process by which an oxygen atom is added to a molecule or a hydrogen atom (or atoms) is removed from a molecule. *Reduction* is the process in which a hydrogen atom (or atoms) is added to a molecule or an oxygen atom is removed from a molecule. The most basic example of oxidation and reduction of organic molecules involves a conversion between an aldehyde and a carboxylic acid.

Figure 9. Oxidation and Reduction

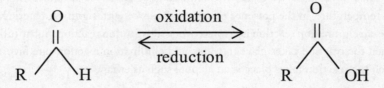

Some commonly used oxidation reagents in organic chemistry are chromic acid, its potassium and sodium salt, and potassium permanganate. Commonly used reducing agents include lithium aluminum hydride, nickel/hydrogen gas mixtures, and sodium borate (sodium tetrahydridoborate).

Esterification

The formation of an ester from an alcohol and a carboxylic acid takes place in the presence of an acid catalyst at high temperature during the process of *esterification*. Esterification reactions are reversible so that an ester can break down into an alcohol and a carboxylic acid under certain conditions. The process of esterification is generally a very slow reaction, but the yields are usually quite good.

Esterification reactions take place in five steps with the formation of four intermediate molecules. The net result of the reaction is that the oxygen atom on the alcohol acts as a nucleophile, and the carbon on the carboxylic acid acts as the electrophile.

1. Protonation of the oxygen of carboxylic acid activates the carbonyl group at the start of the reaction.

2. The molecule now undergoes a nucleophilic addition by an alcohol. This step yields a tetrahedral intermediate.

3. The transfer of a proton from one oxygen atom to another yields another tetrahedral intermediate and converts the hydroxyl group into H_2O, which is a good leaving group.

4. Water leaves the molecule, and the result is a protonated ester.

5. A proton is then lost, leaving a free ester product. The loss of the proton also serves to regenerate the acid catalyst for further use.

Figure 10. Esterification Reaction

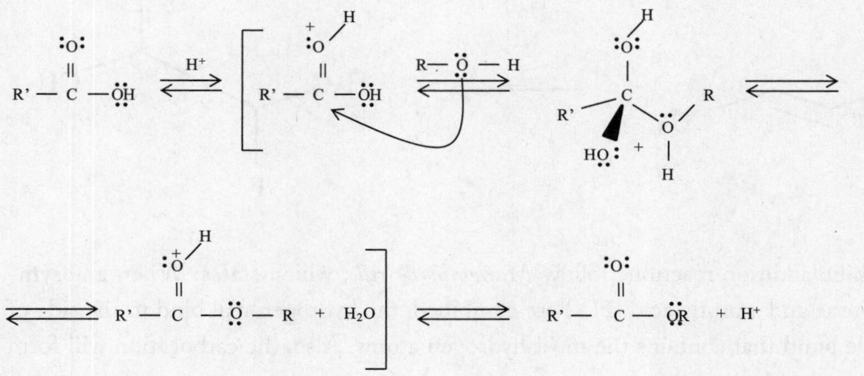

Addition

An *addition reaction* involves two molecules joining together to form a larger molecule. In a sense, an addition reaction is the opposite of an elimination reaction. Addition reactions involve molecules with double- and triple-bonded atoms (alkenes, alkynes, carbonyl, and imine groups). In an addition reaction, a pi bond of the double or triple bond is broken to form a new sigma (single) bond.

An addition reaction can be either nucleophilic or electrophilic. Another type of addition reaction is a free radical addition.

1. **Nucleophilic addition:** As is the case in other reactions involving nucleophiles, molecules such as water or oxygen attack molecules with a low electron density (electrophiles). In many cases, the carbon on either side of a double or triple bond acts as an electrophile. The nucleophilic attack serves to open up the double or triple bond, and the unbound valence electron can then be shared. The negative charge on the molecule attracts a proton (or other positively charged ion) from the solution or environment.

Figure 11. Nucleophilic Addition Reaction

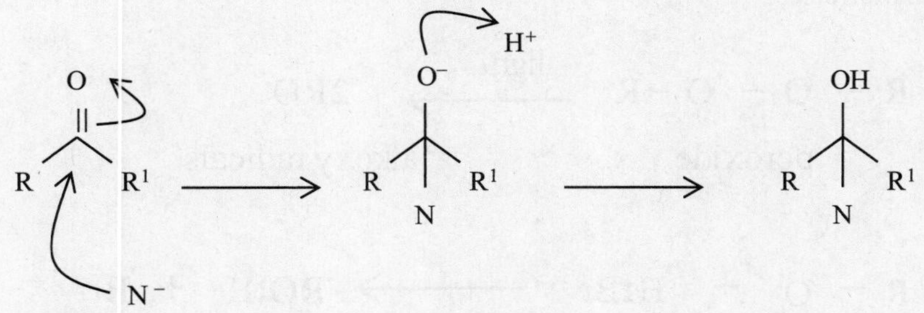

2. **Electrophilic addition:** In an electrophilic addition reaction, the electrons in the π bond bind to an electrophile. The result is that the π bond is broken, leaving a carbocation. The carbocation is then able to covalently bind to a nucleophile or positively charged species. The reaction of hydrogen halide with an alkene is an example of an electrophilic addition reaction.

Figure 12. Electrophilic Addition Reaction

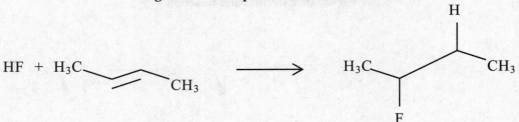

Electrophilic addition reactions follow *Markonikov's rule*, which states: When an asymmetric alkene and a protic acid (HX) are combined, the hydrogen will bind to the side of the double bond that contains the most hydrogen atoms. Also, the carbocation will form on the carbon with the most electron-donating substituents.

3. **Free radical addition:** Free radical addition is different from electrophilic addition in that it does not follow Markonikov's rule. In most cases, what occurs is exactly opposite to Markonikov's rule. For example, when hydrogen bromide reacts with an alkene in a free radical addition reaction in the presence of a peroxide molecule, the bromine radical is added to the opposite carbon as would be predicted by Markonikov's rules. Addition to this carbon produces a more stable product, and the reaction proceeds through this more stable intermediate.

This free radical addition reaction is initiated in two steps. The first step involves a light-induced hemolytic cleavage of the O-O bond in peroxide, which generates two alkoxy radicals (RO˙). In the second step, the alkoxy radical removes the hydrogen atom from HBr, forming a bromine radical (Br). There are two repeating propagation steps in this addition reaction. In the first step, the bromine radical adds to the alkene double bond, forming an alkyl radical. In the second propagation step, the alkyl radical reacts with hydrogen bromide (HBr) to yield a bromine radical and the addition product.

Initiation steps:

$$R - O - O - R \xrightarrow{\text{light}} 2RO˙$$

peroxide   alkoxy radicals

$$R - O˙ \; + \; H\!:\!Br \longrightarrow RO\!:\!H \; + \; Br˙$$

Propagation steps:

$$H_2C=CH-R \;+\; \boxed{Br^{\,\bullet}} \;\longrightarrow\; Br\,CH_2-\overset{\bullet}{C}R$$

$$Br\,CH_2-\overset{\bullet}{C}R \;+\; HBr \;\longrightarrow\; Br\,CH_2-CH_2R \;+\; \boxed{Br^{\,\bullet}}$$

METHODOLOGY

Each time a chemical reaction is run in a laboratory, the products must be isolated and purified. There are several methods for isolating, purifying, and modifying organic compounds. Some of the more common and important methods are extraction, crystallization, distillation, sublimation, chromatography, and combustion analysis. Chromatography can be divided into liquid chromatography, high-pressure liquid chromatography, and gas chromatography.

Extraction

The process of *extraction* involves the separation of a substance from a solution or matrix. An extraction can be a solid-phase extraction in which solids are dissolved in liquid and the components of the solid separated from each other based on their chemical and physical properties. In the case of a solid extraction, the separated solution can be evaporated to dryness such that the extracted solid is left.

A *liquid extraction* is an extraction in which a liquid solute can be separated from a liquid solvent.

Another type of liquid extraction is a *solvent extraction*, in which a substance is separated from a mixture by preferentially dissolving the substance in a suitable solvent so that it is separated from another substance that is insoluble in that particular solvent. This process of solvent extraction separates liquids based on their relative solubilities in two different immiscible liquids, one of which is usually water and the other is an organic solvent.

Liquid–liquid extraction is commonly performed in organic chemical reactions and is carried out in a separatory funnel. The liquid to be extracted and the extraction solvent are both added to the separatory funnel. A stopper is used to block the opening of the funnel, and the mixture is shaken. The build-up of pressure from the shaken mixture is released by opening a stopcock at the end of the funnel. After a given time, layers of liquid are distinguishable, and the bottom layer can be removed via the stopcock on the end of the funnel. In some instances, multiple extractions are necessary to remove completely a liquid from its solvent.

Crystallization

Crystallization is a straightforward and effective way of purifying a solid. A crude sample of the reaction product is dissolved in a minimal amount of liquid solvent and heated to boiling. Once all the product has dissolved in the solvent, the solution is slowly cooled. As the solution cools, pure crystals form and precipitate out of the solution. The formation of crystals can be brought about by the addition of a seed crystal or by scratching the side of the vessel containing the solution. The impurities are left behind in the solution, and the pure crystals are isolated through a process of filtration.

ALERT

Remember that the majority of questions in the science sections involve applying basic principles to solve a problem. You need to be able to do more than recognize facts.

The solvents most commonly used in crystallization processes are water, alcohol, ether, benzene, petroleum ether, ligroin, carbon bisulphide, chloroform, acetone, and glacial acetic acid. The liquid chosen as the mobile phase should be one which yields well-formed crystals and does not evaporate too quickly.

Distillation

The process of *distillation* is a simple and effective method of purifying a volatile liquid. A crude liquid reaction product is heated to its boiling point and as the vapor rises, it is collected and condensed back into a liquid. The nonvolatile impurities in the product are left behind and the result is a purified volatile liquid product. The heating of the distillation flask should enable the condensed liquid to fall in drops from the condenser at a rate of about one drop per second.

In a crude mixture of two or more volatile liquids with different boiling points, a process of *fractional distillation* can separate the liquids. The more volatile liquid with the lower boiling point distills first, and the higher boiling point liquid is then distilled.

Sublimation

A *sublimation point* is the temperature and pressure at which the vapor pressure of a solid equals the applied pressure. The process of sublimation is used when it is necessary to separate a volatile solid substance from substances that do not readily vaporize. The solid product is vaporized by methods of gently heating it and the vapor is then condensed back into a solid state. In the process, the desired volatile solid is separated from less volatile impurities. The temperature of the sublimation chamber must be accurate in order to ensure proper sublimation of the volatile substance. In addition, the apparatus must be heated slowly and the substance cooled slowly and evenly.

Chromatography

Chromatography can be used if crystallization and distillation are not effective. *Chromatography* methods can be used to separate a mixture of organic compounds. The mixture to be separated is dissolved in a liquid or gaseous mobile phase (solvent), and it is passed through a solid adsorbent phase that is packed in a column of varying size. The idea behind chromatography is that different organic compounds in a mixture will adsorb to the stationary phase to different degrees. Therefore, the different compounds will migrate through the stationary phase at different rates and can be separated as they come out of the stationary phase column. There are three types of chromatography that chemists use to purify components in a mixture: liquid chromatography, high-pressure liquid chromatography, and gas chromatography.

Liquid Chromatography

Liquid chromatography is one of the simplest and most frequently used methods of product purification. A mixture of organic compounds is dissolved in a liquid mobile phase. This solution is then adsorbed by the stationary phase packed into a column. In general, the stationary phase is made up of a solid such as alumina (Al_2O_3) or silica gel. Once the solution of compounds is adsorbed onto the column, more mobile phase solvent is passed through the column. At different times and different concentrations of solvent, the organic compounds are removed from, or eluted off, the stationary phase column. The time at which each compound is eluted off the column has to do with the polarity of the compound. Those molecules with polar functional groups are adsorbed more strongly by the stationary phase than those with nonpolar functional groups. Because they are bound to the column more tightly, the more polar compounds move through the column at a slower rate than the nonpolar compounds.

High-Pressure Liquid Chromatography

High-pressure liquid chromatography (HPLC) is a variant of the simple column chromatography technique. If the stationary phase is composed of very small, uniformly sized spherical particles, the efficiency of chromatography is improved. Small-sized spheres create a greater surface area for the adsorption of compounds, and uniform size allows for the particles of the column to be tightly packed. High-pressure pumps are used to force the mobile phase solvent through the tightly packed HPLC columns. Detectors can then monitor the elution of specific compounds from the column.

Today, most modern HPLC techniques employ stationary phases made of non-polar materials instead of the traditional polar materials like silica gel, and this is referred to as *reverse phase HPLC*. Most organic molecules absorb UV radiation and the detectors are built around UV adsorbance changes as the compound elutes from the column.

Gas Chromatography

Gas chromatography employs a carrier gas such as nitrogen as the mobile phase solvent. In this technique, a small amount of sample mixture is dissolved in a small volume of solvent. This solution is then injected through a syringe into a heated block before passing into a coiled chromatographic column that contains the stationary phase. As the sample is injected into the heated block, it is instantly vaporized, and then shuttled into the column by a stream of gas identical to the mobile phase. As pure substances are eluted from the end of the column, they are detected and register as a peak on a recorder chart. Generally, the column is located in a programmable oven where it can be slowly heated to help drive the compounds from the column to the detectors.

Combustion Analysis

Empirical and molecular formulas of organic compounds can be determined through the process of *combustion analysis*. The mass of the product to be analyzed is determined, and then the product is burned completely. If a product only contains one or some atoms of carbon, hydrogen, and oxygen, as is the case in many organic compounds, then the only products of combustion (burning) are carbon dioxide and water. Carbon dioxide and water that result from combustion are collected in separate tubes that contain materials specific to adsorbing either water or CO_2.

The increase in mass of the water collecting tube is due to the mass of water that formed during the combustion reaction. The increase in mass of the tube collecting carbon dioxide is due to the mass of CO_2 formed in the combustion reaction. The mass of carbon in the starting product can be determined by calculating the mass of carbon in the CO_2 collected. The mass of hydrogen in the starting product can be calculated in the same way by determining the mass of H in the H_2O collected. If the compound contains oxygen, the mass of oxygen can be determined by subtracting the calculated mass of carbon and hydrogen from the mass of the original sample. All of this data can be used to calculate the empirical and molecular formulas of the starting compound.

SPECTROSCOPY

After the products of a chemical reaction have been separated and purified, it is necessary to identify and analyze them. Several types of *spectroscopy* are used to determine the structure and composition of chemical compounds and molecules. The four most common types of spectroscopy are mass spectroscopy, infrared spectroscopy, UV-Vis spectroscopy, and NMR spectroscopy.

Mass Spectroscopy

Mass spectroscopy allows for the measurement of the mass, or molecular weight, of an isolated compound or molecule. In determining the mass of a species, it is also possible to gain insight into the structure of the unknown molecule. There are several different kinds of mass spectrometers, but the most common is the electron-impact, magnetic-sector instrument.

A small amount of sample is needed for mass spectroscopy. This sample is placed into the spectrometer and bombarded with a stream of high-energy electrons. When a high-energy electron hits an organic molecule, it dislodges a valence electron from the sample molecule. This produces what is called a cation radical (positively charged, odd number of electrons). The process of electron bombardment also transfers a large quantity of energy to the molecules of the sample. This causes the cation radicals to fly apart (fragment). Some of the fragments retain a positive charge, and other fragments become neutral. The small fragments are passed through a magnetic field and only the positively charged fragments are deflected based on their charge-to-mass ratio. These positively charged fragments are sorted by the mass spectrometer, and each group of a certain charge to mass ratio is recorded as a peak. The peaks represent the masses of the ions. A molecule will have several peaks, depending on how its molecules can fragment. For example, the molecule methane has a molecular mass of 16 g/mol. The number of charges is 1 (as is almost always the case) so that the charge-to-mass ratio, *m/z*, is equal to 16/1, or 16. The largest peak, or the *base peak*, is represented at 16. There are also peaks at 15 and 14 corresponding to the fragmentation of CH_4 into CH_3^+ and CH_2^+. The larger the molecule, the more complex its spectral fragmentation pattern, and the highest (base) peak does not always correspond to the unfragmented molecular ion.

Figure 13. Mass Spectra of Methane, CH_4

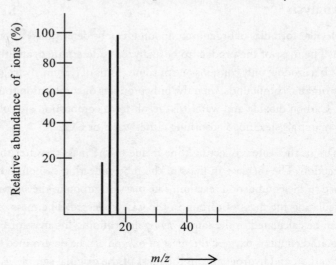

Infrared Spectroscopy

The infrared (IR) region of the electromagnetic spectrum covers the range just beyond the visible light spectrum, and the mid-region of the IR spectra is of particular interest to organic chemists. Molecules are in constant motion, and when a molecule absorbs infrared radiation, the molecular motion of the molecule increases in intensity. Because each radiation frequency corresponds to a different motion, IR spectroscopy reveals the different types of motion within a given molecular sample. Interpreting the IR spectra can help to determine the functional groups in the molecule. However, because most organic molecules are so large, interpretation of the many different bond stretches and bends can be quite complicated. Scientists can look at the most complex region of the spectra, called the *fingerprint region*, and determine if it matches the fingerprint of a known molecule. Each organic molecule will have its own unique spectra. In addition, most functional groups give rise to a characteristic IR absorption pattern. Therefore, knowing where these functional groups' absorption occurs can reveal structural information about different molecules. An IR spectrometer will record this information as peaks at specific wavelength frequencies, and as a result, common functional groups in a molecule can be identified.

Figure 14. IR Spectra for a Hexane Molecule ($CH_3(CH_2)_4CH_3$)

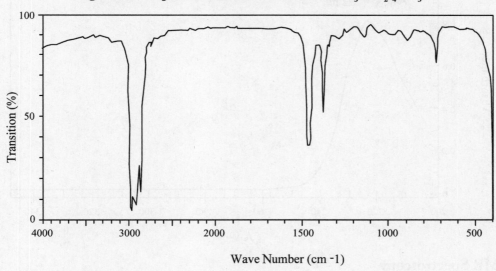

Wave Number (cm -1)

UV-Vis Spectroscopy

One observable physical difference between compounds is their color. For example, ketones range in color from dark red to bright yellow, depending on the conjugation of the double bond. When white light, which contains the entire visible color spectra, passes through a colored substance, as is the case in *UV-Vis spectroscopy*, a characteristic portion of wavelengths is absorbed. Each different color in the spectra corresponds to absorption at a different wavelength.

In order to understand the chemical make-up of a compound with respect to its color and the relationship of bond conjugation to color, it is necessary to make accurate measurements of light absorption at different wavelengths in and near the visible light spectrum. In a UV-Vis spectrometer, a beam of light from a UV and visible light source is separated into wavelength components by a prism or diffraction grating. Each wavelength is then split into two equal intensity beams by a mirror.

One light beam shines through the molecular sample in a given liquid solvent in a transparent container called a *cuvette*. The other beam acts as a reference beam and passes through a second cuvette that contains only the solvent. The intensity of each beam of light is measured and compared. The spectrometer is able to automatically scan all wavelengths, showing peaks at wavelengths where maximum absorption occurs.

Different compounds have very different maximum absorbance wavelength and absorption patterns. Colored compounds can be identified in a solution based on their wavelength absorption. The absorbance of a sample will be proportional to the number of absorbing molecules in the sample. Therefore, if absorbance values are to be compared, they must be corrected so that the concentration of absorbing molecules in the samples is the same. The corrected absorption value is called the *molar absorptivity* (ε) and is defined by the equation: $\varepsilon = A/cl$, where A is absorbance, c is concentration (mol/L), and l is the length of the light path through the sample (that is, the width of the cuvette) in centimeters.

Figure 15. Maximum UV-Vis Wavelength Absorbed in a Sample of Isoprene

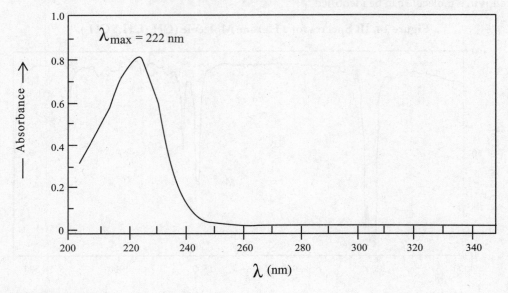

NMR Spectroscopy

Nuclear magnetic resonance (NMR) spectroscopy is a valuable technique in organic chemistry in terms of molecular structure determination. NMR spectroscopy provides information about the carbon-hydrogen framework of an organic molecule. Mass spectroscopy helps to determine the size and molecular formula of a molecule, IR spectroscopy helps to determine the functional groups present, and NMR spectroscopy helps to determine the carbon-hydrogen framework of a molecule.

Certain atomic nuclei have an intrinsic magnetic moment and angular momentum that when placed into a magnetic field absorb electromagnetic radiation of certain frequencies (resonate). For proton and carbon nuclei, only ^1H and ^{13}C isotopes are useful. ^2H (deuterium) and ^{12}C (99% of the carbon atoms) do not resonate, and therefore, do not have a spectrum. For this reason, deuterium solvents are useful for dissolving samples when NMR spectroscopy is used. There are several features of proton and carbon atoms that lead to the NMR phenomenon. The spinning charge of the atomic nuclei generates a magnetic field. The resulting spin-magnet has a magnetic moment, μ, that is proportional to the spin. In the presence of a strong external magnetic field, there are two spin states for a given atom: $+\frac{1}{2}$ and $-\frac{1}{2}$. The lower-energy spin state, $+\frac{1}{2}$, is aligned with the external magnetic field, and the higher-energy spin state, $-\frac{1}{2}$, is opposed to the external field. The difference in energy between the two spin states is dependent on the strength of the external magnetic field, but this difference is always a very small value. When the external field is zero, the two spin states are equal, and this difference increases as the strength of the magnetic field increases. So, NMR spectroscopy requires a strong magnetic field. The difference between two $\frac{1}{2}$ spin states at a given magnetic field strength is proportional to their magnetic moment.

When the oriented nuclei are irradiated with radio waves of a given frequency, energy absorption occurs. This absorption causes the nuclei in the lower-energy spin state to "spin-flip" to the higher-energy state. When this occurs, the nuclei is said to be *in resonance* with the applied radiation. The amount of radio-frequency energy required depends on the strength of the external magnetic field and the type of nucleus being irradiated. Radio frequency energy in the 60 MHz range is required to bring an ^{1}H nucleus into resonance, and 15 MHz is required to bring a ^{13}C nucleus into resonance.

Since all nuclei are surrounded by electron clouds, when a magnetic field is applied to a molecule, its electrons set up tiny local magnetic fields of their own. These local magnetic fields act in opposition to the applied field, so that the overall effect on the nucleus is smaller than that of the actual applied field. The electron cloud in the molecule acts to shield the nucleus. Since each nucleus in a molecular sample is in a slightly different electronic environment (due to each atom's electron cloud), each nucleus is shielded slightly differently. This means that the effective external magnetic field is not the same for each nucleus. These tiny differences can be detected by an NMR spectrometer, and a different NMR signal can be seen for each type of nucleus. Thus, each proton and carbon nucleus in a molecule will give rise to a unique signal. The NMR spectrum of an organic compound can, therefore, provide chemists with a map of the carbon-hydrogen framework of a given molecule.

In order to perform an analysis, an organic sample is dissolved in a suitable solvent, and placed in a glass tube between the poles of the strong magnet. The strong magnetic field causes the ^{1}H and ^{13}C nuclei to align in one of two different orientations. The sample is then irradiated with radio-frequency (rf) energy. The exact amount of rf energy depends on the strength of the external magnetic field and the kind of nucleus being observed. If the frequency of irradiation is held constant and the strength of the external magnetic field varies, each nucleus comes into resonance at a different field strength. A sensitive detector monitors the absorption of rf energy, and the electronic signal is amplified and displayed on a recorder chart as a peak.

^{13}C NMR

Only about one out of every 100 carbons is ^{13}C, thus only 1 percent of the carbons in a sample are observable by NMR. Therefore, the instrument required to perform ^{13}C NMR spectroscopy must be far more sensitive than that for ^{1}H NMR. In its most basic sense, ^{13}C NMR allows chemists to count the number of carbons in an unknown structure. Information about the chemical environment for each ^{13}C atom can be gathered by observing the chemical shift. The chemical shift is the exact place on the recorded chart at which a nucleus absorbs. Many factors affect chemical shift, but in general, sp^3-hybridized carbons absorb in the range of 0–100 δ and sp^2-hybridized carbons absorb in the range of 100–210 δ.

In the spectra of a particular sample, the peaks recorded are not of uniform height. Some peaks are larger than others, even though all may be one-carbon resonances. The relative size of different peaks depends on the mode of spectrometer operation. When the NMR is operated in a gated-decoupled mode, single carbon resonances have the same peak areas. The relative number of carbons in a sample can be determined by the area under each peak. The proton noise-decoupled mode of operation of the spectrometer is more sensitive than the gated-decoupled mode, and so is used almost exclusively, even though there are differences in peak size because of the electronics of the spectrometer.

In the proton noise-decoupled mode, obtaining a spectrum provides a carbon count of the sample molecule and gives information about the environment of each carbon. The number of carbon atoms in a molecule can be determined and their environments can be deduced based on chemical shift.

When more detailed information is needed, the spectrometer can be operated in an off-resonance mode. In this mode, single carbon resonance lines can be split into multiple lines. This phenomenon is known as *spin-spin splitting* and occurs because the nuclear spin of one atom can interact with nearby atoms and is affected by any electron shielding and neighboring nuclei. Thus, the applied field necessary to cause resonance may be different for a group of similar carbon atoms. The consequence is that similar carbon atoms will come into resonance at two slightly different applied field values, and this is seen by the recording of a doublet peak, or a multiplet peak in some cases. A carbon that is bonded to n number of protons gives a peak signal that is split into $n + 1$ peaks. This provides information as to the number of protons to which each carbon atom is bound.

Figure 16. ^{13}C NMR. Off-Resonance Spectrum of Dichloroacetic Acid

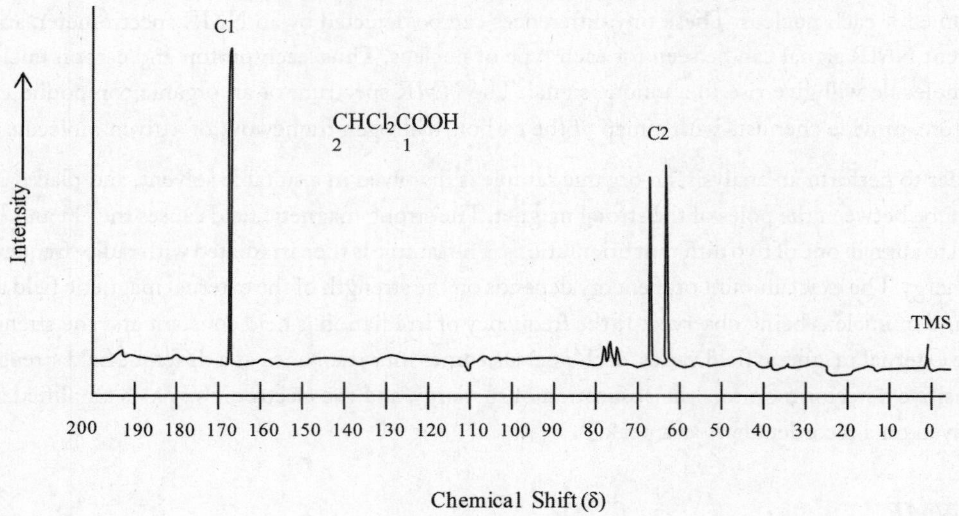

^1H NMR

^{1}H NMR can be used to help identify the product of nearly every reaction in organic chemistry. Proton chemical shifts fall within a narrow range of 0–10 δ. The precise spot of the chemical shift is dependent on the environment of the proton. In proton NMR, spin-spin splitting is due to the interaction or coupling of neighboring spins. The spins of one proton can couple with the spins of neighboring protons. The resultant spin patterns can be complex, but they can provide much information.

The distance between peaks in a multiplet is called the *coupling constant*. The value of a coupling constant, J, is between 0–18 Hz, and the exact value of the coupling constant between two groups of protons depends on several factors, but is independent of spectrometer field strength. *Coupling* is the reciprocal interaction between the spins of two adjacent groups of protons, and it is sometimes possible to determine which multiplets in a spectrum are influenced by one another. If two multiplets have the same coupling constant, then they are most likely related and the protons causing the peaks are likely to be adjacent.

There are three important rules to spin-spin splitting in ^{1}H NMR.

1. Chemically equivalent protons do not exhibit spin-spin splitting. The equivalent protons can be on the same or different carbon atoms. They do not couple and their signal appears as a singlet.

2. A proton with n equivalent neighboring protons gives a signal that is split into $n + 1$ peaks with a coupling constant, J. Protons farther than two carbon atoms apart do not couple.

3. Two groups of protons coupled to each other have the same coupling constant.

Proton NMR is more useful than ^{13}C NMR because the sensitivity of the instrument is very high, and normal spectrometer operating conditions indicate spin-spin splitting. The proton resonances fall in a narrow range of 0–10 δ downfield from the reference peak (TMS), and the exact chemical shift of an absorption indicates the chemical environment of the proton. In addition, the integration of areas under each peak in a proton NMR spectra can give information about the relative number of protons responsible for each peak.

Figure 17. ^{1}H NMR Spectrum for Chloroethane, CH_3CH_2Cl

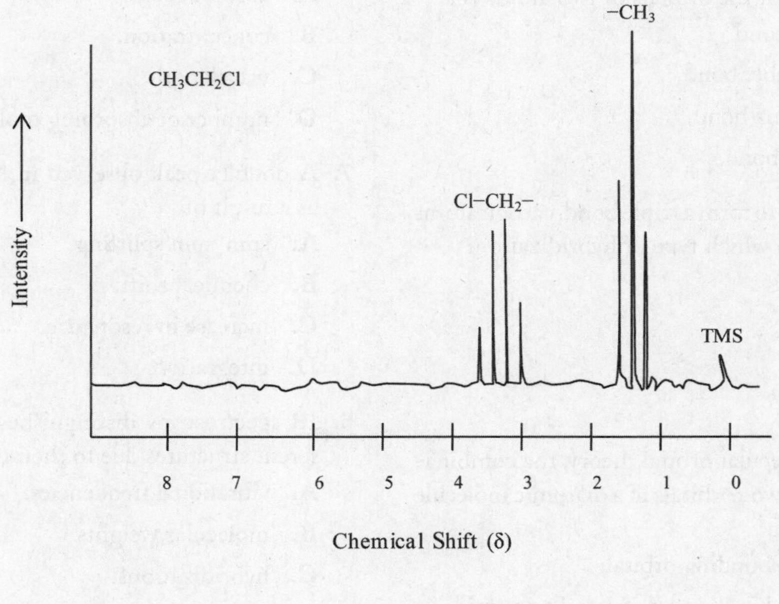

PRACTICE QUESTIONS

Directions: Choose the best answer for each question.

Refer to the following passage for Questions 1–4.

The way carbon atoms bond to one another is dependent on the orbitals that surround them. Single and double bonds involve the overlap of different types of orbitals, and orbital overlap between any two nonmetal atoms becomes even more complex when molecular orbital theory is applied.

1. What type of carbon-carbon bond is present in an ethyne molecule?
   A. Single bond
   B. Double bond
   C. Triple bond
   D. No carbon-carbon bond

2. The type of bond formed by a head-on overlap of the orbitals of two atoms is a
   A. pi bond.
   B. double bond.
   C. sigma bond.
   D. sp^2 bond.

3. In order to form a triple bond, carbon atoms undergo which type of hybridization?
   A. sp
   B. sp^2
   C. sp^3
   D. sp^4

4. Per molecular orbital theory, the combination of two *s* orbitals in a diatomic molecule will form
   A. one bonding orbital.
   B. one bonding orbital and one anti-bonding orbital.
   C. three bonding orbitals.
   D. three bonding orbitals and three anti-bonding orbitals.

Refer to the following passage for Questions 5–8.

IR, UV-Vis, NMR, and mass spectroscopy are used to elucidate the structures of unknown organic compounds. Each of the four techniques focuses on different aspects of compound structures.

5. The various peaks observed when a compound is analyzed by mass spectrometry is due to
   A. fragmentation of the molecule.
   B. functional groups.
   C. the number of carbon molecules.
   D. the number of hydrogen molecules.

6. Molar absorptivity is indirectly proportional to
   A. absorbance.
   B. concentration.
   C. wavelength.
   D. number of absorbing molecules.

7. A doublet peak observed in NMR occurs as a result of
   A. spin-spin splitting.
   B. chemical shift.
   C. increase in resonance.
   D. integration.

8. IR spectroscopy distinguishes among different structures due to their differences in
   A. vibrational frequencies.
   B. molecular weights.
   C. hybridizations.
   D. types of atoms present.

The following questions are standalone and not tied to a passage.

9. Oxygen is an atom with six valence electrons. How many bonds can an oxygen atom form?
   - A. 1
   - B. 2
   - C. 3
   - D. 4

10. The redistribution of electrons such that a ring structure is formed is in
   - A. free radical reaction.
   - B. polar reaction.
   - C. substitution reaction.
   - D. pericyclic reaction.

11. Which type of method is best used for isolating a volatile compound from a mixture of several volatile liquids?
   - A. Distillation
   - B. Fractional distillation
   - C. Sublimation
   - D. Crystallization

12.

The above structures are isomers of which alkane molecule?
   - A. Methane
   - B. Pentane
   - C. Butane
   - D. Ethane

13. A reaction in which a functional group leaves an electrophile at the same time that a nucleophile attacks is an
   - A. S_N1 reaction.
   - B. S_N2 reaction.
   - C. E1 reaction.
   - D. oxidation reaction.

14. HPLC technique utilizes which type of stationary phase?
   - A. A solid such as Al_2O_3
   - B. Nitrogen gas
   - C. Small, uniform-sized spheres
   - D. A volatile solvent

15. The empirical formula of a compound, $C_aH_bO_c$, can be determined by which of the following methods?
   - A. Crystallization
   - B. Distillation
   - C. Sublimation
   - D. Combustion analysis

16. The general formula for an ether molecule is
   - A. R,R'C=O'
   - B. R-O-R'
   - C. R-C-OH
   - D. R'-COO-R

17. Which type of reaction follows Markonikov's rule?
   - A. Free radical addition
   - B. Nucleophilic addition
   - C. Electrophilic addition
   - D. Esterification

18. In ^1H NMR spectroscopy, a proton with 4 equivalent neighboring protons gives a signal that is split into how many peaks?
   - A. 3
   - B. 4
   - C. 5
   - D. 8

19. An amine can be aromatic if it
- **A.** contains a benzene ring as one of its R groups.
- **B.** contains a double bond between its nitrogen and one of its R groups.
- **C.** is tetrahedral in shape.
- **D.** can be crystallized in a buffer solution.

20. The temperature and pressure at which the vapor pressure of a solid equals the applied pressure is called the
- **A.** boiling point.
- **B.** melting point.
- **C.** sublimation point.
- **D.** thermal conductivity.

ANSWER KEY AND EXPLANATIONS

1. C	**5.** A	**9.** B	**13.** B	**17.** C
2. C	**6.** B	**10.** D	**14.** C	**18.** C
3. A	**7.** A	**11.** B	**15.** D	**19.** A
4. B	**8.** A	**12.** C	**16.** B	**20.** C

1. **The correct answer is C.** The molecule ethyne is a hydrocarbon that fits into the category of alkynes. All alkyne molecules have at least one triple bond. Because ethyne only has two carbon atoms, the bond between them must be a triple bond. Choices A, B, and D are, therefore, incorrect.

2. **The correct answer is C.** The type of bond that is formed by the head-on overlap of two orbitals and has a spherical cross-section is called a sigma (σ) bond. Choice A is incorrect because a pi bond is formed by the sideways overlap of orbitals. Choice B is incorrect because the head-on overlap of orbitals forms a sigma bond, which is a single bond. Choice D is incorrect because sp^2 refers to a type of hybridization of electron orbitals, not a bond type.

3. **The correct answer is A.** In order to form a triple bond, carbon forms a type of hybridization orbital called an sp hybrid. In an sp hybrid orbital, two of the p orbitals are used to form a triple bond between two carbon atoms ($C \equiv C$). Choice B is incorrect because formation of sp^2 hybrids allows the formation of double bonds. Choice C is incorrect because the formation of sp^3 hybrid orbitals allows the molecule to form sigma, or single, bonds. Choice D is incorrect because there is no such thing as an sp^4 hybridization because there are only three p orbitals that can hybridize with an s orbital.

4. **The correct answer is B.** The total number of molecular orbitals formed must be the same as the total number of input orbitals. Choices A and C are incorrect because they neglect to indicate the formation of anti-bonding orbitals. Choice D is incorrect because these are the orbitals formed by the combination of three p orbitals from each atom in a diatomic molecule.

5. **The correct answer is A.** A molecule will have several peaks, depending on how its molecules can fragment. The process of electron bombardment also transfers a large quantity of energy to the molecules of the sample. This causes the cation radicals to fly apart (fragment). Choice B is incorrect because IR spectroscopy reveals the different types of motion within a given molecular sample, and interpreting the IR spectra can help to determine what kinds of functional groups are in the molecule. Choice C is incorrect because ^{13}C NMR spectroscopy reveals information about the carbon atoms in a molecule. Choice D is incorrect because ^1H NMR spectroscopy reveals information about the hydrogen atoms in a molecule.

6. **The correct answer is B.** The molar absorptivity (ε) is defined by the equation $\varepsilon = A/cl$, where A is absorbance, c is concentration (mol/L), and l is the length of the light path through the sample. Therefore, molar absorptivity is indirectly proportional to

the concentration and path length of the solution. Choice A is incorrect because ε is directly proportional to absorbance. Choice C is incorrect because ε is proportional to wavelength absorbance, but not the actual wavelength. Choice D is incorrect because the absorbance of a molecule is dependent on the number of absorbing molecules, but the molar absorptivity is inversely related to the concentration.

7. **The correct answer is A.** In the off-resonance mode of NMR, multiplet peaks can be observed due to spin-spin splitting. Neighboring molecules' nuclear spins can couple, splitting the peaks into multiplets. Choice B is incorrect because chemical shift refers to the exact location of a peak on an NMR spectrum. Choice C is incorrect because an increase in resonance would not cause a splitting of peaks. Choice D is incorrect because integration simply refers to the area under an absorption peak.

8. **The correct answer is A.** Different functional groups have different stretching and vibrating frequencies that provide unique signals. Choice B is incorrect because this is more applicable to mass spectroscopy. Choice C is incorrect; it can vaguely be associated with UV-Vis spectroscopy. Choice D is also incorrect; it can also be vaguely associated with NMR spectroscopy.

9. **The correct answer is B.** An oxygen atom has six valence electrons out of a possible eight electrons. Therefore, according to the octet rule, an oxygen atom will seek two shared electrons, and it can form two covalent bonds. Choice A is incorrect because oxygen has two spaces open to form a covalent bond. Choice C is incorrect because there are only two positions open in the valence electron shell so that oxygen is only able to form two

bonds. Choice D is incorrect because oxygen can only form two bonds.

10. **The correct answer is D.** Pericyclic reactions are those that involve the redistribution of bonding electrons in a cyclical manner. Choice A is incorrect because a free radical reaction involves two species called radicals that each donate only one electron to form a bond. Choice B is incorrect because a polar reaction is the result of attractive forces between the positive and negative charges on molecules. Choice C is incorrect because a substitution reaction may form a cyclical product, but it does not always. In a substitution reaction, a nucleophile reacts with an electrophile in a process called nucleophilic attack.

11. **The correct answer is B.** In a crude mixture of two or more volatile liquids with different boiling points, a process of fractional distillation can separate the liquids. The more volatile liquid with the lower boiling point distills first, and the higher boiling point liquid is distilled next. Choice A is incorrect because distillation can purify a single volatile liquid, but fractional distillation is required if there is a mixture of volatile liquids to be separated. Choice C is incorrect because sublimation is used when it is necessary to separate a volatile solid substance from substances that do not readily vaporize. Choice D is incorrect because crystallization is a method used for purifying a solid.

12. **The correct answer is C.** These two four-carbon compounds are known as isomers of butane. Isomers have the same molecular formula, but different structures. The structure on the left is a straight-chain butane, and the one on the right is a branched structure called isobutane. Choice

A is incorrect because methane only has one carbon and therefore does not form isomers. Choice B is incorrect because pentane has five carbon atoms, not four. Choice D is incorrect because ethane has three carbon atoms, not four.

13. **The correct answer is B.** In an S_N2 reaction, the leaving group leaves the electrophile at the same time that the electrophile is attacked by the nucleophile. Choice A is incorrect because in an S_N1 reaction, the two events do not occur simultaneously. The leaving group departs first, and then the nucleophile attacks. Choice C is incorrect because E1 reactions occur by spontaneous dissociation of the leaving group and the loss of a proton from an intermediate carbocation. As in the case of an S_N1 reaction, the loss of the proton (breaking of a C-H bond) occurs after the rate-limiting step of the dissociation of the leaving group. Choice D is incorrect because in organic chemistry, oxidation is the process by which an oxygen atom is added to a molecule or a hydrogen atom (or atoms) is removed from a molecule.

14. **The correct answer is C.** In HPLC, the stationary phase in the column is composed of very small, uniformly sized spherical particles that improve the efficiency of the chromatography. Choice A is incorrect because a solid such as Al_2O_3 is a common stationary phase used in liquid chromatography. Choice B is incorrect because nitrogen is used as a carrier gas in the mobile phase of gas chromatography. Choice D is incorrect because a volatile solvent is not a good choice for HPLC.

15. **The correct answer is D.** Empirical and molecular formulas of organic compounds containing only one or all of the elements C, H, and O can be determined through the process of combustion analysis. Choice A is incorrect because crystallization is the process of purifying a solid compound. Choice B is incorrect because distillation is a simple and effective method of purifying a volatile liquid. Choice C is incorrect because sublimation is a process used to separate a volatile solid from nonvolatile substances.

16. **The correct answer is B.** Ethers are organic compounds containing the general formula R-O-R', where R and R' are functional groups. Choice A is incorrect because R,R'C=O' is the general formula for a carbonyl molecule. Choice C is incorrect because R-C-OH is a general formula for alcohols. Choice D is incorrect because R'-COO-R is a general formula for esters.

17. **The correct answer is C.** Electrophilic addition reactions follow Markonikov's rule that states that when an asymmetric alkene and a protic acid (HX) are combined, the hydrogen will bind to the side of the double bond that contains the most hydrogen atoms. Also, the carbocation will form on the carbon with the most electron-donating substituents. Choice A is incorrect because a free radical addition reaction behaves exactly opposite to Markonikov's rule. Choice B is incorrect because a nucleophilic addition reaction does not follow Markonikov's rule. Choice D is incorrect because esterification is a reaction that involves the formation of an ester from an alcohol and a carboxylic acid and takes place in the presence of an acid catalyst at high temperature. This reaction does not follow Markonikov's rule.

18. **The correct answer is C.** A proton with n equivalent neighboring protons gives a signal that is split into $n + 1$ peaks. Choices A, B, and D are incorrect because they do not follow this rule.

19. The correct answer is A. By definition, an aromatic compound must contain a benzene. The simplest aromatic amine is aniline. Choices B, C, and D contain bits of properties that may be seen in aromatic amines, but they are not requirements of these molecules by any means.

20. The correct answer is C. Sublimation may be used to separate a volatile solid from substances that do not vaporize as easily. Choice A is incorrect because the boiling point describes the conditions under which a liquid is converted to a gas. Choice B is incorrect because the melting describes the conditions under which a solid is converted to a gas. Choice D is incorrect because thermal conductivity is the property of a material that describes its ability to conduct heat.

SUMMING IT UP

- Covalent bonds are the most prevalent bonding type in organic compounds.

- The electron sharing that takes place in a covalent bond tightly binds the atoms; the shared electrons are pulled toward the nucleus of both atoms.

- The *octet rule* states that an atom is in its most favorable, or lowest, energy configuration when it contains eight valence electrons, the maximum number of electrons that can fill a valence shell.

- According to the *molecular orbital theory*, when a covalent bond forms, the atomic orbital on different individual atoms combine to form molecular orbitals. These combined orbitals hold the shared electrons that make up a covalent bond.

- A sigma (σ) bond is formed by the head-on overlap of the atomic orbitals of two atoms. This type of bond has a spherical cross-section.

- A sigma bond can be formed by the combination of two *s* orbitals, two *p* orbitals, or one *s* orbital and one *p* orbital. All single bonds are σ bonds in which two electrons are shared between atoms.

- A strong *pi (π) bond* forms when two *p* orbitals overlap in a sideways fashion.

- When both a sigma bond and a pi bond exist between two atoms, a *double bond* is formed. Furthermore, when a sigma bond and two pi bonds exist, a *triple bond* forms between atoms.

- A combination of an *s* and three *p* orbitals can be mathematically hybridized, or mixed, to form four equivalent orbitals oriented toward the corners of the tetrahedral shape that a carbon molecule adopts. These new tetrahedral orbitals are called *sp^3 hybrid orbitals*.

- The combination of an *s* orbital with only two *p* orbitals (p_x and p_y) forms an *sp^2 hybrid orbital*. In order to form a triple bond, carbon forms a third type of hybridization orbital called an *sp hybrid*. In an *sp* hybrid orbital, two of the *p* orbitals are used to form a triple bond between two carbon atoms (C≡C). The remaining *p* orbital hybridizes with the *s* orbital forming two *sp* hybrid orbitals.

- If the electrons are positioned closer to the nucleus of one atom than the other, the covalent bond is considered to be a *polar bond*. There are different degrees of polarity, depending on the atoms that form the bond.

- *Electronegativity* is the physical property of an atom that describes its relative attraction of the shared electrons in a covalent bond. The electronegativity of an atom is related to the octet rule and the propensity of an atom to fill any unfilled orbitals in its valence shell.

- A *functional group* is composed of atoms or groups of atoms with a known chemical reactivity, and it will behave in much the same way in any molecule to which it is attached.

- *Hydrocarbons*, or compounds with chains of carbon and hydrogen molecules, are named by finding the highest number of carbon-carbon bonds in the molecule.

- *Alkanes* are hydrocarbons that contain only single carbon-carbon bonds. The general molecular formula for alkanes is C_nH_{2n+2}. In this formula, *n* is a positive integer. All alkanes have the suffix *-ane*.

- *Alkenes* are hydrocarbons that contain at least one carbon-carbon double bond. The naming of alkenes is similar to the naming of alkanes, except that the suffix on the end of each compound name is *-ene*. The general molecular formula for alkenes is C_nH_{2n}.

- *Alkynes* are hydrocarbons that contain at least one carbon-carbon triple bond. The naming convention is the same as that of alkanes and alkenes, except that the suffix used is *-yne*. The general formula for alkynes is C_nH_{2n-2}.

- Some unsaturated cyclic hydrocarbon molecules are known as *aromatic rings*. Benzene, C_6H_6, is the parent compound for this type of hydrocarbon.

- All alcohols contain the functional group –OH. Alcohols are named in a similar manner to alkanes with a prefix of *-ol*.

- *Ethers* are organic compounds containing the general formula R-O-R'.

- Carbonyl compounds are those that contain a carbon-oxygen double bond. A C=O bond is referred to as a *carbonyl bond*. Aldehydes, ketones, esters, and carboxylic acids are all carbonyl compounds.

- *Amines* are organic molecules with properties of a base. They have the general formula, R_3N, where R is an H atom or a hydrocarbon group.

- *Polar reactions* are the result of attractive forces between the positive and negative charges on molecules. In a polar reaction, bonds are formed when an electron-rich substance called a nucleophile donates a pair of electrons to an electron-poor substance called an electrophile. The bond is broken when one of the two nuclei leaves with the electron pair and separates from the other atom. In a radical reaction, the species contain an odd number of electrons, and the single unpaired electrons are donated to form a bond in what is called a *homogenic process*. When bonds are broken between radicals, each species leaves the bonding relationship with only one of the bonding electrons. This type of bond breakage is called a *hemolytic breakage*.

- Radical substitution reactions generally occur in three steps: the initiation step, the propagation steps, and the termination steps. Note that the last two are multiple steps.

- *Pericyclic reactions* are those that involve the redistribution of bonding electrons in a cyclical manner.

- In a *substitution reaction*, a nucleophile reacts with an electrophile in a process called *nucleophilic attack*. There are two main categories of substitution reactions: S_N2 and S_N1.

- An *elimination reaction* involves the removal of an atom or functional group from a molecule. This type of reaction usually involves an increase in the number of double or triple bonds in the final product compared to the reactant. Elimination reactions can be divided into two types: E1 and E2 reactions.

- An *organic condensation reaction* is one in which two molecules are united as they expel a smaller molecule such as water. Most condensation reactions take place through substitution, addition, or elimination processes.

- *Dehydration reactions* are special types of elimination reactions in which the leaving group is always a water molecule.

- In organic chemistry, *oxidation* is the process by which an oxygen atom is added to a molecule or a hydrogen atom (or atoms) is removed from a molecule. *Reduction* is the process in which a hydrogen atom (or atoms) is added to a molecule or an oxygen atom is removed from a molecule.

- *Esterification reactions* take place in five steps with the formation of four intermediate molecules. The net result of the reaction is that the oxygen atom on the alcohol acts as a nucleophile, and the carbon on the carboxylic acid acts as the electrophile.

- An *addition reaction* involves two molecules joining together to form a larger molecule. An addition reaction can be either nucleophilic, or electrophilic, or a free radical addition.

- The process of *extraction* involves the separation of a substance from a solution or matrix. An extraction can be a solid phase extraction in which solids are dissolved in liquid and the components of the solid separated from each other based on their chemical and physical properties or a liquid extraction from a liquid solvent.

- *Crystallization* is a straightforward and effective way of purifying a solid. The formation of crystals can be brought about by the addition of a seed crystal or by scratching the side of the vessel containing the solution. The impurities are left behind in the solution, and the pure crystals are isolated through a process of filtration.

- The process of distillation is a simple and effective method of purifying a volatile liquid. A crude liquid reaction product is heated to its boiling point, and as the vapor rises, it is collected and condensed back into a liquid.

- The process of *sublimation* is used when it is necessary to separate a volatile solid substance from substances that do not readily vaporize.

- *Chromatography* methods can be used to separate a mixture of organic compounds. The mixture to be separated is dissolved in a liquid or gaseous mobile phase (solvent), and it is passed through a solid adsorbent phase that is packed in a column of varying size. Different organic compounds in a mixture will adsorb to the stationary phase to different degrees. Therefore, the different compounds will migrate through the stationary phase at different rates and can be separated as they come out of the stationary phase column.

- *Liquid chromatography* is one of the simplest and most frequently used methods of product purification. A mixture of organic compounds is dissolved in a liquid mobile phase. *High-pressure liquid chromatography* (HPLC) is a variant of the simple column chromatography technique. If the stationary phase is composed of very small, uniformly sized spherical particles, the efficiency of chromatography is improved. Gas chromatography employs a carrier gas such as nitrogen as the mobile phase solvent.

- Empirical and molecular formulas of organic compounds can be determined through the process of *combustion analysis*. The mass of the product to be analyzed is determined, and then the product is burned completely. If a product only contains one or some carbon, hydrogen, and oxygen atoms, as is the case in many organic compounds, then the only products of combustion (burning) are carbon dioxide and water.

- *Mass spectroscopy* allows for the measurement of the mass, or molecular weight, of an isolated compound or molecule.

- *IR spectroscopy* reveals the different types of motion within a given molecular sample. Interpreting the IR spectra can help to determine what kinds of functional groups are in the molecule.

- *UV-Vis spectroscopy* is used to understand the chemical make-up of a compound with respect to its color, the relationship of bond conjugation to color, and also when it is necessary to make accurate measurements of light absorption at different wavelengths in and near the visible light spectrum.

- *NMR spectroscopy* provides information about the carbon-hydrogen framework of an organic molecule.

- In its most basic sense, ^{13}C *NMR* allows chemists to count the number of carbons in an unknown structure. Information about the chemical environment for each ^{13}C atom can be gathered by observing the chemical shift.

- When the NMR is operated in a *gated-decoupled mode*, single carbon resonances have the same peak areas. The relative number of carbons in a sample can be determined by the area under each peak. In the *proton noise-decoupled* mode, obtaining a spectrum provides a carbon count of the sample molecule and gives information about the environment of each carbon. When more detailed information is needed, the spectrometer can be operated in an *off-resonance mode*. In this mode, single carbon resonance lines can be split into multiple lines due to spin-spin splitting.

- A carbon that is bonded to *n* number of protons gives a peak signal that is split into *n* + 1 peaks. This gives information as to how many protons each carbon atom is bound to.

- *Proton NMR* is more useful than ^{13}C NMR because the sensitivity of the instrument is very high, and normal spectrometer operating conditions indicate spin-spin splitting. In proton NMR, spin-spin splitting is due to the interaction or coupling of neighboring spins. The spins of one proton can couple with the spins of neighboring protons.

- The integration of areas under each peak in a proton NMR spectra can give information as to the relative number of protons responsible for each peak.

Biochemistry

OVERVIEW

- **Carbohydrates**
- **Lipids**
- **DNA and RNA**
- **Proteins**
- **Practice Questions**
- **Answer Key and Explanations**
- **Summing It Up**

The four classes of biomolecules are carbohydrates, lipids, nucleic acids, and proteins. These biological molecules provide the building blocks of life, however, a basic understanding of carbohydrates is crucial to answering many of the other test items. Approximately 20% questions on the PCAT will test your knowledge of biochemistry.

CARBOHYDRATES

Of the four classes of biomolecules, carbohydrates represent the only class of biomolecules on which the PCAT specifications do not focus, but this class is worth some attention because they are so important to life. Carbohydrates serve as the major energy source for most cells, and they are critical in the synthesis of lipids and proteins. The three key elements that make up carbohydrates are carbon, hydrogen, and oxygen, which are actually the three elements that comprise nearly 99% of the human body.

Carbohydrates have the general empirical formula of $(CH_2O)_n$. In general, carbohydrates consist of a set of carbons arranged in a linear or ring structure, with a number of hydroxyl (-OH), keto (-[C=O]-), or aldehyde (-[CH=O]) groups attached to them. **Monosaccharides** are simple sugars and represent the monomer of carbohydrates. They tend to have 3-6 carbons, and they are named accordingly, per the table below.

Number of Carbons	Name
3	triose
4	tetrose
5	pentose
6	hexose

Chapter 10

Glucose is a well-known example of a monosaccharide, a hexose, and has the chemical formula $C_6H_{12}O_6$. Note that this formula corresponds with the empirical formula noted above. The linear form of glucose is shown in the image below.

While glucose can take on a number of three-dimensional forms called **stereoisomers**, the one that exists in nature is called D-glucose. Glucose is critical to the function of cells because it is the major input carbohydrate for cellular respiration, the process by which cells aerobically use oxygen to produce significant quantities of ATP, or cellular energy. Glucose is an aldose monosaccharide because it features an aldehyde group, shown at the top of the image above.

Fructose, in contrast, is a ketose monosaccharide because it features a ketone. Its structure is shown below.

Fructose is found in a wide array of plants and, like glucose and fellow monosaccharide galactose, is absorbed directly into the bloodstream during digestion. When fructose and glucose bond together, they form sucrose, whose ring structure is shown below.

Sucrose is a **disaccharide**, which means that it consists of two monosaccharides linked together through a bond called a **glycosidic linkage**. Another fairly simple disaccharide is maltose, which is made up of two glucose monosaccharides. The linkage shown above is specifically a (1-4) glycosidic linkage, named for the two carbons that are connected by the intermediary oxygen. Glycosidic linkages can form through condensation reactions and break through hydrolysis reactions.

Maltose is an example of a **reducing sugar**, which means that it possesses an aldehyde group (or can form an aldehyde group via isomerization). Sucrose, on the other hand, lacks this feature and is a **non-reducing sugar**.

Complexity can increase beyond monosaccharides and disaccharides. **Oligosaccharides** consist of 3-6 monosaccharides, while **polysaccharides** consist of more than six monosaccharides. As usual, these monosaccharides are all linked via glycosidic bonds.

Homopolysaccharides consist of the same monosaccharide repeated numerous times. A common example is starch, composed of many glucose units. Glycogen and cellulose are also examples of homopolysaccharides. Glycogen is a molecule in humans that stores energy long term. It is mostly produced by the muscles and liver, but can also be made in the brain and stomach. Glycogen can be quickly mobilized if there is an immediate need for energy. Cellulose is the key component of plant cell walls but is useless in humans, as it is a fiber that cannot be digested. **Heteropolysaccharides**, in contrast, are composed of different kinds of monosaccharides.

LIPIDS

Lipids cover a wide expanse of molecules that include waxes, oils, phospholipids, triglycerides, and fatty acids. In general, they are important for energy storage, cell signaling, and cell membrane structure, as well as hormone regulation. Many lipids can be acquired from one's diet, but some lipids can only be made in the cell. Lipids are formed via fatty acid synthesis, the elongation of hydrocarbon chains that end with a carboxylic acid termination group. A **saturated** fatty acid consists of a hydrocarbon chain consisting entirely of single bonds, while an **unsaturated** fatty acid has at least one double bond that causes a "kink" in the chain. During fatty acid synthesis, NADPH is used as an energy source to polymerize fatty acid chains. The hydrocarbon chains within lipids represent nonpolar regions, while carbonyl and charged portions of lipids represent polar regions.

The three main classes of lipids are triglycerides, steroids, and phospholipids. **Triglycerides** consist of a glycerol head group with three attached fatty acids. **Steroids** tend to be hydrophobic and insoluble in water. Examples of steroids are cholesterol and testosterone. **Phospholipids** consist of a polar head group and a number of fatty acid tails. These tend to have both hydrophobic and hydrophilic parts, and these are the lipids found in membranes. The structure of a lipid bilayer is shown below. The central portion of a membrane bilayer is hydrophobic due to the presence of the hydrophobic tails interacting with one another, while the head groups that face water and the surrounding solution are hydrophilic.

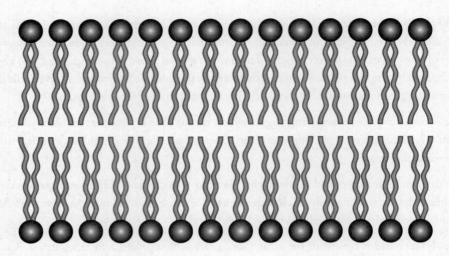

An ester bond is the bond between a head group and a fatty acid in a lipid. As in carbohydrates, condensation reactions form ester bonds. The formation of an ester bond via a condensation reaction is shown below.

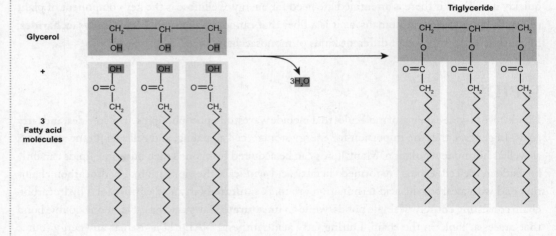

DNA AND RNA

DNA and RNA represent nucleic acids, which store genetic information. The monomer of a nucleic acid is the **nucleotide**, which consists of three parts: a nitrogenase base, a pentose sugar, and a phosphate group. Nucleotides are connected via phosphodiester bonds, which can again form via condensation reactions.

DNA and RNA have a number of similarities and differences. Deoxyribonucleic acid (DNA) and ribonucleic acid (RNA) are named for their pentose sugars, which are deoxyribose and ribose, respectively. DNA and RNA both consist of nucleotides, and nearly the same ones—the nucleotides of DNA are adenine (A), cytosine (C), guanine (G), and thymine (T), while those of RNA are adenine (A), cytosine (C), guanine (G), and uracil (U). DNA takes on the structure of a double helix and is consequently double-stranded. The two strands of DNA are held together by hydrogen bonds between bases; the sugar and phosphate groups make up the backbone of each strand, with the bases centrally holding the strands together. Within DNA, C and G pair up, and A and T pair up. That means that in DNA, for every C in one strand, there is a G in the opposite strand. The same goes for A and T, and vice versa for each. RNA, on the other hand, is single-stranded, but if RNA pairs up with DNA or another nucleic acid, the same pairings occur, with U in place of T.

Among the nitrogenous bases in nucleic acids, the five can be categorized as purines or pyrimidines. Purines have two rings in their structure, while pyrimidines only have one ring in their structure. Purines and pyrimidines always pair up with one another, keeping the strands of DNA (or in some cases, RNA) consistently far apart. The structures of the bases are shown in the image below.

| Purines | Pyrimidines |
| Adenine (A) (DNA and RNA) | Guanine (G) (DNA and RNA) | Cytosine (C) (DNA and RNA) | Thymine (T) (DNA only) | Uracil (U) (RNA only) |

DNA and RNA are involved in a number of key cellular processes. Because they are key components of genetic information in humans (and other organisms) **gene expression** is a key function of nucleic acids. Gene expression refers to the use of DNA to generate proteins for use by the cell. Proteins are coded for by the DNA sequence. However, DNA cannot be directly used to make proteins. First, DNA has to be converted into an RNA sequence. During the process of **transcription**, an RNA strand is constructed by bringing in RNA nucleotides that are complementary to the nucleotides in the DNA template sequence. This developing RNA strand is called **messenger RNA**, or mRNA, because its purpose is to carry the genetic message to a different part of the cell, the ribosome, for protein production. Once a single-stranded mRNA molecule is constructed, it is ready for transport. Transcription consists of initiation, elongation, and termination steps, and the main enzyme involved in the process is **RNA polymerase**.

In eukaryotic cells, however, there is one extra step that produces mature mRNA. This step is called **RNA splicing**. During RNA splicing, a **spliceosome** complex removes noncoding nucleotides from the mRNA strand and leaves behind coding nucleotides. The noncoding sequences are known as **introns**, while the coding sequences are **exons**. The exons are reassembled together after intron removal to form mature mRNA. This process of RNA splicing does not happen in prokaryotic cells; in prokaryotes, the mRNA produced during transcription is the mature mRNA that moves directly to protein synthesis.

Once mature mRNA is prepared, it is transported to the ribosome for **translation**, the process of synthesizing proteins from mRNA. During translation, the ribosome binds to the mRNA and links together amino acids, the building blocks of proteins, using **transfer RNA (tRNA)** molecules. tRNA molecules are RNA molecules that have several main parts, shown below.

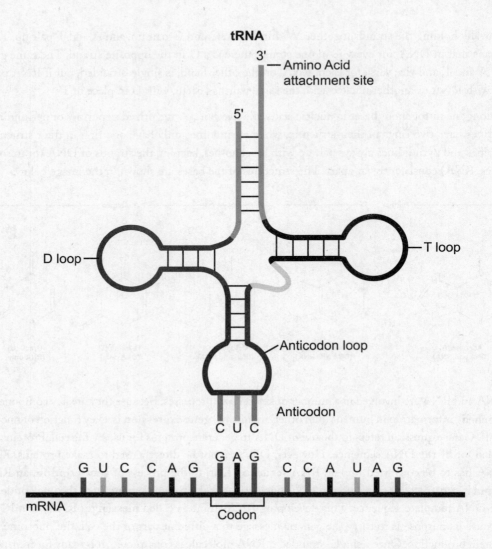

The **anticodon** portion of tRNA is a three-nucleotide sequence that recognizes a complementary mRNA sequence, the **codon**. On the other end of the tRNA is an attached amino acid, which is then added to a growing chain. Ribosomes continually bring in tRNA molecules to add to the growing strand until one of three specific stop codons (UAG, UAA, or UGA) terminates the process and releases the completed protein strand. Like transcription, translation consists of an initiation, elongation, and termination step, and the E, P, and A regions of the ribosome serve as entry, elongation, and exit points for the tRNA molecules as the protein is constructed. The structure of the ribosome is shown below.

In eukaryotes, the produced protein can then undergo posttranslational modifications to form a completed, functional protein. This step usually does not occur in prokaryotic cells.

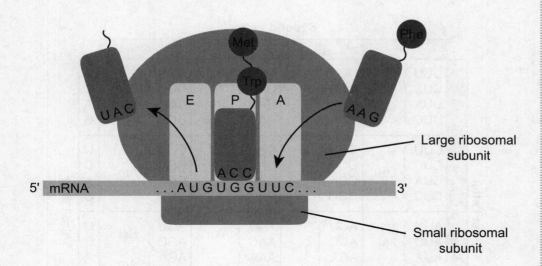

A summary of the process of gene expression in eukaryotes is shown below:

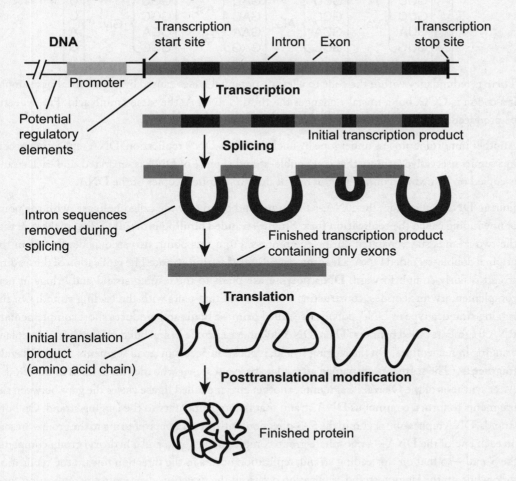

The genetic code is shown below, based on the mRNA sequence produced.

Second Letter

		U	C	A	G	
First Letter	**U**	UUU } Phe UUC } UUA } Leu UUG }	UCU } UCC } UCA } Ser UCG }	UAU } Tyr UAC } **UAA** **Stop** **UAG** **Stop**	UGU } Cys UGC } **UGA** **Stop** UGG Trp	U C A G
	C	CUU } CUC } CUA } Leu CUG }	CCU } CCC } CCA } Pro CCG }	CAU } His CAC } CAA } Gin CAG }	CGU } CGC } CGA } Arg CGG }	U C A G
	A	AUU } AUC } Ile AUA } AUG Met	ACU } ACC } ACA } Thr ACG }	AAU } Asn AAC } AAA } Lys AAG }	AGU } Ser AGC } AGA } Arg AGG }	U C A G
	G	GUU } GUC } GUA } Val GUG }	GCU } GCC } GCA } Ala GCG }	GAU } Asp GAC } GAA } Glu GAG }	GGU } GGC } GGA } Gly GGG }	U C A G

Third Letter (right side)

There is redundancy within the code to alleviate potential issues caused by mutations. For example, if a codon is CCC, but a mistake changes the third C to an A, the same amino acid, Pro, will still be produced.

Another important process undergone by nucleic acids is DNA replication. DNA replication occurs in a semiconservative fashion; that is, a double-stranded piece of DNA is separated, and each strand is copied on its own, becoming part of one of the two identical copies of the DNA.

During DNA replication, the DNA is first unwound by an enzyme called **helicase**, with the point of unwinding called the **replication fork**. **Single-stranded binding proteins** (SSBs) make sure that the two strands stay separated during the process. From this point, two strands develop from the original double-stranded DNA: a **leading strand** and a **lagging strand**. The replication of the leading strand is fairly straightforward: **DNA polymerase** binds to the leading strand and brings in new complementary nucleotides, constructing a new strand that pairs with the leading strand. On the lagging strand, a type of DNA polymerase called **primase** binds and produces short complementary RNA fragments called **primers**. Then, DNA polymerases come in and build off that initial template, bringing in nucleotides. On the lagging strand, replication occurs in small segments called **Okazaki fragments**. (The segments are named after a Japanese researcher who identified them in the 1960s.) After synthesis of the Okazaki fragments , another enzyme called **ligase** closes the gaps between the fragments to form a continuous DNA strand that is complementary to the lagging strand. On both strands, DNA replication occurs in the 5'-3' direction, with the numbers referring to the groups present on each end of the DNA—a phosphate group completes the 5' end and a hydroxyl group completes the 3' end—so that on the leading strand, replication occurs in the direction toward the replication fork, while on the lagging strand, replication occurs in the direction away from the replication fork.

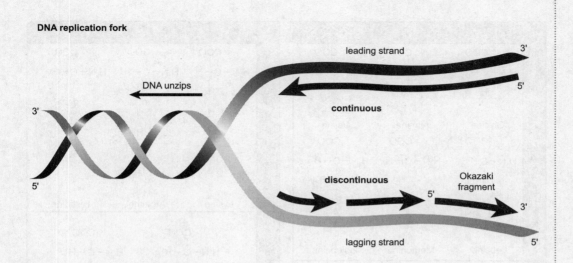

PROTEINS

Proteins, the products of translation, have a vast array of functions. Proteins play both structural and functional roles in the cell. Hemoglobin, for example, is found in the blood and binds oxygen, allowing for its circulation and subsequent use throughout the body. Actin and myosin are key players in muscle contraction. Antibodies are produced by the immune system to target antigens. Many proteins are **enzymes**, which catalyze chemical reactions by lowering the **activation energy** required to get the reaction started, converting **substrates** to **products**. Enzymes are almost exclusively proteins, though ribozyme is a ribonucleic acid that acts as an enzyme to catalyze specific reactions.

The monomer of a protein is the **amino acid**. The generalized structure of an amino acid is shown below.

An amino acid consists of a central carbon surrounded by four main functional groups: a simple hydrogen atom, a carboxylic acid group (-COOH), an amino group ($-NH_2$), and a variable R group. There are twenty naturally occurring amino acids that have unique R groups. R groups can be polar or nonpolar, charged or uncharged, small or large—this variety allows for a wide array of different kinds of proteins to be formed.

AMINO ACID		

Amino acids can join together through condensation reactions, also known as **dehydration synthesis**, to form longer polymeric chains of amino acids. The type of bond that forms between amino acids is called the peptide bond, forming between the carboxyl group of one amino acid and the amino group of the next amino acid.

peptide bond

When two amino acids join together, a **dipeptide** forms. A **polypeptide** consists of 2-30 amino acids, and any longer amino acid chain is called a **protein**.

Proteins have four levels of structure:

1. The **primary structure** of a protein consists simply of its sequence of amino acids. Because there are twenty naturally occurring amino acids, there are many different combinations of amino acids that can come together to form a protein, so the primary structure is the level of protein structure that generally introduces the greatest amount of diversity in proteins.

2. The **secondary structure** of a protein consists of localized motifs such as alpha helices and beta sheets. These localized structures can often be seen within the context of the overall three-dimensional shape of a protein. These structures are held together by hydrogen bonds.

3. The **tertiary structure** refers to the overall three-dimensional shape of a protein. This involves more complex folding beyond the signature alpha helices and beta sheets. Included in tertiary structure are **disulfide bonds**, S-S bonds that form between cysteine amino acids, and **ionic** interactions between charged components of the protein.

4. The **quaternary structure** refers to the combination of multiple peptide subunits that come together to form a large protein complex.

Not all proteins have all four levels of structure. Proteins that consist of one folded amino acid chain may have primary, secondary, and tertiary, but not quaternary structure because there are no other chains in complex with the protein.

Proteins fold by a variety of mechanisms, but the way proteins fold is extremely important to their function. Much of protein folding is directed by the **hydrophobic effect**, which indicates that hydrophobic molecules tend to interact with each other rather than with water. As a result, many of the hydrophobic amino acids in a protein will tend toward the inside of the protein, avoiding contact as much as possible with the surrounding solution. On the other hand, hydrophilic amino acids are more likely to be found on the external surface of a protein because they favorably interact with water.

Proteins can be finicky with regard to the types of conditions in which they can survive. **Buffers** can help to resist changes in the pH of solutions to ensure that proteins are maintained at favorable, functional pH levels. Dramatic pH increases or decreases can result in the unfolding of a protein and the loss of its function; this is called **denaturation**. Denaturation can also result from changes in temperature, particularly a dramatic increase in temperature. High temperatures can weaken the intramolecular forces holding proteins together, which could then result in the unfolding of the protein and the loss of function. Other chemicals can destroy protein function by influencing the way they fold or by chemically changing the functional groups found within the structure of the proteins.

PRACTICE QUESTIONS

Directions: Choose the best answer for each question.

Use the following passage to answer questions 1–4.

Passage 1

The enzyme catalase is found in plant and animal tissues, including humans. This enzyme prevents the toxic buildup of hydrogen peroxide in cells by breaking it down into oxygen gas and water. A group of students tested the effects of temperature on human catalase, testing bubble formation (i.e., oxygen gas) at 20°C, 30°C, 40°C, and 50°C. Human catalase consists of four polypeptide chain subunits. They saw that bubble formation increased as temperature increased from 20 to 40°C, but then bubble formation declined at the 50°C temperature mark.

1. Which monomer makes up catalase?
   A. Monosaccharide
   B. Amino acid
   C. Fatty acid
   D. Nucleotide

2. The most complex level of structure seen in catalase is:
   A. primary structure.
   B. secondary structure.
   C. tertiary structure.
   D. quaternary structure.

3. Why does bubble formation decrease above 40°C?
   A. The higher temperature has begun to denature the enzyme.
   B. The higher temperature promotes oxygen formation.
   C. The higher temperature increases the strength of intramolecular bonds within proteins.
   D. The higher temperature breaks the peptide bonds between amino acids.

4. By what mechanism does catalase break down hydrogen peroxide?
   A. It increases the amount of heat released in the reaction.
   B. It lowers the activation energy of the reaction.
   C. It decreases substrate usage in the reaction.
   D. It unfolds to maximize its activity during the reaction.

Use the following passage to answer questions 5–8.

A sequence of mature mRNA in Organism 1 has the sequence CCC AAA GCU. A sequence of mature mRNA in a related organism, Organism 2, has the sequence CCC AAG GCU.

5. What is the first amino acid coded for by the mRNA sequence in Organism 2?
   A. Leu
   B. Lys
   C. Pro
   D. Tyr

6. How do the amino acids in the peptide chain differ between Organism 1 and Organism 2?
   A. The amino acid chains are the same.
   B. The amino acid chains differ by one amino acid.
   C. The amino acid chains differ by two amino acids.
   D. The amino acid chains differ by three amino acids.

7. By what process will each mRNA be converted to protein?

A. DNA replication

B. RNA splicing

C. Transcription

D. Translation

8. If Organisms 1 and 2 are animals, which type of sequences are present in the provided mRNA sequence?

A. Exons, the coding sequences

B. Introns, the coding sequences

C. Exons, the noncoding sequences

D. Introns, the noncoding sequences

These questions are not linked to a passage.

9. The enzyme that unwinds DNA during DNA replication is

A. DNA polymerase.

B. helicase.

C. ligase.

D. RNA polymerase.

10. Raffinose is composed of a galactose, a fructose, and a glucose. Accordingly, raffinose is a(n)

A. disaccharide.

B. monosaccharide.

C. oligosaccharide.

D. polysaccharide.

11. Disulfide bonds are included in which level of protein structure?

A. Primary

B. Secondary

C. Tertiary

D. Quaternary

12. Single-stranded binding proteins

A. generate mRNA during transcription.

B. hold DNA strands apart during replication.

C. construct proteins during translation.

D. remove noncoding mRNA sequences during RNA splicing.

13. A double-stranded piece of DNA is composed of 40% G. What is the composition of A?

A. 10%

B. 20%

C. 40%

D. 80%

14. Alpha helices are held together by

A. ester bonds.

B. hydrogen bonds.

C. peptide bonds.

D. phosphodiester bonds.

15. The pieces of a nucleotide that make up the backbone of DNA are

A. sugar and phosphate.

B. phosphate and nitrogenous base.

C. nitrogenous base and sugar.

D. phosphate, sugar, and nitrogenous base.

16. Unsaturated hydrocarbon chains have "kinks" due to the presence of

A. double bonds.

B. oxygen atoms.

C. aldehyde groups.

D. rings.

17. Buffers resist changes in

A. solute concentration.

B. solvent type.

C. pH.

D. temperature.

18. A tRNA molecule brings in the appropriate amino acid during translation due to

A. the specificity of its anticodon for the mRNA codon.

B. the properties of the R group on the amino acid.

C. the shape of the tRNA molecule.

D. the specificity of its anticodon for the DNA codon.

19. Which of the following formula represent a carbohydrate?
- **A.** $C_{12}H_{24}O_{12}$
- **B.** $C_6H_6O_6$
- **C.** CH_2O_2
- **D.** $C_2H_5O_3N$

20. Oxygen gas passes through the plasma membrane easily because
- **A.** O_2 and the inside of the plasma membrane are polar.
- **B.** O_2 and the inside of the plasma membrane are nonpolar.
- **C.** O_2 is polar and the inside of the plasma membrane is nonpolar.
- **D.** O_2 is nonpolar and the inside of the plasma membrane is polar.

ANSWER KEY AND EXPLANATIONS

1. B	**5.** C	**9.** B	**13.** A	**17.** C
2. D	**6.** A	**10.** C	**14.** B	**18.** A
3. A	**7.** D	**11.** C	**15.** A	**19.** A
4. B	**8.** A	**12.** B	**16.** A	**20.** B

1. **The correct answer is B.** The amino acid is the monomer of a protein. Choice A is incorrect because the monosaccharide is the monomer of a carbohydrate. Choice C is incorrect because the fatty acid is a subunit of a lipid. Choice D is incorrect because the nucleotide is the monomer of a nucleic acid.

2. **The correct answer is D.** Because catalase consists of four polypeptide chain subunits, the most complex level of protein structure is quaternary structure. Choices A, B, and C are incorrect because the quaternary structure is the most complex level observed in catalase and is more complex than primary, secondary, or tertiary structure.

3. **The correct answer is A.** At the higher temperature, catalase starts to denature and unfold a bit, resulting in lower oxygen production and fewer bubbles. Choice B is incorrect because the opposite is true, based on the scenario. Choice C is incorrect because higher temperatures tend to decrease the strength of intramolecular forces within proteins. Choice D is incorrect because proteins unfold at higher temperatures; peptides are not physically broken apart from one another.

4. **The correct answer is B.** By lowering the activation energy, enzymes are able to increase the rate of chemical reactions. Choice A is not relevant to enzyme activity, and choices C and D express opposite effects of enzymes on chemical reactions.

5. **The correct answer is C.** Per the genetic code chart, CCC codes for Pro, the amino acid proline. Choices A, B, and D are incorrect

because they do not correspond with CCC on the chart.

6. **The correct answer is A.** There was one nucleotide change, but it did not alter the identity of the second amino acid. Choice B is incorrect because one is the number of nucleotides that is different in the mRNA. Choices C and D are incorrect because no amino acids differ between the amino acids in the two organisms' mRNA sequences.

7. **The correct answer is D.** Translation is the process by which mRNA is converted into protein. Choice A is incorrect because DNA replication is the process by which DNA is duplicated. Choice B is incorrect because RNA splicing is the mechanism by which eukaryotes remove non-coding bases from mRNA. Choice C is incorrect because transcription is the conversion of DNA to mRNA.

8. **The correct answer is A.** Exons are coding sequences for protein products. Choices B and C are incorrect because they reverse the definitions of exons and introns. Choice D is incorrect because introns are removed from mRNA as it becomes mature.

9. **The correct answer is B.** Helicase unwinds DNA during replication. Choice A is incorrect because DNA polymerase adds new nucleotides to the growing strands. Choice C is incorrect because ligase closes the gaps between Okazaki fragments on the lagging strand. Choice D is incorrect because RNA polymerase generates mRNA from DNA during transcription.

10. **The correct answer is C.** An oligosaccharide consists of 3-6 monosaccharides. Choice A is incorrect because a disaccharide consists of 2 monosaccharides. Choice B is incorrect because each component of raffinose is a monosaccharide. Choice D is incorrect because polysaccharides consist of more than 6 monosaccharides.

11. **The correct answer is C.** Disulfide bonds contribute to the overall three-dimensional structure of a protein. Choice A is incorrect because the primary structure of a protein is its amino acid sequence. Choice B is incorrect because the secondary structure of a protein is its localized structures, like alpha helices and beta sheets. Choice D is incorrect because the quaternary structure involves polypeptide chains complexed together.

12. **The correct answer is B.** Single-stranded binding proteins, or SSBs, help to keep DNA strands apart after helicase unwinds them. Choice A is incorrect because it describes RNA polymerase. Choice C is incorrect because it describes the ribosome. Choice D is incorrect because it describes the spliceosome.

13. **The correct answer is A.** If 40% is G, then 40% is C, leaving 20% to be A and T. 10% must then be A and 10% is T, since they must be even. Choice B is incorrect because this is the combined percentage for A and T. Choice C is incorrect because this is the percentage of G or C. Choice D is incorrect because this is the combined percentage of C and G.

14. **The correct answer is B.** Hydrogen bonds are intermolecular forces that hold secondary structures together. Choice A is incorrect because ester bonds hold pieces of lipids together. Choice C is incorrect because peptide bonds hold amino acids together. Choice D is incorrect because phosphodiester bonds hold nucleotides together.

15. **The correct answer is A.** The DNA backbone alternates between sugar and phosphate. The nitrogenous bases appear between the strands, not in the DNA backbone, so choices B, C, and D are incorrect.

16. **The correct answer is A.** "Kinks" in the hydrocarbon chains are caused by double bonds. Choice B is incorrect because oxygens do not appear in a hydrocarbon chain. Choices C and D are incorrect because neither of these is present in a hydrocarbon chain.

17. **The correct answer is C.** Buffers help to maintain a consistent pH in solution. Choices A, B, and D are simply other physical properties of solutions, but they are not relevant specifically to the purpose of buffers.

18. **The correct answer is A.** tRNA indeed has an anticodon that matches up with the corresponding mRNA codon. Choice B is incorrect because the R group itself does not influence the order in which tRNAs come in. Choice C is incorrect because the tRNA molecule shape is not related to its specificity for the mRNA sequence. Choice D is incorrect because tRNAs target mRNA, not DNA.

19. **The correct answer is A.** It has an empirical formula of (CH_2O). Choice B is incorrect; it has an empirical formula of CHO. Choice C is incorrect; it has an empirical formula of CH_2O_2. Choice D is incorrect; its empirical formula is $C_2H_5O_3N$.

20. **The correct answer is B.** O_2 is a small, nonpolar molecule, and it interacts favorably with the nonpolar internal region of the lipid bilayer. Choice A and C are incorrect because O_2 is nonpolar, not polar. Choice D is incorrect because the inside of a plasma membrane bilayer is nonpolar.

SUMMING IT UP

- The four classes of biomolecules are carbohydrates, lipids, nucleic acids, and proteins. They are key components of cells and provide materials for the building blocks of life.

- Carbohydrates have the general empirical formula of $(CH_2O)_n$, serve as a major energy source for cells, and are important for lipid and protein synthesis. The monomer of a carbohydrate is the monosaccharide, and carbohydrates are linked by glycosidic bonds.

- Lipids include triglycerides, phospholipids, and steroids, and they are essential for energy storage, cell signaling, cell membrane structure, and hormone regulation. Saturated and unsaturated fatty acids are key components of lipids and are attached to head groups through ester bonds.

- DNA and RNA are nucleic acids, the holders of genetic information. Nucleotides are the monomers of nucleic acids, consisting of a nitrogenous base, a pentose sugar, and a phosphate group. Nucleotides are connected by phosphodiester bonds.

- Per the central tenets of molecular biology, DNA is transcribed into messenger RNA via transcription. In eukaryotes, messenger RNA is spliced by a spliceosome complex to convert pre-mRNA to mature mRNA. mRNA that is ready for translation then heads to the ribosome, where transfer RNA molecules supply the building blocks to generate an amino acid chain.

- DNA replicates via the semiconservative mode of replication, with each daughter DNA molecule receiving one original strand from the parental DNA.

- Proteins are very diverse functionally, with structural, enzymatic, and other types of roles. The monomer of a protein is an amino acid. Amino acids are linked by peptide bonds.

- The four main levels of protein structure are primary structure, the amino acid sequence; secondary structure, the localized three-dimensional structures; tertiary structure, the overall 3D structure; and quaternary structure, the complex formed by multiple polypeptide chains.

PART VI
QUANTITATIVE REASONING

Arithmetic

Chapter 11

OVERVIEW

- **Number Types**
- **Number Operations**
- **Fractions**
- **Ratios**
- **Proportions**
- **Decimals**
- **Percents**
- **Moving Between Fractions, Decimals, and Percents**
- **Logarithms**
- **Practice Questions**
- **Answer Key and Explanations**
- **Summing It Up**

The purpose of the Quantitative Ability subtests is to assess test-takers' ability to reason through and understand quantitative concepts and relationships," according to the PCAT test-maker. Candidates may not bring calculators, but a nonscientific standard calculator will be available by clicking the icon in the upper left corner of each item during the Quanititative Reasoning test. The biggest focus of this test, however, is on your ability to reason. This chapter reviews basic arithmetic concepts that will underlie many of the questions.

NUMBER TYPES

There are different types of numbers:

1. *Natural numbers* are all the positive whole numbers: $\{1, 2, 3, 4, 5, \ldots\}$.

2. *Integers* include positive and negative whole numbers and zero: $\{\ldots -3, -2, -1, 0, 1, 2, 3, \ldots\}$. All natural numbers are also integers.

3. *Rational numbers* are all the numbers that can be expressed as fractions where the numerator and denominator are both integers and the denominator is not 0. Examples of fractions are $-\frac{3}{4}$, $\frac{0}{6}$ and $\frac{7}{1}$. All integers are also rational numbers.

4. *Irrational numbers* are real numbers that cannot be expressed as the quotient of two integers. These are nonterminating, nonrepeating decimals, such as $\sqrt{2}$

(which equals 1.41421 . . .), $\sqrt{3}$ (which equals 1.73205 . . .) and π (which equals 3.14159 . . .).

5. *Real numbers* are all numbers other than complex numbers. The set of all real numbers includes all natural numbers, integers, and rational and irrational numbers.

Number Line

Sometimes, it is useful to visualize all real numbers (integers and rational and irrational numbers) as if lying on a line that extends infinitely in both directions.

Numbers increase in value as we move to the right and decrease as we move to the left. Thus, between any two numbers, the one farther to the right is the greater one.

NUMBER OPERATIONS

Number operations include addition, subtraction, multiplication, and division.

Order of Operations

When simplifying an expression involving several operations, the order in which you perform these operations is critical. The acronym **PEMDAS** can help you remember the correct order.

1. **P**arentheses: First, perform the operations within parentheses (working from the inside to the outside, if there are parentheses within parentheses).

2. **E**xponents: Next, simplify any exponents.

3. **M**ultiplication and **D**ivision: Next, perform any multiplications and divisions, from left to right.

4. **A**ddition and **S**ubtraction: Finally, perform any additions and subtractions, again from left to right.

Example: Simplify $(5-3)^3 \times 6 - (16 \div 2) \div 2^2$

$(5-3)^3 \times 6 - (16 \div 2) \div 2^2$	Perform operations within parentheses
$2^3 \times 6 - 8 \div 2^2$	Simplify exponents
$8 \times 6 - 8 \div 4$	Perform multiplication and division
$48 - 2$	Perform the remaining subtraction
46	

TIP

When you add positive numbers, the answer is positive. When you add negative numbers, the answer is always negative. When you add a negative and a positive number, the answer is negative or positive, depending on which is the larger number.

TIP

When you subtract a positive number from a negative number, the answer is negative. When you subtract a negative number from a positive number, the answer is positive. When you subtract a negative number from a negative number, the answer may be either negative or positive, depending on which number is larger.

Commutative Law of Addition and Multiplication

Addition and multiplication are *commutative operations;* that is, you may change the order of the numbers in a sum or product without changing the result:

$$a + b = b + a$$

$$a \times b = b \times a$$

Subtraction and division are NOT commutative. Subtracting 2 from 6 is not the same as subtracting 6 from 2; similarly, dividing 6 by 2 is not the same as dividing 2 by 6.

Associative Law of Addition and Multiplication

Addition and multiplication are also *associative operations;* that is, you may change the manner in which numbers are grouped in a sum or product without changing the result:

$$(a + b) + c = a + (b + c)$$

$$(a \times b) \times c = a \times (b \times c)$$

Subtraction and division are NOT associative. The manner in which the numbers are grouped affects the result. For instance, $3 - (5 - 1)$ is different from $(3 - 5) - 1$. The former equals -1, whereas the latter equals -3.

Distributive Law of Multiplication

Multiplication is distributive with respect to addition and subtraction. That is, when you have a set of parentheses within which several numbers are added or subtracted, and that entire quantity is multiplied by another number, you may either 1) perform the operations within the parentheses first and then multiply the resulting number by the number outside the parentheses, or 2) you may first distribute the number outside the parentheses by each of the numbers within the parentheses, and then perform the resulting additions and subtractions:

$$a \times (b + c) = ab + ac$$

$$a \times (b - c) = ab - ac$$

Identity Property of Addition

The number zero is called the identity element of addition because adding zero to any real number leaves that number unchanged:

$$a + 0 = 0 + a = a$$

This property does not hold for subtraction, because subtracting any number from zero changes the number into its opposite $(0 - a = -a)$, which does NOT equal the original number unless the original number is zero.

When you divide a positive number by a positive number, the answer is always positive.

When you divide a negative number by a negative number, the answer is always positive.

When you divide a negative number by a positive number or vice versa, the answer is always negative.

When you multiply positive numbers, the answer is always positive.

When you multiply negative numbers, the answer is always positive.

When you multiply a negative number and a positive number, the answer is always negative.

Identity Property of Multiplication

The number 1 is called the identity element of multiplication because multiplying any real number by 1 leaves that number unchanged:

$$a \times 1 = 1 \times a = a$$

This property does not hold for division because dividing 1 by any number changes that number into its inverse or reciprocal $\left(1 \div a = \dfrac{1}{a}\right)$, which does NOT equal the original number unless that number is 1 or −1.

FRACTIONS

Fractions are rational numbers written in the form $\dfrac{a}{b}$, where a and b are the fraction's numerator and denominator, respectively. Every integer a can be written as a fraction with a denominator of 1: $\dfrac{a}{1}$. The fraction $\dfrac{a}{b}$ represents the division of a by b; division by zero is undefined, so b cannot be zero. You can also think of fraction $\dfrac{a}{b}$ as the ratio of the number a to the number b.

Many different fractions may be equal to one another if they all represent the same ratio. For instance, the fractions $\dfrac{1}{3}$, $\dfrac{10}{30}$, and $\dfrac{250}{750}$ are all equal to one another, since each fraction's denominator equals three times that fraction's numerator.

Adding and Subtracting Fractions

You can add or subtract two or more fractions, all of which have the same denominator, by adding or subtracting the numerators and leaving the denominator unchanged:

$$\frac{a}{b} + \frac{c}{b} + \frac{d}{b} = \frac{a + c + d}{b}$$

$$\frac{a}{b} + \frac{c}{b} - \frac{d}{b} = \frac{a + c - d}{b}$$

If you must add fractions that do not have the same denominator, you must convert some or all of them into new fractions (but equal to the original ones), so all fractions being added have the same denominator. For instance, in order to add $\dfrac{1}{4}$ and $\dfrac{3}{2}$, you must first convert $\dfrac{3}{2}$ into its equivalent $\dfrac{6}{4}$.

In order to arrive at a common denominator for all fractions in a sum, you must 1) first find the least common multiple of all the denominators. 2) Next, you must convert each fraction to a new one that has this least common multiple as its denominator. You do that by multiplying both the numerator and the denominator of the original fraction by that number, which will convert the original denominator to the least common multiple. (Multiplying both the numerator and the denominator of a fraction by the same number is the same as multiplying the fraction by 1, an action that does not change the fraction's value, since 1 is the identity element of multiplication.) 3) Finally, you can add the resulting fractions:

Example: $\frac{1}{4} + \frac{2}{3} + \frac{5}{6} = ?$

The least common multiple of 4, 3, and 6 is 12.

$$\frac{1}{4} + \frac{2}{3} + \frac{5}{6} = \frac{1 \times 3}{4 \times 3} + \frac{2 \times 4}{3 \times 4} + \frac{5 \times 2}{6 \times 2}$$

$$= \frac{3}{12} + \frac{8}{12} + \frac{10}{12}$$

$$= \frac{3 + 8 + 10}{12}$$

$$= \frac{21}{12}$$

If you're dealing with two fractions, the easiest way to find a common denominator is to multiply each fraction's numerator and denominator by the other fraction's denominator:

$$\frac{m}{n} + \frac{p}{q} = \frac{m \times q}{n \times q} + \frac{p \times n}{q \times n}$$

$$= \frac{mq + pn}{qn}$$

This might not be the least common denominator, but it always works.

Multiplying Fractions

To compute a product of fractions, multiply all the numerators together and all the denominators together in order to get the numerator and denominator, respectively, of the result:

$$\frac{a}{b} \times \frac{m}{n} \times \frac{p}{q} = \frac{a \times m \times p}{b \times n \times q}$$

Dividing Fractions

Division by a fraction is the same as multiplication by that fraction's inverse. That is, in order to divide a number (fraction or otherwise) by a fraction, invert the fraction by which you're dividing, and then multiply:

$$\frac{a}{b} \div \frac{m}{n} = \frac{a}{b} \times \frac{n}{m} = \frac{a \times n}{b \times m}$$

Sometimes, you may encounter division by a fraction in the form of a single complex fraction, that is, a fraction that has one fraction in the numerator and another in the denominator:

$$\frac{\frac{a}{b}}{\frac{m}{n}}$$

This is computed as follows:

$$\frac{\dfrac{a}{b}}{\dfrac{m}{n}} = \frac{a}{b} \div \frac{m}{n} = \frac{a}{b} \times \frac{n}{m} = \frac{a \times n}{b \times m}$$

Reducing Fractions

We have already seen that some fractions are equal to one another even if their numerators and denominators are different. In fact, for each fraction, there is an infinite number of other fractions that are equal to it. You can create such fractions by taking the original fraction and multiplying both its numerator and its denominator by the same nonzero integer. For instance, $\frac{1}{2} = \frac{1 \times 2}{2 \times 2} = \frac{1 \times 3}{2 \times 3}$, $= \frac{1 \times 100}{2 \times 100} = \frac{1 \times 5,300}{2 \times 5,300}$ and so on.

Sometimes, it is useful to reduce a fraction to the lowest terms, that is, to remove from both its numerator and its denominator their greatest common factor. Do this by dividing both the numerator and the denominator by that factor. If you do not immediately see what the greatest common factor is, start by dividing both numerator and denominator by any factor you can tell is common to both, and continue the process a few times until you've arrived at a fraction that cannot be reduced further.

Example: Reduce $\frac{36}{84}$.

$$\frac{36}{84} = \frac{36 \div 2}{84 \div 2} = \frac{18}{42} = \frac{18 \div 2}{42 \div 2} = \frac{9}{21} = \frac{9 \div 3}{21 \div 3} = \frac{3}{7}$$

Improper Fractions and Mixed Numbers

Improper fractions are fractions that have a numerator whose absolute value is greater than the absolute value of the denominator, that is, fractions whose absolute value is greater than 1. (Absolute value is the value of a number without regard to its sign.) For instance, $\frac{8}{3}$ and $-\frac{8}{3}$ are improper fractions.

Mixed numbers are numbers that have an integer part and a proper fraction part. You can write any improper fraction as a mixed number, and vice versa. For instance, $\frac{8}{3}$ is equal to the mixed number $2\frac{2}{3}$, "two and two-thirds." Since there are six thirds in the number 2, the total number of thirds in $2\frac{2}{3}$ is 8, and so this mixed number is equal to $\frac{8}{3}$.

To convert a mixed number to an improper fraction, multiply the integer part by the denominator, and add to that the numerator. The resulting number becomes the numerator of the improper fraction. The denominator of the improper fraction is the same as the denominator of the original fraction.

Example: Convert $5\frac{3}{7}$ to a fraction.

$$5\frac{3}{7} = \frac{5 \times 7 + 3}{7} = \frac{38}{7}$$

To convert an improper fraction to a mixed number, divide the numerator by the denominator. The quotient becomes the integer part of the mixed number, and the remainder becomes the numerator of the fraction part. For instance, to convert the fraction $\frac{38}{7}$, divide 38 by 7. Doing so yields a quotient of 5 and a remainder of 3. Thus, $\frac{38}{7}$ converts to $5\frac{3}{7}$.

RATIOS

A *ratio* is a fraction that expresses the numerical relationship between two "like" objects or quantities, such as boys and girls in a class, or milk and sugar in a cup of coffee. A ratio does not tell you the exact numbers of each item; rather it gives only the relationship between the two. So, if there are 6 boys for every 7 girls in a class, you know that the ratio of boys to girls is 6:7 (or $\frac{6}{7}$, or "six to seven"). Although, you won't know if there are exactly 6 boys and 7 girls, or exactly 12 boys and 14 girls, and so on. On the other hand, if, instead of a ratio, you are given exact numbers, then you can find the ratio: A class with 12 boys and 14 girls has a boy-to-girl ratio of 12:14, which, reduced to lowest terms, equals 6:7.

Example: A sock drawer contains 4 pairs of black socks, 6 pairs of white socks, and 5 pairs of brown socks. Reduced to lowest terms, what are the ratios of pairs of black socks to pairs of white socks; of pairs of brown socks to pairs of black socks; and of pairs of black socks to pairs of white socks to pairs of brown socks?

Since there are 4 pairs of black socks and 6 pairs of white socks, the ratio of pairs of black socks to pairs of white socks is 4:6, or 2:3, in lowest terms. Similarly, the ratio of pairs of brown socks to pairs of black socks is 5:4, while the ratio of pairs of black socks to pairs of white socks to pairs of brown socks is 4:6:5.

Part-to-Part and Part-to-Whole Ratios

There are two types of ratios: 1) part-to-part and 2) part-to-whole. The above examples, socks in a drawer and boys and girls in a class, are part-to-part ratios, that is, ratios of one part of the whole to another part of the whole. We could just as well have found the ratios of one part of the whole to the whole itself.

Example: If in a certain class there are 6 boys for every 7 girls, what is the ratio of the number of boys to the total number of students in the class?

Here, you are given the ratio of boys to girls in the class, but you do not know the total number of students. Is that a problem? No! You can find the ratio of boys to students (or girls to students) without knowing how many students there are. Since there are 6 boys for every 7 girls, then there are 6 boys for every 6 + 7 students. Thus, the ratio is 6:13.

TIP

Always read questions carefully. This, plus turning confusing word problems into ones with concise wording minus extraneous details, are two of the best strategies that you can use.

TIP

Make sure you are answering the question being asked. That means you need to read the questions carefully.

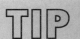

TIP

Be careful to cancel only factors that are common to both denominators, or factors that are common to both numerators, but not factors that one denominator shares with the other numerator!

PROPORTIONS

A *proportion* is an equation relating two ratios, and it is written as $a{:}b = c{:}d$, or $\frac{a}{b} = \frac{c}{d}$. To solve a proportion, use the fraction notation and cross-multiply: $\frac{a}{b} = \frac{c}{d} \Rightarrow ad = bc$. Setting up a proportion is often very useful in solving a ratio problem.

Example: A certain chemical solution contains 7 milliliters of substance A for every 9 milliliters of substance B. There are no other substances in the solution. If the total volume of the solution is 144 milliliters, what is the volume of substance A in the solution?

For every 7 + 9 milliliters of the solution, there are 7 milliliters of substance A. Set up and solve a proportion:

$$\frac{7}{7+9} = \frac{x}{144}$$

$$\frac{7}{16} = \frac{x}{144}$$

$$7 \times 144 = 16x$$

$$1{,}008 = 16x$$

$$x = 63$$

When solving proportions, you can make your life easier by canceling common factors from both sides of the equation. For instance, when you arrived at $\frac{7}{16} = \frac{x}{144}$, if you had noticed that 144 is a multiple of 16, then you could have multiplied each side of the equation by 16 in order to arrive at $\frac{7}{1} = \frac{x}{9}$. If you did not realize that 144 equals 16 times 9, then you could have multiplied each side by 2, and repeated this process as many times as necessary until there were no more common factors to cancel.

DECIMALS

Decimal notation is another way of representing rational numbers. *Decimal numbers* consist of a sequence of digits (the numbers 0, 1, 2, . . . , 9, in any order) and one decimal point. The digits to the left of the decimal point make up the whole number part of the number, while the digits to the right of the decimal point make up the fraction part of the number. Each position to the right and left of the decimal point corresponds to a certain power of ten; and each digit placed in that position corresponds to the factor by which that power of ten is multiplied in the particular decimal number you're looking at. Consider the following (partial) table of place values and names:

Place	Name	Place Value
4 spots to the left of the decimal point	Thousands	$10^3 = 1{,}000$
3 spots to the left of the decimal point	Hundreds	$10^2 = 100$
2 spots to the left of the decimal point	Tens	$10^1 = 10$
1 spot to the left of the decimal point	Ones	$10^0 = 1$
1 spot to the right of the decimal point	Tenths	$10^{-1} = 0.1$
2 spots to the right of the decimal point	Hundredths	$10^{-2} = 0.01$
3 spots to the right of the decimal point	Thousandths	$10^{-3} = 0.001$

So, for instance, the number 1,325.678 has "1" in the thousands place, "2" in the tens place, and "6" in the tenths place. In this number, the third power of ten ($10^3 = 1,000$) is multiplied by 1; the first power of ten ($10^1 = 10$) is multiplied by 2; and the -1 power of ten ($10^{-1} = 0.1$) is multiplied by 6. More fully, you can write the number 1,325.678 as follows:

$$1,325.678 = (1 \times 1,000) + (3 \times 100) + (2 \times 10) + (5 \times 1) + (6 \times 0.1) + (7 \times 0.01) + (8 \times 0.001)$$

Adding and Subtracting Decimals

You can add or subtract decimals the same way you add or subtract integers. Make sure all the decimal points line up vertically. If one of the decimal numbers has fewer digits to the right of the decimal point, you may want to add one or more zeros after the final digit on the right side of that number so that all decimals have the same number of digits to the right of the decimal point.

Example: 2,015.3 + 456.139 + 7.88 = ?

$$
\begin{array}{r}
2,015.300 \\
456.139 \\
+\quad 7.880 \\
\hline
2,479.319
\end{array}
$$

Multiplying Decimals

You can multiply decimals the same way you multiply integers. This time, you do not need to add extra zeros or line up the decimal points. In fact, you can ignore the decimal point while you perform the multiplication until the last step. At that point, count all the digits to the right of the decimal point in all the numbers you are multiplying. Then, place the decimal point that many places from the right in your result.

Example: 3.2 × 2.11 = ?

$$
\begin{array}{r}
3.2 \\
\times\, 2.11 \\
\hline
32 \\
32 \\
64 \\
\hline
6.752
\end{array}
$$

There are a total of three digits to the right of the decimal point in the numbers being multiplied, so count three numbers from the right of the number, moving left, and place the decimal point.

Dividing Decimals

In order to divide a decimal by another decimal, it is easiest to first convert them both to integers by multiplying them by an appropriate power of ten. Be sure to multiply both numbers by the same power of ten in order to preserve the ratio between the two. For instance, in order to divide 45.66 by 3.2, multiply each by 100, turning them into 4,566 and 320. Then divide one integer by the other.

Rounding Decimals

Sometimes, you need to round decimals to a particular place, such as the nearest tenth or nearest hundredth. To do so, first determine the place to which you should round—for instance, the tenths place, if you're asked to round to the nearest tenth. Then, consider the digit to the right of that place.

1) If this digit is 5 or greater, then increase the digit immediately to its left by 1 and ignore everything to the right of this increased digit. For instance, 4.352 rounded to the nearest tenth equals 4.4.

2) If, on the other hand, the digit to the right of the place to which you must round is less than 5, leave as is the digit in the place to which you have to round and delete everything to the right of this digit. For instance, 5.2738 rounded to the nearest hundredth equals 5.27.

PERCENTS

Percents are ratios whose denominator is 100. Think of "per cent" as "out of 100." So, when we say that a certain country exports 25% of its olive oil production, we mean that it exports 25 out of every 100 bottles (or casks, etc.) of olive oil it produces.

Percent Change Problems

You often need to deal with percent change problems, such as questions regarding revenue or population increases or decreases from year to year. Think of these problems in terms of proportions.

Example: In 2012, Mary earned $10,000 more than she did in 2011. In 2011, she earned $35,000. What was the percent increase in her earnings in 2012 compared to 2011, rounded to the nearest hundredth?

Out of $35,000, Mary's earnings increased by $10,000, and you are asked to find what that increase was "out of 100." Set up and solve the following proportion:

$$\frac{10,000}{35,000} = \frac{x}{100}$$
$$35,000x = 1,000,000$$
$$x = \frac{1,000,000}{35,000}$$
$$x \approx 28.57$$

MOVING BETWEEN FRACTIONS, DECIMALS, AND PERCENTS

Sometimes, problems will give you information in different formats. In order to solve the problem, you will need to convert a number into another format, for example, a percent to a fraction, or a fraction to a decimal.

Converting Fractions to Decimals

To convert a fraction to a decimal, divide the numerator by the denominator. If the fraction is proper, then the absolute value of the decimal will be less than 1 (that is, the digit to the left of the decimal point will be 0).

If the fraction is improper, then the absolute value of the decimal will be greater than 1.

Some fractions represent repeating, nonterminating decimals. For instance, $\frac{1}{3}$ equals 0.33333... and $\frac{2}{11}$ equals 0.181818.... An elegant way to write such decimals is with a horizontal line over the repeating digit(s): $0.\overline{3}$ and $0.\overline{18}$.

Converting Decimals to Fractions

You can write any terminating decimal as a mixed number. The mixed number's integer part will be the same as the decimal's whole number part. Next, think of the decimal number's digits to the right of the decimal point as multiplied by the power of 10 represented by the place of the right-most digit. For instance, the number 0.15 is equivalent to 15×10^{-2}, which equals $\frac{15}{10^2}$, or $\frac{15}{100}$. This fraction becomes the fraction part of the mixed number. So, for example, 7.15 becomes $7\frac{15}{100}$. Then you can convert the mixed number into a fraction as you saw earlier in the chapter.

Converting Percents to Fractions

To convert a percent to a fraction, divide the percent by 100%. This eliminates the percent sign and places "100" as the denominator. For instance, 45% equals $\frac{45}{100}$.

Note that 100% literally means $\frac{100}{100}$, which equals 1, so division by 100% does not alter the value of the starting number.

Converting Percents to Decimals

Once you have converted a percent to a fraction, you can then convert it further to a decimal. In the case of a fraction that represents a percent, this conversion is particularly easy, because the denominator is always 100. For instance, 45% equals $\frac{45}{100}$, which in turn equals 0.45.

Converting Fractions to Percents

You can convert a fraction to a percent by multiplying the fraction by 100%. For instance:

$$\frac{7}{4} = \frac{7}{4} \times 100\%$$
$$= 7 \times 25\%$$
$$= 175\%$$

Converting Decimals to Percents

Similarly, you can convert a decimal to a percent by multiplying the decimal by 100%. This amounts to moving the decimal point two places to the right and adding the percent sign. Moving the decimal point two places to the right is the result of multiplication by 100; adding the percent sign next to a number is equivalent to dividing that number by 100. By performing both of these actions—multiplying and dividing by 100—the original number is unaltered. For instance, 3.2 = 320%.

Common Conversions

Certain fractions, decimals, and percents occur frequently, so it is wise to remember how they convert from one format to another, rather than figuring out how to derive them from scratch on test day.

Fraction	Decimal	Percent
$\frac{1}{100}$	0.01	1%
$\frac{1}{50}$	0.02	2%
$\frac{1}{25}$	0.04	4%
$\frac{1}{20}$	0.05	5%
$\frac{1}{10}$	0.1	10%
$\frac{1}{9}$	$0.\overline{1}$	$11.\overline{1}$%
$\frac{1}{8}$	0.125	12.5%
$\frac{1}{6}$	$0.1\overline{6}$	$16.\overline{6}$%
$\frac{1}{5}$	0.2	20%
$\frac{1}{4}$	0.25	25%
$\frac{1}{3}$	$0.\overline{3}$	$33.\overline{3}$%
$\frac{3}{8}$	0.375	37.5%
$\frac{2}{5}$	0.4	40%

Fraction	Decimal	Percent
$\frac{1}{2}$	0.5	50%
$\frac{3}{5}$	0.6	60%
$\frac{5}{8}$	0.625	62.5%
$\frac{2}{3}$	$0.\overline{6}$	$66.\overline{6}$%
$\frac{3}{4}$	0.75	75%
$\frac{4}{5}$	0.8	80%
$\frac{5}{6}$	$0.8\overline{3}$	$83.\overline{3}$%
$\frac{7}{8}$	0.875	87.5%
$\frac{1}{1}$	1	100%

Unit Conversions

Knowing how to convert from one to another is assessed in different ways on the PCAT. Below are some common conversion factors with which you should be familiar.

Type of Quantity	Some Useful Conversion Factors
Length	1 foot = 12 inches 1 yard = 3 feet = 36 inches 1 mile = 1,760 yards = 5,280 feet
Time	1 minute = 60 seconds 1 hour = 60 minutes = 3,600 seconds 1 day = 24 hours
Area	1 square foot = 12^2 square inches 1 square yard = 3^2 square feet
Volume	1 cubic foot = 12^3 cubic inches 1 cubic yard = 3^3 cubic feet

If converting from a smaller unit of measure to a larger one, you divide by the conversion factor, whereas if you are converting from a larger unit of measure to a smaller one, you multiply by the conversion factor.

Example: Nick's racecar can reach the speed of 65 miles per hour in about 4 seconds. What is this speed in feet per minute?

First, note that the "in about 4 seconds" is superfluous information. We are simply asked to convert the speed from miles per hour. Since there are 5,280 feet in 1 mile and 60 minutes in 1 hour, we have the following:

$$\frac{65 \text{ miles}}{1 \text{ hour}} \times \frac{1 \text{ hour}}{60 \text{ minutes}} \times \frac{5,280 \text{ feet}}{1 \text{ mile}} = \frac{65 \times 5,280}{60} \text{ feet per minute} = 5,720 \text{ feet per minute}$$

LOGARITHMS

A logarithm is just an exponent. Specifically, we write $\log_a b = c$ whenever $a^c = b$, and we read $\log_a b$ as "log base a of b."

Example: Simplify $\log_2 16$.

Using the definition, $\log_2 16 = c$ whenever $2^c = 16$. Since $2^4 = 16$, it follows that $\log_2 16 = 4$.

When simplifying expressions involving logarithms it is convenient to think of $\log_a b$ in the following sense: "To what power must a be raised to get b?" For instance, in the above example, we have $a = 2$ and $b = 16$. So, we would ask the question, "To what power must 2 be raised to get 16?"

Example: Simplify these logarithms.

i. $\log_3 9$

ii. $\log_7 7$

iii. $\log_2 1$

i. Since $3^2 = 9$, it follows that $\log_3 9 = 2$.

ii. Since $7^1 = 7$, it follows that $\log_7 7 = 1$.

iii. Since $2^0 = 1$, it follows that $\log_2 1 = 0$.

There are two special bases for logarithms, namely 10 and e. When the base is the natural exponential e, it is typical to write $\ln x$ for $\log_e x$. When the base is 10, we usually omit the subscript and simply write $\log x$ for $\log_{10} x$.

Example: Simplify these logarithms.

i. $\log 100$

ii. $\ln e^2$

i. $\log 100 = \log_{10} 100 = 2$

ii. $\ln e^2 = \log_e e^2 = 2$

PRACTICE QUESTIONS

Directions: Choose the best answer for each question.

1. Compute: $-4^2(1-3)$.
   A. -32
   B. -16
   C. 16
   D. 32

2. Compute: $\dfrac{16 - 8 \times 2 \div 4}{4^2 - 4}$.
   A. 0
   B. $\dfrac{1}{3}$
   C. 1
   D. 3

3. Compute: $1 - 2\,(-1 - 2(1-2))^2$.
   A. -5
   B. -1
   C. 1
   D. 3

4. $\dfrac{\frac{2}{3}}{4} + \dfrac{5}{6} - \dfrac{1}{2} =$
   A. 3
   B. $\dfrac{3}{2}$
   C. $\dfrac{3}{4}$
   D. $\dfrac{1}{2}$

5. Multiply and simplify: $\dfrac{16}{81} \times \dfrac{27}{8} \times \dfrac{4}{3}$.
   A. $\dfrac{8}{9}$
   B. $\dfrac{4}{9}$
   C. $\dfrac{9}{10}$
   D. 1

6. Divide and simplify: $\dfrac{5}{4} \div 10$.
   A. $\dfrac{25}{2}$
   B. $\dfrac{1}{8}$
   C. $\dfrac{2}{25}$
   D. 8

7. Which of the following, when added to 0.65, yields 2?
   A. 0.35
   B. $\dfrac{2.6}{2}$
   C. 135%
   D. 2.65

8. What is $\dfrac{1}{4}\%$ of 60?
   A. 15
   B. 1.5
   C. 0.15
   D. 0.015

9. In his grocery bag, John is carrying three items whose weights are 450 grams (g), 600 g, and 1.20 kilograms (kg). What is the total weight of the items that John is carrying?
   A. $1{,}051.20$ kg
   B. 2.25 kg
   C. $1{,}140$ g
   D. $1{,}051.20$ g

10. A company is participating in a corporate trivia challenge with a team consisting of 6 married men, 2 married women, 4 unmarried men, and 5 unmarried women. What is the ratio of unmarried individuals on the team to the total number of team members?
    A. $4{:}17$
    B. $8{:}17$
    C. $9{:}17$
    D. $9{:}8$

11. Of the 120 people on a company's Research and Development team, 60% are men. If 20 women and 10 men are hired and nobody leaves the team, approximately what is the percentage of women on the new team?
    A. 45%
    B. 52%
    C. 57%
    D. 68%

12. Which of the following is equivalent to 0.8%?
    A. 0.008
    B. 0.08
    C. 0.8
    D. 8

13. On a high school football team with 54 players, the ratio of freshmen to sophomores to juniors to seniors is 4:5:5:4. How many non-freshmen are on the team?
    A. 4
    B. 12
    C. 14
    D. 42

14. According to the census, a city's population had increased by 10% by the year 2000 compared to the city's population in 1990. In 2010, the city's population decreased by 20% compared to its population in 2000. What percent of the city's population in 1990 was its population in 2010?
    A. 72%
    B. 88%
    C. 90%
    D. 130%

15. Jack Carson spends 25% of his monthly income on rent, 15% on food, and 7% on utilities. If he earns $3000 per month, how much does he spend each month on food and utilities?
    A. $210
    B. $450
    C. $660
    D. $750

16. Which of the following computations is used to determine the number of seconds equivalent to 3 hours?
    A. $\dfrac{3 \text{ hours}}{1} \times \dfrac{60 \text{ minutes}}{1 \text{ hour}} \times \dfrac{60 \text{ seconds}}{1 \text{ minute}}$

    B. $\dfrac{3 \text{ hours}}{1} \times \dfrac{1 \text{ hour}}{60 \text{ minutes}} \times \dfrac{1 \text{ minute}}{60 \text{ seconds}}$

    C. $\dfrac{3 \text{ hours}}{1} \times \dfrac{1 \text{ hour}}{3,600 \text{ seconds}}$

    D. $\dfrac{3 \text{ hours}}{1} \times \dfrac{1 \text{ hour}}{60 \text{ minutes}} \times \dfrac{60 \text{ seconds}}{1 \text{ minute}}$

17. Convert 2.5 square feet to square inches.
    A. 30 square inches
    B. 288 square inches
    C. 360 square inches
    D. 4,320 square inches

18. Convert 90 feet per second to yards per minute.
    A. 0.5 yard per minute
    B. 4.5 yards per minute
    C. 1,800 yards per minute
    D. 16,200 yards per minute

19. Compute: $\log\left(\dfrac{1}{1,000}\right)$.
    A. −3
    B. −2
    C. 2
    D. 3

20. Compute: $\log\left(\sqrt[3]{100,000}\right)$.
    A. $\dfrac{3}{5}$
    B. $\dfrac{5}{3}$
    C. 3
    D. 5

ANSWER KEY AND EXPLANATIONS

1. D	**5.** A	**9.** B	**13.** D	**17.** C
2. C	**6.** B	**10.** C	**14.** B	**18.** C
3. B	**7.** C	**11.** A	**15.** C	**19.** A
4. D	**8.** C	**12.** A	**16.** A	**20.** B

1. **The correct answer is D.** Use the order of operations:

$$-4^2(1-3) = -16(1-3)$$
$$= -16(-2)$$
$$= 32$$

2. **The correct answer is C.** Use the order of operations:

$$\frac{16 - 8 \times 2 \div 4}{4^2 - 4} = \frac{16 - 16 \div 4}{16 - 4}$$
$$= \frac{16 - 4}{16 - 4}$$
$$= 1$$

3. **The correct answer is B.** Use the order of operations:

$$1 - 2\left(-1 - 2(1-2)\right)^2 = 1 - 2\left(-1 - 2(-1)\right)^2$$
$$= 1 - 2\left(-1 + 2\right)^2$$
$$= 1 - 2(1)^2$$
$$= 1 - 2$$
$$= -1$$

4. **The correct answer is D.** Simplify the complex fraction, find the least common multiple of the resulting denominators (which is 6), convert all fractions so they all have 6 as the denominator, and then add:

$$\frac{\frac{2}{3}}{4} + \frac{5}{6} - \frac{1}{2} = \frac{1}{6} + \frac{5}{6} - \frac{1}{2} =$$
$$\frac{1}{6} + \frac{5}{6} - \frac{3}{6} = \frac{1 + 5 - 3}{6} = \frac{3}{6} = \frac{1}{2}$$

5. **The correct answer is A.** Factor all numerators and denominators. Then, combine terms with the same base in the numerator and denominator, separately. Finally, use the exponent rules to simplify:

$$\frac{16}{81} \times \frac{27}{8} \times \frac{4}{3} = \frac{2^4}{3^4} \times \frac{3^3}{2^3} \times \frac{2^2}{3}$$
$$= \frac{2^6 \times 3^3}{2^3 \times 3^5}$$
$$= \frac{2^3}{3^2}$$
$$= \frac{8}{9}$$

6. **The correct answer is B.** Convert to a product, then simplify:

$$\frac{5}{4} \div 10 = \frac{5}{4} \times \frac{1}{10} = \frac{\cancel{5}}{4} \times \frac{1}{\cancel{10}_2} = \frac{1}{8}$$

7. **The correct answer is C.** 2 minus 0.65 equals 1.35. Among the answer choices, only 135% (that is, $\frac{135}{100}$) equals 1.35.

8. **The correct answer is C.** Evaluate $\frac{1}{4}\%$ of 60:

$$\left(\frac{1}{4}\%\right)60 = \frac{\frac{1}{4}}{100}60 = \frac{60}{400} = 0.15$$

9. **The correct answer is B.** One kilogram equals 1,000 grams. Convert all quantities either to kg or to g and then add:

$$450 \text{ g} + 600 \text{ g} + 1,200 \text{ g} = 2,250 \text{ g} = 2.25 \text{ kg}$$

10. **The correct answer is C.** The team has a total of 6 plus 2 plus 4 plus 5 members, that is, 17 members. Of those, 4 plus 5, or 9, are unmarried. Thus, the ratio of unmarried individuals to the total number of team members is 9:17.

11. **The correct answer is A.** If at first 60% of the team members are men, then 40% are women. So, initially the number of women is:

$$40\%(120) = \frac{40}{100}120 = 48$$

On the new team, there are 48 plus 20 women, that is, 68 women. The total number of members on the new team is 120 plus 20 plus 10, or 150. Set up a proportion and calculate the percentage of women on the new team:

$$\frac{68}{150} = \frac{x}{100}$$

$$\frac{68}{15} = \frac{x}{10}$$

$$15x = 680$$

$$x = 45\frac{1}{3}$$

Therefore, the correct answer is about 45.

12. **The correct answer is A.** Divide 0.8 by 100:

$$0.8\% = \frac{0.8}{100} = 0.008.$$

13. **The correct answer is D.** If there are 5 + 5 + 4, or 14, non-freshmen out of every 4 + 5 + 5 + 4, or 18, football players, then how many non-freshmen are there out of the 54 total players on the team? Set up and solve this proportion:

$$\frac{5+5+4}{4+5+5+4} = \frac{x}{54}$$

$$\frac{14}{18} = \frac{x}{54}$$

$$\frac{7}{9} = \frac{x}{54}$$

$$\frac{7}{1} = \frac{x}{6}$$

$$x = 42$$

14. **The correct answer is B.** In problems such as this one, it is useful to pick the number 100 to represent the starting value: in this case, the city's population in 1990. From 1990 to 2000, the city's population increased by 10%. Thus, the city's population in 2000 was 110. From 2000 to 2010, the city's population decreased by 20%. So, from 110 in 2000, it decreased to 110 minus 22, which is 88, in 2010. Thus, in 2010 the city's population was $\frac{88}{100}$, or 88% of its population in 1990.

15. **The correct answer is C.** If, out of the $3,000 he earns each month, Jack Carson spends 15% plus 7% on food and utilities, then he spends the following on food and utilities:

$$(15+7)\%(\$3,000) = 22\%(\$3,000) =$$
$$\frac{22}{100}(\$3,000) = \$660$$

16. **The correct answer is A.** There are 60 minutes in 1 hour and 60 seconds in 1 minute. When converting units, you want to make certain the units with which you begin cancel and that the units to which you want to convert remain at the end of the computation. Here, this means you need to have "hours" in the denominator and "seconds" in the numerator:

$$\frac{3 \text{ hours}}{1} \times \frac{60 \text{ minutes}}{1 \text{ hour}} \times \frac{60 \text{ seconds}}{1 \text{ minute}}$$

17. **The correct answer is C.** Since there are 12 inches in 1 foot, it follows that there are 12^2, or 144, square inches in 1 square foot. Use this fact to convert the units as follows:

$$\frac{2.5 \text{ square feet}}{} \times \frac{144 \text{ square inches}}{1 \text{ square foot}} =$$

(2.5×144) square inches = 360 square inches

18. **The correct answer is C.** Use the fact that there are 60 seconds in 1 minute and 3 feet in 1 yard to perform the conversion, as follows:

$$\frac{90 \text{ feet}}{1 \text{ second}} \times \frac{60 \text{ seconds}}{1 \text{ minute}} \times \frac{1 \text{ yard}}{3 \text{ feet}} = 1,800$$ yards per minute

19. **The correct answer is A.**

$$\log\left(\frac{1}{1,000}\right) = \log\left(10^{-3}\right) = -3$$

20. **The correct answer is B.**

$$\log\left(\sqrt[3]{100,000}\right) = \log\left(\sqrt[3]{10^5}\right) =$$
$$\log\left(10^{\frac{5}{3}}\right) = \frac{5}{3}$$

SUMMING IT UP

- Remember the acronym **PEMDAS** to perform operations within an expression in the correct order: 1) perform operations within parentheses, 2) simplify exponents, 3) multiply and divide from left to right, and 4) add and subtract from left to right.

- Addition and multiplication are commutative and associative operations, whereas subtraction and division are neither commutative nor associative. That is, the order of the numbers you are adding or multiplying, as well as the manner in which they are grouped, does not matter. However, these do matter in subtraction and division.

- A fraction's denominator can never be zero, since division by zero is undefined.

- Fractions can be added or subtracted directly only when they have the same denominator. If they do not, one or more of them must be converted so that all fractions have the same denominator.

- Do not confuse part-to-part ratios with part-to-whole ratios.

- Proportions are useful when solving ratio and percent change problems.

- To convert a fraction to a decimal, divide the numerator by the denominator.

- To convert a decimal to a fraction, first convert the decimal to a mixed number and then the mixed number to a fraction.

- To convert a percent to a fraction, divide the percent by 100%.

- To convert a percent to a decimal, first convert it to a fraction and then convert the fraction to a decimal.

- To convert a fraction to a percent, multiply the fraction by 100%.

- To convert a decimal to a percent, multiply the decimal by 100%.

- If converting from a smaller unit of measure to a larger one, you divide by the conversion factor, whereas if you are converting from a larger unit of measure to a smaller one, you multiply by the conversion factor.

- $\log_a b = c$ whenever $a^c = b$.

- Think of $\log_a b$ in the sense: "To what power must a be raised to get b?"

- When the base is the natural exponential e, we write $\ln x$ for $\log_e x$, and when the base is 10, we omit the subscript and simply write $\log x$ for $\log_{10} x$.

Algebra

OVERVIEW

The Quantitative Ability subtest contains 48 questions, and you have 40 minutes to answer them. You also will not have a calculator to use, but the good news is that wrong answers do not count against your score. Estimation and the process of elimination can help you if time starts running out.

EXPONENTS AND RADICALS

Exponents and radicals play a key role in algebra, so we'll begin this chapter by defining them and reviewing their properties.

Integer Exponents

For any number a and positive integer n, a^n equals the number a multiplied by itself for a total of n factors of a, that is:

$$a^n = a \times a \times a \times \ldots \times a$$

a repeats n times

For instance:

$$a^2 = a \times a$$
$$y^3 = y \times y \times y$$
$$3^5 = 3 \times 3 \times 3 \times 3 \times 3 = 243$$

Chapter 12

Remember these four important test-taking strategies: 1. use the clock to stick to your pacing plan, 2. skip and return to difficult questions, 3. eliminate answers that you know are wrong, and 4. use educated guessing if you're not sure.

We say that a is the *base*, n is the *exponent*, a^n is the *n*th *power* of a, and a is raised to the *n*th power. We define zero and negative exponents, as follows:

$a^0 = 1$ for all nonzero numbers a. Zero raised to the zero power is undefined.

$a^{-n} = \dfrac{1}{a^n}$ for all nonzero numbers a (since division by zero is undefined).

The following rules of exponents are very important, so you should memorize them:

Rules	Examples
$a^n a^m = a^{n+m}$ and $\dfrac{a^n}{a^m} = a^{n-m}$	$a^5 a^{-2} = a^3$ and $\dfrac{a^5}{a^{-2}} = a^7$
$\left(a^n\right)^m = a^{n \times m}$	$\left(a^5\right)^{-2} = a^{-10}$
$(ab)^n = a^n b^n$ and $\left(\dfrac{a}{b}\right)^n = \dfrac{a^n}{b^n}$	$(3x)^2 = 3^2 x^2 = 9x^2$ and $\left(\dfrac{y}{3}\right)^3 = \dfrac{y^3}{3^3} = \dfrac{y^3}{27}$

These rules can be expanded to beyond two factors. For instance, $a^n a^m a^p = a^{n+m+p}$ and $(abcde)^n = a^n b^n c^n d^n e^n$.

Make sure you do not confuse the first two rules: When you multiply powers with the same base, you ADD the exponents; but when you raise a power to an exponent, you MULTIPLY the exponents. Also, be careful to note correctly which numbers or variables are raised to which exponents; for example, $3x^{-3}$ equals $\dfrac{3}{x^3}$, not $\dfrac{1}{3^3 x^3}$. However, $(3x)^{-3}$ does equal $\dfrac{1}{3^3 x^3}$.

Rational Exponents and Radicals

A rational exponent is of the form $\dfrac{m}{n}$, where n and m are integers and n is not zero. Of particular interest are rational exponents of the form $\dfrac{1}{n}$, where n is a nonzero integer. Consider the equation $a^{\frac{1}{n}} = b$. If we raise both sides of the equation to the *n*th power, we get $a = b^n$. We call $a^{\frac{1}{n}}$ the *n*th *root of a*.

All the rules of exponents discussed above hold for rational exponents, as well. In particular:

$$a^{\frac{n}{m}} = \left(a^{\frac{1}{m}}\right)^n = \left(a^n\right)^{\frac{1}{m}}$$

Another way to write rational exponents is in radical notation: $\sqrt[n]{a} = a^{\frac{1}{n}}$. Most familiar is the square root, $\sqrt[2]{a}$, which is written simply as $\sqrt{a}$. For any number, a, there are two other numbers which, when squared, equal a. One of these numbers is positive, and the other is negative—and the two are opposite of each other. They have the same absolute value, but opposite signs. $\sqrt{a}$ refers to the positive one of these numbers and is called the *principal square root* of a. For instance, $\sqrt{4}$ equals 2, not −2, even though both 2 squared and −2 squared equal 4. This holds true for all even roots, not just the square root.

Note also that an even root of a negative number does not exist in the real number set. In other words, for all even n, the expression $\sqrt[n]{a}$ or $a^{\frac{1}{n}}$ has a real solution only if a is not negative.

- If $a^{\frac{1}{n}} = b$, then b is the number that, when raised to the *n*th power, equals a. When n is even, b^n is a product with an even number of terms, all of which are equal to one another.

- If all of them are positive—that is, if b is positive—then their product will also be positive.

- If all of them are negative—that is, if b is negative—then their product will be positive because the product of an even number of negative numbers is positive.

- If all of them are zero, then their product is zero. Thus, a itself has to be either positive or zero.

Example: Evaluate $\dfrac{5^3 \left(4^2 \times 3^4\right)^{\frac{1}{2}}}{15 \times 2^{-1}}$

First, start with the numerator: Distribute the exponent to each term of the product inside the parenthesis:

$$\frac{5^3 \left(4^2 \times 3^4\right)^{\frac{1}{2}}}{15 \times 2^{-1}} = \frac{5^3 \times 4^{2 \times \frac{1}{2}} \times 3^{4 \times \frac{1}{2}}}{15 \times 2^{-1}} = \frac{5^3 \times 4 \times 3^2}{15 \times 2^{-1}}$$

Next, move to the denominator: Factor the number 15, and bring the denominator to the numerator using a negative exponent:

$$\frac{5^3 \times 4 \times 3^2}{15 \times 2^{-1}} = \frac{5^3 \times 4 \times 3^2}{3 \times 5 \times 2^{-1}} = 5^3 \times 4 \times 3^2 \times \left(3 \times 5 \times 2^{-1}\right)^{-1} = 5^3 \times 4 \times 3^2 \times 3^{-1} \times 5^{-1} \times 2^1$$

Finally, combine powers with the same base and simplify:

$$5^3 \times 4 \times 3^2 \times 3^{-1} \times 5^{-1} \times 2^1 = 5^{3+(-1)} \times 4 \times 3^{2+(-1)} \times 2 = 5^2 \times 4 \times 3 \times 2 = 600$$

Example: Simplify $\left(\sqrt[4]{x^3 y^2}\right)^{-8}$

$$\left(\sqrt[4]{x^3 y^2}\right)^{-8} = \frac{1}{\left(\sqrt[4]{x^3 y^2}\right)^8} = \frac{1}{\left(\left(x^3 y^2\right)^{\frac{1}{4}}\right)^8} = \frac{1}{\left(x^3 y^2\right)^{\frac{8}{4}}} = \frac{1}{\left(x^3 y^2\right)^2} = \frac{1}{x^6 y^4}$$

ALGEBRAIC EXPRESSIONS

Algebraic expressions are mathematical phrases that contain numbers, variables (e.g., x, y, a, or b), and operators (e.g., $+$, $-$, $\times$, and $\div$). A statement that equates two algebraic expressions is called an *equation*.

Translating Language into Algebra

In your daily life, as well as on the PCAT, you frequently have to translate regular language into algebraic expressions and equations. Consider a few examples.

Everyday Statement	Algebraic Expression or Equation
Twice as large as a certain number	$2x$ [Note: You can use any letter, such as x, y, a, b, n, m, etc., for the variable.]
Three less than a certain number	$a - 3$ [Again, you may use a letter other than a.]
Three consecutive even integers added together	$2n + (2n + 2) + (2n + 4)$ [Note: "$2n$" and "$2n + 1$" are convenient ways to signify an even and an odd integer, respectively.]
Twice the sum of three numbers is eight	$2 \times (a + b + c) = 8$

TIP

Remember the importance of turning abstract questions into concise and concrete language to help you understand a problem.

Everyday Statement	Algebraic Expression or Equation
Evan is three years older than Andrew	$E = A + 3$ [where E and A represent the ages of Evan and Andrew, respectively]
Two apples and three bottles of water together cost \$7	$2A + 3W = 7$ [where A and W represent the prices of each apple and bottle of water, respectively]
A shoe store sold twice as many men's shoes in September as it did in August	$M_S = 2M_A$ [where M_S and M_A stand for the number of men's shoes sold in September and August, respectively]

Example: What is the value of $2x + 6y$ when x equals 3 and y equals 1?

Substitute the values of x and y in the expression and solve: $2 \times 3 + 6 \times 1 = 12$.

POLYNOMIALS

Each individual product of numbers and variables within an algebraic expression is a *term* of the expression. An expression that includes variables raised to nonnegative integer exponents is called a *polynomial*. A polynomial with one term is called a *monomial*; one with two terms is called a *binomial*; and one with three terms is called a *trinomial*. The *degree* of a polynomial in one variable is the largest exponent to which the variable is raised in the polynomial. For instance, the degree of $3x^2 + 2x - 5$ is two because the largest exponent to which x is raised is 2.

Adding and Subtracting Polynomials

The *coefficient* of a term of a polynomial is the real number by which the variable is multiplied. So, in the polynomial $3x^2 + \frac{2}{3}x - 5$, the coefficient of x^2 is 3, and the coefficient of x is $\frac{2}{3}$. *Like terms* are terms featuring the same variable(s) raised to the same power. For instance, in the expression $3x^3 + 2x^2 + 4x - 3x^2 - 5$, $2x^2$ and $-3x^2$ are like terms.

Add and subtract polynomials by combining like terms. For instance, in order to add $3x^2 + 2x - 5$ and $x + 3$, combine $2x$ with x, and -5 with 3, while keeping $3x^2$ unaltered. In order to combine like terms, add together their coefficients, and multiply the result by the variable that these like terms have in common.

Example: Subtract $4x - 2xy + 3y - 2$ from $2x^2 + xy + 2y$.

$$(2x^2 + xy + 2y) - (4x - 2xy + 3y - 2) = 2x^2 + xy + 2y - 4x + 2xy - 3y + 2$$
$$= 2x^2 - 4x + (xy + 2xy) + (2y - 3y) + 2$$
$$= 2x^2 - 4x + 3xy - y + 2$$

Multiplying Polynomials

Multiply polynomials by multiplying each term in one polynomial by each term in the other polynomial. The laws of exponents discussed at the beginning of the chapter are used here.

Example: Multiply $4x - 2$ by $2x^2 + x + 2$.

$$(4x - 2)(2x^2 + x + 2) = 4x(2x^2 + x + 2) - 2(2x^2 + x + 2)$$
$$= (4x \times 2x^2 + 4x \times x + 4x \times 2) + (-2 \times 2x^2 - 2 \times x - 2 \times 2)$$
$$= 8x^3 + 4x^2 + 8x - 4x^2 - 2x - 4$$

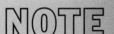

NOTE

One way the test-maker may assess your facility with algebraic equations is to ask you to evaluate an algebraic expression for given values of the variables.

At this point, simplify further by combining like terms:

$$8x^3 + 4x^2 + 8x - 4x^2 - 2x - 4 = 8x^3 + (4x^2 - 4x^2) + (8x - 2x) - 4$$
$$= 8x^3 + 6x - 4$$

Factoring Polynomials

Factoring is the process by which a polynomial is broken down to its individual factors, that is, to the polynomials of lower degree which, when multiplied by one another, yield the original polynomial.

Factoring Out the Greatest Common Divisor

One way of factoring a polynomial is by factoring out the greatest divisor common to all the terms of the polynomial—if there is such a common divisor, of course.

Example: Factor $4x^3(5x - 8) + 2x^2(5x - 8) - (5x - 8)12x$.

It's rather easy to notice that $(5x - 8)$ is common to all terms of the polynomial, so it must be part of these terms' greatest common divisor. However, $2x$ also divides each of the terms of the polynomial. So, the greatest common divisor is $2x(5x - 8)$. Factor this out of each term to arrive at the following:

$$4x^3(5x - 8) + 2x^2(5x - 8) - (5x - 8)12x = 2x(5x - 8)(2x^2 + x - 6)$$

Factoring Quadratic Polynomials

A *quadratic* is a second-degree polynomial. For instance, x^2, $1 - 3x^2$, and $(x + 2)(1 - 3x)$ are examples of quadratics. (The last one appears in factored form, but in distributed form will have $-3x^2$ as the highest power term, as the result of the multiplication of x by $-3x$.) In standard form, a quadratic is written as: $ax^2 + bx + c$, where a, b, and c are real numbers, a is nonzero, and x is a variable.

When factored, a quadratic with integer coefficients will be of the form $(mx + p)(nx + q)$, where m, n, p, and q are integers. The product of mx and nx will produce the second-degree term of the quadratic; the sum of mx multiplied by q and nx multiplied by p will produce the first-degree term; and the product of p and q will produce the constant term.

A quadratic in which a equals 1, that is, the distributed form of the quadratic is $x^2 + bx + c$, is a little easier to work with. The factored form of such a quadratic is $(x + p)(x + q)$, where $pq = c$ and $(p + q) = b$.

Example: Factor $x^2 + 3x + 2$.

Since the coefficient of x^2 is 1, the factored form of the quadratic will be $(x + p)(x + q)$. The trick is to determine p and q. We know that pq must equal 2 because multiplying p by q is the only way to arrive at the constant term, 2, of the distributed form of the quadratic. There are two pairs of integers whose product is 2: (1 and 2) and (−1 and −2). So, which of these is correct? The correct pair features the two integers whose sum is 3, the coefficient of the linear term. The sum of −1 and −2 is not 3; however, the sum of 1 and 2 is 3. Thus, $x^2 + 3x + 2$ must equal $(x + 1)(x + 2)$.

In this case, we do not care whether p is 1 and q is 2, or vice versa. In other examples, however, we'll have to be more specific.

Special Products

Three particular products of binomials occur frequently.

Factored Form	Distributed Form
$(a + b)(a + b)$ or $(a + b)^2$	$a^2 + 2ab + b^2$
$(a - b)(a - b)$ or $(a - b)^2$	$a^2 - 2ab + b^2$
$(a + b)(a - b)$	$a^2 - b^2$

You should be able to recognize these and go from the factored form to the distributed form, and vice versa, quickly. For instance, you should be able to recognize that $4x^2 - 20x + 25$ equals $(2x - 5)^2$, or that $36 - 49x^2$ equals $(6 + 7x)(6 - 7x)$, without having to actually perform lengthy calculations. This will save you time on the test.

EQUATIONS

Equations are statements equating two mathematical expressions. For instance, $x - 1 = 0$, $p^2 + 4 = 4p$, and $\frac{1 - K}{3} = 0$ are equations. Solving an equation—finding its solution(s)—means finding the value(s) of the unknown, or variable, that satisfies the equation. For instance, if $x - 1 = 0$, then x must equal 1. That is, 1 is the only value of x for which $x - 1 = 0$.

As a general rule, when manipulating an equation, you must perform the same action to both sides of the equation. That way, the equality between the statements to the left and right of the equals sign is preserved. For instance, you can add or subtract the same number to or from both sides of the equation; multiply both sides by the same number; or divide both sides by the same nonzero number.

Linear Equations

A *linear equation* is one whose variable is raised to no power other than 1. In standard form, a linear equation is written as $ax + b = 0$, where x is the variable, a is the coefficient of x, and b is a constant.

In order to solve a linear equation, you must isolate the variable with the coefficient of 1 on one side, and everything else on the other side.

Example: Solve $\dfrac{x + 5}{2} = 3(2 - x) + 7$

$\dfrac{x + 5}{2} = 3(2 - x) + 7$	Distribute 3 over the two terms inside the parentheses in order to remove the parentheses.
$\dfrac{x + 5}{2} = 6 - 3x + 7$	Multiply both sides by 2 in order to get rid of the denominator.
$x + 5 = 12 - 6x + 14$	Add "$6x - 5$" to both sides of the equation in order to move all variables to the left and all constants to the right.
$x + 6x = 12 + 14 - 5$	Add the variables together and the constants together.
$7x = 21$	Divide both sides by 7.
$x = 3$	

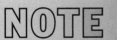

NOTE

If you decide to skip a question, make sure you click the bookmark box so you can return to it later.

You can verify your answer by plugging the result in the original equation. If doing so produces an obviously wrong equality (such as 5 = 7), then you've made a mistake:

$$\frac{3+5}{2} = 3(2-3) + 7$$

$$\frac{8}{2} = -3 + 7$$

$$4 = 4$$

So, $x = 3$ is a solution.

Equations Involving Rational Expressions

Rational expressions are fractions that feature a polynomial in the numerator and the denominator. If you see a variable in the denominator, proceed as you would if there were only numbers in the denominator. Find the least common denominator of all fractions in the equation in order to get rid of the fractions. However, you must make sure that whatever solution you end with is not one that, when plugged into the original equation, will yield a denominator of 0.

Example: Solve $\dfrac{3-a}{9+a^2-6a} + 5 = \dfrac{7}{2}$.

First, factor the denominator on the left side, recognizing that it is the distributed form of one of the three special products we mentioned earlier in this chapter:

$$\frac{3-a}{9+a^2=6a} + 5 = \frac{7}{2}$$

$$\frac{3-a}{(3-a)^2} + 5 = \frac{7}{2}$$

Now, you can cancel out a factor of $(3-a)$ from both the numerator and the denominator, keeping in mind that the denominator cannot be zero, hence a cannot equal 3:

$$\frac{1}{3-a} + 5 = \frac{7}{2}$$

The least common denominator for the three terms in this equation is $2(3-a)$. Multiply each term by $2(3-a)$ in order to get rid of the denominators, and continue solving:

$$\frac{2(3-a) \times 1}{(3-a)} + 5 \times 2(3-a) = \frac{7 \times 2(3-a)}{2}$$

$$2 \times 1 + 10(3-a) = 7(3-a)$$

$$2 + 30 - 10a = 21 - 7a$$

$$2 + 30 - 21 = 10a - 7a$$

$$11 = 3a$$

$$a = \frac{11}{3}$$

Note that $\dfrac{11}{3}$ is different from 3, which you noted earlier cannot be the value of a, so $\dfrac{11}{3}$ is indeed the solution of the original equation.

Solving for One Unknown in Terms of Another Unknown

If a question asks you to find the value of one unknown in terms of another unknown, proceed exactly as you would if you were asked to find an exact numerical value. Just expect that your answer will equate the one unknown to one that contains the other unknown.

Example: If $3n - m = 2m + 6$, what is n in terms of m?

Isolate n on one side of the equation, and everything else on the other:

$$3n - m = 2m + 6$$
$$3n - m + m = 2m + m + 6$$
$$3n = 3m + 6$$
$$\frac{3n}{3} = \frac{3m + 6}{3}$$
$$n = m + 2$$

Simultaneous Equations

Sometimes, you are asked to solve a system of equations. There are two useful methods for solving simultaneous equations: **substitution** and **elimination**.

Example: If $2x + y = 3$ and $x + 1 = 4y$, what is the value of y?

Substitution method:

First, solve the second equation for x in terms of y:

$$x + 1 = 4y$$
$$x = 4y - 1$$

Now, substitute this expression for x into the first equation:

$$2x + y = 3$$
$$2(4y - 1) + y = 3$$
$$8y - 2 + y = 3$$
$$9y = 5$$
$$y = \frac{5}{9}$$

Example: If $2y - x = 4$ and $2x - y = 1$, what is x?

Elimination method:

Since you are looking for x, try to eliminate y. To do so, multiply the second equation by 2 so that the coefficient of y in that equation is the opposite of the coefficient of y in the first equation:

$$2(2x - y) = 2(1)$$
$$4x - 2y = 2$$

Next, rewrite the first equation as $-x + 2y = 4$, add the two equations, and solve for x:

$$\begin{array}{r} -x + 2y = 4 \\ +\ 4x - 2y = 2 \\ \hline 3x + 0y = 6 \\ x = 2 \end{array}$$

The notion of a "solution of the system" remains unchanged when the system is comprised of three equations and three unknowns: we hunt for values of x, y, and z which satisfy all the equations in the given system.

We can still use the analytical techniques used for 2×2 systems, but with minor modifications.

Example: Solve the following system:

$$\begin{cases} 4x - 3y + 5z = 8 \\ x + y - 3z = -3 \\ 5x - 3y - 2z = -5 \end{cases}$$

Eliminate x in Equations 1 and 2:

Multiply the second by -4 and then, add them together to obtain:

$$\begin{aligned} 4x - 3y + 5z &= 8 \\ -4x - 4y + 12z &= 12 \\ \hline -7y + 17z &= 20 \quad \text{Equation A} \end{aligned}$$

Eliminate x in Equations 2 and 3:

Multiply the second by -10 and the third by 2; then, add the results to obtain:

$$\begin{aligned} -10x - 10y + 30z &= 30 \\ 10x - 6y - 4z &= -10 \\ \hline -16y + 26z &= 20 \quad \text{Equation B} \end{aligned}$$

Dividing both sides of Equation B by 2 yields the simplified equation $-8y + 13z = 10$.

Next, we must solve this system of two equations and two unknowns:

$$\begin{cases} -7y + 17z = 20 \quad \text{Equation A} \\ -8y + 13z = 10 \quad \text{Equation B} \end{cases}$$

Again, we use the elimination method.

Multiply Equation A by 8 and Equation B by -7; then, add them together:

$$\begin{aligned} -56y + 136z &= 160 \\ 56y - 91z &= -70 \\ \hline 45z &= 90 \end{aligned}$$

Thus, $z = 2$. Substituting this value back into either Equation A or Equation B for z, we $y = 2$. Finally, substituting both $z = 2$ and $y = 2$ back into any one of the three equations of the original system yields $x = 1$. Therefore, we conclude that the solution to the system is $(1, 2, 2)$.

Note: Using this notation, the first coordinate is the value for x, the second is the value for y, and the third is the value for z.

Quadratic Equations

A *quadratic equation* is a second-degree equation. In standard form, a quadratic equation is written as $ax^2 + bx + c = 0$, where a, b, and c are real numbers, a is nonzero, and x is a variable. In order to solve a quadratic equation, you must first write it in standard form. Then, 1) either write the left side as a product of two factors and then set each factor equal to zero, or 2) use the quadratic formula.

Solving Quadratics by Factoring

If a product equals zero, at least one of its factors must be zero. So, when you factor a quadratic into two linear factors, at least one of these factors equals zero.

Example: What is the solution set of the equation $x^2 + x = 2$?

Write the equation in standard form, and factor:

$$x^2 + x = 2$$
$$x^2 + x - 2 = 0$$
$$(x - 1)(x + 2) = 0$$

At least one of the two factors equals zero:

$$(x - 1) = 0 \text{ OR } (x + 2) = 0$$
$$x = 1 \qquad\qquad x = -2$$

So, the solution set is {1,–2}.

Solving Quadratics by Using the Quadratic Formula

Solving quadratics by factoring is often the simpler way to work, but you may not always be able to use it. Using the quadratic formula always works, though working with the formula involves a fair amount of arithmetic. If $ax^2 + bx + c = 0$ (with a not equal to zero), then the equation's solutions are given by the following formula:

$$x = \frac{-b \pm \sqrt{b^2 - 4ac}}{2a}$$

The quantity under the radical, $b^2 - 4ac$, is called the *discriminant*. A quadratic equation has the following number and type of roots (solutions):

- Two distinct real roots if the discriminant is greater than zero.
- One double root if the discriminant equals zero. This happens when the quadratic is factorable into a perfect square, such as $(x + 1)^2$ or $(3x - 2)^2$.
- No real roots, but two complex conjugate roots if the discriminant is less than zero.

Example: Solve the equation $3x^2 + 5x + 1 = 0$.

Proceed straight to the quadratic formula on this one:

$$x = \frac{-5 \pm \sqrt{5^2 - 4 \times 3 \times 1}}{2 \times 3}$$
$$x = \frac{-5 \pm \sqrt{13}}{6}$$

Equations Involving Radicals

If the unknown is under a square root, isolate the radical on one side of the equation and then remove the root by squaring both sides of the equation. When you've finished solving, check the solution against the original equation to see if it is valid. It may not be—squaring both sides of the equation may have changed the original equation and introduced an extra solution that does not satisfy the original equation.

Example: Solve $\sqrt{x+1} + 1 = x$.

$\sqrt{x+1} + 1 = x$	Isolate the radical on the left side of the equation.
$\sqrt{x+1} = x - 1$	Square both sides.
$\left(\sqrt{x+1}\right)^2 = (x-1)^2$	Solve the quadratic equation.
$x + 1 = x^2 - 2x + 1$ $x^2 - 3x = 0$ $x(x-3) = 0$	
$x = 0$ OR $x = 3$	

The final step is to check these solutions against the original equation. If $x = 0$:

$$\sqrt{0+1} + 1 = 0$$
$$\sqrt{1} + 1 = 0$$
$$2 = 0 \quad \text{This solution is invalid.}$$

Next, if $x = 3$:

$$\sqrt{3+1} + 1 = 3$$
$$\sqrt{4} + 1 = 3$$
$$3 = 3 \quad \text{This solution is valid.}$$

Solving equations containing two radicals is like solving those containing a single radical expression in that the strategy is the same: get rid of the radical expressions. The difference lies in the fact that we cannot get rid of both radical terms at the same time. The process is illustrated in the following example.

Example: Solve $\sqrt{x+4} + \sqrt{x+1} = 3$.

First, isolate one of the radical terms. It does not matter which one: $\sqrt{x+4} = 3 - \sqrt{x+1}$

Square both sides to get rid of the radical you isolated:

$$\left(\sqrt{x+4}\right)^2 = \left(3 - \sqrt{x+1}\right)^2$$
$$x + 4 = \left(3 - \sqrt{x+1}\right)^2$$

Expand the squared binomial on the right side and then, isolate the remaining radical:

$$x + 4 = 9 - 6\sqrt{x+1} + x + 1$$
$$x + 4 = -6\sqrt{x+1} + x + 10$$
$$-6 = -6\sqrt{x+1}$$
$$1 = \sqrt{x+1}$$

Now, square both sides to get rid of the radical. Then, solve for x:

$$1 = x + 1$$
$$0 = x$$

Generally, not all x-values that result from this process will satisfy the original equation. So, you should always substitute them back into the original equation to ensure it is actually a solution. Doing so here shows that it is indeed a solution.

INEQUALITIES

Inequalities are statements about the relative size of two mathematical expressions. For instance, $x > 2$ means that "x is greater than 2," whereas $2 - y \leq 5$ means that "two minus y is less than or equal to five." Solving an inequality means finding the range of values of the unknown that satisfy the inequality.

The solution sets for inequalities are sometimes given in terms of intervals.

- In interval notation, the solution set of the inequality $x > 2$ is $(2, \infty)$. This means that all numbers from 2 (but not including 2) up to infinity are included in the solution. The parenthesis to the left of the number 2 indicates that 2 is not part of the solution.

- On the other hand, the solution set for $x \geq 2$ is $[2, \infty)$. The bracket indicates that 2 is included in the solution. Infinity itself is never included in the solution set, so it is always bounded by a parenthesis.

- In addition, the symbol $\cup$ stands for the union of two sets. For instance, if the solution is $x < 3$ or $x > 5$, then the solution set is $(-\infty, 3) \cup (5, \infty)$.

Here are a few other examples:

Inequality	Solution Set in Interval Notation
$x < 5$	$(-\infty, 5)$
$-2 < x \leq 17$	$(-2, 17]$
$x \leq a$ OR $x > -b$	$(-\infty, a] \cup (-b, \infty)$

Linear Inequalities

Solving a linear inequality is similar to, but not entirely the same as, solving a linear equation. Just as with equations, 1) you can add or subtract the same number from both sides of an inequality, and 2) you can multiply or divide both sides by the same positive number. 3) However, if you multiply or divide by a negative number, you must reverse the direction of the inequality.

Example: What values of z satisfy the inequality $(4 - 3z)2 \geq \dfrac{z+1}{-3}$?

$(4 - 3z)2 \geq \dfrac{z+1}{-3}$	Multiply both sides by −3, remembering to reverse the direction of the inequality.
$(4 - 3z)2 \times (-3) \leq z + 1$ $(4 - 3z)(-6) \leq z + 1$ $-24 + 18z \leq z + 1$ $18z - z \leq 1 + 24$ $17z \leq 25$ $z \leq \dfrac{25}{17}$	Continue solving as you would an equation.

If you are manipulating a double inequality, make sure you take the same action on all three portions of the inequality. For instance, in order to solve the inequality $3 < \dfrac{x}{2} < 5,$ you must multiply all three parts by 2, thus arriving at the correct $2(3) < 2(\frac{x}{2}) < 2(5)$, or $6 < x < 10$.

Inequalities Involving Rational Expressions

Inequalities that include fractions with a polynomial in the denominator add an extra level of complexity. In an inequality, you cannot multiply by a number if you do not know whether it is positive or negative. Because you do not know whether the polynomial in the denominator is positive or negative, you cannot remove the denominator by multiplying all terms of the inequality by it. You have to proceed differently.

Example: What is the solution set of the inequality $\dfrac{4x - 2}{x + 3} > 3$?

First, manipulate the inequality so it follows the format $\dfrac{\text{Something}}{\text{Something else}} > 0$ (or less than zero, or greater than or equal to zero, or less than or equal to zero, as the case may be):

$$\frac{4x - 2}{x + 3} > 3$$

$$\frac{4x - 2}{x + 3} - 3 > 0$$

$$\frac{4x - 2 - 3(x + 3)}{x + 3} > 0$$

$$\frac{4x - 2 - 3x - 9}{x + 3} > 0$$

$$\frac{x - 11}{x + 3} > 0$$

From this point on, you can solve using a trick. Recall that one number divided by another number is positive if both of the numbers are positive, or if both of them are negative. Find the values of x for which the numerator and the denominator are positive or negative, and then create a table.

- In the top row, list number intervals determined by the values of x at which the various factors in the numerator and denominator are zero.

- In this case, the numerator equals zero when $x = 11$, and the denominator equals zero when $x = -3$, so you need to consider three intervals: $x < -3$, $-3 < x < 11$, and $x > 11$.

- In the left-most column, list each of the factors that appear in the numerator and denominator, with the last row corresponding to the entire fraction, itself.

- In the remaining cells, determine whether each factor, and the fraction itself, are positive or negative. In order to determine whether the fraction is positive or negative for each interval, see whether the fraction is the result of the multiplication of positive or negative factors, and how many of them there are, and then apply what you know about the products of positive and negative numbers.

	$x < -3$	$-3 < x < 11$	$x > 11$
$(x - 11)$	Negative	Negative	Positive
$(x + 3)$	Negative	Positive	Positive
$\dfrac{x - 11}{x + 3}$	**Negative × Negative = Positive**	Negative × Positive = Negative	**Positive × Positive = Positive**

The fraction is positive when x is less than -3 or when x is greater than 11, so the solution set for this inequality is $(-\infty, 3) \cup (11, \infty)$. Keep in mind that the factors in the denominator can never equal zero.

Quadratic Inequalities

Solving quadratic inequalities is similar to solving inequalities involving rational expressions. Factor the quadratic and create a table as in the previous example.

Example: Solve the inequality $2x^2 + 3 \leq 5x$.

Move all terms to the left side and factor:

$$2x^2 + 3 \leq 5x$$
$$2x^2 - 5x + 3 \leq 0$$
$$(x - 1)(2x - 3) \leq 0$$

For the expression on the left side to be less than zero, one of the factors must be positive while the other is negative. For the expression to equal zero, either factor must equal zero.

$(x - 1)$ equals 0 when x equals 1.

$(2x - 3)$ equals 0 when x equals $\dfrac{3}{2}$.

	$x < 1$	$1 < x < \dfrac{3}{2}$	$x > \dfrac{3}{2}$
$(x - 1)$	Negative	Positive	Positive
$(2x - 3)$	Negative	Negative	Positive
$(x - 1)(2x - 3)$	Positive	**Negative**	Positive

Since you need the expression to be "less than or equal to zero," the values that make either factor zero are part of the solution. Thus, the solution set is $[1, \frac{3}{2}]$.

Inequalities Involving Radicals

When you encounter a radical in an inequality, first determine the values of the unknown for which the radical has a real value. Once you have determined this, solve the inequality as you would an equation. Then combine the result you get from solving the inequality and the result you got when you considered the quantity under the radical to arrive at the complete solution.

Example: Solve the inequality $6 - \sqrt{x+3} > 2$.

For the radical to have real values, $x + 3$ must be nonnegative:

$$x + 3 \geq 0$$
$$x \geq -3$$

Now, solve the inequality:

$$6 - \sqrt{x+3} > 2$$
$$6 - 2 > \sqrt{x+3}$$
$$\sqrt{x+3} < 4$$
$$\left(\sqrt{x+3}\right)^2 < 4^2$$
$$x + 3 < 16$$
$$x < 13$$

Combining $x \geq -3$ with $x < 13$ results in the double inequality $-3 \leq x < 13$. To make sure this interval is correct, check a value less than -3, one between -3 and 13, and one greater than 13. Indeed, only the values in the set $[-3, 13)$ satisfy the inequality.

Equations and Inequalities Involving Absolute Value

The *absolute value*, $|n|$, of any real number n is the distance of n from zero in the number line. For instance, $|3| = 3$, and $|-3| = 3$ because both 3 and -3 are three units away from zero. The absolute value of any number is nonnegative. In general,

$$|n| = n, \text{ if } n \geq 0, \text{ and } |n| = -n, \text{ if } n < 0$$

Absolute Value Equations

Since every nonzero number and its opposite have the same absolute value, most linear equations featuring an absolute value have two solutions:

If $|n| = a$, where a is a nonnegative number, then $n = a$ or $n = -a$.

Example: If $|x + 1| = 3 + 2x$, what is x?

$$|x + 1| = 3 + 2x$$

Remember that whenever you're dealing with an even root, the number under the radical cannot be negative.

Working backwards from the answer choices can help. Start with the second answer. That way you'll know if the answer is more or less than the second answer. If it's less, you don't have to do any work. Just choose the first answer. If it's more than the second answer, try the fourth answer. If it's not the fourth answer, then it's the third and you are finished either way.

$$x + 1 = 3 + 2x \quad \text{OR} \quad x + 1 = -3 - 2x$$
$$x = -2 \qquad\qquad 3x = -4$$
$$x = -\frac{4}{3}$$

Now, check the two solutions against the original equation to see whether they are valid. For $x = -2$:

$$|-2 + 1| = 3 + 2(-2)$$
$$|-1| = 3 - 4$$
$$1 = -1$$

This equation is incorrect, so $x = -2$ is not a valid solution. For $x = -\frac{4}{3}$:

$$\left|-\frac{4}{3} + 1\right| = 3 + 2\left(-\frac{4}{3}\right)$$
$$\left|-\frac{1}{3}\right| = 3 - \frac{8}{3}$$
$$\frac{1}{3} = \frac{1}{3}$$

This result is correct, so the solution is valid.

Absolute Value Inequalities

Absolute value inequalities must be broken down into two cases: "less than" and "greater than" inequalities. For any nonnegative number a:

$$\text{If } |n| \le a, \text{ then } -a \le n \le a.$$

(Why? Well, if the absolute value of n is less than or equal to a, then on the number line, n is closer to 0 than either a or $-a$, so n must lie between $-a$ and a.)

Next, for any nonnegative number a:

$$\text{If } |n| \ge a, \text{ then } n \le -a \text{ or } n \ge a.$$

(Why? If the absolute value of n is greater than or equal to a, then on the number line, n must lie either to the left of $-a$ or to the right of a.)

Example: Solve $|2x + 3| < 4$.

$$|2x + 3| < 4$$

$$-4 < 2x + 3 < 4$$
$$-7 < 2x < 1$$
$$-\frac{7}{2} < x < \frac{1}{2}$$

Example: Solve $|2x + 3| \geq 4$.

$$|2x + 3| \geq 4$$

$$2x + 3 \leq -4 \quad \text{OR} \quad 2x + 3 \geq 4$$

$$2x \leq -7 \qquad\qquad 2x \geq 1$$

$$x \leq -\frac{7}{2} \qquad\qquad x \geq \frac{1}{2}$$

FUNCTIONS

A *function* is a relation between two sets: the domain and the range. A function associates each element in the domain with exactly one element in the range. Typically, a function is represented in an equation such that each x for which the equation is defined yields a unique value for y, based on a certain formula, such as:

$$y = 2x, \, y = 3 + \sqrt{2x}, \text{ or } y = 4x^2 + 4x + 1$$

In function notation, replace y with $f(x)$ (to read as "f of x," not "f times x") to indicate that y, the dependent variable, varies based on the values of (or is a function of) x, the independent variable.

The *domain* of a function is the set of numbers for which the function is defined—that is, the set of all x for which the function has a real value. For instance, the domain of $f(x) = \sqrt{x}$ consists of all nonnegative numbers, since the square root of a negative number is not defined in the set of real numbers. Similarly, a function that features a variable in the denominator is defined only for those values of the variable for which the denominator is nonzero.

Example: Determine the domain of these functions.

(i) $f(x) = \sqrt{1 - 4x}$

(ii) $g(x) = \dfrac{2x + 1}{(x - 5)\left(x^2 + 1\right)}$

(i) The radicand of a square root must be nonnegative. Otherwise, the result is an imaginary number. So, the domain is the set of all x-values for which $1 - 4x \geq 0$. Solving for x yields

$$1 - 4x \geq 0$$

$$1 \geq 4x$$

$$\frac{1}{4} \geq x$$

Or, equivalently, $x \leq \dfrac{1}{4}$. Using interval notation, the domain is $\left(-\infty, \dfrac{1}{4}\right]$.

(ii) The denominator of a fraction cannot equal zero. Here, the only x-value that makes the denominator equal to zero is 5. So, the domain is $\left(-\infty, 5\right) \cup \left(5, \infty\right)$.

The *range* of a function is the set containing the values of y that are produced when all the values of x in the domain are entered into the formula of the function.

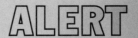

This example and explanation offer important information about function test questions.

An elementary way for the test-maker to assess your facility with functions is to ask you to evaluate a function for given values of the independent variable.

Example: If $f(x) = 2x + 6$, what is $f(3)$?

Substitute 3 for x in the function and solve: $f(3) = 2 \times 3 + 6 = 12$.

Example: If $g(x) = \dfrac{x^2 - 2x}{1 - x}$, compute $g(-3)$.

Substitute -3 in for x everywhere it appears in the formula. Then, simplify using the order of operations:

$$g(-3) = \frac{(-3)^2 - 2(-3)}{1 - (-3)} = \frac{9 + 6}{1 + 3} = \frac{15}{4}$$

Operations on Functions

Functions can be added or multiplied together, one can be subtracted from the other, and one can be divided by the other:

$$(f + g)(x) = f(x) + g(x)$$
$$(f - g)(x) = f(x) - g(x)$$
$$(fg)(x) = f(x)g(x)$$
$$\left(\frac{f}{g}\right)(x) = \frac{f(x)}{g(x)}, \text{ for } g(x) \neq 0$$

Let $f(x)$ and $g(x)$ be two functions.

To compute any of the arithmetic combinations $f(x) + g(x), f(x) - g(x)$ and $f(x) \cdot g(x)$ at a specific x-value, you must be able to compute both $f(x)$ and $g(x)$, individually, at that x-value. As such, the domain of these three arithmetic combinations is the set of x-values at which *both* $f(x)$ and $g(x)$ are defined. This means an x-value must belong to both of their domains. This is typically written as the *intersection* of the two domains, $dom(f) \cap dom(g)$.

The x-values for which the quotient function $\dfrac{f(x)}{g(x)}$ is defined must also belong to $dom(f) \cap dom(g)$, with the additional restriction that the denominator does not equal zero. So, any x-value for which $g(x) = 0$ must be excluded from the domain of $\dfrac{f(x)}{g(x)}$.

Example: If $f(x) = x + 6$ and $g(x) = 1 - x^2$, what is $(fg)(x)$?

$$\begin{aligned}
(fg)(x) &= f(x)g(x) \\
&= (x + 6)(1 - x^2) \\
&= x - x^3 + 6 - 6x^2 \\
&= -x^3 - 6x^2 + x + 6
\end{aligned}$$

Functions may also be combined via *function composition*. The composition of functions $f(x)$ and $g(x)$ is denoted by $(f \circ g)(x) = f[g(x)]$ and pronounced "f of g of x." This is different from the multiplication of the two functions. Also, the order in which the functions are listed is important; usually, $(f \circ g)(x) \neq (g \circ f)(x)$.

In order to evaluate $(f \circ g)(x)$, substitute $g(x)$ for x in $f(x)$—that is, treat $g(x)$ as the independent variable in $f(x)$.

Example: If $f(x) = x + 6$ and $g(x) = 1 - x^2$, what is $(g \circ f)(x)$?

$$
\begin{aligned}
(g \circ f)(x) &= g(x + 6) \\
&= 1 - (x + 6)^2 \\
&= 1 - (x^2 + 12x + 36) \\
&= -x^2 - 12x - 35
\end{aligned}
$$

Example: Let $f(x) = \dfrac{2}{x + 1}$. Compute and simplify $\dfrac{f(x + h) - f(x)}{h}$.

$$
\begin{aligned}
\frac{f(x + h) - f(x)}{h} &= \frac{\dfrac{2}{(x + h) + 1} - \dfrac{2}{x + 1}}{h} \\[2em]
&= \frac{\dfrac{2(x + 1) - 2(x + h + 1)}{(x + h + 1)(x + 1)}}{h} \\[2em]
&= \frac{2(x + 1) - 2(x + h + 1)}{h(x + h + 1)(x + 1)} \\[1em]
&= \frac{2x + 2 - 2x - 2h - 2}{h(x + h + 1)(x + 1)} \\[1em]
&= \frac{-2h}{h(x + h + 1)(x + 1)} \\[1em]
&= \frac{-2}{(x + h + 1)(x + 1)}
\end{aligned}
$$

When computing the composition $(f \circ g)(x) = f(g(x))$ at a given x-value, that x must satisfy two criteria. First, $g(x)$ must be defined, meaning x must belong to the domain of g. If that is the case, then the value $g(x)$ must belong to the domain of f. Putting these two conditions together, we have:

The domain of $\left(f \circ g\right)$ is the set of all x-values in the domain of g for which $g(x)$ itself belongs to the domain of f.

Example: Suppose $f(x) = \dfrac{1}{x}$ and $g(x) = \sqrt{x}$. What is the domain of $\left(g \circ f\right)$?

First, an x-value must belong to the domain of $f(x)$. This means that x cannot be zero. Now, of all nonzero values of x, the expression $\dfrac{1}{x}$ cannot be negative since the radicand of a square root cannot be negative. Therefore, the domain of the composition function $\left(g \circ f\right)$ is the set of all positive x-values.

Inverses of Functions

If each element in the range corresponds to exactly one element in the domain—that is, if each value of the dependent variable y is produced by one and only one value of the independent variable x—then the function is called *one-to-one*.

Two one-to-one functions, $f(x)$ and $g(x)$, are *inverses* of each other if $(f \circ g)(x) = (g \circ f)(x) =$ for all values of x in their domain.

Notate the inverse of $f(x)$ as $f^{-1}(x)$.

Make sure you do not treat the "−1" as an exponent: $f^{-1}(x)$ does NOT equal $\dfrac{1}{f(x)}$!

In order to find the inverse of a function, switch the y and x in the function and solve for y. If you have not made any mistakes, this will be the inverse, $f^{-1}(x)$.

To be sure, verify that $(f \circ f^{-1})(x) = x$ and $(f^{-1} \circ f)(x) = x$.

Example: What is the inverse of the function defined as $f(x) = x + 1$?

First, replace $f(x)$ with y, to simplify the notation.

Then, switch x and y and solve for y.

So, if $y = x + 1$, then the "switched" function is $x = y + 1$.

Solving for y, yields $y = x − 1$. This is the inverse you're looking for because:

$$(f \circ f^{-1})(x) = (x - 1) + 1 = x$$

$$(f^{-1} \circ f)(x) = (x + 1) - 1 = x$$

Quadratic Functions

A *quadratic function* is a function of the form $f(x) = a(x - h)^2 + k$, where a, h, and k are real numbers and $a \neq 0$.

The graph of the most basic quadratic function is as follows:

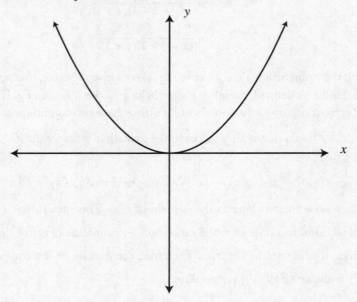

The graph is U-shaped; such a graph is called a *parabola*. The graph appears to be symmetric about the y-axis. Also, the point $(0, 0)$ is the minimum of the graph. For quadratic functions, this point is called the *vertex*.

If a quadratic function is expressed in the form $F(x) = Ax^2 + Bx + C$, we must first transform this function into the form $f(x) = a(x - h)^2 + k$ by *completing the square*. We illustrate the process of completing the square with an example.

Example. Rewrite $f(x) = x^2 + 16x + 3$ in standard form. Then, identify the vertex.

Complete the square to rewrite the function in the form $f(x) = a(x - h)^2 + k$.

Step 1: Group the x-terms together: $f(x) = (x^2 + 16x) + 3$.

Step 2: Determine what number could be added inside the parentheses so that the resulting trinomial is of the form $(x - h)^2$ for some number h.

It turns out that you find this number by dividing the coefficient of 16 by 2, and then squaring that result; doing so yields 64. Indeed, observe $x^2 + 16x + 64 = (x + 8)^2$.

Step 3: Now, add and subtract the number 64 from the right side of $f(x) = (x^2 + 16x) + 3$, and simplify as follows:

$f(x) = (x^2 + 16x + 64) + 3 - 64$

$f(x) = (x + 8)^2 - 61$

The final expression above is the desired form with $a = 1$, $h = -8$, and $k = -61$. The vertex is $(-8, -61)$.

Quadratic functions arise in various applications. One such example is as follows:

Example: Suppose that a ball is launched from ground-level (meaning a height of 0 feet) at time $t = 0$ seconds and then lands when $t = 10$ seconds later. Assuming the path of the ball is parabolic and that the height of the ball when $t = 2$ seconds is 10 feet, determine the maximum height achieved by the ball.

Since the path is parabolic, we can use a quadratic function to model it. Also, we know the times at which the height is 0, namely at $t = 0$ seconds and $t = 10$ seconds; these are the intercepts. Since a quadratic function can have at most two distinct factors, the quadratic function has the form $f(t) = a(t - 0)(t - 10)$.

We need to find a using the fact that $f(2) = 10$. Substituting this value in yields the equation $10 = a(2 - 0)(2 - 10) = -16a$, so that $a = -\dfrac{5}{8}$. So, the function is given by $f(t) = -\dfrac{5}{8}(t - 0)(t - 10)$.

The vertex occurs halfway between the two intercepts, namely when $t = 5$. And, the height at this time is $f(5) = -\dfrac{5}{8}(5 - 0)(5 - 10) = \dfrac{125}{8}$. Since the coefficient of the squared term is negative, we know that the maximum height of the ball occurs at the vertex and so, the maximum height the ball achieves is $\dfrac{125}{8}$ feet.

COMMON WORD PROBLEMS

Word problems whose solution involve solving an algebraic equation, or system thereof, come in several varieties. We give a sample of some common word problems below.

Example: Bianca orders 5 pizzas and 4 six-packs of soda for a small get-together. The cost of each of the pizzas is 8 dollars more than the cost of a six-pack. If Bianca pays for the refreshments with a 100-dollar bill and receives 15 dollars change, find the price of a six-pack and the price of the pizza.

Let x be the cost of one six-pack of soda. Then, the cost of one pizza is $8 + x$. Since Bianca buys 5 pizzas and 4 six-packs, the total cost is $5(8 + x) + 4x$ dollars. Further, since she gets $15 change after paying with $100-bill, the total cost is $85. Equating these two expressions yields the equation $5(8 + x) + 4x = 85$. Solve for x:

$$5(8 + x) + 4x = 85$$
$$40 + 5x + 4x = 85$$
$$9x = 45$$
$$x = 5$$

So, one six-pack of soda is $5 and one pizza is $13.

Example: Kari invested some money at 10% interest and $1500 more than that amount at 11% interest. Her total yearly interest was $795. How much did she invest at each rate?

Let x be the amount Kari invested at 10%. Then, she invested $1500 + x$ at 11%. The total interest for one year on these two investments, combined, is $0.10x + 0.11(1500 + x)$. Since this equals $795, we get the equation $0.10x + 0.11(1500 + x) = 795$. Solve for x:

$$0.10x + 0.11(1,500 + x) = 795$$
$$10x + 11(1,500 + x) = 79,500$$
$$10x + 16,500 + 11x = 79,500$$
$$21x = 63,000$$
$$x = 3,000$$

So, Kari invested $3,000 at 10% and $4500 at 11%.

Example: A boat can travel 15 miles upstream and 15 miles back downstream in a total of 4 hours. If the speed of the current is 5 mph, set up a system of equations that could be used to find the speed of the boat in still water and the time it takes it to complete the trip upstream.

Let x be the time (in hours) it takes the boat to complete the trip upstream. Then, the time (in hours) it takes the boat to complete the trip downstream is $4 - x$. Let y be the speed of the boat in still water. Then, the speed of the boat when traveling upstream against the current is $y - 5$ mph, and the speed of the boat when traveling downstream with the current is $y + 5$ mph. Using the formula *distance = rate times time*, we get two equations: one for the upstream trip and one for the downstream trip:

Upstream: $15 = (y - 5)x$

Downstream: $15 = (y + 5)(4 - x)$

PRACTICE QUESTIONS

Directions: Choose the best answer for each question.

1. Mindy won $2.5 million in the lottery. Forty percent of that amount was deducted for taxes, and Mindy spent $600,000 of the remainder to buy a house. How much of the $2.5 million does she have left?

    A. $1,500,000
    B. $900,000
    C. $600,000
    D. $400,000

2. If $2a - 6b = 3d$ and $c = d + 2b$, what is $2a - 3c$?

    A. 0
    B. $-12b$
    C. $12b + 6d$
    D. $4b + 2d$

3. Solve the system:
$$\begin{cases} y - 3x = 1 \\ 4z = -16 \\ 2x + 3z = 6 \end{cases}$$

    A. $x = 9, y = 28, z = -4$
    B. $x = 3, y = 10, z = 0$
    C. $x = 9, y = -26, z = -4$
    D. $x = -3, y = -8, z = -4$

4. If $25z^2 = 64$, which of the following is a solution to the equation?

    A. $z = 8$
    B. $z = \dfrac{5}{8}$
    C. $z = -\dfrac{5}{8}$
    D. $z = -\dfrac{8}{5}$

5. What is the factored form of $6x^2 - 11x + 4$?

    A. $(3x + 4)(2x - 1)$
    B. $(3x - 4)(2x + 1)$
    C. $(3x - 4)(2x - 1)$
    D. $(3x + 4)(2x + 1)$

6. Which of the following equations has no real solution?

    A. $\dfrac{x + 3}{2} = 6$
    B. $4x^2 - 9 = 0$
    C. $(18 - 7x)^3 = 0$
    D. $x^2 + x + 1 = 0$

7. What is x, if $\dfrac{(2 - x)(x^2 + x - 6)}{(x - 2)} = 0$?

    A. -3
    B. -2
    C. 2
    D. 3

8. If $\sqrt{x + 4} + 4 = x + 2$, which of the following is a value of x?

    A. -5
    B. -4
    C. 0
    D. 5

9. Solve for x: $\sqrt{x - 10} + \sqrt{x - 3} =$

    A. 7
    B. 11
    C. 19
    D. No solution

10. For which values of x is the expression $\dfrac{39}{\sqrt{x^2 - 4}}$ defined and real?

    A. $(-\infty, -2] \cup (2, \infty)$

    B. $(-\infty, -2) \cup (2, \infty)$

    C. $(-\infty, -2)$

    D. $(2, \infty)$

11. If $2 + |x - 2| = 2x$, what is x?

    A. $-\dfrac{4}{3}$

    B. 0

    C. $\dfrac{4}{3}$

    D. 2

12. Find all values of x that satisfy the inequality $|x + 2| - x \le 4$.

    A. $x \ge -3$

    B. $x \le -3$

    C. $-3 \le x \le 0$

    D. $x \ge 0$

13. Determine the domain of the function $f(x) = \dfrac{x}{x^2 + 4}$.

    A. $(-\infty, 0) \cup (0, \infty)$

    B. $(-\infty, -2) \cup (-2, 2) \cup (2, \infty)$

    C. $(-\infty, -2) \cup (-2, 0) \cup (0, 2) \cup (2, \infty)$

    D. All real numbers

14. Determine the range of the following function:

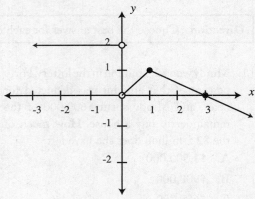

    A. $(-\infty, 1) \cup \{2\}$

    B. $(-\infty, 1] \cup \{2\}$

    C. $(-\infty, 1)$

    D. $(-\infty, 0) \cup (0, \infty)$

15. If $g(x) = \dfrac{2}{x + 1} - 3$ and $h(x) = \dfrac{x}{x - 1} - 5$, which of the following equals $(g - h)(x)$?

    A. $\dfrac{4 - x}{2x}$

    B. $\dfrac{x^2 + x - 4}{x^2 - 1}$

    C. $\dfrac{-x^2 + x - 2}{x^2 - 1}$

    D. $\dfrac{x^2 - 4}{x^2 - 1}$

16. If $f(x) = \dfrac{x}{x^2 - 4}$ and $g(x) = \sqrt{x + 4}$, what is the domain of $\left(\dfrac{f}{g}\right)(x)$?

    A. $(-4, -2) \cup (-2, 2) \cup (2, \infty)$

    B. $(-2, 2) \cup (2, \infty)$

    C. $(4, \infty)$

    D. $(-\infty, -4) \cup (-4, -2) \cup (-2, 2) \cup (2, \infty)$

17. The sum of three consecutive even integers is 132. What are the three integers?
    A. 41, 43, 45
    B. 40, 42, 44
    C. 42, 44, 46
    D. 42, 43, 44

18. A man left Nelsonville traveling by motorcycle at an average speed of 40 miles per hour 3.5 hours after his son left Nelsonville on a bicycle. If the man travels the same road as his son and overtakes him in 1.5 hours, set up and solve an equation to find the average speed of the bicycle.
    A. 10 mph
    B. 12 mph
    C. 14 mph
    D. 16 mph

19. Mike took three Physics exams and has an average score of 88. His second exam was 10 points better than his first and his third exam was 4 points better than his second exam. What was the highest of the three exam scores?
    A. 80
    B. 88
    C. 90
    D. 94

20. A rectangle has length in feet that is three less than twice the width. If the rectangle has an area of 14 square feet, find its dimensions.
    A. 3.5 feet by 4 feet
    B. 1 foot by 2 feet
    C. 3.5 feet by 10 feet
    D. 7 feet by 8 feet

ANSWER KEY AND EXPLANATIONS

1. B	**5.** C	**9.** C	**13.** D	**17.** C
2. A	**6.** D	**10.** B	**14.** B	**18.** B
3. A	**7.** A	**11.** C	**15.** B	**19.** D
4. D	**8.** D	**12.** A	**16.** A	**20.** A

1. **The correct answer is B.** If 40 percent are deducted for taxes, then Mindy kept 60% of the $2.5 million. Set up an equation and solve for x:

$$x = \frac{60}{100}(\$2,500,000) - \$600,000$$
$$x = \$1,500,000 - \$600,000$$
$$x = \$900,000$$

2. **The correct answer is A.** Use the elimination method. First, multiply the equation $c = d + 2b$ by -3, to arrive at $-3c = -6b - 3d$. Next, add $6b$ to the left and right side of the other equation so that $2a$ is by itself on the left of the equal sign. Then add the two equations:

$$2a = 6b + 3d$$
$$+ (-3c = -6b - 3d)$$
$$\overline{2a - 3c = 0}$$

3. **The correct answer is A.** First, solve the second equation for z: $z = -4$

Substitute this into the third equation to find x:

$$2x + 3(-4) = 6$$
$$2x = 18$$
$$x = 9$$

Substitute this value of x into the first equation to find y: $y - 3(9) = 1$, so that $y = 28$.

So, the solution is $x = 9$, $y = 28$, $z = -4$.

4. **The correct answer is D.** Write the equation in standard form and factor, noting that you're dealing with a difference of two squares, which is the distributed form of one of the three special products reviewed in this chapter:

$$25x^2 = 64$$
$$25x^2 - 64 = 0$$
$$(5z - 8)(5z + 8) = 0$$
$$5z - 8 = 0 \quad \text{OR} \quad 5z + 8 = 0$$
$$z = \frac{8}{5} \qquad\qquad z = -\frac{8}{5}$$

5. **The correct answer is C.** You can use the quadratic formula in order to factor the roots of this expression (as if you were trying to solve the equation $6x^2 - 11x + 4 = 0$), or you can use a shortcut by working from the answer choices. In particular, check the linear term for each of the answer choices, in order to see which of them is correct. If you perform the operations on the first answer choice, you get a $5x$ for the linear term; likewise, from the second choice you get $-5x$. The third choice yields $-11x$ and the fourth yields $11x$. Only the third answer choice produces the correct linear term, thus choice C is correct.

6. **The correct answer is D.** The first equation, a linear equation with the variable in the numerator, has a real solution. The second equation is a difference of squares, and factors into $(2x + 3)(2x - 3) = 0$; this one has two real solutions. The third equation is already factored, and it has one triple real solution: $18 - 7x = 0 \Rightarrow x = \dfrac{18}{7}$. The last equation is a quadratic equation written in the form $ax^2 + bx + c = 0$, with $a = b = c = 1$. Recall that the discriminant of a quadratic equation, which equals $b^2 - 4ac$, tells you how many, if any, real roots the equation has. So, you can check the discriminant of the equation in choice D in order to see whether this equation has any real solutions:

$b^2 - 4ac = 1^2 - 4 \times 1 \times 1 = -3 < 0$

Since the discriminant is less than zero, the equation has no real solutions.

7. **The correct answer is A.** Simplify the expression and then solve:

$$\frac{(2 - x)(x^2 + x - 6)}{(x - 2)} = 0$$

$$\frac{-(x - 2)(x^2 + x - 6)}{(x - 2)} = 0$$

$$-(x^2 + x - 6) = 0$$

$$x^2 + x - 6 = 0$$

$$(x - 2)(x + 3) = 0$$

$x = 2$ or $x = -3$

$x = 2$ makes the original denominator equal to zero, so it is not a solution of the equation. Thus, $x = -3$.

8. **The correct answer is D.** First, solve the equation:

$$\sqrt{x + 4} + 4 = x + 2$$

$$\sqrt{x + 4} = x - 2$$

$$x + 4 = (x - 2)^2$$

$$x + 4 = x^2 - 4x + 4$$

$$x^2 - 5x = 0$$

$$x(x - 5) = 0$$

$x = 0$ or $x = 5$

Then plug both values of x into the original equation. If $x = 0$, the equation becomes $6 = 2$, which is incorrect. If $x = 5$, the equation becomes $7 = 7$, which is correct. Thus, the correct answer is choice D.

9. **The correct answer is C.** Isolate one of the radical expressions: $\sqrt{x - 10} = 7 - \sqrt{x - 3}$ Square both sides and then simplify the right side:

$$x - 10 = \left(7 - \sqrt{x - 3}\right)^2$$

$$x - 10 = 49 - 14\sqrt{x - 3} + x - 3$$

$$-10 = 46 - 14\sqrt{x - 3}$$

$$-56 = -14\sqrt{x - 3}$$

$$4 = \sqrt{x - 3}$$

$$16 = x - 3$$

$$19 = x$$

This is a solution of the original equation.

10. **The correct answer is B.** The denominator cannot be zero; in addition, the expression under the radical sign cannot be negative. Therefore:

$$x^2 - 4 > 0$$

$$(x + 2)(x - 2) > 0$$

Check the values of x in the intervals $x < -2$, $-2 < x < 2$, and $x > 2$. You'll find that x must be greater than 2 or less than -2.

11. **The correct answer is C.** Solve the equation:

$$2 + |x - 2| = 2x$$
$$|x - 2| = 2x - 2$$

$$x - 2 = 2x - 2 \text{ OR } x - 2 = -2x + 2$$
$$x = 0 \qquad\qquad 3x = 4$$
$$x = \frac{4}{3}$$

Now, check the two solutions against the original equation to see whether they are valid. For $x = 0$:

$$0 + |-2| = 0 \Rightarrow 0 = 2$$

This equation is incorrect, so $x = -2$ is not a valid solution. For $x = \frac{4}{3}$:

$$2 + \left|\frac{4}{3} - 2\right| = 2 \times \frac{4}{3}$$
$$2 + \left|\frac{-2}{3}\right| = \frac{8}{3}$$
$$2 + \frac{2}{3} = \frac{8}{3}$$
$$\frac{8}{3} = \frac{8}{3}$$

This result is correct, so the solution is valid.

12. **The correct answer is A.** Solve the inequality:

$$|x + 2| - x \le 4$$
$$|x + 2| \le x + 4$$

$$-(x + 4) \le x + 2 \le x + 4$$

$$-(x + 4) \le x + 2 \text{ OR } x + 2 \le x + 4$$

$$-x - 4 \le x + 2 \qquad 0x \le 2$$

$$2x \ge -6 \qquad\qquad 0 \le 2$$

$$x \ge -3$$

The inequality 0 (insert less than or equal to sign) 2 is a true statement for any value of x. So, all real numbers are solutions to this

inequality. However, extraneous solutions (solutions that don't work when plugged back into the original equation) arise in absolute value inequalities and solutions must be checked. Check values less than −3, between −3 and 0, and greater than 0 to find the true solution. In this case, only those solutions greater than −3 will be correct in the original inequality

.13. **The correct answer is D.** For a rational function, the only restrictions on the domain come from the denominator being 0. However, $x^2 + 4$ is never equal to zero. So, the domain is the set of all real numbers.

14. **The correct answer is B.** The range is the set of all y-values attained at at least one point on the graph. This set is $(-\infty, 1] \cup \{2\}$.

15. **The correct answer is B.** Let $g(x) = \frac{2}{x + 1} - 3$ and $h(x) = \frac{x}{x - 1} - 5$. Subtract the functions and simplify by getting a common denominator, as follows:

$$(g - h)(x) = \left(\frac{2}{x + 1} - 3\right) - \left(\frac{x}{x - 1} - 5\right)$$

$$= \frac{2(x - 1) + 2(x + 1)(x - 1) - x(x + 1)}{(x + 1)(x - 1)}$$

$$= \frac{2x - 2 + 2x^2 - 2 - x^2 - x}{(x + 1)(x - 1)}$$

$$= \frac{x^2 + x - 4}{x^2 - 1}$$

16. **The correct answer is A.** The domain of a quotient function $\left(\frac{f}{g}\right)(x)$ consists of those x-values that satisfy three criteria: they must belong to the domain of f and the domain of g, and $g(x)$ must not equal zero. For $f(x) = \frac{x}{x^2 - 4}$ and $g(x) = \sqrt{x + 4}$, the domain of $f(x)$ is the set of all real numbers except -2 and 2, and the x-values in the domain of g for which $g(x)$ does not equal zero are the real numbers strictly

larger than -4. Hence, the domain is $(-4, -2) \cup (-2, 2) \cup (2, \infty)$.

17. **The correct answer is C.** Let x be the smallest of three consecutive even integers. Then, the two successively larger integers are $x + 2$ and $x + 4$. Since the sum is 132, we have the equation $x + (x + 2) + (x + 4) = 132$. Solve for x, as follows:

$3x + 6 = 132$

$3x = 126$

$x = 42$

So, the three integers are 42, 44, and 46.

18. **The correct answer is B.** Let x be the speed of the bike. At the time when the motorcycle catches the bike, the motorcycle has traveled 1.5 hours at a rate of 40 mph, and the bike has traveled 5 hours at an unknown rate of x mph. At the moment when the motorcycle catches up to the bike, they have traveled the same distance. Using the formula *distance equals rate times time*, we have $40(1.5) = 5x$. Solving for x yields $x = 12$ mph.

19. **The correct answer is D.** Let x be the score on the first exam. Then, the score on the second exam is $x + 10$ and the score on the third exam is $x + 14$. Using the fact that their average is 88 gives rise to the equation $\frac{x + (x + 10) + (x + 14)}{3} = 88$.
Solve for x, as follows:

$3x + 24 = 264$

$3x = 240$

$x = 80$

So, the three exam scores are 80, 90, and 94. Thus, the highest of the three scores is 94.

20. **The correct answer is A.** Let x be the width of the rectangle (in feet). Then, the length is $(2x - 3)$ feet. Since the area is 14 square feet, we get the equation $x(2x - 3) = 14$. Solve for x, as follows:

$x(2x - 3) = 14$

$2x^2 - 3x - 14 = 0$

$(2x - 7)(x + 2) = 0$

$x = \frac{7}{2}, \cancel{-2}$

So, the width is $\frac{7}{2}$, or 3.5 feet, and the length is $2(\frac{7}{2}) - 3 = 4$ feet. So, the dimensions of the rectangle are 3.5 feet by 4 feet.

SUMMING IT UP

- $a^n a^m = a^{n+m}$ and $\dfrac{a^n}{a^m} = a^{n-m}$

- $\left(a^n\right)^m = a^{n \times m}$

- $(ab)^n = a^n b^n$ and $\left(\dfrac{a}{b}\right)^n = \dfrac{a^n}{b^n}$

- $\sqrt[n]{a} = a^{\frac{1}{n}}$. If n is even, then a must be nonnegative.

- A quadratic of the form $x^2 + bx + c$ factors into $(x + p)(x + q)$, where $pq = c$ and $(p + q) = b$.

- If $(x + a)(x + b) = 0$, then either $(x + a) = 0$ or $(x + b) = 0$ or both.

- You can also solve a quadratic equation via the quadratic formula: $x = \dfrac{-b \pm \sqrt{b^2 - 4ac}}{2a}$.

- Always perform the same action to both sides of an equation.

- In multiplying or dividing both sides of an inequality by a negative number, reverse the direction of the inequality.

- If an inequality contains a polynomial in the denominator, both sides of the inequality cannot be multiplied by that polynomial in order to remove the denominator because whether the polynomial is positive or negative is unknown.

- When solving a double inequality, take the same action on all three parts of the inequality, not just two of the three.

- If $(x + a) (x + b) \geq 0$, then either $(x + a) \geq 0$ and $(x + b) \geq 0$ OR $(x + a) \leq 0$ and $(x + b) \leq 0$. The same is true if $\dfrac{x + a}{x + b} \geq 0$, but remember that the factors in the denominator can never equal zero.

- If $(x + a) (x + b) \leq 0$, then either $(x + a) \geq 0$ and $(x + b) \leq 0$ OR $(x + a) \leq 0$ and $(x + b) \geq 0$. The same is true if $\dfrac{x + a}{x + b} \leq 0$, but remember that the factors in the denominator can never equal zero.

- $|n| = n$, if $n \geq 0$, and $|n| = -n$, if $n < 0$

- If $|n| = a$, where a is a nonnegative number, then $n = a$ or $n = -a$.

- If $|n| \leq a$, where a is a nonnegative number, then $-a \leq n \leq a$.

- If $|n| \geq a$, where a is a nonnegative number, then $n \leq -a$ or $n \geq a$.

- The notion of a "solution of the system" remains unchanged when the system is comprised of three equations and three unknowns: we hunt for values of x, y, and z which satisfy all the equations in the given system.

- A *quadratic function* is a function of the form $f(x) = a(x - h)^2 + k$, where a, h, and k are real numbers and $a \neq 0$.

- A quadratic function expressed in the form $F(x) = Ax^2 + Bx + C$ is transformed into the form $f(x) = a(x - h)^2 + k$ by completing the square.

- $(f + g)(x) = f(x) + g(x)$

- $(f - g)(x) = f(x) - g(x)$

- $(fg)(x) = f(x)g(x)$

- $\left(\dfrac{f}{g}\right)(x) = \dfrac{f(x)}{g(x)}$, for $g(x) \neq 0$

- In order to evaluate $(f \circ g)(x)$ or $f[g(x)]$, substitute $g(x)$ for x in $f(x)$.

- Two one-to-one functions, $f(x)$ and $g(x)$, are *inverses* of each other if $(f \circ g)(x) = (g \circ f)(x) = x$. In order to find the inverse of a function, switch the y and x in the function and solve for y.

- If $a^x = a^y$, then $x = y$.

- The slope-intercept form of a line is $y = mx + b$.

Probability and Statistics

OVERVIEW

- **Probability of a Single Event**
- **Probability of Compound Events**
- **Measures of Central Tendency: Mean, Median, and Mode**
- **Measures of Variation: Range, Standard Deviation, and Variance**
- **Graphical Representations**
- **Practice Questions**
- **Answer Key and Explanations**
- **Summing It Up**

PROBABILITY OF A SINGLE EVENT

Probability is the measure of the likelihood that an event will happen. For instance, the probability that one will get an outcome of tails in a single coin toss is 0.5; the probability that rolling a regular, six-sided die will produce a number greater than 4 is $33.\overline{3}\%$; and the probability that one will select a face card on a single, random draw of one card from a deck of 52 playing cards is $\frac{12}{52}$. We write the probability of an event happening as a decimal or fraction (with values between 0 and 1) or as a percent (with values between 0% and 100%). An impossible event has a probability of 0, or 0%. A certain event has a probability of 1, or 100%.

If all outcomes can be counted and are equally likely, the probability P of event A happening is expressed thus:

$$P(A) = \frac{\text{Number of desired outcomes}}{\text{Number of possible outcomes}}$$

For instance, on a single coin flip, the possible outcomes are heads and tails, so the number of possible outcomes is 2. If the desired outcome is tails, then the number of desired outcomes is 1. Therefore:

$$P(tails) = \frac{1}{2} = 0.5 = 50\%$$

To find the probability of selecting a face card on a single, random draw of one card from a deck of 52 playing cards, consider the desired and possible outcomes. There are 52 possible outcomes, since any card in the deck may be selected. There are 12 desired outcomes, since there are 4 suits and each suit has 3 face cards. Thus:

$$P(\textit{face card}) = \frac{12}{52} = \frac{3}{13}$$

501

Chapter 13

PROBABILITY OF COMPOUND EVENTS

Sometimes we need to find the probability that multiple events will occur—for instance, events that can or cannot occur together and events that do or do not depend on one another. In such cases, we need to know how to combine the probabilities of the individual events in order to find the desired result.

Independent Events

Two or more events are called *independent* if none of them affects any of the others. For instance, five coin flips in a row are independent of one another: the result of any of the flips does not affect the results of any of the other flips. Rolling a die and picking a playing card are also independent of each other: the chances of getting any single outcome on the roll of the die are not affected by the card picked, and vice versa.

To find the probability that two independent events both occur, multiply the probabilities that each one occurs:

$$P(A \text{ and } B) = P(A) \times P(B), \text{ when events } A \text{ and } B \text{ are independent}$$

Example: What is the probability that each of four consecutive rolls of a regular, six-sided die will produce an even number?

The die has 3 even numbers and 6 numbers in total. Thus, the probability that any given roll will produce an even number is $\frac{3}{6}$, or $\frac{1}{2}$. Since each roll of the die is independent of the others, the probability that four rolls will produce four even numbers is $\frac{1}{2} \times \frac{1}{2} \times \frac{1}{2} \times \frac{1}{2}$, or $\frac{1}{16}$.

Dependent Events: Conditional Probability

Two or more events are called *dependent* if the outcome of one event affects the outcome of subsequent ones. For instance, picking four cards in a row from a deck of cards without replacement (that is, without putting back in the deck each card that is picked) are dependent events. Let $P(B|A)$ be the probability of event B happening given that event A has already happened. Then:

$$P(A \text{ and } B) = P(A) \times P(B|A)$$

Example: Jason picks 2 cards in a row and at random from a deck of 52 cards without replacing the first card. What is the probability that the first card will be a 6 and the second card will be an ace?

Let event A be the selection of a six on the first try, and let event B be the selection of an ace on the second try. On the first pick, there are four "6" cards available out of 52 total cards. Once a 6 has been picked, there are 4 aces available out of 51 remaining cards. Thus:

$$\begin{aligned}
P(A \text{ and } B) &= P(A) \times P(B \mid A) \\
&= \frac{4}{52} \times \frac{4}{51} \\
&= \frac{1}{13} \times \frac{4}{51} \\
&= \frac{4}{663}
\end{aligned}$$

Example: Jason picks 2 cards in a row and at random from a deck of 52 cards without replacing the first card. What is the probability that the second card will be an ace?

This is a little trickier. Jason may pick 2 aces, an ace only on the first pick, an ace only on the second pick, or no aces at all. Of all these combinations, we are interested in two: "ace on first pick AND ace on second pick" and "no ace on first pick AND ace on second pick." A tree diagram can help organize these options:

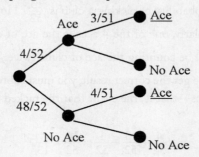

Two of the four paths lead to an ace in the second pick: Ace-Ace and No Ace-Ace. Let's trace the first path first. The probability that Jason will pick an ace on the first draw is $\frac{4}{52}$; the probability that he will then pick an ace on the second draw is $\frac{3}{51}$, since 3 of the remaining 51 cards are aces. Next, let's look at the second path. The probability that Jason will not pick an ace on the first draw is $\frac{48}{52}$; the probability that he will then pick an ace on the second draw is $\frac{4}{51}$, since 4 of the remaining 51 cards are aces.

Thus, the probability that he will pick an ace as his second card is:

$$\frac{4}{52} \times \frac{3}{51} + \frac{48}{52} \times \frac{4}{51} = \frac{1}{13} \times \frac{3}{51} + \frac{1}{13} \times \frac{48}{51}$$

$$= \frac{1}{13}\left(\frac{3}{51} + \frac{48}{51}\right)$$

$$= \frac{1}{13}$$

Mutually Exclusive and Non-Mutually Exclusive Events

Two events are called *mutually exclusive* if they cannot happen at the same time. For instance, on a single roll of a die, rolling an even number and rolling an odd number are mutually exclusive: if the number rolled is even, then it cannot be odd. On the other hand, rolling an even number and rolling a 4 are not mutually exclusive: if the number rolled is even, it may, in fact, be a 4.

If events A and B are mutually exclusive, then by definition $P(A \text{ and } B)$ equals 0. On the other hand, the probability of one event or the other occurring is found by the following formula:

$P(A \text{ or } B) = P(A) + P(B)$, when events A and B are mutually exclusive

A more general version of this formula applies not only to events that are mutually exclusive but also to those that are NOT mutually exclusive:

$P(A \text{ or } B) = P(A) + P(B) - P(A \text{ and } B)$

For non-mutually exclusive events, you must subtract the probability of A and B occurring at the same time, because otherwise you will be counting the outcomes for this event twice.

Example: Jason picks 1 card at random from a deck of 52 playing cards. What is the probability that the card is either an ace or a club?

There are 4 aces in the deck, so the probability of picking an ace is $\frac{4}{52}$. There are 13 clubs in the deck, so the probability of picking a club is $\frac{13}{52}$. However, one of these 13 clubs is the ace of clubs. Similarly, one of the 4 aces is the ace of clubs. Thus, if you simply add $\frac{4}{52}$ and $\frac{13}{52}$, you will be counting the ace of clubs twice. These events are not mutually exclusive, so in order to get the correct result, you must subtract one time the probability of getting the ace of clubs—that is, the event that the picked card is both an ace and a club. The answer, then, is:

$$\frac{4}{52} + \frac{13}{52} - \frac{1}{52} = \frac{16}{52} = \frac{4}{13}$$

Complementary Events

The complement of "an event happening" is "that event not happening." For instance, if "rolling a 4 on a regular six-sided die" is the event, then its complement is "rolling anything but a 4." The probabilities of two complementary events sum to 1:

$$P(\text{event happens}) + P(\text{event doesn't happen}) = 1$$

Sometimes, when you need to find the probability that an event happens, it may be easier to calculate the probability that the event does not happen:

$$P(\text{event doesn't happen}) = 1 - P(\text{event happens})$$

Example: Marlee picks at random 3 pairs of socks, one after the other, out of her sock drawer. If the drawer contains 3 pairs of blue socks, 4 pairs of red socks, 3 pairs of black socks, and 6 pairs of white socks, what is the probability that Marlee picks at least 1 pair of red socks?

This looks a little complicated. Marlee's three picks may be "red-other-other," "other-red-other," "other-other-red," "red-red-other," and so on. Instead of trying to find all the combinations of picks that will lead to at least 1 red pair, calculate the probability that Marlee does not pick a red pair at all, and subtract that number from 1. There are 16 total pairs, 4 of which are red and 12 of which are not red. Thus:

$$P(\text{1 red or more}) = 1 - P(\text{no red})$$
$$= 1 - \frac{12}{16} \times \frac{11}{15} \times \frac{10}{14}$$
$$= 1 - \frac{11}{28}$$
$$= \frac{17}{28}$$

MEASURES OF CENTRAL TENDENCY: MEAN, MEDIAN, AND MODE

Statistics is the branch of mathematics that deals with the collection, organization, analysis, and interpretation of numerical data. In the remainder of this chapter, we will discuss measures of central tendency, including the mean (or average), median, and mode; measures of variation, including range, standard deviation, and variance; and some graphical representations of statistical data.

The *mean* of a set of numbers is the arithmetic average of all the numbers. This average is the sum of all the terms in the set divided by the number of terms in the set:

$$\text{Mean} = \frac{\text{Sum of terms}}{\text{Number of terms}}$$

For instance, if a certain baseball team scored 3, 4, 3, and 7 runs in 4 games, then the average number of runs the team it scored over these 4 games was $\frac{3+4+3+7}{4}$, or 4.25.

The average formula is useful not only for finding the average of a set of numbers, but also for finding individual terms if one of the terms is unknown but the average itself and the number of terms are known.

Example: If the average of the numbers 3, 7, 4, 1, and x is 4, what is x?

You know the mean (4) and the number of terms (5). Apply the average formula to find x:

$$4 = \frac{3+7+4+1+x}{5}$$
$$20 = 15 + x$$
$$x = 5$$

The *median* is the "middle" value of a set of numbers. It is determined in one of two ways, depending on whether the set contains an even or an odd number of terms. When the terms are arranged in increasing (or decreasing) order, the median is:

- The middle term if the set contains an odd number of terms;
- The arithmetic average of the two middle terms if the set contains an even number of terms.

The *mode* of a set of terms is the term that occurs most frequently in the set. A set may have more than one mode or no mode if none of the terms occurs more than once.

Example: The 10 students in a biology class received the following scores on a particular exam: 75, 79, 69, 83, 96, 75, 89, 83, 78, and 94. What are the median and the mode of the students' scores?

First, write the scores in increasing order: {69, 75, 75, 78, 79, 83, 83, 89, 94, 96}. Since the set has an even number of terms, the median is the average of the middle two terms, 79 and 83. Thus, the median score is 81. Next, two scores, 75 and 83, are repeated twice each. Thus, these two scores are the two modes of the set.

MEASURES OF VARIATION: RANGE, STANDARD DEVIATION, AND VARIANCE

The *range* of a set of numbers is the difference between the greatest and the smallest numbers in the set. In the above example, the students' biology scores varied from a low of 69 to a high of 96. Thus, the range of the set of scores was 96 − 69, or 27.

Standard deviation and *variance* are measures of dispersion in a frequency distribution: They tell you how spread out the data points are from the mean. The variance of a set of data points equals the square of the standard deviation. Both are computed via a somewhat complicated formula; however, for the PCAT, you need mainly to understand the concept of standard deviation and variance rather than to be able to compute them directly.

Consider the following two sets of five numbers: {18, 19, 20, 21, 22} and {10, 15, 20, 25, 30}. Both sets have a mean of 20, yet the two are very different. The elements in the second set are much more spread out from the mean than are those in the first set. Thus, the second set has a higher standard deviation than the first set.

Example: Which set has the higher standard deviation: {1, 3, 5, 7} or {82, 84, 86, 88}?

> The terms in the two sets are equally spread out. The mean of the first set is 4, and the elements in the set are, respectively, −3, −1, 1 and 3 away from the mean. The mean of the second set is 85, and the elements in the set are −3, −1, 1 and 3 away from the mean. Thus, while the two sets have different means, they have the same standard deviation. (They also have the same range, since in both sets the difference between the smallest and the greatest elements is 6.)

GRAPHICAL REPRESENTATIONS

Data are frequently displayed in graphs or tables, rather than as a series of numbers. Such displays can reveal patterns in the data quickly and clearly.

Box Plots

A *box plot* (or *box-and-whisker plot*, or *five-point summary*) is a graph of the distribution of certain data that clearly identifies the lowest and highest data point, the median, and the 25th and 75th percentiles. Box plots may be drawn vertically or horizontally, but in both cases, they tell the same story. The rectangular box stretches from the lower quartile (the 25th percentile) to the upper quartile (the 75th percentile), and thus contains the middle 50% of the data. This is called the *interquartile range*. Somewhere inside the box is another line that marks the median. To the right and left of the box (or above and below it, in the case of a vertical display) are two lines (or whiskers), which stretch out from the lower and upper quartiles to the smallest and greatest data point, respectively. The difference between the endpoints of the two whiskers equals the range of the data.

Example: Which of the following box plots represents data with the greatest variance?

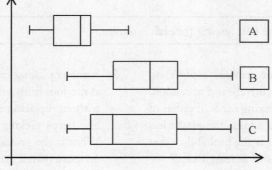

Box plot A has the smallest range (the difference between the right endpoint of the right whisker and the left endpoint of the left whisker), as well as the smallest interquartile range. Thus, it has the least variance of the three plots. Box plots B and C have the same range, but the interquartile range in plot C is greater than that in plot B. Thus, box plot C represents data with the greatest variance.

Frequency Tables

A *frequency table* is a table with two columns that shows how often each data point occurs in a data set. The left column lists the data points and the right column the frequency.

Example: On the twentieth reunion of a certain high school graduating class, the class secretary wrote down the number of children that each member of the class has and compiled the frequency table below. How many children do the class' members have on average, and what is the mode of the data set?

Number of Children	Frequency
0	2
1	6
2	8
3	5
4	2
5	1

The table shows that 2 members of the class have 0 children; 6 members have 1 child; and so on. Thus, the average number of children is:

$$Ave = \frac{0 \times 2 + 1 \times 6 + 2 \times 8 + 3 \times 5 + 4 \times 2 + 5 \times 1}{2 + 6 + 8 + 5 + 2 + 1}$$

$$= \frac{50}{24}$$

$$= 2.08\overline{3}$$

More members of the class have 2 children than any other number of children, so the mode is 2.

PRACTICE QUESTIONS

> **Directions:** Choose the best answer for each question.

1. A certain card game requires a player to select 2 cards consecutively and at random from a deck of 52 playing cards. If either of the selected cards is a king, the player has to set it aside. What is the probability that the player will set aside at least 1 card?

   A. $\dfrac{1}{221}$

   B. $\dfrac{33}{221}$

   C. $\dfrac{188}{221}$

   D. $\dfrac{220}{221}$

2. A high school class of 11 boys and 14 girls is electing a president and vice-president. The president is elected first. President and vice-president cannot be of the same gender. What is the probability that a girl will be vice-president?

   A. $\dfrac{11}{14}$

   B. $\dfrac{11}{25}$

   C. $\dfrac{14}{25}$

   D. $\dfrac{77}{300}$

3. Suma is picking cards, one card at a time, at random from a deck of 52 playing cards, without replacing each card that she picks. She keeps picking until she picks an ace. What is the probability that she will pick no more than 2 cards?

   A. $\dfrac{1}{221}$

   B. $\dfrac{16}{221}$

   C. $\dfrac{33}{221}$

   D. $\dfrac{188}{221}$

4. During its 22-game season, a university's basketball team won 13 games, averaging p points per win. If it averaged q points for the games it lost, which of the following equals the number of points the team scored on average per game during the season?

   A. $\dfrac{13p + 9q}{22}$

   B. $13p + 9q$

   C. $22(13p + 9q)$

   D. $\dfrac{13q + 9p}{22}$

5. The students in a college Linear Algebra class received the following grades on an exam: A, C, C, B, A, A, A, C, D, C, B, C, B, and F. What is the mode of these grades?

   A. A

   B. B

   C. C

   D. D

6. The frequency table below shows the number of goals scored in a set of soccer matches for a country's national league.

Number of Goals	Frequency
0	2
1	3
2	5
3	4
4	2
7	1

What was the median score?

A. 3.5

B. 3

C. 2.5

D. 2

7. A contestant participating in a talent show needs to receive an average score of at least 8.5 from the seven judges on the panel in order to advance to the next round. The first five judges have given him the following scores: 7, 9, 9, 8, 10. If each judge's score must be an integer, which of the following is the lowest combined score the contestant must receive from the last two judges in order to advance?

A. 14

B. 15

C. 16

D. 17

8. Last year a small consulting company paid each of its five managers $41,000, two statistical analysts $80,000 each, and the senior statistician $220,000. What number of employees earns no more than the mean salary?

A. 0

B. 4

C. 5

D. 6

9. Consider the output obtained when analyzing the percent nitrogen composition of soil collected in farms near a septic facility in 2017.

Number of Cases = 55

Mean = 23.01

Median = 24.26

Standard Deviation = 4.131

Minimum = 12.05

Maximum = 31.49

75th Percentile = 30.12

Which of these statements is correct?

A. The 25th percentile is approximately 18.4.

B. The IQR is 19.44.

C. About 10% of the data values are between 30.12 to 31.49.

D. Some outliers appear to be present.

10. To study the relationship between county and support for a certain amendment concerning school taxes, 200 registered voters were surveyed with the following results:

	For amendment	Against amendment	Neutral
County A	40	2	8
County B	62	35	3
County C	6	39	5

What percentage of those surveyed were against the amendment and were residents of County C?

A. 19.5%

B. 51.3%

C. 78%

D. 80.5%

11. The following statistics were collected on two groups of bison:

	Group I	Group II
sample size	45	30
sample mean	1,000 lbs.	800 lbs.
sample std. dev.	80 lbs.	70 lbs.

Which of the following statements is correct?

A. Group I is less variable than Group II because Group I's standard deviation is larger.

B. Group I is more variable than Group B because Group II's standard deviation is smaller.

C. Group I is relatively more variable than Group II since the sample mean is larger.

D. Group I is more variable than Group II since the sample size is larger.

12. The number of goal shots made (out of 30 shots attempted) by 13 hockey players is recorded as follows: 4, 7, 8, 9, 11, 11, 11, 17, 17, 20, 21, 21, 28.

An error was discovered when the coach started to conduct the analysis. Specifically, it was found that one of the 11s should have been a 21. Which measures of central tendency will change as a result?

A. Median only

B. Mean only

C. Mode only

D. Mean, median, and mode

13. According to the following box plot, what was the upper quartile of the number of chicken wings consumed during the chicken wing eating contest at a college-town university during Homecoming weekend?

Chicken Wings Consumed

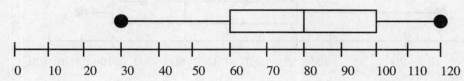

A. 40

B. 60

C. 100

D. 120

14. Suppose a single fair die is rolled. What is the probability that it lands on a 2, given that the number rolled is odd?

A. 0

B. $\frac{1}{6}$

C. $\frac{1}{2}$

D. 1

15. The following table provides data on two bus companies that have a terminal in a mid-sized rural town:

	Number of late arrivals this month	Number of on-time arrivals this month
Speed Z Us	11	43
A+ Bussers	6	27

If a bus trip is selected randomly, what is the probability that it will arrive late?

A. $\frac{17}{70}$

B. $\frac{6}{27}$

C. $\frac{11}{43}$

D. $\frac{17}{87}$

16. According to the following frequency histogram, what is the approximate mode heart rate (measured at rest) of athletes who work out at a local gym?

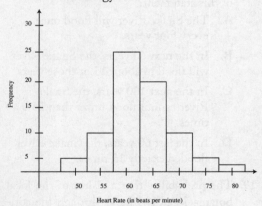

A. 50

B. 55

C. 60

D. 65

17. According to the following box plot, what is the interquartile range of squash weights recorded by judges at the Annual Tri-county Autumn Festival this year?

Squash Weights (in pounds)

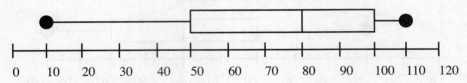

0   10   20   30   40   50   60   70   80   90   100   110   120

    A. 30

    B. 70

    C. 80

    D. 100

18. The probability that Snake River will flood in any given year has been estimated from 180 years of historical data to be 0.25. Which of the following is an accurate interpretation of this statement?

    A. The Snake River will flood once every four years.

    B. In the next 60 years, the Snake River will flood in about 15 of those years.

    C. In the next 100 years, the Snake River cannot flood fewer than 25 times.

    D. In the last 60 years, the Snake River flooded exactly 15 times.

19. The probability that a visitor of the local botanical gardens walks through the conservatory is 0.65, and the probability that a visitor meanders through the new meadow is 0.45. The probability that a visitor does both activities on the same day is 0.32. What is the probability that a visitor does at least one of the activities on a given day?

    A. 0

    B. 0.22

    C. 0.50

    D. 0.78

20. The weights (in ounces) of 10 randomly selected New York Strip steaks are listed below. What is the range of the data set?

12.2, 10.3, 14.6, 12.0, 13.4, 9.8, 16.4, 11.3, 8.9, 15.5

    A. 7.5

    B. 8.9

    C. 14.0

    D. 16.4

ANSWER KEY AND EXPLANATIONS

1. B	**5.** C	**9.** D	**13.** C	**17.** B
2. B	**6.** D	**10.** A	**14.** A	**18.** B
3. C	**7.** D	**11.** B	**15.** D	**19.** D
4. A	**8.** C	**12.** D	**16.** C	**20.** A

1. **The correct answer is B.** This probability is equal to 1 minus the probability that the player will not set aside either card—that is, the probability that the player will select no kings (K) at all:

$$P(\text{More than 1K}) = 1 - P(\text{No K})$$
$$= 1 - \frac{48}{52} \times \frac{47}{51}$$
$$= 1 - \frac{12}{13} \times \frac{47}{51}$$
$$= 1 - \frac{4}{13} \times \frac{47}{17}$$
$$= \frac{33}{221}$$

2. **The correct answer is B.** For a girl to be elected vice-president, a boy must have been elected president first. Thus, the probability of a girl being vice-president is equal to the probability of a boy being president:

$$\frac{11}{11+14} = \frac{11}{25}$$

3. **The correct answer is C.** Suma may pick an ace on her first try, in which case she stops picking, or she may pick a different card on her first try and an ace on her second try. Thus, the probability that she will pick no more than 2 cards equals the probability, $P(A1)$, of her picking an ace on the first try, plus the probability, $P(A2)$, of her picking an ace on the second try:

$$P(A1) + P(A2) = \frac{4}{52} + \frac{48}{52} \times \frac{4}{51}$$
$$= \frac{1}{13} + \frac{1}{13} \times \frac{48}{51}$$
$$= \frac{1}{13} + \frac{1}{13} \times \frac{16}{17}$$
$$= \frac{1}{13} + \frac{16}{13 \times 17}$$
$$= \frac{17 + 16}{13 \times 17}$$
$$= \frac{33}{221}$$

4. **The correct answer is A.** During the games it won, the team scored $13p$ points in total. The team lost $22 - 13$, that is, 9 games, scoring $9q$ points in total. Thus, over the 22 games, it averaged $\frac{13p + 9q}{22}$ points.

5. **The correct answer is C.** The mode of a set is the value that appears most frequently in the set. The students received 4 As, 3 Bs, 5 Cs, 1 D, and 1 F, so the mode of their grades is C.

6. **The correct answer is D.** Arrange the number of goals per match in increasing order:

0, 0, 1, 1, 1, 2, 2, 2, 2, 2, 3, 3, 3, 3, 4, 4, 7

There were 17 matches in total, so the median number of goals is the ninth term in the list: 2.

7. **The correct answer is D.** The five scores the contestant has received add up to 43. Let x be the combined score he receives from the last two judges. Then:

$$\frac{43 + x}{7} = 8.5$$
$$43 + x = 59.5$$
$$x = 16.5$$

That is, the contestant must receive at least 16.5 from the last two judges. Since the judges' scores must be integers, the contestant must receive 17 or better from the last two judges.

8. **The correct answer is C.** The mean of the 8 salaries listed is

$$\frac{5(41,000) + 2(80,000) + 220,000}{8} =$$

73,125 .

So, 5 employees earn no more than the mean salary.

9. **The correct answer is D.** An outlier is a data point that is more than two standard deviations from the mean. There appear to be such values beyond the 75th percentile.

10. **The correct answer is A.** The event of interest is "against amendment AND lives in County C." The number of respondents satisfying this criterion is in the lower left cell of the table. Hence, the percentage satisfying this criterion is $\frac{39}{200}$ = 19.5%.

11. **The correct answer is B.** The larger the standard deviation, the more variability.

12. **The correct answer is D.** The mean changes because the sum of all 13 values has now increased. The median, which it the data value in the 7th position from the left in the ascending data set, will become 17 after the change. The mode will now become 21 (whereas it *was* 11 before the change).

13. **The correct answer is C.** The upper quartile is the rightmost vertical bar in the box portion of the box plot. This value is 100.

14. **The correct answer is A.** This is a conditional probability.

$P(\text{roll a 2}) =$

$$\frac{P\left(\text{roll a 2 AND roll is odd}\right)}{P\left(\text{roll is odd}\right)} = \frac{0}{\frac{1}{2}} = 0$$

because 2 is even, not odd.

15. **The correct answer is D.** Divide the total number that have arrived late by the total number of bus trips used in the entire table. The former is the sum of the entries in the first column and the latter is the sum of all entries in the table. Doing so yields a probability of $\frac{17}{87}$.

16. **The correct answer is C.** The mode is the most commonly occurring data value. Here, the best approximation that can be made is to use the class corresponding to 60 beats per minute.

17. **The correct answer is B.** The interquartile range is the difference between the first quartile (30) and the third quartile (100), which is 100 − 30 = 70.

18. **The correct answer is B.** In the long run, this statement means that the Snake River floods about 25% of the time. Since 25% of 60 is 15, we expect it to flood about 15 times in the next 60 years.

19. The correct answer is D. Let A be the event "walks through the conservatory" and B the event "meanders through the new meadow." We must compute $P(A \cup B)$. To do so, use the addition formula, as follows:

$$P(A \cup B) = P(A) + P(B) - P(A \cap B)$$
$$= 0.65 + 0.45 - 0.32 = 0.78$$

20. The correct answer is A. The range is the difference between the largest and smallest data values, namely $16.4 - 8.9 = 7.5$.

SUMMING IT UP

- The probability P of event A happening is $P(A) = \dfrac{\text{Number of desired outcomes}}{\text{Number of possible outcomes}}$

- For independent events A and B, $P(A \text{ and } B) = P(A) \times P(B)$.

- If event B is dependent on event A, then $P(A \text{ and } B) = P(A) \times P(B \,|\, A)$, where $P(B|A)$ is the probability of event B happening given that event A has already happened.

- The probability that event A or event B (or both) happens is
$P(A \text{ or } B) = P(A) + P(B) - P(A \text{ and } B)$. If A and B are mutually exclusive, then
$P(A \text{ or } B) = P(A) + P(B)$.

- $P(\text{event doesn't happen}) = 1 - P(\text{event happens})$

- $\text{Mean} = \dfrac{\text{Sum of terms}}{\text{Number of terms}}$

- When the terms in a set are arranged in increasing (or decreasing) order, the median is the middle term if the set contains an odd number of terms or the arithmetic average of the two middle terms if the set contains an even number of terms.

- The mode of a set of terms is the term that occurs most frequently in the set. A set may have more than one mode or no mode, if none of the terms occurs more than once.

- The range of a set of numbers is the difference between the greatest and the smallest numbers in the set.

- Standard deviation and variance are measures of dispersion in a frequency distribution. They tell you how spread out the data points are from the mean.

- A box plot (or box-and-whisker plot, or five-point summary) is a graph of the distribution of certain data that clearly identifies the lowest and highest data point, the median, and the 25th and 75th percentiles. The difference between the endpoints of the two whiskers equals the range of the data. The rectangular box itself contains the middle 50% of the data.

Precalculus

OVERVIEW

- **Graphs**
- **Exponential and Logarithmic Equations**
- **Logarithmic and Exponential Functions**
- **Trigonometric Functions**
- **Vectors**
- **Complex Numbers**
- **Practice Questions**
- **Answer Key and Explanations**
- **Summing It Up**

According to the PCAT information booklet, 22 percent of the quantitative ability questions will assess your knowledge and understanding of precalculus. That amounts to 10 or 11 questions. Only calculus has the same number of questions, and no other math section has as many. In this chapter, we will review the main precalculus topics tested on the PCAT.

GRAPHS

The *graph* of a function is a visual way to represent the function as a set of points, often forming a line or curve, which represents the values of the function.

The Cartesian Coordinate System

The Cartesian coordinate system consists of two lines, called axes, which meet at a 90° angle. The horizontal axis is the x-axis, and the vertical one is the y-axis. The four different areas, called quadrants, into which the axes divide the coordinate system correspond to:

- **Quadrant I:** positive values of both x and y
- **Quadrant II:** negative values of x and positive values of y
- **Quadrant III:** negative values of both x and y
- **Quadrant IV:** positive values of x and negative values of y

You can plot points in this system, which are written as ordered pairs of an x-value and a y-value. For instance, the ordered pair (2,1) corresponds to the point with an x-value of 2

Chapter 14

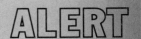

Two-dimensional graphs are drawn in the Cartesian, or rectangular, coordinate system. You will see these graphs on the PCAT.

and a *y*-value of 1—that is, a point whose *x*- and *y*-coordinates are 2 and 1, respectively. The two axes meet at the point (0,0), called the origin.

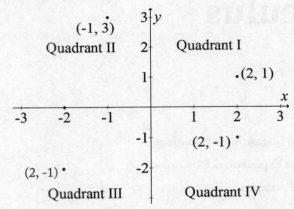

The graph of a function is the set of all points that satisfy the function. If point *P* lies on the graph of function $f(x)$, then, when $f(x)$ is evaluated for point *P*'s *x*-coordinate, the function's value equals point *P*'s *y*-coordinate. For instance, the graph of the function $f(x) = x$ is a line that includes all the points (x, y) such that $x = y$.

Common Graphs

The following are common graphs that you may find on the PCAT:

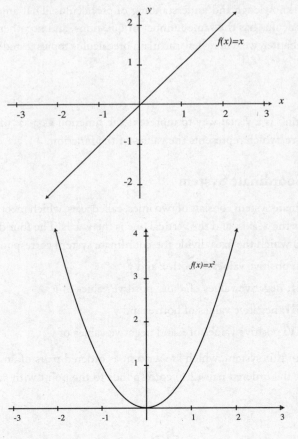

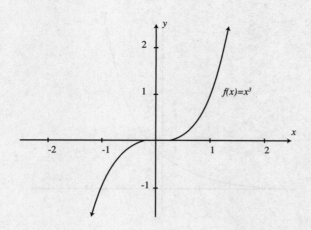

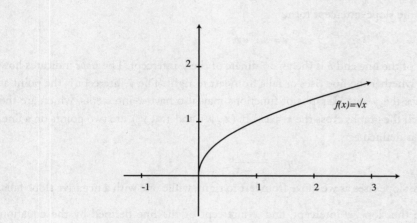

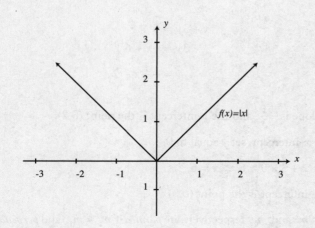

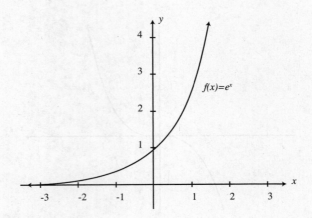

Slope and Intercept of Lines

The graph of a *linear equation* (that is, an equation in which each term is either a constant or the product of a constant and the first power of a single variable) is a line. One way to write a linear equation is by using the slope-intercept form:

$$y = mx + b$$

where m is the slope of the line and b is the y-coordinate of the y-intercept. The *slope* indicates how steep the line is and whether the line rises or falls from left to right. The y-intercept is the point at which the line crosses the y-axis. (Graphs of functions may also have x-intercepts, which are the points, if any, at which the graphs cross the x-axis.) If (x_1, y_1) and (x_2, y_2) are two points on a line, then the line's slope is defined as:

$$m = \frac{y_2 - y_1}{x_2 - x_1}$$

A line with a positive slope rises as we move from left to right, while one with a negative slope falls.

Example: What are the slope, y-intercept, and x-intercept of the line defined by the equation $x + 3y = 6$?

Write the equation in slope-intercept form:

$$x + 3y = 6$$
$$3y = -x + 6$$
$$y = -\frac{1}{3}x + 2$$

Thus, the slope is $-\frac{1}{3}$, and the y-intercept is the point $(0,2)$.

To find the x-intercept, set y equal to 0.

Solve for x: $x + 3 \times 0 = 6 \Rightarrow x = 6$.

Thus, the x-intercept is the point $(6,0)$.

Two lines with slopes m_1 and m_2, respectively, are *parallel* if $m_1 = m_2$, and *perpendicular* if $m_1 = -\frac{1}{m_2}$.

Example: What is the equation of the line that passes through the point (–1,2) and is perpendicular to the line defined by $2x + y = 1$?

Write the given equation in slope-intercept form:
$$2x + y = 1$$
$$y = -2x + 1$$

This line's slope is –2, so you're looking for the equation of a line whose slope is $\frac{1}{2}$. Since the slope equals $\frac{y_2 - y_1}{x_2 - x_1}$, let (x_1, y_1) be the point (–1,2), drop the subscripts for x_2 and y_2, and solve:

$$\frac{1}{2} = \frac{y - 2}{x + 1}$$
$$\frac{1}{2}x + \frac{1}{2} = y - 2$$
$$y = \frac{1}{2}x + \frac{5}{2}$$

EXPONENTIAL AND LOGARITHMIC EQUATIONS

What are logarithms? Think of this question: How many 2s do you need to multiply together in order to get 16? The answer is four: the product of four 2s equals 16. So, "the logarithm base 2 of 16" is 4.

In general, $\log_a b$ is the exponent to which a must be raised to get b.

Further, saying $x = \log_a b$ is equivalent to saying $a^x = b$.

Example: Evaluate the following logarithms: (a) $\log_3 27$; (b) $\log_{27} 3$; (c) $\log_{\frac{1}{3}} 3$.

Convert these to exponential form:

(a) $\log_3 27 = x$ (b) $\log_{27} 3 = x$ (c) $\log_{\frac{1}{3}} 3 = x$

$3^x = 27$ $27^x = 3$ $\left(\frac{1}{3}\right)^x = 3$

$3^x = 3^3$ $\left(3^3\right)^x = 3$ $\left(3^{-1}\right)^x = 3$

$x = 3$ $3^{3x} = 3^1$ $3^{-x} = 3^1$

   $3x = 1$ $-x = 1$

   $x = \frac{1}{3}$ $x = -1$

Two logarithms appear very frequently: the *common logarithm* (whose base is 10, and which is written as $\log_{10} x$ or simply $\log x$) and the *natural logarithm* (whose base is e, and which is written as $\ln x$).

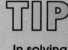

In solving some simple exponential and logarithmic equations, the following property to know comes in handy:

If $a^x = a^y$, then $x = y$.

You should commit the following rules of logarithms to memory:

$\log_a (xy) = \log_a x + \log_a y$

$\log_a \left(\frac{x}{y}\right) = \log_a x - \log_a y$

$\log_a x^r = r \log_a x$

The following results, derived directly from the definition of a logarithm, are also useful to remember:

$\log_a 1 = 0$, since $a^0 = 1$

$\log_a a = 1$, since $a^1 = a$

If $\log_a x = \log_a y$, then $x = y$

The number e, not a variable but an irrational number equal to 2.7182818..., plays an important role in many areas of mathematics.

Example: Simplify the following expressions: (a) $\log\left(10m^2n^3\right)$ (b) $\log_6\left(10\dfrac{m^2}{n^3p}\right)$; (c) $\ln\left(\dfrac{10}{x^e}\right)$.

(a) $\log\left(10m^2n^3\right) = \log 10 + \log m^2 + \log n^3$

$= 1 + 2\log m + 3\log n$

(b) $\log_6\left(10\dfrac{m^2}{n^3p}\right) = \log_6 10m^2 - \log_6 n^3p$

$= \log_6 10 + \log_6 m^2 - \left[\log_6 n^3 + \log_6 p\right]$

$= \log_6 10 + 2\log_6 m - 3\log_6 n - \log_6 p$

(c) $\ln\left(\dfrac{10}{x^e}\right) = \ln 10 - \ln x^e$

$= \ln 10 - e\ln x$

We review some basic techniques used for solving equations involving exponential and logarithmic terms.

The following property is helpful when solving many exponential equations:

If a, x, and y are real numbers, then $a^x = a^y$ if and only if $x = y$.

One strategy that often works for solving exponential equations is to express each side of the equation as a power of the same base. Then, use the above property to equate the exponents and solve the resulting equation.

Example: Solve the exponential equation: $2^{x-5} = 8$.

Using the fact that $8 = 2^3$, we see that

$2^{x-5} = 8$

$2^{x-5} = 2^3$

Applying the given property yields $x - 5 = 3$. So $x = 8$ is the solution.

Logarithms are useful when solving equations for which the above procedure is inapplicable.

Example: Solve the exponential equation: $2^{x-5} = 7$.

There is no base common to both sides of the equation. So, take log base 2 of both sides, and use the logarithm properties to simplify:

$2^{x-5} = 7$

$\log_2 2^{x-5} = \log_2 7$

$x - 5 = \log_2 7$

$x = 5 + \log_2 7$

When solving equations involving logarithms, the logarithm rules are very useful.

Example: Solve this logarithmic equation: $\log x + \log(x - 15) = 2$

Rewrite the left-hand-side as a single logarithm. Then, convert this to an equivalent exponential equation and solve for x.

$$\log x + \log(x - 15) = 2$$
$$\log\left[x(x - 15)\right] = 2$$
$$x(x - 15) = 10^2$$
$$x^2 - 15x - 100 = 0$$
$$(x - 20)(x + 5) = 0$$
$$x = -5,\ 20$$

But, $x = -5$ cannot be a solution because -5 is not in the domain of $\log x$. Thus, $x = 20$ is the only solution. (see page 8).

LOGARITHMIC AND EXPONENTIAL FUNCTIONS

Exponential functions are functions in which the base is fixed, and the exponent is the variable quantity, such as $f(x) = 3^x$ and $g(x) = \left(\dfrac{3}{2}\right)^{-x}$. The general shape of the graphs of exponential functions come in two related varieties which depend on the value of the base. Precisely, the graph of $F(x) = b^x$ is as follows:

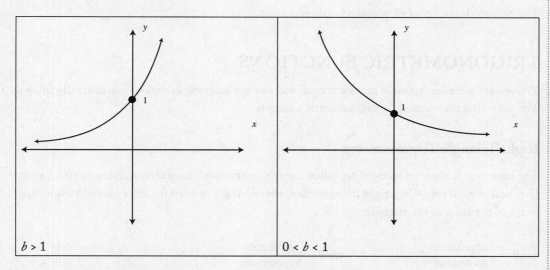

The following are characteristics of the graphs of exponential functions.

If $b > 1$, the graph of $y = b^x$ gets closer to the x-axis as the x-values move to the left, and then grows very rapidly as the x-values move to the right.

If $0 < b < 1$, the graph of $y = b^x$ gets closer to the x-axis as the x-values move to the right, and grows very rapidly as the x-values move to the left.

If $b > 0$, then $b^x > 0$, for any value of x. Consequently, the equation $b^x = 0$ has no solutions.

Logarithmic Functions

Next, we examine the graphs of logarithmic functions. The general shape of $f(x) = \log_b x$, where $b > 1$, is as follows:

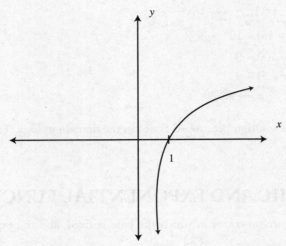

As the x-values decrease toward zero, the graph continues downward toward negative infinity.

As the x-values move to the right, the graph increases, albeit very slowly.

The domain is the set of all positive x-values.

TRIGONOMETRIC FUNCTIONS

Trigonometry means "triangle measurement" and has applications in various scientific disciplines. The following are some main trigonometric concepts.

Right Triangle Trigonometry

The basic trigonometric functions are called *sine (sin), cosine (cos), tangent (tan), cotangent (cot), secant (sec),* and *cosecant (csc)*. On a right triangle, these functions are defined for any non-right angle, θ, in terms of the sides of the triangle:

$$\sin\theta = \frac{\text{opposite}}{\text{hypotenuse}} \qquad\qquad \cos\theta = \frac{\text{adjacent}}{\text{hypotenuse}}$$

$$\tan\theta = \frac{\text{opposite}}{\text{adjacent}} = \frac{\sin\theta}{\cos\theta} \qquad\qquad \cot\theta = \frac{\text{adjacent}}{\text{opposite}} = \frac{\cos\theta}{\sin\theta} = \frac{1}{\tan\theta}$$

$$\sec\theta = \frac{\text{hypotenuse}}{\text{adjacent}} = \frac{1}{\cos\theta} \qquad\qquad \csc\theta = \frac{\text{hypotenuse}}{\text{opposite}} = \frac{1}{\sin\theta}$$

So, for example, for the triangle ABC, below, $\cos\theta = \dfrac{BC}{AC}$, $\sin\theta = \dfrac{AB}{AC}$, and so on.

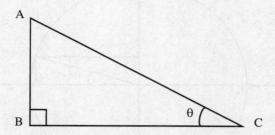

The table below gives the values of the sine and cosine of some common angles. These are tested frequently, so you should learn them by heart. You may see angles measured in either degrees or *radians*. The latter is a very common unit of angle measurement, so you should have experience working with it.

Measure of angle θ (degrees)	0°	30°	45°	60°	90°
Measure of angle θ (radians)	0	$\dfrac{\pi}{6}$	$\dfrac{\pi}{4}$	$\dfrac{\pi}{3}$	$\dfrac{\pi}{2}$
sinθ	0	$\dfrac{1}{2}$	$\dfrac{\sqrt{2}}{2}$	$\dfrac{\sqrt{3}}{2}$	1
cosθ	1	$\dfrac{\sqrt{3}}{2}$	$\dfrac{\sqrt{2}}{2}$	$\dfrac{1}{2}$	0

The Unit Circle

Note the symmetry of the sine and cosine values in the above table: As the angle measure increases from 0° to 90°, the value of the sine function increases from 0 to 1, while the value of the cosine function decreases from 1 to 0. This is even more evident if you envision these angles drawn on the unit circle (a circle with radius of 1 unit, drawn on the Cartesian coordinates). Any line segment between the origin and some point, *P*, on the circle forms an angle, θ, whose cosine and sine are the *x*- and *y*-coordinates of *P*, respectively. You can see that cosθ decreases as the angle increases from 0° to 90°, while sinθ increases. When the angle is 45°, that is, when the line segment is part of the line *y* = *x*, then the angle's sine and cosine are equal (and measure $\dfrac{\sqrt{2}}{2}$).

A complete revolution equals an angle of measure 360°, or 2π. Any pair of angles that differ by some multiple of 2π have the same trigonometric functions. For example, the angles with measure $\dfrac{\pi}{3}$, $\dfrac{\pi}{3} + 2\pi$, and $\dfrac{\pi}{3} - 4\pi$ have the same sine, cosine, and so on.

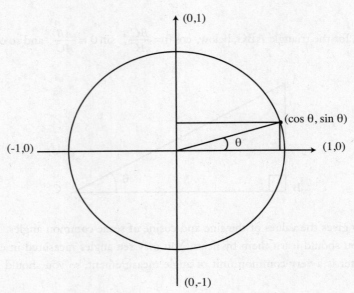

Example: What is the value of $\cos\left(\dfrac{3\pi}{4}\right)$?

This angle is not among the common values that you should commit to memory, but you can use to your advantage the unit circle and this angle's symmetry with the angle of measure $\dfrac{\pi}{4}$. The lines that form these two angles intersect the unit circle at points that are symmetrical about the y-axis. That is, these points have the same y-coordinate (so the angles have the same sine) and opposite x-coordinates (so the angles have opposite cosines). The cosine of an angle of measure $\dfrac{\pi}{4}$ is $\dfrac{\sqrt{2}}{2}$, so the cosine of an angle of measure $\dfrac{3\pi}{4}$ is $-\dfrac{\sqrt{2}}{2}$.

This example illustrates why it is so important to know the sine and cosine values of the common angles between 0 and $\dfrac{\pi}{2}$ radians (that is, angles in the first quadrant of the unit circle):

- You can find the values of all other trigonometric functions if you know the sine and cosine.
- You can find the values of these functions for any angles that do not lie in the first quadrant, but which are symmetric to any of the angles in the first quadrant.

Graphs of Trigonometric Functions

Trigonometric functions are periodic—in other words, their values repeat in regular intervals. The graphs of the main trigonometric functions are:

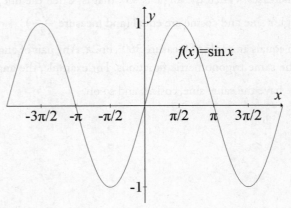

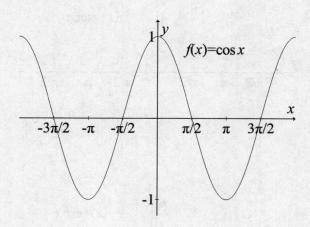

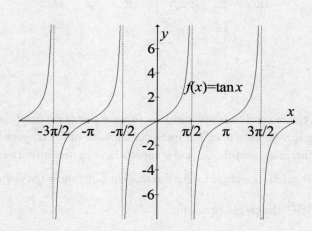

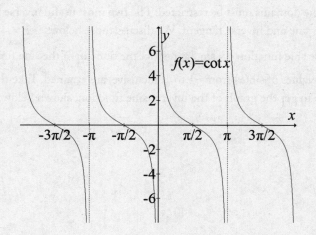

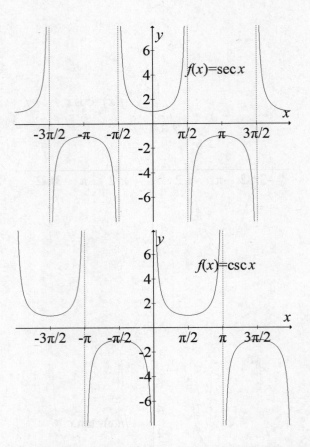

Note that for the tan, cot, sec, and csc, the vertical lines are not part of the graph, but rather asymptotes drawn to make the graph easier to read. For instance, the value of the tangent function approaches infinity as the angle increases towards $\frac{\pi}{2}$, and it approaches negative infinity as the angle decreases towards $\frac{\pi}{2}$. However, when the angle is $\frac{\pi}{2}$, the tangent function is not defined (remember that $\tan x = \frac{\sin x}{\cos x}$, and at $\frac{\pi}{2}$ the cosine equals 0).

Inverse Trigonometric Functions

Trigonometric functions are periodic and so, their graphs are not one-to-one. So, to define an inverse function for them, the domains must be restricted. The two most useful inverse trigonometric functions are the inverse sine and inverse tangent. We discuss those below.

To define the inverse sine function $y = \sin^{-1}x$, restrict the domain of the sine function to $\left[-\frac{\pi}{2}, \frac{\pi}{2} \right]$. On this interval, all values of $\sin(x)$ from −1 to 1, inclusive, are attained. Take this graph and reflect it over the $y = x$ line to get the graph of the inverse sine function, shown below:

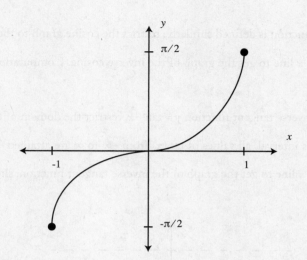

Using the definition of an inverse function, the following is true:

$$y = \sin^{-1} x \quad \text{means} \quad x = \sin y \quad \text{and} \quad -\frac{\pi}{2} \le y \le \frac{\pi}{2}$$

That is, y is an angle whose sine is x and y is in quadrant I or IV.

Example: Compute the following:

i.) $\sin^{-1}\left(\dfrac{1}{2}\right)$

ii.) $\sin^{-1}\left(-\dfrac{\sqrt{3}}{2}\right)$

iii.) $\sin^{-1}\left(\sin\left(\dfrac{3\pi}{4}\right)\right)$

The thought process used to compute these is always the same.

i.) $\sin^{-1}\left(\dfrac{1}{2}\right) = y$ means $\sin(y) = \dfrac{1}{2}$. So, we must find a y-value in the interval $\left[-\dfrac{\pi}{2}, \dfrac{\pi}{2}\right]$ whose sine is $\dfrac{1}{2}$. Using the unit circle, this value is $\dfrac{\pi}{6}$.

ii.) $\sin^{-1}\left(-\dfrac{\sqrt{3}}{2}\right) = y$ means $\sin y = -\dfrac{\sqrt{3}}{2}$. So, we must find a y-value in the interval $\left[-\dfrac{\pi}{2}, \dfrac{\pi}{2}\right]$ whose sine is $-\dfrac{\sqrt{3}}{2}$. Using the unit circle, this value is $-\dfrac{\pi}{3}$.

iii.) This one is tricky! It is tempting to use the property that $f^{-1}(f(x)) = x$ here, but you must keep in mind that it only applies for x values in the restricted domain of $f(x)$, which here is $\left[-\dfrac{\pi}{2}, \dfrac{\pi}{2}\right]$. Since $\dfrac{3\pi}{4}$ does not belong to this interval, you cannot use this property. Rather, start by computing $\sin\left(\dfrac{3\pi}{4}\right)$; this value is $\dfrac{\sqrt{2}}{2}$. Now, compute $\sin^{-1}\left(\dfrac{\sqrt{2}}{2}\right)$. Call this value y. This means we must find y in $\left[-\dfrac{\pi}{2}, \dfrac{\pi}{2}\right]$ such that $\sin y = \dfrac{\sqrt{2}}{2}$. This value is $\dfrac{\pi}{4}$.

The inverse cosine function is defined similarly: restrict the cosine graph to the interval $[0, \pi]$ and reflect it over the $y = x$ line to get the graph of the inverse cosine. Computations are performed in the same manner.

Next, to define the inverse tangent function $y = \tan^{-1}x$, restrict the domain of the tangent function to $\left(-\dfrac{\pi}{2}, \dfrac{\pi}{2}\right)$. On this interval, all values of $\tan(x)$ from $-\infty$ to ∞ are attained. Take this graph and reflect it over the $y = x$ line to get the graph of the inverse tangent function, shown below:

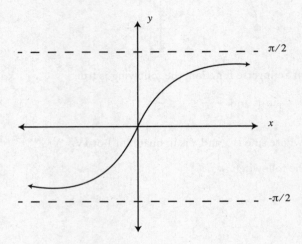

Using the definition of an inverse function, it follows that $y = \tan^{-1}x$ means $x = \tan y$ and $-\dfrac{\pi}{2} < y < \dfrac{\pi}{2}$.

That is, y is an angle whose tangent is x and y is in quadrant I or IV.

Example: Compute $\tan^{-1}(-1)$.

$\tan^{-1}(-1) = y$ means $\tan(y) = -1$. So, we must find a y-value in the interval $\left(-\dfrac{\pi}{2}, \dfrac{\pi}{2}\right)$ whose tangent is -1. Remember, $\tan y = \dfrac{\sin y}{\cos y}$. For this quotient to be equal to -1, the numerator and denominator must be opposites of each other. Using the unit circle, this occurs only when $y = -\dfrac{\pi}{4}$.

The inverse cotangent, inverse secant, and inverse cosecant can all be defined in a similar manner, but are rarely used, primarily because for most situations, one can model a scenario to make use of the inverse sine or inverse tangent. So, being comfortable with these two functions is sufficient.

VECTORS

A *vector* is a quantity that has both magnitude and direction. Examples of such quantities are the velocity or acceleration of a moving object, or the force exerted by an object. A vector is represented by an arrow whose direction indicates the vector's direction, and whose length indicates the vector's magnitude.

There are several ways to notate this vector, such as $\vec{AB}$, $\overline{AB}$, or **a**.

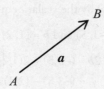

Two vectors are equal to each other if they have the same magnitude and direction. Two vectors are negatives of each other if they have the same magnitude, but opposite directions.

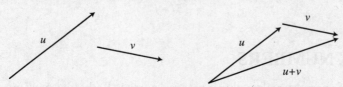

$$\vec{AB} = -\vec{PQ}$$
$$\vec{AB} = \vec{CD}$$

Vectors can be manipulated in a variety of ways, including the following six methods:

1. In order to add vectors graphically, connect them head-to-tail.

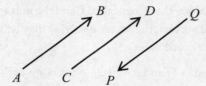

2. In order to subtract vector *v* from vector *u* graphically, first reverse the direction of *v*, and then add this new vector head-to-tail with vector *u* (add the negative of *v*):

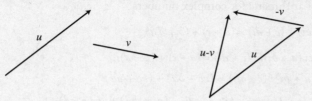

3. Vectors may also be broken down into horizontal and vertical components:

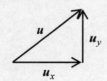

The above vector may be expressed as the ordered pair (x, y), where x is the magnitude of the vector's horizontal component and y is the magnitude of its vertical component.

4. In order to add vectors expressed using components algebraically, add the first components together and the second components together:

If $a = (x, y)$ and $b = (u, v)$, then $a + b = (x + u, y + v)$.

5. In order to multiply a vector by a *scalar*—that is, a quantity with magnitude only and no direction—multiply each component of the vector by the scalar:

The product of vector $a = (x, y)$ by the scalar c equals (cx, cy).

Example: Given vectors $a = (-3, 5)$ and $b = (1, 2)$, what is $a - 2b$?

$$a - 2b = (-3,5) - 2(1,2)$$
$$= (-3,5) - (2,4)$$
$$= (-3 - 2, 5 - 4)$$
$$= (-5,1)$$

6. Consider vectors plotted in the rectangular coordinate system, with the unit vector (that is, the vector of magnitude 1) along the x-axis called i, and the unit vector along the y-axis called j. In terms of these unit vectors, the vector $a = (x, y)$ may be written as $a = xi + yj$, with x and y being the vector's coordinates.

Example: Given vectors $a = -3i + 5j$ and $b = i + 2j$, what is $a - 2b$?

$$a - 2b = (-3i + 5j) - 2(i + 2j)$$
$$= (-3i + 5j) - (2i + 4j)$$
$$= -3i + 5j - 2i - 4j$$
$$= -5i + j$$

COMPLEX NUMBERS

The square root of a negative real number is *not* a real number. Rather, it is *imaginary*, meaning that it involves i, where $i^2 = -1$. Using this fact, we can write, for instance, $\sqrt{-49} = \sqrt{-1} \cdot \sqrt{49} = i \cdot 7 = 7i$.

A *complex number* is a number of the form $a + bi$, where a and b are both real numbers. The following are the basic rules of arithmetic for complex numbers:

Sum: $(a + bi) + (c + di) = (a + c) + (b + d)i$

Difference: $(a + bi) - (c + di) = (a - c) + (b - d)i$

Product: $(a + bi) \cdot (c + di) = (ac - bd) + (bc + ad)i$

Quotient: $\dfrac{a + bi}{c + di} = \dfrac{a + bi}{c + di} \cdot \dfrac{c - di}{c - di} = \dfrac{(ac + bd) + (bc - ad)i}{c^2 + d^2}$

Example: Compute the following:

i.) $(2 - 3i) + (-5i) - (-1 - 3i)$

ii.) $(2 + 3i)(2 - 5i)$

iii.) $\dfrac{2i}{1 - 2i}$

i.) Simplification of such an arithmetic expression is like simplifying a polynomial expression. Distribute any constants and then add like terms. Doing so here yields

$$(2 - 3i) + (-5i) - (-1 - 3i) = 2 - 3i - 5i + 1 + 3i$$
$$= (2 + 1) + (-3i - 5i + 3i)$$
$$= 3 - 5i$$

ii.) Multiplying complex numbers is done by FOILing the two expressions:

$$(2 + 3i)(2 - 5i) = 2(2) + 2(-5i) + (3i)(2) + (3i)(-5i)$$
$$= 4 - 10i + 6i - 15i^2$$
$$= 4 - 10i + 6i + 15$$
$$= 19 - 4i$$

iii.) To divide two complex numbers, multiply the numerator and denominator by the so-called *conjugate* of the denominator—that is, the complex number obtained by simply switching the sign of the imaginary part. Here, the complex conjugate of the denominator is $1 + 2i$. Doing so yields

$$\frac{2i}{1 - 2i} = \frac{2i}{1 - 2i} \cdot \frac{1 + 2i}{1 + 2i}$$
$$= \frac{2i + 4i^2}{1 - 4i^2}$$
$$= \frac{2i - 4}{1 + 4}$$
$$= \frac{-4 + 2i}{5}$$
$$= -\frac{4}{5} + \frac{2}{5}i$$

PRACTICE QUESTIONS

Directions: Choose the best answer for each question.

1. If $f(z) = \dfrac{z-1}{2}$ and $g(z) = z^2 + 3$, what is $(f - g)(2)$?

   A. $-\dfrac{13}{2}$

   B. -2

   C. $\dfrac{1}{2}$

   D. $\dfrac{13}{2}$

2. Let $f(x) = 1 - 2x$ and $g(x) = 3 - x^2$. Compute $(f \cdot g)(-2)$.

   A. -5

   B. -3

   C. 3

   D. 35

3. What is the domain of the function $f(x) = \dfrac{x(x-1)}{\sqrt{x+2}}$?

   A. All real numbers except -2

   B. All real numbers except -2, 0, and 1

   C. $(-2, \infty)$

   D. $[-2, \infty)$

4. If $f(x) = e^{x+1} - 2$ and $g(x) = 2x - 1$, what is $(f \circ g)(x)$?

   A. $2e^{x+1} - 5$

   B. $e^{x+1}(2x-1) - 4x + 2$

   C. $e^{2x+1} - 3$

   D. $e^{2x} - 2$

5. Let $f(x) = \dfrac{2}{x+1}$ and $g(x) = 3x$. What is the domain of $(f \circ g)$?

   A. $(-\infty, -1) \cup (-1, \infty)$

   B. $\left(-\infty, -\dfrac{1}{3}\right) \cup \left(-\dfrac{1}{3}, \infty\right)$

   C. $(-\infty, -1) \cup \left(-1, -\dfrac{1}{3}\right) \cup \left(-\dfrac{1}{3}, \infty\right)$

   D. $(-\infty, -1) \cup (-1, 0) \cup (0, \infty)$

6. Given $f(x) = 2x + 3$, what is $f^{-1}(x)$?

   A. $\dfrac{1}{2x+3}$

   B. $\dfrac{x-3}{2}$

   C. $\dfrac{x}{2x+3}$

   D. $3x + 2$

7. Evaluate $\log\left(\sqrt{1,000}\right)$.

   A. 1

   B. $\dfrac{2}{3}$

   C. $\dfrac{3}{2}$

   D. 3

8. If $\log_4(x^2) = 6$, what is $\log_4\left(\dfrac{x}{2}\right)$?

   A. 6

   B. $\dfrac{5}{2}$

   C. $\dfrac{\sqrt{6}}{2}$

   D. $\dfrac{3}{2}$

9. Which of the following is equivalent to $\frac{1}{2} \ln 64 - \ln 4$?

  A. $\ln 2$

  B. $\ln 4$

  C. $\ln 8$

  D. $\frac{1}{2} \ln 60$

10. Solve for x: $36^{2-x} = \left(\frac{1}{6}\right)^{-4x}$.

  A. $-\frac{2}{3}$

  B. $\frac{2}{3}$

  C. $-\frac{2}{5}$

  D. $\frac{2}{5}$

11. Solve for x: $3^{x^2} = 6$.

  A. $\left\{\log_3 6\right\}$

  B. $\left\{\log_3 \sqrt{6}\right\}$

  C. $\left\{-\log_3 \sqrt{6}, \log_3 \sqrt{6}\right\}$

  D. $\left\{\sqrt{\log_3 6}, -\sqrt{\log_3 6}\right\}$

12. Solve for x: $\ln x + \ln(x + 1) = \ln 12$.

  A. $\{3\}$

  B. $\{11\}$

  C. $\{11, 12\}$

  D. $\{-4, 3\}$

13. Which of the following lines is parallel to $3x + 2y = 6$?

  A. $y + \frac{3}{2}x = 8$

  B. $y = \frac{2}{3}x + 3$

  C. $y = -3x + 6$

  D. $2x + 3y = 6$

14. Which of the following is the graph of $y = 3^{x+2} - 3$?

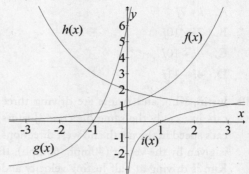

  A. $f(x)$

  B. $g(x)$

  C. $h(x)$

  D. $i(x)$

15. For what values of x, if any, in the interval $[0, 2\pi]$ does $\sin x = -\frac{1}{2}$?

  A. $\frac{5\pi}{6}, \frac{7\pi}{6}$

  B. $\frac{2\pi}{3}, \frac{4\pi}{3}$

  C. $\frac{7\pi}{6}, \frac{11\pi}{6}$

  D. There are no such values.

16. Compute: $\sec\left(\frac{5\pi}{6}\right)$.

  A. $-\frac{2\sqrt{3}}{3}$

  B. -2

  C. $\sqrt{2}$

  D. $-\sqrt{2}$

17. Compute: $\tan^{-1}\left(-\frac{\sqrt{3}}{3}\right)$.

  A. $-\frac{\pi}{3}$

  B. $-\frac{\pi}{6}$

  C. $\frac{5\pi}{6}$

  D. $\frac{2\pi}{3}$

18. If $a = (-2, 3)$ and $b = 3i + 4j$, what is $2a + b$?

    A. $i + 7j$

    B. $7i + 10j$

    C. $-i + 10j$

    D. $4i + 11j$

19. Justin, Kim, and Annie are driving three cars in exactly the same direction. Justin's car's speed in the north and west directions is given by the vector (40mph, 60mph). If Kim is driving at half Justin's velocity and Annie is driving at 1.5 times Kim's velocity, which vector represents Annie's velocity?

    A. (10,15)

    B. (20,30)

    C. (30,45)

    D. (60,90)

20. Compute: $(3 - 4i)(2 - 3i)$.

    A. $18 - 17i$

    B. -11

    C. $-6 - 17i$

    D. 17

ANSWER KEY AND EXPLANATIONS

1. A	**5.** B	**9.** A	**13.** A	**17.** B
2. A	**6.** B	**10.** B	**14.** B	**18.** C
3. C	**7.** C	**11.** D	**15.** C	**19.** C
4. D	**8.** B	**12.** A	**16.** A	**20.** C

1. **The correct answer is A.** To find $(f-g)(2)$, evaluate $f(2) - g(2)$:

$$f(2) = \frac{2-1}{2} = \frac{1}{2}$$
$$g(2) = 2^2 + 3 = 7$$
$$(f-g)(2) = \frac{1}{2} - 7 = \frac{1-14}{2}$$
$$= -\frac{13}{2}$$

2. **The correct answer is A.** Substitute $x = -2$ into $f(x) = 1 - 2x$ and $g(x) = 3 - x^2$ to see that $f(-2) = 1 - 2(-2) = 1 + 4 = 5$ and $g(-2) = 3 - (-2)^2 = 3 - 4 = -1$. Thus, $(f \cdot g)(-2) = f(-2) \cdot g(-2) = 5 \cdot (-1) = -5$

3. **The correct answer is C.** There are two restrictions of note when determining the domain of the function $f(x) = \frac{x(x-1)}{\sqrt{x+2}}$. One, the denominator cannot be zero. And two, the radicand of the radical in the denominator cannot be negative. Taking both conditions simultaneously, we infer that any member x of the domain must satisfy the inequality $x + 2 > 0$, or equivalently $x > -2$. So, the domain is $(-2, \infty)$.

4. **The correct answer is D.** Substitute $2x - 1$ for x into $f(x)$ and solve:

$$(f \circ g)(x) = e^{(2x-1)+1} - 2 = e^{2x} - 2$$

5. **The correct answer is B.** Given that $f(x) = \frac{2}{x+1}$ and $g(x) = 3x$, the composition equals $(f \circ g) = f(g(x)) = f(3x) = \frac{2}{3x+1}$. Any member x of the domain must satisfy two criteria. First, the value $3x$ must be well-defined and not imaginary. Since x is a real number, $3x$ must also be a real number. So, there is no restriction on x at this point; it could be any real number. Next, once the expression $3x$ is substituted in for x the formula for $f(x)$, the result is $\frac{2}{3x+1}$. For this to be well-defined, the denominator cannot be zero. Specifically, $3x + 1$ cannot be zero, so x cannot be $-\frac{1}{3}$. This is the only restriction on x. Hence, the domain is $\left(-\infty, -\frac{1}{3}\right) \cup \left(-\frac{1}{3}, \infty\right)$.

6. **The correct answer is B.** To find $f^{-1}(x)$, switch y and x in $f(x)$ and solve for y:

$$x = 2y + 3 \Rightarrow 2y = x - 3 \Rightarrow y = \frac{x-3}{2}$$

Verify that $(f \circ f^{-1})(x) = x$ in order to be sure that these two functions are inverses of each other:

$$\left(f \circ f^{-1}\right)(x) = 2\left(\frac{x-3}{2}\right) + 3 = x - 3 + 3 = x$$

7. **The correct answer is C.**

$$\log\left(\sqrt{1,000}\right) = \log\left(\sqrt{10^3}\right) = \log\left(10^{\frac{3}{2}}\right) = \frac{3}{2}.$$

8. **The correct answer is B.** Find x:

$$\log_4\left(x^2\right) = 6$$
$$2\log_4 x = 6$$
$$\log_4 x = 3$$
$$x = 4^3$$
$$x = 64$$

Now, evaluate $\log_4\left(\dfrac{x}{2}\right)$:

$$\log_4\left(\dfrac{x}{2}\right) = \log_4 x - \log_4 2$$
$$= \log_4 64 - \log_4 2$$
$$= 3 - \dfrac{1}{2}$$
$$= \dfrac{5}{2}$$

9. **The correct answer is A.** Use the properties of logarithms to simplify the expression:

$$\dfrac{1}{2}\ln 64 - \ln 4 = \ln\left(64^{\frac{1}{2}}\right) - \ln 4$$
$$= \ln 8 - \ln 4$$
$$= \ln\dfrac{8}{4}$$
$$= \ln 2$$

10. **The correct answer is B.** Express both sides as powers of 6 and then equate the exponents and solve for x:

$$36^{2-x} = \left(\dfrac{1}{6}\right)^{-4x}$$
$$6^{2(2-x)} = 6^{-1(-4x)}$$
$$2(2-x) = 4x$$
$$4 - 2x = 4x$$
$$4 = 6x$$
$$\dfrac{2}{3} = x$$

11. **The correct answer is D.** Take the log base 3 of both sides, apply the logarithm property for powers and solve for x:

$$3^{x^2} = 6$$
$$\log_3 3^{x^2} = \log_3 6$$
$$x^2 = \log_3 6$$
$$x = \pm\sqrt{\log_3 6}$$

12. **The correct answer is A.** Express the left side as the natural logarithm of a single quantity using the property governing the sum of logs. Then, take the exponential of both sides and solve for x:

$$\ln x + \ln(x+1) = \ln 12$$
$$\ln(x(x+1)) = \ln 12$$
$$x(x+1) = 12$$
$$x^2 + x = 12$$
$$x^2 + x - 12 = 0$$
$$(x+4)(x-3) = 0$$
$$x = \cancel{-4}, 3$$

Note that -4 is not a solution of the original equation because you cannot take the log of a negative number. So, the only solution is $x = 3$.

13. **The correct answer is A.** Two parallel lines have the same slope. Write $3x + 2y = 6$ in slope-intercept form in order to find its slope:

$$3x + 2y = 6$$
$$2y = -3x + 6$$
$$y = -\dfrac{3}{2}x + 3$$

So, its slope is $-\dfrac{3}{2}$. The only equation in the answer choices with the same slope is choice A.

14. **The correct answer is B.** Check the function's intercepts. When $x = 0$:

$$y = 3^{0+2} - 3$$
$$= 3^2 - 3$$
$$= 6$$

Therefore, the y-intercept is (0,6).

Next, when $y = 0$:

$$0 = 3^{x+2} - 3$$
$$3^1 = 3^{x+2}$$
$$1 = x + 2$$
$$x = -1$$

Therefore, the x-intercept is (–1,0). These two points are a match only with the points at which the graph of $g(x)$ intercepts the two axes, so $g(x)$ is the correct answer.

15. **The correct answer is C.** To solve $\sin x = -\frac{1}{2}$, use the unit circle. The sine is negative in quadrants III and IV, and you want multiples of the angle x in the first quadrant whose sine equals $\frac{1}{2}$. That value is $\frac{\pi}{6}$. Using the symmetry of the circle, conclude that the values of x are $\frac{7\pi}{6}$ and $\frac{11\pi}{6}$.

16. **The correct answer is A.** Use the definition of the secant function with the unit circle, as follows:

$$\sec\left(\frac{5\pi}{6}\right) = \frac{1}{\cos\left(\frac{5\pi}{6}\right)} = \frac{1}{-\frac{\sqrt{3}}{2}} =$$

$$-\frac{2}{\sqrt{3}} = -\frac{2}{\sqrt{3}} \cdot \frac{\sqrt{3}}{\sqrt{3}} = -\frac{2\sqrt{3}}{3}$$

17. **The correct answer is B.** $\tan^{-1}\left(-\frac{\sqrt{3}}{3}\right) = y$

means $\tan y = -\frac{\sqrt{3}}{3}$. Now, observe that

$$-\frac{\sqrt{3}}{3} = -\frac{1}{\sqrt{3}} = -\frac{\frac{1}{2}}{\frac{\sqrt{3}}{2}}.$$

The reason for doing this is to help us identify a standard angle. Using the facts that $\tan y = \frac{\sin y}{\cos y}$ and $\cos(y)$ are positive values of y in $\left(-\frac{\pi}{2}, \frac{\pi}{2}\right)$, answering this question reduces to identifying the value of y for which $\sin y = -\frac{1}{2}$ and $\cos y = \frac{\sqrt{3}}{2}$. This value is $-\frac{\pi}{6}$.

18. **The correct answer is C.** Convert the two vectors to the same notation and calculate:

$$2a + b = 2(-2i + 3j) + (3i + 4j)$$
$$= (-4i + 6j) + (3i + 4j)$$
$$= -4i + 6j + 3i + 4j$$
$$= -i + 10j$$

19. **The correct answer is C.** If Kim is driving at half Justin's velocity, then:

$$\vec{K} = \frac{1}{2}\vec{J}$$
$$\vec{K} = \frac{1}{2}(40, 60)$$
$$\vec{K} = (20, 30)$$

Similarly, if Annie is driving at 1.5 times Kim's velocity, then:

$$\vec{A} = 1.5\vec{K}$$
$$\vec{A} = 1.5(20, 30)$$
$$\vec{A} = (30, 45)$$

20. **The correct answer is C.** FOIL as follows:

$(3 - 4i)(2 - 3i) = 6 - 8i - 9i + 12i^2 = 6 - 17i$
$- 12 = -6 - 17i$

SUMMING IT UP

- If (x_1, y_1) and (x_2, y_2) are two points on a line, then the line's slope is defined as $m = \dfrac{y_2 - y_1}{x_2 - x_1}$. A line with positive slope rises as we move from left to right, while one with negative slope falls.

- Two lines with slopes m_1 and m_2 are *parallel* if $m_1 = m_2$, and *perpendicular* if $m_1 = -\dfrac{1}{m_2}$.

- $\tan \theta = \dfrac{\sin \theta}{\cos \theta}$

- $\cot \theta = \dfrac{\cos \theta}{\sin \theta} = \dfrac{1}{\tan \theta}$

- $\sec \theta = \dfrac{1}{\cos \theta}$

- $\csc \theta = \dfrac{1}{\sin \theta}$

- In order to add vectors graphically, connect them head-to-tail.

- If $a = (x, y)$ and $b = (u, v)$, then $a + b = (x + u, y + v)$.

- The product of vector $a = (x, y)$ by the scalar c equals (cx, cy).

- The vector $a = (x, y)$ may be written as $a = x\boldsymbol{i} + y\boldsymbol{j}$, with x, y being the vector's coordinates and $\boldsymbol{i}, \boldsymbol{j}$ the unit vectors.

- If a, x, and y are real numbers, then $a^x = a^y$ if and only if $x = y$.

- If $b > 1$, the graph of $y = b^x$ gets closer to the x-axis as the x-values move to the left, and grows very rapidly as the x-values move to the right.

- If $0 < b < 1$, the graph of $y = b^x$ gets closer to the x-axis as the x-values move to the right, and grows very rapidly as the x-values move to the left.

- If $b > 0$, then $b^x > 0$, for any value of x. Consequently, the equation $b^x = 0$ has no solutions.

- As the x-values decrease toward zero, the graph of $f(x) = \log_b x$, where $b > 1$, continues downward toward negative infinity.

- As the x-values move to the right, the graph of $f(x) = \log_b x$, where $b > 1$, increases, albeit very slowly.

- The domain of $f(x) = \log_b x$, where $b > 1$, is the set of all positive x-values.

- $y = \sin^{-1} x$ means $x = \sin y$ and $-\dfrac{\pi}{2} \le y \le \dfrac{\pi}{2}$. That is, y is an angle whose sine is x and y is in quadrant I or IV.

- $y = \tan^{-1} x$ means $x = \tan y$ and $-\dfrac{\pi}{2} < y < \dfrac{\pi}{2}$. That is, y is an angle whose tangent is x and y is in quadrant I or IV.

- A *complex number* is a number of the form $a + bi$, where a and b are both real numbers, and $i^2 = -1$.

- Sum: $(a + bi) + (c + di) = (a + c) + (b + d)i$

- Difference: $(a + bi) - (c + di) = (a - c) + (b - d)i$

- Product: $(a + bi) \cdot (c + di) = (ac - bd) + (bc + ad)i$

- Quotient: $\dfrac{a + bi}{c + di} = \dfrac{a + bi}{c + di} \cdot \dfrac{c - di}{c - di} = \dfrac{(ac + bd) + (bc - ad)i}{c^2 + d^2}$

Calculus

Remember that calculus questions represent 22 percent of the quantitative ability questions, which translates into 10 or 11 questions. The questions will test your understanding of basic calculus concepts and applications. A nonscientific standard calculator will be available by clicking on the icon in the upper left corner of each item during the Biological Processes, Chemical Processes, and Quantitative Reasoning subtests. Test-takers are also given erasable boards to work out problems.

LIMITS

We often need to know how a function behaves near a certain value of x. With simple functions, such as lines, this is easy enough to do: Plug the value of x into the equation and get a value for the function itself. With more complex functions, however, plugging in will not work. In those cases, you must take the limit of the function at that value of x in order to discern the function's behavior. The limit of $f(x)$ as x approaches a equals L if, as x gets increasingly closer to a, from either side, then $f(x)$ gets increasingly closer to L. This is written as:

$$\lim_{x \to a}(x) = L$$

Note that the function doesn't need to actually be defined as $x = a$ for the limit of the function at that point to exist. However, for certain functions (called *continuous* at $x = a$), $\lim_{x \to a} f(x) = f(a)$.

Example: Evaluate $\lim_{x \to 2}\left(x^2 - 3\right)$

Substitute $x = 2$ into the function and evaluate:

$$\lim_{x \to 2}\left(x^2 - 3\right) = 2^2 - 3 = 1$$

The previous example was easy to evaluate because the function is continuous at $x = a$. Not all functions are continuous however, so direct substitution won't always work.

Example: Evaluate $\lim\limits_{x \to 2} \left(\dfrac{x^2 - 4}{x - 2} \right)$.

This function is not defined at $x = 2$, because at that point, the denominator becomes zero. However, you can still find the function's limit as x approaches 2. To do so, factor the numerator, and then cancel the common factor from numerator and denominator:

$$\lim\limits_{x \to 2} \left(\frac{x^2 - 4}{x - 2} \right) = \lim\limits_{x \to 2} \left(\frac{(x + 2)(x - 2)}{x - 2} \right)$$
$$= \lim\limits_{x \to 2} (x + 2)$$

You could not have eliminated the denominator if you were trying to simplify the function. However, for the purposes of taking the limit, eliminating the denominator is all right to do because $g(x) = x + 2$ is the same as $f(x) = \dfrac{x^2 - 4}{x - 2}$ at all points except at $x = 2$; all you're interested in is how $f(x)$ behaves close to 2 on both sides. You can now substitute $x = 2$ into the limit and evaluate:

$$\lim\limits_{x \to 2} (x + 2) = 2 + 2 = 4$$

You can see that this is the case by evaluating $f(x) = \dfrac{x^2 - 4}{x - 2}$ for values of x increasingly close to 2, from both sides:

x	$f(x)$	x	$f(x)$
1.9	3.9	2.1	4.1
1.95	3.95	2.05	4.05
1.99	3.99	2.01	4.01

Limits at Infinity

Sometimes, you must find $\lim\limits_{x \to \infty} f(x)$. To evaluate such limits, you will often need to use the fact that $\lim\limits_{x \to \infty} \dfrac{c}{x^n} = 0$ for any real number c and positive rational number n. (This makes sense: As the denominator gets increasingly larger while the numerator stays constant, the fraction approaches zero.)

Example: Evaluate $\lim\limits_{x \to \infty} \left(\dfrac{x + 3}{2x - 1} \right)$

Direct substitution leads to $\dfrac{\infty}{\infty}$, which is indeterminate. Also, you cannot factor this in any of the usual ways. The trick here, odd though it may seem, is to change the numerator and the denominator so they include fractions with x in the denominator.

Specifically, multiply both numerator and denominator by $\dfrac{1}{x}$. (This is chosen such that the "x" is the largest degree term in the denominator of the given fraction.)

$$\lim\limits_{x \to \infty} \left(\frac{x + 3}{2x - 1} \right) = \lim\limits_{x \to \infty} \left(\frac{x \left(1 + \dfrac{3}{x} \right)}{x \left(2 - \dfrac{1}{x} \right)} \right)$$
$$= \lim\limits_{x \to \infty} \left(\frac{1 + \dfrac{3}{x}}{2 - \dfrac{1}{x}} \right)$$

As x gets larger, both $\frac{3}{x}$ and $\frac{1}{x}$ become negligibly small, while 1 and 2 stay as they are. As such:

$$\lim_{x \to \infty}\left(\frac{1 + \frac{3}{x}}{2 - \frac{1}{x}}\right) = \frac{1 + 0}{2 - 0} = \frac{1}{2}$$

In general, the following two rules can be used to compute limits of polynomials and rational functions:

1. If p is a polynomial of degree n, then the limit of p as the variable approaches ∞ (or $-\infty$) equals the limit of the term with the nth power of the variable:

$$\lim_{x \to \infty}\left(a_n x^n + a_{n-1} x^{n-1} + ... + a_0 x^0\right) = \lim_{x \to \infty} a_n x^n, \text{ where } a_n \neq 0$$

2. The limit of a quotient of two polynomials as the variable approaches ∞ (or $-\infty$) equals the limit of the quotient of the highest degree terms in each polynomial:

$$\lim_{x \to \infty}\left(\frac{a_n x^n + a_{n-1} x^{n-1} + ... + a_0 x^0}{b_m x^m + b_{m-1} x^{m-1} + ... + b_0 x^0}\right) = \lim_{x \to \infty}\left(\frac{a_n x^n}{b_m x^m}\right), \text{ where } a_n, b_m \neq 0$$

Using these facts, the limit in the above example becomes

$$\lim_{x \to \infty}\left(\frac{x + 3}{2x - 1}\right) = \lim_{x \to \infty}\left(\frac{x}{2x}\right) = \lim_{x \to \infty}\left(\frac{1}{2}\right) = \frac{1}{2}.$$

One-Sided Limits

Consider the graph of the function $f(x) = \frac{1}{x}$:

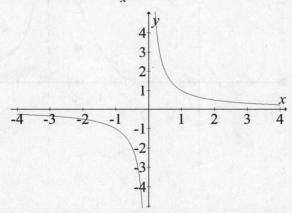

What is this function's limit as x approaches 0? Well, as x approaches 0 "from the right," the function approaches infinity, while as x approaches 0 "from the left," the function approaches negative infinity. The definition of the limit of a function requires the function to be approaching the same value from both sides, so the limit of $f(x) = \frac{1}{x}$ does not exist as x approaches 0. However, the function does have one-sided limits even as x approaches 0.

The *right-hand limit*, $\lim_{x \to a^+} f(x)$, of function $f(x)$ is the function's limit as x approaches a, with $x > a$.

The function's *left-hand limit*, $\lim_{x \to a^-} f(x)$, is its limit as x approaches a, with $x < a$.

NOTE

Not all math problems will require long drawn-out math calculations. Some will require clear thinking using a variety of math concepts.

Example: Evaluate $\lim_{x \to 0^-} \left(\frac{1}{x^2} \right)$.

Think through this problem. As x approaches 0 from the side of the negative numbers, x^2 also approaches 0—but as an ever-decreasing positive number, since squaring the variable turns it positive. So, $\frac{1}{x^2}$ is always positive, and the denominator approaches 0, while the numerator is constant. Thus, the left-hand limit that you're looking for is ∞: $\lim_{x \to 0^-} \left(\frac{1}{x^2} \right) = \infty$ (Incidentally, in this case, the right-hand limit at 0 is also ∞, so the limit of this function as x approaches 0 exists and is itself, ∞.)

The notions of a limit of a function at an x-value and continuity at an x-value can be interpreted graphically.

For a function to have a limit at $x = a$, there can be no jumps, vertical asymptotes, or wild oscillations at that value. Open holes do not prevent a limit from existing, though.

Continuity is more restrictive than the mere existence of a limit. Specifically, a function f is continuous at $x = a$ if it has a limit at $x = a$ (so that the above restrictions apply) AND this limit must equal the functional value $f(a)$. This effectively implies that there is no open hole in the graph at $x = a$.

Example: Consider the following graph:

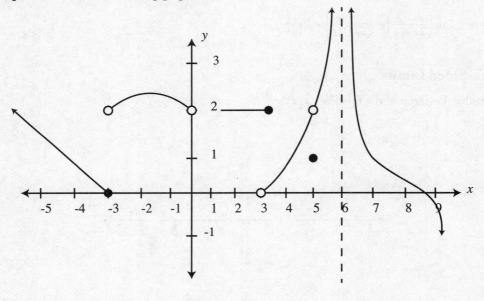

$g(x)$ does not have a limit at -3 or at 3 because there is a jump in the graph. As such, g cannot be continuous at these values.

$g(x)$ *does* have a limit at $x = 0$, and this value is 2, despite the open hole in the graph. However, the function is not continuous at 0 since the limit value does not equal the functional value, which is non-existent.

$g(x)$ has a limit at $x = 5$, which is 2, but it is not continuous here because of the open hole. Specifically, $g(5) = 1$ does not equal the limiting value of 2.

$g(x)$ does not have a limit at $x = 6$ because of the vertical asymptote here.

DIFFERENTIATION

Calculus is the study of how one quantity changes with relation to another. It has two main branches: differential calculus and (2) integral calculus. *Differentiation*, the process of finding the derivative of a function, is the main concern of differential calculus.

First Derivative

The notation for the first derivative of a function $f(x)$ with respect to x tells how the function changes with respect to x. Written as $f'(x)$ ("f prime of x"), the first derivative is defined as:

$$f'(x) = \lim_{h \to 0} \frac{f(x + h) - f(x)}{h}$$

The first derivative may be written in other ways, too, such as y', $\frac{dy}{dx}$, or $\frac{df(x)}{dx}$.

The slope of a line expresses this type of concept: Given a linear function, its slope relates how y (the value of the function) changes as x changes ($m = \frac{y_2 - y_1}{x_2 - x_1}$). This is handy for lines, but for nonlinear functions, it is insufficient. The first derivative needs to be used instead.

The formula in the definition of the derivative can be tedious to work with, but luckily there are five rules that simplify the differentiation process:

1. If $f(x) = c$, where c is a constant, then $f'(x) = 0$. (Think of the slope of a line with equation $f(x) = c$.)

2. If $f(x) = x^n$, where n is any number, then $f'(x) = nx^{n-1}$. This is known as the *Power Rule*.

3. Given two functions $f(x)$ and $g(x)$, then $(f(x) \pm g(x))' = f'(x) \pm g'(x)$.

4. Given a function $f(x)$ and a constant c, then $(cf(x))' = cf'(x)$.

5. If two functions $f(x)$ and $g(x)$ are differentiable—that is, if their derivatives exist—then $(fg)' = f'g + fg'$ *(Product Rule)* and $\left(\frac{f}{g}\right)' = \frac{f'g - fg'}{g^2}$ *(Quotient Rule)*.

Example: If $f(x) = 4x^3 + \frac{3}{x^6}$, what is $f'(x)$?

In order to use the power rule on the second term, the numerator must be brought to x:

$$f(x) = 4x^3 + \frac{3}{x^6}$$

$$f(x) = 4x^3 + 3x^{-6}$$

Find the derivative of each term (as if each term of $f(x)$ were a function itself, and $f(x)$ were the sum of two functions), and add the two:

$$f'(x) = 3 \times 4x^2 + 3(-6)\,x^{-7}$$
$$= 12x^2 - 18\,x^{-7}$$

Example: What is the derivative of $f(x) = \dfrac{\sqrt{x} - 1}{x^2 + 1}$?

Treat the two quantities in the numerator and denominator as individual functions and use the quotient rule:

$$f'(x) = \frac{\left[\frac{d}{dx}\left(\sqrt{x} - 1\right)\right]\left(x^2 + 1\right) - \left(\sqrt{x} - 1\right)\left[\frac{d}{dx}\left(x^2 + 1\right)\right]}{\left(x^2 + 1\right)^2}$$

$$= \frac{\left(\frac{1}{2}x^{-\frac{1}{2}}\right)\left(x^2 + 1\right) - \left(x^{\frac{1}{2}} - 1\right)2x}{\left(x^2 + 1\right)^2}$$

$$= \frac{\frac{1}{2}x^{\frac{3}{2}} + \frac{1}{2}x^{-\frac{1}{2}} - 2x^{\frac{3}{2}} + 2x}{\left(x^2 + 1\right)^2}$$

$$= \frac{-\frac{3}{2}x^{\frac{3}{2}} + 2x + \frac{1}{2}x^{-\frac{1}{2}}}{\left(x^2 + 1\right)^2}$$

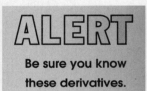

Be sure you know these derivatives.

Derivatives of Trigonometric, Inverse Trigonometric, Exponential, and Logarithmic Functions

You may find a question that asks you to differentiate trigonometric, inverse trigonometric, exponential, and logarithmic functions. The proofs of these derivatives are interesting but lengthy, and beyond the scope of this review. For the purposes of review, here are the derivatives:

$\dfrac{d}{d\theta}\left(\sin\theta\right) = \cos\theta$	$\dfrac{d}{d\theta}\left(\cos\theta\right) = -\sin\theta$
$\dfrac{d}{d\theta}\left(\tan\theta\right) = \sec^2\theta$	$\dfrac{d}{d\theta}\left(\cot\theta\right) = -\csc^2\theta$
$\dfrac{d}{d\theta}\left(\sec\theta\right) = \sec\theta\tan\theta$	$\dfrac{d}{d\theta}\left(\csc\theta\right) = -\csc\theta\cot\theta$
$\dfrac{d}{dx}\left(e^x\right) = e^x$	$\dfrac{d}{dx}\left(\ln x\right) = \dfrac{1}{x}$
$\dfrac{d}{dx}\left(a^x\right) = a^x\ln a$	$\dfrac{d}{dx}\left(\log_a x\right) = \dfrac{1}{x\ln a}$
$\dfrac{d}{dx}\sin^{-1}x = \dfrac{1}{\sqrt{1 - x^2}}$	$\dfrac{d}{dx}\cos^{-1}x = \dfrac{-1}{\sqrt{1 - x^2}}$
$\dfrac{d}{dx}\tan^{-1}x = \dfrac{1}{1 + x^2}$	

The Chain Rule and Implicit Differentiation

Functions such as $f(x) = (3x - 1)^5$ or $f(x) = \sin(x^2 + x)$, are compositions of functions. The *chain rule* is used to differentiate such functions, as follows:

If $f(x)$ and $g(x)$ are differentiable functions and $F(x) = (f \circ g)(x)$, then $F'(x) = f'(g(x))g'(x)$.

Alternatively, if $y = f(u)$ and $u = g(x)$, then $\dfrac{dy}{dx} = \dfrac{dy}{du}\dfrac{du}{dx}$.

Example: If $f(x) = \sin(x^2 + x)$, what is $f'(x)$?

Let $u = x^2 + x$, and apply the chain rule:

$$\frac{d}{dx}\left[\sin\left(x^2 + x\right)\right] = \frac{d}{du}\left(\sin u\right)\frac{d}{dx}\left(u\right)$$
$$= \left(\cos u\right)\frac{d}{dx}\left(x^2 + x\right)$$
$$= \left(\cos u\right)\left(2x + 1\right)$$
$$= \left(2x + 1\right)\cos\left(x^2 + x\right)$$

This rule applies for more complicated functions formed by composing more than two functions.

Example: Compute the derivative using the chain rule: $\dfrac{d}{dx}\sin^{-1}\left(\sqrt[3]{e^x - 1}\right)$

Decompose the function as follows: Let $y = \sin^{-1}(u)$, $u = \sqrt[3]{v}$, $v = w - 1$, $w = e^x$

Then, $\sin^{-1}\left(\sqrt[3]{e^x - 1}\right) = y(u(v(w(x))))$. So, the chain rule is $\dfrac{dy}{dx} = \dfrac{dy}{du} \cdot \dfrac{du}{dv} \cdot \dfrac{dv}{dw} \cdot \dfrac{dw}{dx}$. Here,

$$\frac{dy}{du} = \frac{1}{\sqrt{1 - u^2}} = \frac{1}{\sqrt{1 - \left(\sqrt[3]{e^x - 1}\right)^2}}$$

$$\frac{du}{dv} = \frac{1}{3}v^{-\frac{2}{3}} = \frac{1}{3}\left(e^x - 1\right)^{-\frac{2}{3}}$$

$$\frac{dv}{dw} = 1$$

$$\frac{dw}{dx} = e^x$$

So, $\dfrac{dy}{dx} = \dfrac{1}{\sqrt{1 - \left(\sqrt[3]{e^x - 1}\right)^2}} \cdot \dfrac{1}{3}\left(e^x - 1\right)^{-\frac{2}{3}} \cdot e^x$

Sometimes, you are presented with functions, such as $y^3 - xy^2 + xy = 3 - x^3$, which are not explicit expressions of one variable in terms of another (e.g., $y = f(x)$). In such cases, use *implicit differentiation* in order to find y'—a process during which both sides of an equation as given are differentiated with respect to x, and then solved for y':

Example: If $x^2 + y^2 = 4$, what is $\dfrac{dy}{dx}$?

This is the equation of a circle with radius 2. In differentiating each term with respect to x, remember that because you're differentiating in terms of x, y must be treated as a function of x. Thus, when it comes to the y^2-term, use the chain rule:

$$x^2 + y^2 = 4$$

$$\frac{d}{dx}\left(x^2 + y^2\right) = \frac{d}{dx}(4)$$

$$2x + 2y\frac{dy}{dx} = 0$$

$$2y\frac{dy}{dx} = -2x$$

$$\frac{dy}{dx} = \frac{-x}{y}$$

Derivative at a Point

Questions may ask you to find the derivative of a function at a particular point. To do this, find the general formula for the derivative, and then evaluate it for a particular value of x.

There are two common types of questions requiring you to find the derivative at a point: questions asking for the rate of change of a function (such as a function describing an object's velocity) at a given point in time, and questions asking for the slope of a line that is a tangent to the graph of a particular function at a given point—the slope of such a tangent being equal to the function's derivative at that point.

Example: What is the slope of the line tangent to $f(x) = x^3 - 2x$ at $x = 3$?

Find the derivative: $f'(x) = 3x^2 - 2$.

Evaluate $f'(3)$: $f'(3) = 3 \times 3^2 - 2 = 25$.

The derivative of $f(x)$, and thus the slope of the tangent to $f(x)$, at $x = 3$ is 25.

Higher-Order Derivatives

The derivative of a function is also a function, so it can be differentiated. The derivative of a function's derivative is called the original function's *second derivative* and is notated as $f''(x)$ or $\dfrac{d^2y}{dx^2}$. For that matter, a function may also have a *third derivative, fourth derivative*, and so on. All the differentiation rules and techniques discussed so far apply in finding higher derivatives, as well.

Example: If $f(x) = \ln(x^2 + 3)$. Compute $f'''(-1)$.

To compute a third derivative, differentiate $f(x)$ to get $f'(x)$. Then, differentiate $f'(x)$ to get $f''(x)$, and finally differentiate $f''(x)$ to get $f'''(x)$. Once you have the formula, *then* you substitute $x = -1$, but not before!

$$f(x) = \ln(x^2 + 3)$$

$$f'(x) = \frac{1}{x^2 + 3} \cdot 2x = \frac{2x}{x^2 + 3}$$

$$f''(x) = \frac{(x^2 + 3)(2) - (2x)(2x)}{(x^2 + 3)^2} = \frac{-2x^2 + 6}{(x^2 + 3)^2}$$

$$f'''(x) = \frac{(x^2 + 3)^2 (-4x) - (-2x^2 + 6) \cdot 2(x^2 + 3)(2x)}{(x^2 + 3)^4}$$

$$= \frac{-4x(x^2 + 3)\big((x^2 + 3) + (-2x^2 + 6)\big)}{(x^2 + 3)^4}$$

$$= \frac{-4x(x^2 + 3)(-x^2 + 9)}{(x^2 + 3)^4}$$

$$= \frac{-4x(-x^2 + 9)}{(x^2 + 3)^3}$$

Thus, $f'''(-1) = \dfrac{-4(-1)\big(-(-1)^2 + 9\big)}{\big((-1)^2 + 3\big)^3} = \dfrac{4(8)}{4^3} = \dfrac{32}{64} = \dfrac{1}{2}.$

Mean Value Theorem for Derivatives: If f is a function that is continuous on $[a,b]$ and differentiable on (a,b), then there is at least one value c in (a,b) for which $f'(c) = \dfrac{f(b) - f(a)}{b - a}$.

Geometrically, this means that there is at least one point on the curve over the interval (a,b) at which the tangent line is parallel to the secant line passing through the points $(a, f(a))$ and $(b, f(b))$, as shown below:

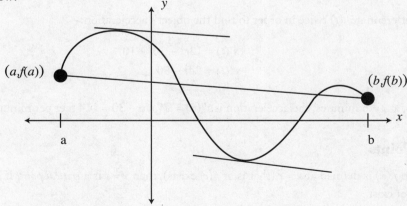

Example: Consider the function $f(x) = x^2 - x^3$ on the interval $(0,2)$. Find a value of c in the interval $(0,2)$ that illustrates the Mean Value Theorem.

The Mean Value Theorem applies in this case because the function $f(x)$ is a polynomial and so, is continuous and differentiable for all real numbers, in particular on the given interval. Observe that $f'(x) = 2x - 3x^2$. To verify the conclusion of the Mean Value Theorem, we must determine a real number c in $(0,2)$ for which $f'(c) = \dfrac{f(2) - f(0)}{2 - 0}$.

Since $f'(c) = 2c - 3c^2$, $f(0) = 0$, and $f(2) = 2^2 - 2^3 = 4 - 8 = -4$, this equation becomes $2c - 3c^2 = \dfrac{-4 - 0}{2 - 0} = -2$, or equivalently $3c^2 - 2c - 2 = 0$. Using the quadratic formula yields the following two solutions:

$$c = \frac{2 \pm \sqrt{4 - 4(3)(-2)}}{2(3)} = \frac{2 \pm \sqrt{28}}{6} \approx 1.22, -0.55$$

So, the c-value in $(0,2)$ that illustrates the conclusion of the Mean Value Theorem is approximately 1.22.

APPLICATIONS OF THE DERIVATIVE

Differentiation has various applications. This section looks at what derivatives tell about rates of change, as well as about the graphs of functions. We will also cover contextual problems involving related rates.

Rates of Change

For any function $f(x)$, $f'(a)$ represents the function's instantaneous rate of change at $x = a$. One example of a rate of change problem that you may encounter on the PCAT concerns an object's motion: If $s(t)$ is the function giving the position of an object with respect to time, then the object's velocity, $v(t)$, equals $s'(t)$ (velocity is the derivative of position), while the object's acceleration, $a(t)$, equals $v'(t)$ (acceleration is the derivative of velocity).

Example: Suppose the position of an object (measured in feet) with respect to time (measured in minutes) is given by the equation $s(t) = 4t^3 - 15t^2 + 10t + 5$. What is the object's acceleration when $t = 6$?

Differentiate $s(t)$ twice in order to find the object's acceleration:

$$s'(t) = 12t^2 - 30t + 10$$
$$s''(t) = 24t - 30$$

So, at $t = 6$ minutes, the acceleration is $s''(6) = 24 \times 6 - 30 = 114$ feet per minute.

Critical Points

If a function $f(x)$ is defined at $x = c$ (that is, if $f(c)$ exists), then $x = c$ is a *critical point* if $f'(c) = 0$ or $f'(c)$ does not exist.

Example: What are the critical points of the function $f(x) = x^3 - 3x^2 + 3x + 1$?

Find the first derivative: $f'(x) = 3x^2 - 6x + 3$.

Set $f'(x)$ equal to zero and solve for x:

TIP

Remember to use the computer clock to keep track of time and work at a steady pace.

$$3x^2 - 6x + 3 = 0$$
$$x^2 - 2x + 1 = 0$$
$$(x - 1)^2 = 0$$

So, at $x = 1$, $f(x)$ has a critical point.

Relative Extrema, Concavity, and Inflection Points

A function's first derivative at any given point equals the slope of a line tangent to the graph of the function at that point.

- A line with positive slope increases from left to right (as x increases).
- A line with negative slope decreases from left to right.
- A line with zero slope is horizontal.

Knowing this, for any function, you can use the sign of the first derivative in order to determine whether the function is increasing, decreasing, or constant. Given an interval in the domain of a function $f(x)$, then:

- If $f'(x) > 0$ for all x in the interval, then $f(x)$ is *increasing* over the interval.
- If $f'(x) < 0$ for all x in the interval, then $f(x)$ is *decreasing* over the interval.
- If $f'(x) = 0$ for all x in the interval, then $f(x)$ is *constant* over the interval.

Local *extrema* are extreme values (maximum or minimum) of a function within a given interval. A function $f(x)$ has a *local maximum* at $x = c$, if $f(x) \leq f(c)$ for all x in some interval (a,b) such that $a < c < b$. $f(x)$ has a *local minimum* at $x = c$, if $f(x) \geq f(c)$ for all x in some interval (a,b) such that $a < c < b$. To the left of a local maximum, $f(x)$ is increasing, while to its right, $f(x)$ is decreasing. Conversely, to the left of a local minimum, $f(x)$ is decreasing, while to its right, $f(x)$ is increasing.

You can use the *First Derivative Test* in order to find local extrema. If $x = c$ is a critical point of $f(x)$, then:

- If $f'(x) > 0$ to the left of $x = c$ and $f'(x) < 0$ to the right of $x = c$, then $f(x)$ has a *relative maximum*.
- If $f'(x) < 0$ to the left of $x = c$ and $f'(x) > 0$ to the right of $x = c$, then $f(x)$ has a *relative minimum*.
- If $f'(x)$ has the same sign on both sides of $x = c$, then $f(x)$ does not have a relative extremum.

In addition to local extrema, another important feature of graphs is concavity. A function is *concave up* on a given interval if it is shaped like a bowl over that interval; it is *concave down* if a function is shaped like a dome. Note that a function may be increasing or decreasing over an interval, regardless of whether it is concave up or down. Further, a point on the graph of a function is an *inflection point* if the function is continuous at that point and the concavity of the graph changes at that point.

The figure below illustrates the concepts of local extrema, concavity, inflection points, and increasing/decreasing functions. The dotted vertical lines are not part of the graph of the function; they're only drawn to highlight the points at which the direction or concavity of the function changes.

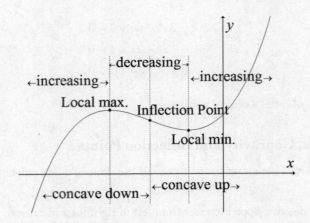

Just as the first derivative helps determine whether a function is increasing or decreasing, the second derivative helps determine the function's concavity. Given an interval in the domain of a function $f(x)$, then:

- If $f''(x) > 0$ for all x in the interval, then $f(x)$ is *concave up* over the interval.
- If $f''(x) < 0$ for all x in the interval, then $f(x)$ is *concave down* over the interval.

The *Second Derivative Test* is another way of finding local extrema. If $x = c$ is a critical point of $f(x)$, with $f''(c) = 0$, and $f''(c)$ is continuous near c, then:

- If $f''(c) < 0$, then $f(x)$ has a *relative maximum* at $x = c$. This makes intuitive sense, since the function is concave down over this interval.
- If $f''(c) > 0$, then $f(x)$ has a *relative minimum* at $x = c$. Again, this makes intuitive sense, since the function is concave up over this interval.
- If $f''(c) = 0$, then we cannot draw a conclusion about this behavior of $f(x)$ at $x = c$.

A function's second derivative can be used to help find inflection points. If $x = c$ is a point on $f(x)$ such that $f''(c) = 0$ or $f''(c)$ is undefined, and if the sign of $f''(c)$ to the left of c is different from the sign of $f''(c)$ to the right of c, then $(c, f(c))$ is an *inflection point*.

Example: Find the local extrema and inflection points, if any, of the function $f(x) = 2x^3 + 5x^2 + 3x + 2$.

The first derivative is $f'(x) = 6x^2 + 10x + 3$.

Set it equal to 0 in order to find the function's critical points:

$$f'(x) = 0$$
$$6x^2 + 10x + 3 = 0$$
$$x = \frac{-10 \pm \sqrt{100 - 72}}{12}$$
$$x = \frac{-10 \pm 2\sqrt{7}}{12}$$
$$x = \frac{-5 \pm \sqrt{7}}{6}$$

The square root of 7 is approximately 2.65, so x equals approximately -0.39, or approximately -1.275. Perform the first derivative test, using 0, -1, and -2 as test values of x:

	$x = -2$	$x = \dfrac{-5 - \sqrt{7}}{6} \approx -1.275$	$x = -1$	$x = \dfrac{-5 + \sqrt{7}}{6} \approx -0.39$	$x = 0$
$f'(x)$	$7 > 0$	0	$-1 < 0$	0	$3 > 0$
Critical Point		Local Maximum		Local Minimum	

Find the second derivative: $f''(x) = 12x + 10$.

This is equal to 0 when x equals $-\dfrac{5}{6}$.

Test the second derivative for values to the right and left of $-\dfrac{5}{6}$:

$$f''(-1) = -2 < 0$$

$$f''(0) = 10 > 0$$

Since the sign of the second derivative changes, $x = -\dfrac{5}{6}$ is an inflection point.

Related rate problems require one to determine the rate of change of a quantity that is linked in some way to the rate of change of some other quantity. Often, the link between the two quantities is a known formula—area, volume, distance formula, trigonometric ratio, etc. The strategy used to solve such problems is illustrated in following example:

Example: A child is standing still and flying a kite. The kite remains at an altitude of 30 feet above the child's hand while traveling parallel to the ground at a rate of 10 feet per second. When the kite is 50 feet away from the child, how fast is the kite string leaving the child's hand?

The first step of solving these problems is to draw a labeled diagram, identify given information and what you need to find. To this end, we have the following diagram:

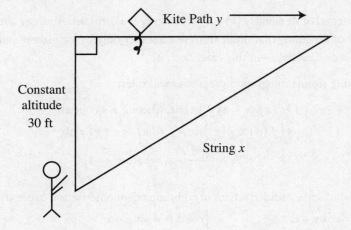

We are given $\dfrac{dy}{dt} = 10$ feet per second, and we must determine $\dfrac{dx}{dt}$ when $x = 50$ feet.

Next, the formula that relates y to x is naturally the Pythagorean theorem in this scenario, since it is a right triangle. Applying this gives the equation $30^2 + y^2 = x^2$.

Both x and y depend on time t. So, implicitly differentiate both sides with respect to t to get $2y\dfrac{dy}{dt} = 2x\dfrac{dx}{dt}$, or more simply, $y\dfrac{dy}{dt} = x\dfrac{dx}{dt}$.

At this point, we can plug in known information and solve for the desired unknown. Doing so, though, we see that we need to have the value of y at the instant when $x = 50$. To find this value, use the Pythagorean theorem with $x = 50$. This results in a 30-40-50 right triangle, so that $y = 40$ feet.

Now, plug in all known information into $y\frac{dy}{dt} = x\frac{dx}{dt}$ and solve for $\frac{dx}{dt}$:

$$(40 \text{ feet})(10 \text{ feet}/_{sec}) = (50 \text{ feet})\frac{dx}{dt}$$

$$\frac{dx}{dt} = 8 \text{ feet}/_{sec}$$

INTEGRATION

Integral calculus is the other major branch of calculus. *Integration* is the opposite process of differentiation. Integration helps you recover a function from its derivative.

The Indefinite Integral

An *antiderivative* of a function $f(x)$ is any function $F(x)$, such that $F'(x) = f(x)$. The *indefinite integral* of $f(x)$ refers to any antiderivative of $f(x)$ and is notated as follows:

$$\int f(x)dx = F(x) + c, \text{ where } c \text{ is a constant}$$

Why is it "*any* antiderivative" instead of "*the* antiderivative"? Consider the two functions $f(x) = x^2$ and $g(x) = x^2 + 5$. The derivative of both functions is $2x$. So then, if the process were to be reversed—that is, if $2x$ were integrated—which of the two functions would be the correct answer? Which of the two is the antiderivative of $2x$? They both are, so each of them is *a* rather than *the* antiderivative of $2x$.

The indefinite integral of $2x$ equals $f(x) = x^2 + c$, where c is a constant. Adding c allows us to include the entire family of functions that differ from one another only by a constant and which have the same derivative as one another—in this case, $2x$.

Learn the following simple integration properties and rules:

$$\int kf(x)\,dx = k\int f(x)\,dx, \text{ where } k \text{ is a constant}$$
$$\int (f(x) \pm g(x))\,dx = \int f(x)\,dx \pm \int g(x)\,dx$$
$$\int x^n dx = \frac{x^{n+1}}{n+1} + c, \text{ where } n \neq -1$$

TIP

It may help you remember the last rule if you think of it as the reverse of differentiation's power rule.

Also, learn the list of some antiderivatives of common trigonometric and exponential functions:

$$\int \sin x dx = -\cos x + c \qquad \int \cos x dx = \sin x + c$$
$$\int \sec^2 x dx = \tan x + c \qquad \int \csc^2 x dx = -\cot x + c$$
$$\int \sec x \tan x dx = \sec x + c \qquad \int \csc x \cot x dx = -\csc x + c$$
$$\int e^x dx = e^x + c \qquad \int a^x dx = \frac{a^x}{\ln a} + c \qquad \int \frac{1}{x} dx = \ln|x| + c$$

Example: What is $\int\left(3x^3 + \sqrt{x^5} - x^{-1}\right)dx$?

Rewrite the second term in fractional exponent form and integrate the sum:

$$\int\left(3x^3 + \sqrt{x^5} - x^{-1}\right)dx = \int\left(3x^3 + x^{\frac{5}{2}} - \frac{1}{x}\right)dx$$

$$= 3\frac{x^4}{4} + \frac{x^{\frac{7}{2}}}{\frac{7}{2}} - \ln|x| + c$$

$$= \frac{3}{4}x^4 + \frac{2}{7}x^{\frac{7}{2}} - \ln|x| + c$$

Integration Methods: Substitution Rule and Integration by Parts

For more complicated integrals, the rules above may not suffice. However, you will probably encounter few, if any, such integrals on the PCAT. Nevertheless, it's worth introducing two integration methods that can help you if you do.

First, consider integrals that are of, or may be written in, the form $\int f(g(x))g'(x)dx$. The *Substitution Rule,* through which you may evaluate such integrals, allows you to replace the given integral with an integral that is easier to evaluate:

$$\int f\left(g\left(x\right)\right)g'\left(x\right)dx = \int f\left(u\right)du,$$
$$\text{where } u = g\left(x\right) \text{ and } du = g'\left(x\right)dx$$

Here, du is called the differential of function u. Given $u = g(x)$, then $du = g'(x)dx$.

Example: Evaluate $\int x(x^2+5)^3\, dx$.

Let $u = x^2 + 5$, in which case $du = 2xdx$. Then:

$$\int x\left(x^2 + 5\right)^3 dx = \int u^3 \frac{1}{2}du = \frac{1}{2}\frac{u^4}{4} + c = \frac{1}{8}\left(x^2 + 5\right)^4 + c$$

The *Integration by Parts Rule* is anti-differentiation's product rule and is useful when no substitution can help evaluate an integral. Given functions $f(x)$ and $g(x)$, then:

$$\int f(x)g'(x)dx = f(x)g(x) - \int f'(x)g(x)dx$$

Example: Evaluate $\int x\sin 2xdx$.

First, find the derivative of $\cos 2x$, using the chain rule with $u = 2x$:

$$\left(\cos 2x\right)' = \frac{d}{du}\left(\cos u\right)\frac{du}{dx}$$
$$= \left(-\sin u\right)2$$
$$= -2\sin 2x$$

Therefore, $\sin 2x = -\frac{1}{2}\left(\cos 2x\right)'$ and the integral becomes:

$$\int x \sin 2x\, dx = \int x \left[-\frac{1}{2}\left(\cos 2x\right)' \right] dx$$

$$= -\frac{1}{2} x \cos 2x - \int (x)' \left(-\frac{1}{2} \right) \cos 2x\, dx$$

$$= -\frac{1}{2} x \cos 2x + \frac{1}{2} \int \cos 2x\, dx$$

In order to evaluate $\int \cos 2x\, dx$, use the substitution rule with $u = 2x$ and $du = 2dx$. Then:

$$-\frac{1}{2} x \cos 2x + \frac{1}{2} \int \cos 2x\, dx = -\frac{1}{2} x \cos 2x + \frac{1}{2} \left(\frac{1}{2} \int \cos u\, du \right)$$

$$= -\frac{1}{2} x \cos 2x + \frac{1}{4} \sin u + c$$

$$= -\frac{1}{2} x \cos 2x + \frac{1}{4} \sin 2x + c$$

Sums and Sigma Notation

Sigma notation is a handy way to notate certain large sums. Given a list of numbers, $a_n, a_{n+1}, a_{n+2}, \ldots,$ a_m, where n and m are integers such that $n < m$, the sum of all the numbers in the list can be written as $\sum_{i=n}^{m} a_i$. Read this as "the sum of a_i for all integer values of i between, and including, n and m." Suppose you are considering the sum of all expressions of the form $(k^2 + k)$, for values of k between, and including, 2 and 10. You can write this sum as $\sum_{k=2}^{10} (k^2 + k)$ In expanded form, this would be:

$$\sum_{k=2}^{10} \left(k^2 + k \right) = \left(2^2 + 2 \right) + \left(3^2 + 3 \right) + \left(4^2 + 4 \right) + \ldots + \left(10^2 + 10 \right)$$

So, sigma notation is an elegant way of expressing large sums such as this one. In addition, formulas such as the following ones simplify considerably the calculation of certain sums:

$$\sum_{i=1}^{n} c = cn, \text{ where } c \text{ is a constant}$$

$$\sum_{i=1}^{n} i = \frac{n(n+1)}{2}$$

$$\sum_{i=1}^{n} i^2 = \frac{n(n+1)(2n+1)}{6}$$

Suppose on the PCAT you are asked to calculate a very manageable sum written in sigma notation—something like $\sum_{k=1}^{3} (k^2 + k)$. Do this by listing all the terms of the sum one by one and performing the calculations directly. For instance, you can calculate the aforementioned sum as follows:

$$\sum_{k=1}^{3} \left(k^2 + k \right) = \left(1^2 + 1 \right) + \left(2^2 + 2 \right) + \left(3^2 + 3 \right) = 1 + 1 + 4 + 2 + 9 + 3 = 20$$

Approximate Areas Bounded by Curves

Say that you have a function $f(x)$ and a closed interval $[a, b]$ on which the formula is defined and positive, and you want to calculate the area bounded by the graph of the function and the x-axis over that interval. For example, say that you are considering the area under the graph of the function $f(x) = x^2 - 2x + 2$ over the interval $[1, 3]$:

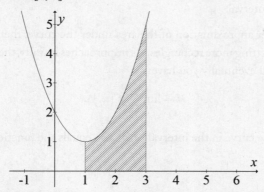

You cannot calculate this area precisely with simple algebra and geometry only. However, you can estimate it. For instance, divide the interval $[1, 3]$ into four subintervals, each having a width of 0.5. Then, in each interval, form a rectangle whose height equals the value of the function at the left endpoint of the interval (shown on the figure on the left, below) or the value of the function at the right endpoint of the interval (shown on the figure on the right, below). The sum of the areas of these rectangles provides an estimate of the area below the curve.

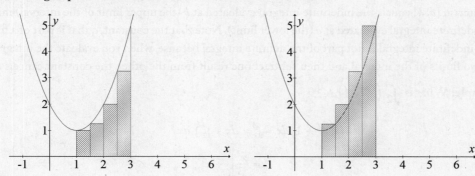

As you can see, because the function is increasing on the interval $[1, 3]$, if you use the left endpoints of each subinterval to calculate the heights of the rectangles, then you are underestimating the area; and using the right endpoints yields an overestimate.

Alternatively, you could use some intermediate value of the function in each subinterval in order to calculate the height of the rectangle corresponding to that subinterval. For instance, for the rectangle whose base is the subinterval $[1, 1.5]$, you could use the value of the function at $x = 1.25$.

In general, if you have a function $f(x)$ and a closed interval $[a, b]$ on which the formula is defined and positive, you may subdivide the interval into n subintervals, each of length $\Delta x = \dfrac{b - a}{n}$.

Then, you may choose a point x_i in each interval.

Let the height of the rectangle that corresponds to that interval be equal to $f(x_i)$.

Thus, the area under the curve will be approximately equal to the sum of the areas of all these rectangles:

$$A \approx f(x_1)\Delta x + f(x_2)\Delta x + \dots + f(x_n)\Delta x \approx \sum_{i=1}^{n} f(x_i)\Delta x$$

This sum is called a *Riemann sum*. Sometimes, you may encounter an "upper" or "lower" Riemann sum—that is, a Riemann sum in which each $f(x_i)$ corresponds to the right endpoint or left endpoint, respectively, of each subinterval.

If you wish to get a better approximation of the area under the curve, then divide the interval into more subintervals, thus getting more rectangles. As n approaches infinity, the approximation becomes increasingly accurate, and eventually you have:

$$A = \lim_{n \to \infty} \sum_{i=1}^{n} f(x_i)\Delta x$$

Finally, the area under the curve in the interval $[a, b]$ also equals the function's definite integral over this interval.

The Definite Integral

The *definite integral* of a function is the function's indefinite integral evaluated over a specific interval. If $f(x)$ is a function that is continuous on an interval $[a, b]$, and if $F(x)$ is any antiderivative of $f(x)$, then:

$$\int_a^b f(x)dx = F(x)\Big|_a^b = F(b) - F(a)$$

This is called the *Fundamental Theorem of Calculus*, and it says that the definite integral of $f(x)$ over the interval $[a, b]$ equals the indefinite integral evaluated at b (the upper limit of the interval) minus the indefinite integral evaluated at a (the lower limit). Note that the constant, c, that is part of a function's indefinite integral is not part of the definite integral because, when you evaluate the integral at the two limits of the interval and then subtract one result from the other, the constant cancels out.

Example: What is $\int_2^4 (x^2 + 1)\,dx$?

$$\int_2^4 (x^2 + 1)\,dx = \int_2^4 x^2 dx + \int_2^4 1\,dx$$

$$= \frac{x^3}{3}\Big|_2^4 + x\Big|_2^4$$

$$= \left(\frac{4^3}{3} - \frac{2^3}{3}\right) + (4 - 2)$$

$$= \left(\frac{64}{3} - \frac{8}{3}\right) + 2$$

$$= \frac{56}{3} + \frac{6}{3}$$

$$= \frac{62}{3}$$

PRACTICE QUESTIONS

Directions: Choose the best answer for each question.

1. What is $\lim\limits_{x \to -3^-}\left(\dfrac{17}{x+3}\right)$?
   - **A.** $-\infty$
   - **B.** 0
   - **C.** 17
   - **D.** ∞

2. What is $\lim\limits_{x \to \infty}\left(\dfrac{x^2+3}{2-x}\right)$?
   - **A.** ∞
   - **B.** 0
   - **C.** $-\infty$
   - **D.** $\dfrac{3}{2}$

Use the following graph for Questions 3 – 6:

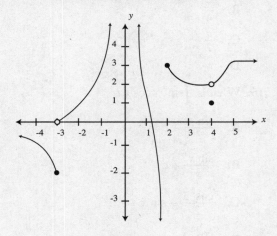

3. Compute $\lim\limits_{x \to 4} f(x)$.
   - **A.** 1
   - **B.** 2
   - **C.** 3
   - **D.** Does not exist

4. Compute $\lim\limits_{x \to -3^+} f(x)$.
   - **A.** -2
   - **B.** -1
   - **C.** 0
   - **D.** Does not exist

5. Compute $\lim\limits_{x \to 2^-} f(x)$
   - **A.** -1
   - **B.** 3
   - **C.** ∞
   - **D.** $-\infty$

6. At which of these x-values is the graphed function continuous?
   - **A.** -3
   - **B.** 0
   - **C.** 4
   - **D.** 6

7. If $f(x) = x^2 - \dfrac{3}{x^2}$, what is $f'(2)$?
   - **A.** 7
   - **B.** 2
   - **C.** 5
   - **D.** $\dfrac{19}{4}$

8. If $f(x) = [\cos(x)]^2 + \sin(x^2)$, what is $f'(x)$?
   - **A.** $2\cos(x) - \sin(x^2)$
   - **B.** 0
   - **C.** $2x\cos(x^2) - 2\sin(x)\cos(x)$
   - **D.** $2\cos(x) + \sin(x^2)$

9. If $f(x) = \tan^{-1}\left(x^2\right)$, compute $f''(x)$.

   A. $f''(x) = \dfrac{-1}{\left(1 + x^4\right)^2}$

   B. $f''(x) = \dfrac{2x}{1 + x^4}$

   C. $f''(x) = \dfrac{2 - 6x^4}{\left(1 + x^4\right)^2}$

   D. $f''(x) = \dfrac{1}{1 + x^4}$

10. Suppose a curve in the xy-plane is described by the implicit equation $xy^3 = y$. Determine $\dfrac{dy}{dx}$.

    A. $\dfrac{dy}{dx} = \dfrac{y^3}{1 - 3xy^2}$

    B. $\dfrac{dy}{dx} = y^3$

    C. $\dfrac{dy}{dx} = y^3 + 3xy^2$

    D. $\dfrac{dy}{dx} = \dfrac{y^3}{3xy^2 - 1}$

11. If $g(x) = \ln(1 + xe^x)$, compute $g'(x)$.

    A. $g'(x) = \dfrac{1}{1 + xe^x}$

    B. $g'(x) = \dfrac{e^x}{1 + xe^x}$

    C. $g'(x) = \dfrac{xe^x}{1 + xe^x}$

    D. $g'(x) = \dfrac{e^x(x + 1)}{1 + xe^x}$

12. A snowball is melting at the rate of 2 cubic feet per hour. If it remains spherical, at what rate is the radius decreasing when the radius of the snowball is 18 inches, accurate to two decimal places?

    A. 0.33 foot per hour

    B. 0.22 foot per hour

    C. 0.11 foot per hour

    D. 0.07 foot per hour

13. If an object's position with respect to time is given by the equation $s(t) = t^3 - 9t^2 + 24t$, at which of the following values of t will the object be at rest?

    A. 0

    B. 3

    C. 4

    D. 6

14. Which of the following is a critical point of the function $f(x) = \dfrac{x^2 - 4}{x^2 - 2x - 3}$?

    A. $x = -1$

    B. $x = 0$

    C. $x = 3$

    D. This function has no critical points.

15. At which of the following points does the graph of $f(x) = \sin(2x)$ have a local maximum?

    A. 0

    B. $\dfrac{\pi}{4}$

    C. $\dfrac{\pi}{2}$

    D. π

16. What is $\displaystyle\int \sin^2 x \cos x\, dx$?

    A. $\dfrac{\sin^3 x}{3} + c$

    B. $\dfrac{\sin x^3}{3} + c$

    C. $\dfrac{\cos^2 x}{2} + \sin x + c$

    D. $\dfrac{\cos^2 x}{2} - \sin x + c$

17. What is the approximate area bounded by the graph of the function $f(x) = x^3$ and the x-axis over the interval $[1, 3]$, when the right Riemann sum with four subintervals is used?

    A. 18

    B. 27

    C. 50

    D. 100

18. What is $\int_1^2 \left(4x^{-3} + 3x^{-2} \right) dx$?

    A. -7

    B. $-\dfrac{35}{16}$

    C. $\dfrac{13}{4}$

    D. 3

19. Compute $\int x^4 \cdot \ln x \, dx$.

    A. $\dfrac{4}{3} x^3 \left(3 \ln x - 1 \right) + C$

    B. $\dfrac{1}{25} x^5 \left(5 \ln x - 1 \right) + C$

    C. $\dfrac{1}{5} x^4 + C$

    D. $x^3 \left(1 + 4 \ln x \right) + C$

20. Compute $\int_{\pi/4}^{\pi/2} \cos x \cdot \sin^2 x \, dx$.

    A. $\dfrac{1}{12}$

    B. $\dfrac{1}{3} \left(1 - \dfrac{\sqrt{3}}{8} \right)$

    C. $-\dfrac{\sqrt{2}}{12}$

    D. $\dfrac{1}{3} \left(1 - \dfrac{\sqrt{2}}{4} \right)$

ANSWER KEY AND EXPLANATIONS

1. A	**5.** D	**9.** C	**13.** C	**17.** B
2. C	**6.** D	**10.** A	**14.** D	**18.** D
3. B	**7.** D	**11.** D	**15.** B	**19.** B
4. C	**8.** C	**12.** D	**16.** A	**20.** D

1. **The correct answer is A.** Since this is a left-hand limit, check values of x less than -3. When $x < -3$, then $x + 3 < 0$. Also, $x + 3 = 0$ when $x = 3$. In other words, the denominator is negative and tends towards 0. As x tends towards -3 from the left, the fraction has a positive number in its numerator that is being divided by an increasingly smaller negative number in its denominator, so the left-hand limit is negative infinity.

2. **The correct answer is C.**
$$\lim_{x \to \infty} \frac{x^2 + 3}{2 - x} = \lim_{x \to \infty} \frac{x^2 + 3}{2 - x} \cdot \frac{\frac{1}{x}}{\frac{1}{x}} = \lim_{x \to \infty} \frac{x + \frac{3}{x}}{\frac{2}{x} - 1}$$
$$= \lim_{x \to \infty} \frac{x}{-1} = -\infty, \text{ where we have used the}$$
fact that $\lim_{x \to \infty} \frac{3}{x} = \lim_{x \to \infty} \frac{2}{x} = 0$.

3. **The correct answer is B.** The functional values get close to 2, the location of the open hole, as the input x-values get closer to 4. So, $\lim_{x \to 4} f(x) = 2$.

4. **The correct answer is C.** The functional values get close to 0 as the input x-values, all taken to the right of -3, get closer to -3. So, $\lim_{x \to -3^+} f(x) = 0$.

5. **The correct answer is D.** The functional values become more negative, without bound, as the input x-values, all taken to the left of 2, get closer to 2. So, $\lim_{x \to 2^-} f(x) = -\infty$.

6. **The correct answer is D.** Graphically, a function is continuous at an x-value $x = a$ if the limit as x approaches a, from both sides, is equal to the functional value $f(a)$. As such, there can be no open holes, jumps, or vertical asymptotes at such a value a. Using the given graph, the function cannot be continuous at -3, 0, or 4, but it is continuous at 6.

7. **The correct answer is D.** Find the general function of the derivative:
$$f(x) = x^2 - \frac{3}{x^2}$$
$$f(x) = x^2 - 3x^{-2}$$
$$f'(x) = 2x + 6x^{-3}$$
$$= 2x + \frac{6}{x^3}$$

Calculate it at $x = 2$:
$$f'(2) = 4 + \frac{6}{8} = 4 + \frac{3}{4} = \frac{19}{4}.$$

8. **The correct answer is C.** Use the chain rule on each term:
$$\frac{dy}{dx} = 2\cos(x)\frac{d}{dx}(\cos(x)) + \cos(x^2)\frac{d}{dx}(x^2)$$
$$= 2\cos(x)(-\sin(x)) + 2x\cos(x^2)$$
$$= 2x\cos(x^2) - 2\sin(x)\cos(x)$$

9. **The correct answer is C.** Use the chain rule and differentiate twice, in succession to get the first derivative: $f'(x) = \dfrac{1}{1 + (x^2)^2} \cdot 2x = \dfrac{2x}{1 + x^4}$. To get the second derivative, differentiate *this* function using the quotient rule:

$$f''(x) = \frac{\left(1 + x^4\right) \cdot 2 - 2x\left(4x^3\right)}{\left(1 + x^4\right)^2}$$

$$= \frac{2 + 2x^4 - 8x^4}{\left(1 + x^4\right)^2} = \frac{2 - 6x^4}{\left(1 + x^4\right)^2}$$

10. **The correct answer is A.** Implicitly differentiate both sides with respect to x:

$$xy^3 = y$$

$$x \cdot 3y^2 \frac{dy}{dx} + y^3 \cdot 1 = \frac{dy}{dx}$$

$$x \cdot 3y^2 \frac{dy}{dx} - \frac{dy}{dx} = -y^3$$

$$\left(3xy^2 - 1\right)\frac{dy}{dx} = -y^3$$

$$\frac{dy}{dx} = \frac{-y^3}{3xy^2 - 1}$$

$$\frac{dy}{dx} = \frac{y^3}{1 - 3xy^2}$$

11. **The correct answer is D.** Use the chain rule and product rule, as follows:

$$g'(x) = \frac{1}{1 + xe^x}\left(xe^x + e^x\right) = \frac{e^x\left(x + 1\right)}{1 + xe^x}$$

12. **The correct answer is D.** The volume V of a sphere with radius r is given by the formula $V = \dfrac{4}{3}\pi r^3$. We are given that $\dfrac{dV}{dt} = -2$ cubic feet per hour (since the snowball is melting) and are asked to find $\dfrac{dr}{dt}$ (in feet per hour) at the instant when the radius of the snowball is $r = 18$ inches $= 1.5$ feet.

Implicitly differentiate both sides of the volume formula with respect to t and then, substitute in known information:

$$\frac{dV}{dt} = 4\pi r^2 \cdot \frac{dr}{dt}$$

$$-2 \;{}^{\text{ft}^3}\!/_{\text{hour}} = 4\pi(1.5 \text{ ft})^2 \cdot \frac{dr}{dt}$$

$$\frac{-2}{4\pi(1.5)^2}\;{}^{\text{ft}}\!/_{\text{hour}} = \frac{dr}{dt}$$

$$-0.07\;{}^{\text{ft}}\!/_{\text{hour}} = \frac{dr}{dt}$$

So, the radius is decreasing at a rate of 0.07 foot per hour.

13. **The correct answer is C.** The object will be at rest when its velocity is zero. First differentiate the function of the object's position in order to find the function of its velocity:

$$s(t) = t^3 - 9t^2 + 24t$$

$$s'(t) = 3t^2 - 18t + 24$$

Set the velocity equal to zero and solve:

$$3t^2 - 18t + 24 = 0$$

$$t^2 - 6t + 8 = 0$$

$$(t - 2)(t - 4) = 0$$

$$t = 2 \text{ OR } t = 4$$

Only 4 is given as an answer choice.

14. **The correct answer is D.** Find the derivative, using the quotient rule:

$$f\left(x\right) = \frac{x^2 - 4}{x^2 - 2x - 3}$$

$$f'\left(x\right) = \frac{2x\left(x^2 - 2x - 3\right) - \left(x^2 - 4\right)\left(2x - 2\right)}{\left(x^2 - 2x - 3\right)^2}$$

$$= \frac{2x^3 - 4x^2 - 6x - 2x^3 + 2x^2 + 8x - 8}{\left(x^2 - 2x - 3\right)^2}$$

$$= \frac{-2x^2 + 2x - 8}{\left(x^2 - 2x - 3\right)^2}$$

$$= -2\frac{x^2 - x + 4}{\left(x^2 - 2x - 3\right)^2}$$

$$= -2\frac{x^2 - x + 4}{\left[\left(x + 1\right)\left(x - 3\right)\right]^2}$$

The denominator of the derivative is 0 when $x = -1$ and $x = 3$, which means that the derivative does not exist at those points. However, in this case for a critical point to exist at $x = c$, the function itself would have a denominator equal to zero, making $f(x)$ undefined. Thus, $x = -1$ and $x = 3$ are not critical points.

Thus, you have to worry only about values of x for which the first derivative is 0. Set the numerator equal to 0 and solve. The discriminant, $b^2 - 4ac$, equals -15, which means that the polynomial in the numerator does not have real roots. Therefore, this function does not have any critical points.

15. **The correct answer is B.** Find the first derivative:

$$\frac{d}{dx}\left[\sin(2x)\right] = \cos(2x)\frac{d}{dx}(2x)$$
$$= 2\cos(2x)$$

Let the first derivative equal 0:

$$2\cos(2x) = 0$$
$$2x = \pm\frac{\pi}{2} + 2\pi n$$
$$x = \pm\frac{\pi}{4} + \pi n$$

n may be any integer. If we take the "plus" version of the result ($x = +\frac{\pi}{4} + \pi n$), x may be $\frac{\pi}{4}$, $\frac{5\pi}{4}$, $\frac{9\pi}{4}$, and so on, or $-\frac{3\pi}{4}$, $-\frac{7\pi}{4}$, and so on. If we take the "minus" version of the result ($x = -\frac{\pi}{4} + \pi n$), x may be $-\frac{\pi}{4}$, $\frac{3\pi}{4}$, $\frac{7\pi}{4}$, and so on, or $-\frac{5\pi}{4}$, $-\frac{9\pi}{4}$, and so on. Among those, only $\frac{\pi}{4}$ is an answer choice, so it must be the correct answer. You can verify this by using the second derivative test:

$$\frac{d}{dx}\left[2\cos(2x)\right] = -2\sin(2x)\frac{d}{dx}(2x)$$
$$= -4\sin(2x)$$

At $x = \frac{\pi}{4}$,

$$-4\sin(2x) = -4\sin\left(\frac{\pi}{2}\right) = -4 \times 1 < 0.$$

The second derivative at this point is negative, so this point is a local maximum.

16. **The correct answer is A.** Use the substitution rule: Let $u = \sin x$, in which case $du = \cos x\, dx$.

$$\int \sin^2 x \cos x\, dx = \int u^2\, du = \frac{u^3}{3} + c = \frac{\sin^3 x}{3} + c$$

17. **The correct answer is B.** The approximate area will be equal to the sum of the areas of four rectangles, each with width $\frac{3-1}{4} = \frac{1}{2}$. You want the right Riemann sum, so the height of each rectangle will be the value of the function at the right endpoint of the subinterval to which the rectangle corresponds. For the left-most subinterval, that endpoint is $1 + \frac{1}{2}$; for the second subinterval from the left, the right endpoint is $1 + \frac{1}{2} + \frac{1}{2}$; in general, for each subinterval, the right endpoint is $1 + \frac{1}{2}i$, where $i = 1, 2, 3, 4$. Thus, the Riemann sum becomes:

$$\sum_{i=1}^{4}\left[\frac{1}{2}\left(1 + \frac{1}{2}i\right)^3\right] = \frac{1}{2}\left[\left(\frac{3}{2}\right)^3 + 2^3 + \left(\frac{5}{2}\right)^3 + 3^3\right]$$
$$= \frac{1}{2}\left[\frac{27}{8} + 8 + \frac{125}{8} + 27\right]$$
$$= \frac{1}{2}\left[\frac{27}{8} + \frac{64}{8} + \frac{125}{8} + \frac{216}{8}\right]$$
$$= \frac{1}{2} \times \frac{432}{8}$$
$$= 27$$

18. The correct answer is D. The first step in calculating the definite integral is finding the indefinite integral:

$$\int_1^2 \left(4x^{-3} + 3x^{-2}\right) dx = \left(4\frac{x^{-2}}{-2} + 3\frac{x^{-1}}{-1}\right)\Big|_1^2$$

$$= \left(-2x^{-2} - 3x^{-1}\right)\Big|_1^2$$

Next, evaluate this expression at $x = 2$, and from that subtract the evaluation of this expression at $x = -1$:

$$\left(-2x^{-2} - 3x^{-1}\right)\Big|_1^2 = \left(-2 \times 2^{-2} - 3 \times 2^{-1}\right) - \left(-2 \times 1^{-2} - 3 \times 1^{-1}\right)$$

$$= -\frac{1}{2} - \frac{3}{2} - (-2 - 3)$$

$$= -2 + 5$$

$$= 3$$

19. The correct answer is B. Use the integration by parts formula $\int u\, dv = uv - \int v\, du$ with $u = \ln x$, $du = \frac{1}{x}dx$, $dv = x^4 dx$, and $v = \frac{1}{5}x^5$ to see that

$$\int x^4 \cdot \ln x\, dx = \frac{1}{5}x^5 \ln x - \frac{1}{5}\int x^4 dx$$

$$= \frac{1}{5}x^5 \ln x - \frac{1}{25}x^5 + C$$

$$= \frac{1}{25}x^5 \left(5\ln x - 1\right) + C$$

20. The correct answer is D. Use the substitution method. Let $u = \sin(x)$. Then, $du = \cos(x)\, dx$. Changing the limits shows that when $x = \frac{\pi}{4}$, $u = \frac{\sqrt{2}}{2}$, and when $x = \frac{\pi}{2}$, then $u = 1$. So,

$$\int_{\pi/4}^{\pi/2} \cos x \cdot \sin^2 x\, dx = \int_{\sqrt{2}/2}^1 u^2\, du = \frac{1}{3}u^3\Big|_{\sqrt{2}/2}^1 = \frac{1}{3}\left(1 - \left(\sqrt{2}/2\right)^3\right) = \frac{1}{3}\left(1 - \frac{\sqrt{2}}{4}\right)$$

SUMMING IT UP

- If $f(x)$ is continuous at $x = a$, $\lim\limits_{x \to a} f(x) = f(a)$.

- $\lim\limits_{x \to \infty} \dfrac{c}{x^n} = 0$ for any real number c and positive rational number n.

- $\lim\limits_{x \to \infty} \left(a_n x^n + a_{n-1} x^{n-1} + \ldots + a_0 x^0 \right) = \lim\limits_{x \to \infty} a_n x^n$

  $\lim\limits_{x \to \infty} \left(\dfrac{a_n x^n + a_{n-1} x^{n-1} + \ldots + a_0 x^0}{b_m x^m + b_{m-1} x^{m-1} + \ldots + b_0 x^0} \right) = \lim\limits_{x \to \infty} \left(\dfrac{a_n x^n}{b_m x^m} \right)$, where $a_n, b_m \neq 0$

- If $f(x) = c$, where c is a constant, then $f'(x) = 0$.

- If $f(x) = x^n$, where n is any number, then $f'(x) = nx^{n-1}$.

- Given two functions $f(x)$ and $g(x)$, then $(f(x) \pm g(x))' = f'(x) \pm g'(x)$.

- Given a function $f(x)$ and a constant c, then $(cf(x))' = cf'(x)$

- If two functions $f(x)$ and $g(x)$ are differentiable, then $(fg)' = f'g + fg'$ and $\left(\dfrac{f}{g} \right)' = \dfrac{f'g - fg'}{g^2}$.

- $\dfrac{d}{d\theta}\left(\sin \theta \right) = \cos \theta$

- $\dfrac{d}{d\theta}\left(\cos \theta \right) = -\sin \theta$

- $\dfrac{d}{d\theta}\left(\tan \theta \right) = \sec^2 \theta$

- $\dfrac{d}{d\theta}\left(\cot \theta \right) = -\csc^2 \theta$

- $\dfrac{d}{d\theta}\left(\sec \theta \right) = \sec \theta \tan \theta$

- $\dfrac{d}{d\theta}\left(\csc \theta \right) = -\csc \theta \cot \theta$

- $\dfrac{d}{dx} \sin^{-1} x = \dfrac{1}{\sqrt{1 - x^2}}$

- $\dfrac{d}{dx} \cos^{-1} x = \dfrac{-1}{\sqrt{1 - x^2}}$

- $\dfrac{d}{dx} \tan^{-1} x = \dfrac{1}{1 + x^2}$

- $\dfrac{d}{dx}\left(e^x \right) = e^x$

- $\dfrac{d}{dx}\left(\ln x \right) = \dfrac{1}{x}$

- $\dfrac{d}{dx}\left(a^x \right) = a^x \ln a$, $a > 0$ and $a \neq 1$

- $\dfrac{d}{dx}\left(\log_a x \right) = \dfrac{1}{x \ln a}$, $a > 0$ and $a \neq 1$

- **Chain Rule of Differentiation:** If $y = f(u)$ and $u = g(x)$, then $\dfrac{dy}{dx} = \dfrac{dy}{du}\dfrac{du}{dx}$.

- **Implicit Differentiation:** Differentiate both sides of an equation as given (that is, without first solving for y), and then solve for y'.

- For any function $f(x)$, $f'(a)$ represents the function's instantaneous rate of change at $x = a$. In particular, if $s(t)$ is the function giving the position of an object with respect to time, then the object's velocity, $v(t)$, equals $s'(t)$ (velocity is the derivative of position), while the object's acceleration, $a(t)$, equals $v'(t)$ (acceleration is the derivative of velocity).

- **Mean Value Theorem for Derivatives:** If f is a function that is continuous on $[a,b]$ and differentiable on (a,b), then there is at least one value c in (a,b) for which $f'(c) = \dfrac{f(b) - f(a)}{b - a}$.

- If a function $f(x)$ is defined at $x = c$ (that is, if $f(c)$ exists), then $x = c$ is a critical point if $f'(c) = 0$, or $f'(c)$ does not exist.

- Given an interval in the domain of a function $f(x)$, then:
  - If $f'(x) > 0$ for all x in the interval, $f(x)$ is increasing over the interval.
  - If $f'(x) < 0$ for all x in the interval, $f(x)$ is decreasing over the interval.
  - If $f'(x) = 0$ for all x in the interval, $f(x)$ is constant over the interval.

- **First Derivative Test:** If $x = c$ is a critical point of $f(x)$, then:
  - If $f'(x) > 0$ to the left of $x = c$ and $f'(x) < 0$ to the right of $x = c$, $x = c$ is a relative maximum.
  - If $f'(x) < 0$ to the left of $x = c$ and $f'(x) > 0$ to the right of $x = c$, $x = c$ is a relative minimum.
  - If $f'(x)$ has the same sign on both sides of $x = c$, $x = c$ is not a relative extremum.

- A function is *concave* up on a given interval if it is shaped like a bowl over that interval; and it is *concave down* if it shaped like a dome. A point on the graph of a function is an inflection point if the function is continuous at that point and the concavity of the graph changes at that point.

- Given an interval in the domain of a function $f(x)$, then:
  - If $f''(x) > 0$ for all x in the interval, $f(x)$ is concave up over the interval.
  - If $f''(x) < 0$ for all x in the interval, $f(x)$ is concave down over the interval.

- **Second Derivative Test:** If $x = c$ is a critical point of $f(x)$, with $f'(c) = 0$, and $f''(c)$ is continuous near c, then:
  - If $f''(c) < 0$, $x = c$ is a relative maximum.
  - If $f''(c) > 0$, $x = c$ is a relative minimum.
  - If $f''(c) = 0$, we cannot draw a conclusion about $x = c$.

- If $x = c$ is a point on $f(x)$ such that $f''(c) = 0$ or $f''(c)$ is undefined, and if the sign of $f''(c)$ to the left of c is different from the sign of $f''(c)$ to the right of c, then $f(c)$ is an inflection point.

- $\int kf(x)dx = k \int f(x)dx$, where k is a constant

- $\int f(x) \pm g(x)dx = \int f(x)dx \pm \int g(x)dx$

- $\int x^n dx = \dfrac{x^{n+1}}{n+1} + c$, where $n \neq -1$

- $\int \sin x\, dx = -\cos x + c$

- $\int \cos x\, dx = \sin x + c$

- $\int \sec^2 x\, dx = \tan x + c$

- $\int \csc^2 x\, dx = -\cot x + c$

- $\int \sec x \tan x\, dx = \sec x + c$

- $\int \csc x \cot x\, dx = -\csc x + c$

- $\int e^x\, dx = e^x + c$

- $\int a^x\, dx = \dfrac{a^x}{\ln a} + c$

- $\int \dfrac{1}{x}\, dx = \ln|x| + c$

- **Substitution Rule:** $\int f(g(x))g'(x)\, dx = \int f(u)\, du$, where $u = g(x)$ and $du = g'(x)\, dx$

- **Integration by Parts:** $\int f(x)g'(x)\, dx = f(x)g(x) - \int f'(x)g(x)\, dx$

- $\displaystyle\sum_{i=n}^{m} a_i = a_n + a_{n+1} + \ldots + a_{m-1} + a_m$

- $\displaystyle\sum_{i=1}^{n} c = cn$, where c is a constant

- $\displaystyle\sum_{i=1}^{n} i = \dfrac{n(n+1)}{2}$

- $\displaystyle\sum_{i=1}^{n} i^2 = \dfrac{n(n+1)(2n+1)}{6}$

- **Riemann Sum:** $A \approx f(x_1)\Delta x + f(x_2)\Delta x + \ldots + f(x_n)\Delta x \approx \displaystyle\sum_{i=1}^{n} f(x_i)\Delta x$

- **Fundamental Theorem of Calculus:** $\displaystyle\int_a^b f(x)\, dx = F(x)\Big|_a^b = F(b) - F(a)$

PART VII
WRITING

Chapter 16　Writing Skills

SPECIAL FEATURE:
　　　　A Quick Review of Common Errors in
　　　　Grammar, Usage, and Mechanics

Writing Skills

OVERVIEW

- **Understand the Scoring Rubrics**
- **Know and Practice the Task**
- **Take It Step By Step**
- **Common Writing Errors**
- **Follow A Model**
- **Essay Prompt**
- **Model Responses, Scoring, and Analysis**
- **A Writing Study Plan**
- **Sharpening Your Writing Skills Every Day**
- **Summing It Up**

During the PCAT, you will write one problem-solution essay at the very beginning of the test. The prompt will present a problem relating to a health, science, social, cultural, or political issue.

You will have thirty minutes to write the essay. There is no time to lose on test day double-checking the requirements or figuring out the right tone and voice. This chapter describes the essay task and the way it will be scored.

UNDERSTAND THE SCORING RUBRICS

You are writing for a score, so begin by learning how your writing will be evaluated. The following information is based on "How the Writing Subtest is Scored" in the PCAT test booklet at http://pcatweb.info/downloads/Faculty/Interpreting_PCAT_Scores.pdf. There are two rubrics against which your essays will be scored: Conventions of Language and Problem Solving. A top-scoring essay

- **must be clearly and effectively persuasive.** That means it will state a clear argument or thesis at the outset and keep its audience in mind throughout. Never forget that you are writing to persuade, not to inform.

- **must be effectively organized.** It will have a clear introduction, an effective conclusion, and separate paragraphs to present and develop each significant reason for, or explanation of, the proposed solution. It may also have a paragraph that logically and thoughtfully dismisses an alternative or competing solution.

571

- **must use logical reasoning.** The successful essay will not present the reader with faulty causes and effects, either/or thinking, or other fallacies.

- **must be well supported.** Many well-chosen, clearly stated reasons, examples, and other details will explain, develop, and support the writer's points.

- **must have no sentence structure problems.** There will be no sentence fragments. A sentence fragment is a group of words that looks like a sentence, but is not a complete sentence because it lacks a subject (or in some cases an object as well), a complete verb, or a complete thought. A typical fragment presents an incomplete thought, such as: *Being that new legislation is only the beginning of the solution to the problem.* A top-scoring essay will also avoid comma splices. A comma splice occurs when two clauses that could stand alone as sentences are run together, such as: *The solution is a simple one, start funding infrastructure work now.*

- **must have no usage problems.** The standard rules for how to write the English language will be followed. Examples of usage problems include the confusion of words such as *two/too/to, than/then, accept/except, affect/effect.* Problems with subject-verb agreement and pronoun-antecedent agreement are also common usage issues.

- **must have few mechanical errors.** Mechanics includes punctuation and capitalization. (The PCAT rubrics make no mention of spelling, however.)

KNOW AND PRACTICE THE TASK

When you practice the task, focus on getting right to the solutions. It is all right, and it may even be rhetorically effective, to restate or acknowledge the problem, but don't spend more than a sentence or two on that. Remember that you're not being asked to analyze the problem either. You are being asked for a solution. So, for example, if you are answering a prompt about voter apathy, the bulk of your essay might be about ways to persuade people that their vote counts, about how to solve the problem of physically getting people to the polls, about persuading people to fulfill the responsibilities of citizenship, or about how to instill pride in taking part in the democratic process.

According to the official PCAT Test Blueprint (https://www.pcatweb.info/Resources.php), the prompt that states the problem you must address in your essay will deal with one of the following issues:

- **Health,** which involves "issues related to public health, medicine, nutrition, fitness, prevention, treatments, therapies, medications, drugs, attitudes"

- **Science,** which involves "issues related to research, theories, findings, applications, controversies, education, attitudes"

- **Social, Cultural or Political Issues,** which involves "issues related to beliefs, attitudes, behaviors, trends, laws, policies"

In order to help you achieve a top score on your essay, you will now take a look at a sample prompt and a top-scoring essay. After you read both, we'll then walk you through the factors that make this essay so strong.

Writing Prompt Sample

A recent study published in *The Lancet* found that air, water, and workplace pollution caused 9 million premature deaths throughout the world in 2015 with air pollution causing 6.5 million of those deaths, especially in low-income societies and developing nations. Discuss a solution to the problem of pollution-related death.

TAKE IT STEP BY STEP

Let's take a moment to think about our prompt. It relates to a health issue, but it also has social and cultural implications as it deals with world health. It is a complex and consequential issue, so the prompt is essentially asking you to solve a tremendous global problem. You should relax, though. No one at the government level is going to read your essay, and no one is expecting you to solve a major problem like pollution-related deaths in the span of 30 minutes. You just need to come up with a few ideas about how to address the problem and present them in a well-considered, well-organized manner. You can take on this problem with our very effective five-step writing process. Just be sure that you do not omit any of these five steps:

1. **Brainstorm.** Don't just start keyboarding your response. You will be provided with an erasable noteboard and marker. Use these items to jot down, and later cross out, if need be, the first ideas that come to mind about a solution to the problem. Don't stop until you have a reasonable, logical solution that is clearly related to the problem stated in the prompt, as well as at least three good points that support, explain, and/or develop your solution. Not everything you come up with while brainstorming will be a million-dollar idea to include in your essay, but it is helpful to write down absolutely everything you think of while brainstorming. This will help you better separate the great ideas from the ones that might be less useful.

   Also, don't waste time with things like grammar and spelling while brainstorming. Brainstorming is not for finalizing your essay; it is for generating ideas, and since time is a major element, you should just get down your ideas as quickly and simply as possible. As you practice for the Writing subtest, work out how much time each step of the process will take. Allot perhaps four to five minutes for this step.

   Here's a sample brainstorming list in response to our prompt about pollution-related deaths:

pollution
global problem—not just local
handle at global and local level
education
elevate to international priority
monitor
mass deaths bad for developing nations
air pollution is worst

NOTE

Just concentrate on making a valid argument, being sure to provide plenty of support and sensible transitions between points

NOTE

A brainstorming list does not require perfect grammar, punctuation, or even complete sentences.

> nations work together
> restrictions on air travel
> research
> force people to recycle
> more funds!
> fines for polluting nations

As you can see, this brainstorming list is not particularly readable, but it does not need to be readable. It just needs to include some strong ideas, and this list does have some strong ones that could come in handy when composing the essay. Some of the ideas might not be great, though. While recycling and pollution are both environmental issues, *forcing people to recycle* is both unrealistic and irrelevant to the specific topic at hand. Also it might not be helpful to fine polluting nations when so many of the worst polluters are already having financial problems. We do not want to disable nations; we just want to come up with some general solutions to the deadly pollution problem.

2. **Organize.** After generating ideas by brainstorming, make a map, an informal outline, or any kind of diagram to organize those ideas into a logical order. Think of each main piece of support as a separate paragraph that you will develop. Remember that your writing must have a recognizable structure. The good news is that there is a pretty standard three-part essay structure:

Introduction: the opening paragraph of an essay, which in the case of a problem-solving essay, introduces the problem and alludes to a solution or at least acknowledges that a solution is necessary.

Body: the paragraphs that get into deeper detail. Perhaps the first of those paragraphs will give more details about the problem than the introduction, and the following paragraphs will give detailed information about the solution.

Conclusion: the final paragraph, which may provide a little new information but is mostly concerned with wrapping up the discussion and summarizing the essay's findings.

It's important to map out this structure before you begin to write. Use numbers, arrows, or whatever works to organize your ideas quickly and clearly. Allot perhaps two minutes for this step.

Here's a sample outline for our pollution-related death prompt:

Introduction: Discuss pollution as it related to mass deaths throughout world.

Body Paragraph 1: More details on pollution deaths.

Body Paragraph 2: Making pollution international priority.

Monitoring pollution.

Emphasizing deadliness of pollution.

NOTE

A persuasive essay has a standard structure. Be sure to use that structure when composing your essay for the PCAT Writing subtest.

Body Paragraph 3: Handle problem at local and global levels

Funding

Research

Conclusion: Importance of finding solution.

Notice that, like the brainstorming list, matters of grammar and sentence structure do not apply when making an outline. Also notice that many of the ideas from that brainstorming list have found a home in this outline while others have been discarded.

3.   **Write.** The preparation phase is now over and it is time to actually compose your essay. Numerous strategies can make this process go smoothly. A good opening line can restate the problem, acknowledge that the problem exists, or warn readers of the consequences of not solving the problem. Use that opening line to segue—immediately or in a sentence or two—to your solution. Be sure to state your solution very clearly. (Note that you may be able to refer back to that opening line in your conclusion.)

Then begin developing your reasons or explanations in separate paragraphs. Remember, your central task is to persuade the reader of your solution in each paragraph. Present relevant facts in as objective a manner as possible.

Conclude with a separate paragraph. A good way to conclude is with a call to action. Remember that a call to action doesn't necessarily mean taking a physical action such as cleaning up roadside trash. It can also be a call to changing one's way of thinking or mindset about a problem. Allot perhaps fifteen minutes for writing.

Here's an essay that responds to our sample prompt:

> In our public discourse, the pollution problem is often framed as a somewhat abstract problem. We read statistics related to the negative effects of air, water, and workplace pollution, but we rarely consider the very real, every day impacts of those problems, but this abstraction is rapidly becoming all too concrete as more and more people throughout the world are dying because of various types of pollution.

> According to a recent study published in *The Lancet*, it claimed nine million lives in 2015 alone. This situation is most dire in low-income societies that likely do not have protections and limits in place to reduce environmental pollution. Developing nations that may put progress ahead of public health. While water contamination and workplace-related pollution are significant factors in those statistics, air pollution is the most effective killer, being responsible for 6.5 million of those 9 million deaths.

> Sculpting a solution to a problem such as this is especially tricky because of its global nature. It is not enough for a single nation to resolve to tackle its pollution problem, all nations must come together to address it. Because of their varying agendas, many nations may be reluctant to do so despite the objectively disturbing statistics. Perhaps the best way to begin solving this problem is by drawing attention to it by elevating pollution to an international priority and building partnerships between nations to work together to agree to reduce pollution. Even the most cynical leaders who prioritize development over human life must realize that a disappearing populace is at odds with development.

NOTE

Ending with a call to action or a provocative question is a strong way to conclude a persuasive essay.

Ultimately, the pollution problem must be handled at the local level, which could involve working pollution limits into both country and city plans. None of this can be achieved without proper funding, so increased pollution control funding must also be implemented. Funds must also be allocated for further research into both the impacts of pollution and solutions to this grave problem.

No matter what our global nation does to address this problem, we must make it our mission to ensure that something is done. Mass deaths is an issue no nation can take lightly. Since there are some weapons at our disposal as I've detailed, we would be foolish not to use them in our ongoing battle against pollution.

NOTE

Revising involves strengthening ideas; correcting mechanical errors is for the editing/proofreading process.

4. **Revise.** Congratulations! At this point the majority of the work you will do on your essay is done. However, it is not complete yet. You must now make sure that your essay is as strong as it can possibly be, and that means you need to reread it and make revisions if you find any room for improvement. Combine short sentences where it makes sense. Be sure references are clear, and clarify confusing ideas by reworking sentences and parts of paragraphs. Basically, this is the step in the process where you ensure your ideas make sense and your argument is complete.

In the case of our sample essay, there is definitely need for some revision. The opening paragraph has an unnecessarily long sentence that can be split into two more digestible sentences. The second paragraph begins with a sentence that needs a clearer subject than *it*. The third paragraph could use some fleshing out with additional details. Revision should take about four to five minutes.

Here's how the essay should look after a thorough revision:

In our public discourse, the pollution problem is often framed as a somewhat abstract problem. We read statistics related to the negative effects of air, water, and workplace pollution, but we rarely consider the very real, everyday impacts of those problems. While water contamination and workplace-related pollution are significant factors in those statistics. Air pollution is the most effective killer, being responsible for 6.5 million of those 9 million deaths.

According to a recent study published in *The Lancet*, pollution claimed nine million lives in 2015 alone. This situation is most dire in low-income societies that likely do not have protections and limits in place to reduce environmental pollution, and developing nations that may put progress ahead of public health. While water contamination and workplace-related pollution are significant factors in those statistics, air pollution is the most effective killer, being responsible for 6.5 million of those 9 million deaths.

Sculpting a solution to a problem such as this is especially tricky because of its global nature. It is not enough for a single nation to resolve to tackle its pollution problem, all nations must come together to address it. Because of their varying agendas, many nations may be reluctant to do so despite the objectively disturbing statistics. Perhaps the best way to begin solving this problem is by drawing attention to it by elevating pollution to an international priority and building partnerships between nations to work together to agree to reduce pollution. Monitoring pollution is also crucial since this will yield results on the worst problem areas as well as the causes and changes in percentages. Reports should emphasize the deadly effects of pollution, because despite their individual agendas, nations must react to statistics revealing that their populations are dying en mass. Even the most cynical leaders who prioritize development over human life must realize that a disappearing populace is at odds with development.

Ultimately, the pollution problem must be handled at the local level, which could involve working pollution limits into both county and city plans. None of this can be achieved without proper funding, so increased pollution control funding must also be implemented. Funds must also be allocated for further research into both the impacts of pollution and solutions to this grave problem.

No matter what our global "nation" does to address this problem, we must make it our mission to ensure that something is done. Mass deaths is an issue no nation can take lightly. Since there are some weapons at our disposal as I've detailed, we would be foolish not to use them in our ongoing battle against pollution.

5. **Edit and Proofread.** Revision involves finding ways to strengthen your message. The editing and proofreading step is a bit different, because in this final step of the writing process, you will look for mistakes related to grammar, usage, and mechanics rather than meaning.

Editing and proofreading is more important on the PCAT than it is on almost every other test because there is a separate *and equal* score for conventions. Do not just leave two minutes for this step because conventions account for 50 percent of your writing score. Clean up any usage problems, correct any subject-verb errors, and be sure antecedents for pronouns and modifiers are clear.

If you devise a reasonable time allotment for each step, you should have four to five minutes for this last step.

So now it's time to clean up our sample essay, because the second paragraph has a fragment that can be corrected by joining it to the previous sentence, the third paragraph starts with a comma splice, and the fourth paragraph contains a lack of agreement between a subject (the plural *Mass deaths*) and verb (the singular *is*).

Once it is edited and proofread, the sample essay should look like this… and earn a top score!

In our public discourse, the pollution problem is often framed as a somewhat abstract problem. We read statistics related to the negative effects of air, water, and workplace pollution, but we rarely consider the very real, every day impacts of those problems. However, this abstraction is rapidly becoming all too concrete as more and more people throughout the world are dying because of various types of pollution. Consequently, it is imperative that we figure out a solution to this deadly problem.

According to a recent study published in *The Lancet*, pollution claimed nine million lives in 2015 alone. This situation is most dire in low-income societies that likely do not have protections and limits in place to reduce environmental pollution, and developing nations that may put progress ahead of public health. While water contamination and workplace-related pollution are significant factors in those statistics, air pollution is the most effective killer, being responsible for 6.5 million of those 9 million deaths.

NOTE

While the editing/proofreading process is for correcting mechanical and grammar errors, you may still catch issues with your presentation of ideas during this process. If you do, correct them.

ALERT

Remember that conventions account for 50 percent of your writing score.

Sculpting a solution to a problem such is this is especially tricky because of its global nature. It is not enough for a single nation to resolve to tackle its pollution problem; all nations must come together to address it. Because of their varying agendas, many nations may be reluctant to do so despite the objectively disturbing statistics. Perhaps the best way to begin solving this problem is by drawing attention to it by elevating pollution to an international priority and building partnerships between nations to work together to agree to reduce pollution. Monitoring pollution is also crucial since this will yield results on the worst problem areas as well as the causes and changes in percentages. Reports should emphasize the deadly effects of pollution, because despite their individual agendas, nations must react to statistics revealing that their populations are dying on mass. Even the most cynical leaders who prioritize development over human life must realize that a disappearing populace is at odds with development.

Ultimately, the pollution problem must be handled at the local level, which could involve working pollution limits into both country and city plans. None of this can be achieved without proper funding, so increased pollution control funding must also be implemented. Funds must also be allocated for further research into both the impacts of pollution and solutions to this grave problem.

No matter what our global "nation" does to address this problem, we must make it our mission to ensure that something is done. Mass deaths are an issue no nation can take lightly. Since there are some weapons at our disposal as I've detailed, we would be foolish not to use them in our ongoing battle against pollution.

COMMON WRITING ERRORS

Now that you know what to do when planning, writing, and perfecting your essay, it is important to know what you should *not* do. That's because there are some all-too common errors that writers make time and time again. The following section will help you sidestep those errors on the PCAT Writing subtest.

Keep Your Writing Priorities Straight

When writing it is easy to get sidetracked. Unfortunately, you will only have 30 minutes to plan, write, and revise your essay on the PCAT Writing subtest, so you will not have the luxury of wandering off course and finding your way back on it again. You will have to concentrate on keeping your priorities straight since you have a very specific task to accomplish. Remember that your essay is ultimately a persuasive one that must be logical, well organized, and completely adherent to the conventions of English. Here are some tips for keeping your writing priorities straight:

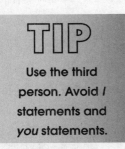

- Include *a clear statement of the solution* at the beginning.
- Make sure you have *a structure.* The PCAT rubric states that, just to score a 3.0, you need at least three distinct paragraphs signaling a beginning, middle, and end. A more sophisticated structure will have 1) a separate paragraph for the introduction; 2) three-to-five body paragraphs, each detailing a separate reason or explanation for your solution (and one alternative to the solution, if you choose this strategy); and 3) an effective conclusion structured as a final paragraph.

- Present *logical reasons or explanations* for your solution. It is a good strategy to state these as the topic sentence of each body paragraph.

- Include *ample support but no filler.* Do not repeat yourself, and do not digress. You do not need to know statistics, but you must include facts. It is not the length of your paragraphs that matters. Instead, your success or failure will lie largely with the quality and relevance of your support.

- Remember *audience and purpose.* You are persuading, not exploring your feelings. Do not get personal. Use formal word choices.

Avoid Questionable Reasoning

Granted, in the span of just 30 minutes it will be a real challenge to construct a perfectly reasoned argument in response to a complex problem, and still have time to revise, edit, and proofread. That does not mean you will be forgiven for lapsing into faulty reasoning. Your argument depends on its reasoning, so this is not something to take lightly. By getting familiar with some of the more common problems in reasoning, you can know what not to do on test day. Be sure to follow the following advice:

- **Do not overstate or exaggerate.** This is sometimes called *faulty generalization, overgeneralization, sweeping generalization,* or *hasty generalization.* Whatever you call the fallacy, do not reach a big conclusion based on too few cases. Also, do not assume that what is true in just a few or some cases is true in all cases. For example, even though the fact that some parents do not vaccinate their children is a very real problem, do not suggest that it is more widespread than it is, or that every child who is not vaccinated will develop dreaded diseases.

- **Do not narrow the possibilities in illogical ways.** This is sometimes called *either/or thinking.* For example, do not suggest that *either* we change this behavior today *or* we will have a full-scale disaster in the future. The real truth in relation to most matters is rarely so reductive or simplistic. Either/or thinking is also called the *false dilemma.* It suggests that one of two outcomes must necessarily ensue, and, sometimes, that both are negative.

- **Do not suggest illogical outcomes or illogical relationships between events.** This is sometimes called false or *faulty cause and effect.* Remember that correlation is not cause. Furthermore, just because there is an increased incidence of something in a particular group or population, it does not necessarily mean that the cause you link with that incidence is the real cause. For example, providing sex education classes for teens is not necessarily the cause of increased sexual activity among teens, even if there is a correlation in some communities.

- **Do not appeal to common sense, to "the crowd," or to tradition.** Calling upon the actions or beliefs of the common person is not a logical way to prove a point. For example, you should not buttress an argument for vaccination with a statement such as, "Everyone knows that vaccination is the right thing to do." Similarly, do not appeal to tradition by saying that because something has always been done in a certain way, it is right or just to keep doing it the same way.

ALERT

PCAT evaluators do not expect you to have expert knowledge. In an essay about vaccinations, you could mention the fact that some children contract grave illnesses when they are not vaccinated. A second fact can be that some parents refuse to vaccinate because they think there is a link between vaccination and autism. Both facts can be found in newspapers and magazine articles.

Avoid Errors in Conventions

As you should know by now, your essay score is not completely dependent on the effectiveness of your argument. You must also follow the conventions of standard English impeccably. That means avoiding the following common convention errors:

1. **Avoid sentence fragments.** A fragment can look like this: *Seeing as fragments will make your score plummet.* It can also look like this: *A poor alternative for a complete sentence.* A sentence fragment can appear to have a subject, verb, or it can appear to express a complete thought, but a sentence must have a complete subject, must have a complete verb, and must express a complete thought to be a sentence. Many sentences often need an object as well as a subject and a verb.

2. **Do not put two complete thoughts together without correct punctuation.** A common sentence error called the *comma splice* looks like this: *Put two sentences together without a period or semicolon, you will lose points.* There are three good ways to correct a comma splice: Separate the two clauses with a semicolon, turn them into two complete sentences, or add an appropriate coordinating conjunction (and, or, for, but, nor, yet, so) between the two clauses.

3. **Know the difference between *it's* and *its*.** *It's* is a contraction meaning *it is*. *Its* is a pronoun showing ownership, as in *its collar*.

4. **Know the difference between *their* and *there*.** *Their* is a possessive pronoun, as in *their house*, and *there* is a word that shows position or place or that serves as a kind of subject placeholder, as in *there is* and *there are*.

5. **Know the difference between *who's* and *whose*.** *Who's* means *who is*, and *whose* is a pronoun showing ownership, as in *whose name*.

6. **Know the difference between *then* and *than*.** *Then* is a word that shows time or sequence; *than* is a word that is used to compare. *By then, scientists knew that the first treatment was more effective than the second.*

7. **Know the difference between *effect* and *affect*.** *Effect* is usually a noun; *affect* is usually a verb. *The drug had some positive effects on the patient's mood, but it did not affect the patient's heart rate.*

8. **Never write *should of, could of, would of, might of,* or *may of*.** The correct constructions for these verb parts use *have*, as in *might have* and *could have*.

9. **Use apostrophes for singular nouns correctly.** Examples include *the study's findings, the child's condition*.

10. **Use apostrophes for plural nouns correctly.** Examples include *the girls' soccer team, the men's club*.

11. **Avoid run-ons and comma splices.** A run-on is a sentence with too many ideas and no proper link between them, such as *A major storm is heading our way be sure to cover the furniture on the patio*. This sentence lacks a proper link between the first clause (*A major storm is heading our way*) and the second (*be sure to cover the furniture on the patio*.). Using a comma alone would create a comma splice, which violates English conventions. It needs a comma and a conjunction such as *so*. This sentence should be corrected so that it reads: *A major storm is heading our way, so be sure to cover the furniture on the patio.* (A semicolon wold also work: A major storm is heading our way; be sure to cover the furniture on the patio.)

12. **Avoid vague pronoun reference**. When you use pronouns, it should always be perfectly clear to what the pronoun refers. Sometimes pronoun reference can be vague, as in this sample sentence: *After the dog sneaked up behind the cat, it pounced.* So which animal pounced: the dog or the cat? If there is more than one word to which a pronoun can refer, perhaps it is best to use a concrete noun rather than a pronoun. This sentence should be corrected so that it reads: *After the dog sneaked up behind the cat, the dog pounced.*

13. **Make sure pronouns and antecedents agree.** A pronoun must match the number or gender of its antecedent. In the sentence *My shoes have been missing ever since my dog snatched it,* the pronoun should refer to the plural antecedent *shoes,* but *it* is a singular pronoun. This sentence should be corrected so that it reads: *My shoes have been missing ever since my dog snatched them.*

14. **Choose the right pronoun case.** Make sure to use the correct case of pronouns: subjective for subjects, as in *you and I, he and I,* or *she and I, they and we,* and objective for objects, as in *between you and me* or *for her and me.*

15. **Avoid unnecessary commas.** One of the most common writing errors involves sprinkling around commas without purpose. If you place a comma in a sentence, make sure that it is serving a function in line with English conventions. Commas should not be used to set off restrictive elements, before or after the last item in a series, between the subject and verb, between a verb and object, or between a preposition and object.

16. **Place commas around nonrestrictive elements**. Forgetting to include commas can be as big of a problem as using unnecessary ones. It is common to forget to include commas around nonrestrictive phrases or clauses, which offer information that is not essential to the sentence's meaning. For example, in the sentence *Mr. Sanders, who lives down the street, is my dad's best friend,* the clause *who lives down the street* is the nonrestrictive clause and needs commas before and after it.

17. **Capitalize correctly**. Capital letters are for beginning sentences, titles, and proper nouns. If you are capitalizing for some other reason, you are capitalizing incorrectly.

18. **Punctuate quotations correctly**. Punctuating quotations can seem tricky since they can appear in sentences in so many different ways. However, the sentence punctuation should always be placed *within* the quotation marks. And if the quotation involves terminal punctuation, such as a question mark or exclamation mark, such marks take the place of a comma.

19. **Do not shift verb tense.** If you change the tense of verbs in a sentence or paragraph, there must be a reason for it, such as a shift in the timeline of events. Otherwise all verbs should be written in the same tense. For example, in the sentence, *I went to the movies, studied for my exam, and will sleep late in the morning,* the first two items in the sentence (*I went to the movies, studied for my exam*) are written in the past tense while the final item (*will sleep late in the morning*) shifts to the future tense without purpose. This sentence should be corrected so that it reads: *I went to the movies, studied for my exam, and slept late in the morning.*

20. **Don't leave out any words.** Omitting words is a common sloppy mistake. Make sure you didn't leave any words out of the sentence you intended to write.

21. **Don't forget your hyphens.** There must be a hyphen between each adjective in a compound adjective, such as *a three-year-old girl.*

FOLLOW A MODEL

Read the model 5.0-point essay that responds to the following prompt. Then read why it scored so high.

Directions: Answer the following prompt in 30 minutes, as if you were taking the actual test.

> In recent years, many parents have become skeptical of the value of vaccinations for diseases such as Influenza B (HiB), diphtheria, and whooping cough largely due to misinformation, and their refusal to vaccinate can have serious repercussions for their children. Discuss a solution to the problem of parents who refuse to vaccinate their children.

Unfortunately, some parents decide not to vaccinate their children because they have read or heard unscientific or unproven information that vaccination will cause autism or will otherwise harm their child. The solution to this terrible problem lies in proper education on the risks and benefits of vaccines; this education should be the responsibility of the patient's primary care team and be dispensed during prenatal care visits.

First, parents need to learn why vaccinations are important for their children. They need to be acquainted with the possible effects of diseases like Influenza B (HiB), diphtheria, and whooping cough. These diseases have by no means been totally eradicated. Parents need to know that, without vaccination, their son or daughter could get these diseases, and they need to learn possible effects of the diseases, such as damage to the heart or even death.

Second, parents need to learn that some misinformation from the past might have contributed wrongly to their unwillingness to vaccinate. For many years, some people labored under the misconception that there were toxic components in vaccines that were responsible for the recent rise in rates of autism. The research that led to these ideas has long since been discredited. Yet, like urban legends that continue to live on or be circulated on the Internet, this idea has hung on despite the truth of the matter. Parents need to be given the facts, and they need access to respected web sites and other authoritative materials that discredit the autism link.

Third, parents need to have opportunities to ask their own questions and receive information specific to their own questions. Health care professionals need to treat the concerns of parents-to-be with professional courtesy and respect. They should not just dismiss the concerns as unfounded. Such treatment of parents-to-be could, in fact, exacerbate the problem.

While some may suggest that the solution to the problem of parents who don't vaccinate their children is mandatory vaccination, this solution will never work in a free society. Instead, parents must be sufficiently educated to make the choice freely that vaccination is in the best interests of their child.

When parents know the true facts about vaccination—as well as the very real and horrible possibilities attendant on a choice of not vaccinating—they will be far more likely to vaccinate. Let's institute a national policy of thoughtful, careful, detailed, and respectful parent education during prenatal visits.

Why This Model Scores 5.0

This model earns a perfect score both for conventions of language and problem solving.

Introductory Paragraph

- The introductory paragraph acknowledges and provides factual background information about the problem, restating information from the prompt (some parents refuse to vaccinate their children due to misinformation) while also fleshing it out with information gleaned from outside reading (parents think vaccination can lead to autism).

- The introductory paragraph also presents a clear and unmistakable solution (*vaccination education should be the responsibility of the patient's primary care team and be dispensed during prenatal care visits*). Notice that the solution is specific and that the body paragraphs stick to this solution and explain it.

Body Paragraphs

- Each of the first three body paragraph deals with one facet of the solution: education (paragraph 2), misinformation (paragraph 3), and asking questions (paragraph 4). That facet is made clear at the beginning of each paragraph in a topic sentence.

- The transitional words *first*, *second*, and *third* set off each of the first three body paragraphs and guide the reader through the explanation in a clear, systematic way.

- Many facts (such as the diseases and their possible effects) and solutions to potential problems (such as the most effective way to deal with parents with vaccination concerns) make the writing cogent and work toward supporting the main idea that parents need better education regarding vaccination. Nothing is repeated. There are no digressions.

- The fourth paragraph discusses, and dismisses, a possible alternative solution (mandatory vaccination), which further fleshes out the essay with a relevant subtopic and a logical explanation for the writer's conclusion on this topic (mandatory vaccination *will never work in a free society*).

- The reasoning throughout the essay is logical.

Concluding Paragraph

- The conclusion summarizes the main point (*When parents know the true facts about vaccination…they will be far more likely to vaccinate*) without repeating wording.

- The conclusion ends with an appropriate call to action (*Let's institute a national policy of thoughtful, careful, detailed, and respectful parent education during prenatal visits*).

Conventions and Style

- There are no errors in sentence structure. Furthermore, the sentences are varied and fluid. Notice the variety of simple (example: *These diseases have by no means been totally eradicated.*), compound (example: *Parents need to be given the facts, and they need access to respected web sites and other authoritative materials that discredit the autism link.*), and complex sentences (example: *Parents need to know that, without vaccination, their son or daughter could get these diseases, and they need to learn possible effects of the diseases, such as damage to the heart or even death.*).

- Words are used correctly and well. There are not only appropriate transitions for mapping out the supporting paragraphs, but the writer fluidly incorporates other words and phrases, such as *in fact*, *indeed*, and *by no means* for added clarity or appropriate emphasis. Sophisticated words such as *dispensed*, *eradicated*, and *exacerbated* are also used with ease and fluency.

- The essay is persuasive; the tone is appropriately serious; the voice of the writer is clear and engaged; and the first and second person are avoided.

- There are mechanical errors.

Now read an example of an essay that responded to the same prompt but only earned a 3.0 score.

> These days a lot of parents won't vaccinate their children. This can be a real problem because vaccination prevents diseases.
>
> Why won't parents vaccinate their children? Misinformation for one. They probably heard that vaccinate is not helpful from some sources and decided not to vaccinate their children because of that. Maybe they got this information off the internet where anyone can publish anything no matter how true it is. Maybe they heard it from some celebrity who chose not to vaccinate their kids but is not a medical authority. Maybe they even read it in a book from a so-called "doctor."
>
> So let's think about why you should vaccinate; to prevent diseases. Not vaccinating can lead to diseases like Influenza B (HiB), diphtheria, and whooping cough. Children who are not vaccinated are susceptible to diseases such as these.
>
> So what is my solution? I think we should begin by making sure that all children are vaccinated no matter what. Take the choice out of the parent's hands. The government should make sure everyone is vaccinated. Then children won't be at risk.
>
> So in conclusion I think that not vaccinating your children is a terrible idea. It can lead to diseases that can be prevented with vaccination. So we should make sure everyone is vaccinated. It is up to the government.

Why This Model Score 3.0

This model earns a satisfactory score for both conventions of language and problem solving.

Introductory Paragraph

- The introductory paragraph addresses the problem in the prompt (*These days a lot of parents won't vaccinate their children. This can be a real problem because vaccination prevents diseases.*), but it does not allude to the writer's solution at all and is generally too brief and insubstantial.

Body Paragraphs

- Each of the three body paragraphs deals with a facet of the problem or solution: misinformation (paragraph 2), the benefits of vaccination (paragraph 3), and a solution to the problem (paragraph 3).

- Body paragraphs do an adequate job of referring to the main topic without any digressions, though they are all short on supporting information and reveal little knowledge outside of what was gleaned from the prompt.

- Paragraph 2 dwells too much on the source of misinformation.

- Paragraph 3 reaches a somewhat simplistic conclusion, failing to deal with the complexity of mandatory vaccines in a free society.

Concluding Paragraph

- Concluding paragraph functions as a clear end to the essay.

- Concluding paragraph does an adequate job of restating the importance of vaccination and the writer's solution. It is clear if not well stated or argued.

- The sentence *It is up to the government* is a choppy and weak way to conclude the essay.

Conventions and Style

- There are few major errors in sentence structure, although there is a fragment in paragraph 2 (*Misinformation for one.*). The essay could use more sentence variety. Writer relies too much on simple sentence structure.

- Words are generally used correctly and well. However, the writer overuses the transitional word *so*, especially when beginning new paragraphs. Vocabulary lacks sophistication.

- The essay would be more persuasive with a more consistent voice; the writer should have avoided the second person.

- There are few mechanical errors, although the writer fails to capitalize *Internet* in paragraph 2 and misuses a semicolon in paragraph 3.

- In the fifth sentence of paragraph 2, there is a lack of agreement between the singular antecedent *celebrity* and the plural pronoun *their*.

Now read an example of an essay that responded to the same prompt but only earned a 1.0 score.

So many people don't get their kids vaccinated these days. They should do this so there kids never get diseases. Without vaccination kids will probably get diseases or they could get them. This could be a serious problem and should be prevented. Right now they should think of a way to do this right now.

Why This Model Score 1.0

This model earns a low score for both conventions of language and problem solving.

Problem Solving

- This essay is woefully inadequate in terms of supporting details and problem solving.

- Essay lacks any discernible structure; there is no introductory paragraph, no body paragraphs, and no concluding paragraph.

- The writer restates the problem but makes no attempt to solve it.

- The idea that all children who are not vaccinated *will probably get diseases* is overly simplistic and unrealistic.

Conventions and Style

- Wording is repetitive (the phrase *right now* is used twice in the final sentence; the idea that failing to vaccinate can lead to disease is repeated).

- Wording is too informal (use of *kids* instead of *children*).

- Writer uses the preposition *there* when the pronoun *their* is needed.

ESSAY PROMPT

Directions: Answer the following prompt in 30 minutes, as if you were taking the actual test.

Many cities are not accommodating to alternative forms of transportation, such as bicycles. Discuss a solution to the problem of cities that rely too heavily on cars.

MODEL RESPONSES, SCORING, AND ANALYSIS

Possible 5.0 Response

Facing both increasing traffic and increasing pollution, most cities need to plan for and foster alternative forms of transportation or simply choke themselves off. To encourage more use of existing public transportation options, more walking, and more bicycling, many major cities should consider instituting a congestion free zone. A congestion free zone cordons off a portion of the central city and and it makes using private vehicles during peak traffic hours very costly. That is, it discourages drivers of private cars from using a typically congested area at typically congested times, thus creating space for walkers, bikers, and faster-moving buses.

First, to encourage alternative forms of transportation, such as bicycles, cities have to make it safer for cyclists. A congestion free zone would help accomplish this by greatly reducing the number of cars going into and out of the central city each day. Cyclists would be less wary of being hit by a car, or hit by a passenger door opened thoughtlessly into a bike lane. Cyclists would be able to navigate city streets more confidently, and perhaps even arrive at work or other destinations more quickly.

In addition, a congestion free zone would also make commuting and other travel in the city more pleasant for those not in private vehicles, such as walkers and cyclists. They would not be breathing in as much exhaust. Furthermore, with the volume of automobile traffic greatly reduced, there would also be less noise pollution. Honking horns, the sounds of motors, and the screeching of brakes would all be greatly curtailed.

Furthermore, a congestion free zone might also help change attitudes toward the automobile that are entrenched in our American way of life. People might begin to see that there is an alternative to the private car, and that cities can function, and people can get from place to place efficiently and pleasantly, without relying exclusively on their own vehicles. As such a huge change in attitude gradually takes place, more and more people might consider walking, or riding a bike, or availing themselves of public transit options. That is, while it is almost unquestioned that the "way to go" now is by private car, with the institution of a congestion free zone, it could be possible that thinking about how to travel would eventually change completely.

Instituting a congestion free zone represents the best hope for decreasing the traffic and pollution problems that plague our major cities. Who is to say that parts of New York, Chicago, and Los Angeles, to name just a few cities, could not be places where, as in Copenhagen, the majority of people ride their bikes to work, to shop, and to play?

Scoring Analysis

This essay scores 5.0 out of 5.0 for of the following reasons:

Introductory Paragraph

- The writer wastes no time in offering a solution to the problem, beginning the essay with a summary of that solution that will be fleshed out in the proceeding paragraphs. This is a strong way to begin the essay.

- Writer effectively explains a key term (*congestion free zone*) that may unfamiliar to the reader.

Body Paragraphs

- Each of the first three body paragraph deals with one facet of the solution: safety (paragraph 2), better quality of life (paragraph 3), and improved attitude (paragraph 4). That facet is made clear at the beginning of each paragraph in a clear topic sentence.

- The transitional words *first*, *In addition*, and *Furthermore* set off each of the body paragraphs and guide the reader through the explanation in a clear, systematic way.

- Many details (such as specific benefits of improved safety, life quality, and attitude) make the writing cogent and work toward supporting the main idea that a congestion free zone is a strong solution to the problem of cities that are not welcoming to alternate forms of transportation. Nothing is repeated. There are no digressions.

- The reasoning throughout the essay is logical.

Concluding Paragraph

- The conclusion ends with an appropriate call to action that also summarizes the main point (*Instituting a congestion free zone represents the best hope for decreasing the traffic and pollution problems that plague our major cities*) without repeating wording.

- Ending the essay with a provocative yet relevant question is always a strong way to conclude an essay.

Conventions and Style

There are no errors in sentence structure. Furthermore, the sentences are varied and fluid. Notice the variety of simple (example: *A congestion free zone would help accomplish this by greatly reducing the number of cars going into and out of the central city each day.*), compound (example: A congestion free zone cordons off a portion of the central city and it makes using private vehicles during peak traffic hours very costly.), and complex sentences (example: Cyclists would be able to navigate city streets more confidently, and perhaps even arrive at work or other destinations more quickly.).

- Words are used correctly and well. There are not only appropriate transitions for mapping out the supporting paragraphs, but the writer fluidly incorporates other words and phrases, such as *That is* and *Furthermore* for added clarity or appropriate emphasis. Sophisticated words such as *wary*, *curtailed*, *entrenched*, and *availing*, and are also used with ease and fluency.

- The essay is persuasive; the tone is appropriately serious; the voice of the writer is clear and engaged; and the first and second person are avoided.
- There are no mechanical errors.

Write Your Observations About the Model

_____

_____

_____

_____

_____

_____

_____

_____

_____

_____

_____

_____

_____

_____

_____

_____

Now read an example of an essay that responded to the same prompt but only earned a 3.0 score.

> For the past century or so, people have relied too much on their automobiles. We drive to the supermarket, to work, to school, even around the corner to mail a letter. Think about the affects this is having on our environment. As we know carbon imissions are big contributing factor to air pollution. This is an even bigger problem when so many people driving so many cars are crammed into a big city. I have a solution.
>
> There should be public bicycles. I know what I'm talking about because there are these kinds of bicycles in my town. Basically, they are lined up and locked up by the street. You pay a few dollars and can rent the bicycle for a few hours or the day or however long you want.
>
> Compared to the high cost of gas, using these public bicycles is very cost efficient alternative. What's more, it reduces traffic on the streets. And this is a real problem in the city. Yes special bike lanes need to be built. That is a problem that cannot be ignored.
>
> People riding on bicycles instead of driving cars reduces traffic, pollution, and costs. It is a very sensible alternative to crowding the streets with gas-guzzling cars. The big solution—every city should install these bicycles and every citizen should forget their cars and bicycle instead.

Why This Model Scores 3.0

This model earns a satisfactory score for both conventions of language and problem solving.

Introductory Paragraph

- The introductory paragraph addresses the problem in the prompt (*For the past century or so, people have relied too much on their automobiles*), but it only alludes to the solution by indicating that there is one and is generally too insubstantial.

Body Paragraphs

- The first body paragraph focuses on one facet of the solution: implementation of a public, pay bicycle system.

- The second paragraph is less focused, beginning with a discussion of cost reduction before moving to traffic reduction. The essay would be better fleshed out if each of these topics were the focus of an individual and more substantial paragraph.

- The third paragraph introduces a *problem that cannot be ignored* but fails to offer a solution to it.

Concluding Paragraph

- Concluding paragraph functions as a clear end to the essay.

- Concluding paragraph does an adequate job of restating the problems of cities without alternate forms of transportation and the writer's solution. It is clear if not well stated or argued.

- The idea that *every citizen should forget their cars and bicycle instead* is overly simplistic and unrealistic.

Conventions and Style

- There are few major errors in sentence structure, although the second sentence is a run-on because it lacks a conjunction before its final phrase. The essay could use more sentence variety.

- There is an adequate level of sentence structure variety.

- Words are generally used correctly and well, although there are some errors, as when the writer uses the verb *affects* when the noun *effects* is needed in the first paragraph.

- The vocabulary lacks sophistication. *The big solution* is a particularly unsophisticated way to introduce the concluding statement of the essay.

- *Emissions* is spelled incorrectly in paragraph 1.

- The essay would be more persuasive with a more consistent voice; the writer should have avoided the first and second person.

- There are a few mechanical errors, as when the writer mistakenly uses an em dash instead of a colon in the final paragraph.

Now read an example of an essay that responded to the same prompt but only earned a 1.0 score.

Possible 1.0 Response

> Alternative forms of transportation already exist in many big cities. Including but not limited to subways and buses. These forms of transportation being underused because people don't get to work or wherever their going fast enough when they are using them. So we need a better form of transportation. Which is going around on a bicycle. For this, though, it is necessary to build many bike lanes, riders will not be safe on city streets without them. I know because I was once on a bike and knocked over by a car, and it was very scary and dangerous. It does cost to construct bike lanes, plus you have to use space that cars need. Making crowded roads even more crowded for cars.
>
> Most people do not think that great idea to have more bike lanes as accidents go up when there are more bike lanes, bicycle riders and cars typically don't get along together on the road and that's all there is to it. It shame that its not a situation as more bike riders would reduce traffic, but there you have it. I have seen this myself while pedaling down roads in the city, it can be a total jungle and survival of the fittest out there.
>
> So, in summary, bike lanes is a solution to the problem of traffic and is an alternative form of transportation that cities need to be much more friendly too. Though it will be difficult to make these needed changes.

Why This Model Scores 1.0

This model earns a low score for both conventions of language and problem solving.

Problem Solving

- This essay is woefully inadequate in terms of supporting details and problem solving. The writer introduces only one idea to support his or her solution and does not explain it in cogent way.

- While the writer shows some insight in the idea selected for analysis, the idea is not explained and developed. The use of personal experience is not enough to support the argument by itself.

- The writer restates the problem but makes no attempt to solve it.

- The idea that all children who are not vaccinated *will probably get diseases* is overly simplistic and unrealistic.

Conventions and Style

- The essay lacks organization. The introductory paragraph veers into support for the writer's solution. There are no transitions to mark organizational development.

- The essay has poorly constructed sentences. Many sentence fragments and filler such as *but there you have it* and *So, in summary* distract from any ideas that the writer may be trying to express.

- There are numerous sentence construction errors and usage errors.

Write Your Observations About the Model

_____

_____

_____

_____

_____

_____

_____

_____

_____

_____

_____

_____

_____

_____

_____

_____

_____

TIP

Ask someone with strong writing skills to score your practice essays using the PCAT writing subtest rubric. Perhaps you can even swap essays with someone else who plans to take the PCAT and score each other's practice essays.

A WRITING STUDY PLAN

Now that you know what to expect on test day, you can start preparing for it. You'll do so by deciding upon the study plan that is most effective for you and sticking to it. In the case of the Writing subtest, the very best way to study is to practice writing essays under test-like conditions. Since this book has a number of PCAT-style sample prompts, it is an excellent place to start.

A Time-Based Plan

But let's not jump into the deep end just yet. Since the PCAT only allots you 30 minutes to plan, write, and revise your essay, you may get a bit discouraged if you try studying according to test-day conditions right from the start. Instead, allow yourself more time to start with. For your first few practice essays, try doubling your allotted time for each step in the process, like this:

1. Brainstorming: 10 minutes

2. Outlining: 4 minutes

3. Writing: 30 minutes

4. Revising: 10 minutes

5. Editing and proofreading: 4 minutes

As you get more comfortable with the time crunch, you can begin reducing the time you spend on each step of the process. However, you should make sure not to exceed the above 60-minute timeline for your first few practice prompts. While it's a good idea to give yourself a little extra time for starters, it may be counterproductive to get too comfortable with having all the time in the world to prepare, write, and revise your work.

Begin by retaking the writing subtest in the diagnostic test in this book. Now that you have a better idea of how to plan your essay and for what the test scorers are looking, you'll probably find that you write a very different essay this time around. Then you can try using the first two prompts in the previous chapters—the ones that ask you to address the problems of pollution-related deaths (page 573) and parents who refuse to vaccinate their children (page 582)—using the 60-minute schedule above.

For your next practice prompts, try reducing the doubled timeline a bit.

1. Brainstorming: 7 minutes

2. Outlining: 3 minutes

3. Writing: 20 minutes

4. Revising: 7 minutes

5. Editing and proofreading: 3 minutes

Using this new 40-minute timeline, respond to the prompts that ask you to address the problem of cities that rely too heavily on cars (page 586) and the practice prompt at the end of the next section of this book (page 611).

Finally, you will use the 30-minute timeline we laid out for you in the previous chapter to respond to each prompt in the two Writing subtests at the end of this book (pages 619 and 699). Once again, that timeline is:

1. Brainstorming: 5 minutes
2. Outlining: 3 minutes
3. Writing: 15 minutes
4. Revising: 5 minutes
5. Editing and proofreading: 2 minutes

You may complete these seven practice prompts and conclude that you still need more practice. If that's the case, circle back to the beginning and start over, using the same prompts again. Once again, you should find yourself writing very different essays than the ones you already wrote. However, you should not backtrack in terms of time. Once you start using the 30-minute schedule, stick to it for the remainder of your study sessions. After all, you're going to have to get comfortable with that limited timeline by test day.

A Skills-Based Plan

If you find that time is not an issue for you, then you may want to focus more on sharpening your basic writing skills during your study sessions. This will involve an intensive rereading of the previous chapter and this present chapter so you can re-familiarize yourself with all of the essentials of mechanics, strategy, organization, style, and structure. If you find that you are having trouble with a particular facet of essay writing, leave yourself extra study time to work out your problems. So, when rereading your essay, ask yourself questions such as:

- Is my essay clearly organized?
- Is my main idea clear?
- Did I support it well with convincing and relevant details?
- Are there an introductory paragraph, at least three body paragraphs, and a concluding paragraph?
- Did I include a thesis statement?
- Does my introductory sentence hook the reader?
- Does each paragraph have a topic sentence?
- Is my concluding sentence effectively strong?
- Did I make convincing and logical appeals to be effectively persuasive?
- Did I undermine my argument at all?
- Did I use transitional words or phrases to improve the flow of my essay?
- Is my tone consistent?
- Did I vary my sentence structures and word choices?
- Did I confuse or misuse any words?
- Is my vocabulary sufficiently advanced?
- Did I misuse any punctuation?
- Did I avoid fragments and run-ons?
- Did I make any pronoun errors?

NOTE

Once you start studying by using the 30-minute schedule, stick to it for the remainder of your study sessions since you're going to have to get comfortable with that limited timeline by test day.

- Did I capitalize correctly?
- Did I shift verb tense at all?

NOTE

If you find that both time and weak skills are issues for you, try using a blended study plan that makes room for both essay writing under strict timelines and skills sharpening.

The problem with studying for any essay test is that evaluating your work can be difficult. Ideally, you would ask a friend who happens to be a writing expert to score your practice essays, but not everyone is acquainted with such a person. If that's the case, you might want to consider hiring a writing tutor or teacher to score your essays. A more cost-saving approach is to write your essays in a word processing program and turn off any auto-correct options in the program. In other words, you want to allow yourself to make errors and be able to see those errors in your completed essay. This should alert you to problem areas that require special attention during your skills-based study plan.

You might also want to form a study group with others who are planning to take the PCAT. Then you would have a set group of people with whom you could swap essays and score each others' work.

SHARPENING YOUR WRITING SKILLS EVERY DAY

Writing is communication, and since medical professionals must communicate with colleagues and patients on a daily basis, writing is an essential skill for you to possess on test day and beyond. Therefore, it is important to not only work on your writing skills to ace the PCAT Writing subtest but to also become a more effective communicator in your everyday life. There are numerous ways you can do this.

Write Often/Write Well

NOTE

Writing short fictional stories is another way to practice writing every day.

There is no better way to become good at something than to do it a lot. In the case of sharpening your writing skills, that obviously means writing a lot. In a culture of texting, social media, and e-mailing, most of us actually do a lot of writing every day, but we often don't think too much about how we write. This might be a good time to start. The next time you compose a text message, comment, or e-mail, really think about what you are writing and write it well. Compose a message to a friend as if you were composing an essay paragraph. Make sure you use strong vocabulary, transitional words and phrases between ideas and paragraphs, vary your sentence structure, and every other element of effective writing you learned about in this book. Also be sure to write complete sentences without falling into the convenient conventions of text messaging and e-mailing. For example, it may be quick and convenient to use acronyms such as *lol*, but it isn't strong writing. For the sake of sharpening your skills, use a complete sentence such as, *That comment made me laugh out loud* to express your delight.

Start a Blog

After all this intense focus on tests and studying, writing may not seem like the ideal way to spend your free time at the moment. But believe it or not, some people really love to write and actually do it for fun. No one is forcing most of the bloggers out there to write. Bloggers do it because they enjoy writing. So start a blog about your favorite topic to get used to writing on a regular basis. Be sure to keep your Comments section open, because there are people who like to play amateur proofreader and point out the grammatical errors on others' blogs. Instead of taking such corrections as personal insults, consider them to be free advice that could actually improve your writing.

Keep a Diary

If you aren't comfortable with the idea of making your writing public, you don't have to. Keep a diary for your eyes only. Since a diary is an account of your own daily activities and thoughts, it is a great way to ensure that you write every day. Again, be sure to not cut any corners in your writing—stick to the conventions of fine writing even though no one but you will read your diary.

Read

The more informed you are, the better writer you'll be. Getting informed starts with reading everything you can get your hands on. Since you know that the prompts on the PCAT Writing subtest will deal with health, science, or social, cultural or political issues, it might be valuable to read about such contemporary issues in newspapers or magazines. You may even get lucky and read some articles that will provide you with relevant information for responding to the particular prompt you will see on test day!

Getting Confident

Are your palms getting a bit sweaty? Are you having trouble catching your breath? Is your heart pounding at the thought of writing a strong essay in only 30 minutes? Don't worry. It's natural to feel some anxiety before taking an exam. There are ways to deal with that, though. The good news is that you should already be on your way to alleviating your anxiety if you follow the advice in this chapter, because being well prepared and having a plan are effective ways of dealing with test-related stress. Here are some more tips for getting confident and keeping that anxiety at bay.

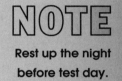

NOTE

Rest up the night before test day.

Manage Your Time

Hopefully, you've allowed yourself plenty of time to study, which should also help reduce some of that anxiety. With a manageable study program of an hour or so a night, you won't have to feel as though you are rushing to learn everything you need to know on test day.

Rest and Exercise

Be sure to keep the night before the exam free. You want to spend that night relaxing and you want to get to bed at a reasonable hour, too, so that you are well rested for test day. You may want to consider making room in your daytime schedule for exercise since it is effective in reducing any kind of stress or anxiety.

Write Away Your Cares

There's another very valuable way for dealing with any kind of anxiety: write about it! That's right—writing about the thing that makes you anxious is a good way to get your concerns out and it is also a proven way of improving test performances. Think of it as another bit of writing practice.

Use This Book!

There's something else that should make you feel confident: you've read this book! Yes, this book is full of proven strategies for navigating the PCAT successfully, and by following our advice about preparing for the test, you should feel confident in your ability to perform well on test day. We believe in you!

SUMMING IT UP

- To earn a 5.0, an essay on the PCAT must
  - be clearly and effectively persuasive.
  - be effectively organized.
  - have logical reasoning.
  - be well supported.
  - have no sentence structure problems.
  - have no usage problems.
  - have few mechanical errors.
- There is one essay prompt about health, science, or social, cultural or political issues.
- Set up a plan for writing your essays: brainstorm, organize, write, revise, and edit and proofread.
- The time limit for answering each prompt is thirty minutes. Set up a plan for using the time. One plan might allot four to five minutes for brainstorming, two minutes for organizing, fifteen minutes for writing, four to five minutes for revising, and four to five minutes for editing and proofreading.
- The most important things to keep in mind are 1) to include a clear statement of the solution; 2) to make sure the essay has a structure; 3) to present logical reasons or explanations; 4) to present support, but not filler; and 5) to write for the appropriate audience and purpose.
- Avoid questionable reasoning in the form of 1) overstatement or exaggeration, 2) narrowing possibilities in illogical ways, 3) suggesting illogical outcomes or illogical relationships between events, and 4) appealing to common sense, to "the crowd," or to tradition.
- Avoid errors in conventions that include 1) sentence fragments, 2) comma splices, 3) usage issues, and 4) mechanics issues.
- Use a time-based or skills-based study plan to prepare for the Writing subtest.
- Sharpen your writing skills every day by writing often in accordance with English conventions.
- Reduce your test anxiety by being well prepared, managing your study time, exercising, being well rested on the night before test day, and using this book.

A Quick Review of Common Errors in Grammar, Usage, and Mechanics

The conventions of language play a larger role in determining a score on the PCAT Writing subtest than they do on most other writing tests. Conventions of language refers to "sentence formation, usage, and mechanics" according to the PCAT candidate information booklet. The booklet notes that a score of 5 indicates that the writer "is in command of the conventions of language. The writer makes very few, if any, mistakes in sentence formation, usage, and mechanics. Some evidence is shown of advanced or innovative techniques." So, even with a 5, a writer may make a "very few . . . mistakes." Notwithstanding this qualifier about allowing very few mistakes, errors in grammar and mechanics, no matter how minor, can create a large problem for the reader: They can hinder the reader's understanding of your ideas. Certain errors can be so egregious they may interrupt the flow of ideas that you want to get across. They can force the reader to reread the sentence or even a couple of sentences to try to figure out what you mean.

Spelling errors can distract the reader, too, and he or she may become confused about what you are trying to say.

"A Quick Review of Common Errors in Grammar, Usage, and Mechanics" is neither extensive nor exhaustive, but focuses on those common problems with sentence construction that trip up many writers, including the best ones occasionally. This information should help you avoid some of the errors that can throw your meaning into question and detract from your analysis. It also highlights some problems with pronouns that, if consistently present, may lower your score. You won't have much time to edit your response, so concentrate on possible problems in the order that you see here:

- Comma splices
- Run-on sentences
- Sentence fragments
- Misplaced modifiers
- Pronoun problems

Errors like the ones described in these pages can make it difficult for the reader to understand your ideas, and that can affect your score.

SENTENCE FAULTS

The most important idea to take away from this section on sentence faults is that fixing these problems is not just a matter of cleaning up grammar; it's a matter of making decisions that will make it easier for your reader to understand your ideas. There are three sentence faults, or problems with sentence constructions, which you should be aware of as you write and proofread your responses. You won't have time to do much editing, so concentrate on finding and correcting these three problems first as you review your responses. They can seriously detract from the meaning of your writing and hinder the reader's understanding of your thesis.

Comma Splice

A comma splice occurs when two or more independent clauses are joined only by a comma.

> Sam decided to go back for his <u>umbrella, Jack</u> thought he would get his, too.

You can fix a comma fault 1. by separating the two clauses completely with a period, or 2. by separating them less completely with a semicolon. In the example sentence, the ideas are so closely related that a semicolon could be considered the better choice.

> Sam decided to go back for his umbrella; Jack thought he would get his, too.

Fixing a comma fault isn't just a matter of grammar; it's a matter of meaning. It's a choice that you, as the writer, need to make. Are the ideas equally important? Or, is there one idea that you want to emphasize over the other? 3. Perhaps you decide that the two ideas are equally important; in that case, use a comma *with a coordinating conjunction* to connect the two ideas/clauses:

> Sam decided to go back for his umbrella, **and** Jack thought he would get his, too.

4. If you decide that one idea is more important than the other, then you need to emphasize that idea by using a subordinating conjunction. The most important idea becomes the main clause of the new sentence, and the second idea becomes the dependent, or subordinate, clause.

> **When** Sam decided to go back for his umbrella, Jack thought he would get his, too.

Coordinating Conjunctions			
and	or	nor	yet
but	for	so	
Subordinating Conjunctions			
after	even though	since	wherever
although	how	so that	whether
as far as	if	though	while
as soon as	in case that	until	why
as if	no matter how	unless	
as though	now that	when	
because	once	whenever	
before	provided that	where	
even if	rather than	whereas	

Run-on Sentence (Also Called Comma Fault and Fused Sentence)

A run-on sentence has two or more independent clauses that are not connected by either punctuation or a conjunction.

> Sam took his wife's yellow <u>umbrella he</u> couldn't find his when he left for work.

Like comma splices, you can fix a run-on sentence 1. by separating the two clauses with a period if the ideas are equal in importance. 2. If the ideas are equal in importance and closely related, then use a semicolon between the two clauses.

> Sam took his wife's yellow umbrella; he couldn't find his when he left for work.

3. If the sentences are not equal in importance, the easiest way to correct the problem is with a subordinating conjunction.

> Sam took his wife's yellow umbrella *because* he couldn't find his when he left for work.

However, there are additional ways to solve the problem of a run-on sentence. You could use 4. a conjunctive adverb or 5. a transitional phrase. Both may require some rewriting of the original sentence.

> With a conjunctive adverb:

> Sam couldn't find his umbrella when he left for work, and *consequently,* he had his wife's yellow umbrella.

> With a transitional phrase:

> Sam couldn't find his umbrella when he left for work, and *as a result,* he had his wife's yellow umbrella.

<table>
<tr><td colspan="4" align="center">Conjunctive Adverbs</td></tr>
<tr><td>also</td><td>furthermore</td><td>moreover</td><td>similarly</td></tr>
<tr><td>anyhow</td><td>however</td><td>nevertheless</td><td>still</td></tr>
<tr><td>anyway</td><td>incidentally</td><td>next</td><td>then</td></tr>
<tr><td>besides</td><td>indeed</td><td>nonetheless</td><td>therefore</td></tr>
<tr><td>consequently</td><td>likewise</td><td>now</td><td>thus</td></tr>
<tr><td>finally</td><td>meanwhile</td><td>otherwise</td><td></td></tr>
<tr><td colspan="4" align="center">Transitional Phrases</td></tr>
<tr><td>after all</td><td>by the way</td><td colspan="2">in other words</td></tr>
<tr><td>as a consequence</td><td>even so</td><td colspan="2">in the first place, in the</td></tr>
<tr><td>as a result</td><td>for example</td><td colspan="2">second place, etc.</td></tr>
<tr><td>at any rate</td><td>in addition</td><td colspan="2">on the contrary</td></tr>
<tr><td>at the same time</td><td>in fact</td><td colspan="2">on the other hand</td></tr>
</table>

Like fixing comma splices, fixing run-on sentences is not just a matter of cleaning up a grammar problem. It's a matter of deciding what you want to say—what's important—and choosing the best solution to make your meaning clear.

Sentence Fragment

A sentence fragment is a group of words that has a period at the end, but does not express a complete thought. 1. It may have a verb form, that is, a verbal such as a participle, but that's not the same as a verb.

> Sam *carrying* a yellow umbrella to the office.

The following are possible corrections of the problem, depending on timing:

> Sam *is carrying (or carries)* a yellow umbrella to the office.
>
> Sam *was carrying* a yellow umbrella to the office.
>
> Sam *carried* a yellow umbrella to the office.

There are several types of sentence fragments in addition to the example above and several ways to correct them.

You may have 2. a subordinate clause alone:

> *Because he thought it would rain.* Sam was carrying his umbrella.

This, you could rewrite as a subordinate clause:

> ***Because he thought it would rain,*** Sam was carrying his umbrella.

You may have just 3. a phrase:

> Sam was ready for rain. *First, his umbrella and then his raincoat.*

This, you could rewrite as a sentence:

> Sam was ready for rain. ***First, he took out his umbrella and then his raincoat.***

You might have 4. a prepositional phrase like this one:

> Sam was impatient for the bus to come. *Kept looking up the street for it.*

This, you could combine and rewrite as a single new sentence:

> ***Sam, impatient for the bus to come, kept looking up the street for it.***

This last one is another example of a writer's judgment. The writer decided that being impatient was less important to the context of what the writer wanted to say than looking up the street for the bus.

Misplaced Modifier

A misplaced modifier is any word, phrase, or clause that does not refer clearly and logically to other words or phrases in the sentence. There are two problems involving misplaced modifiers.

The first occurs when a word, phrase, or clause is not close to the part of the sentence that it refers to, thus confusing the reader.

> At the bus stop, Sam didn't see the bus trying to stay dry under his umbrella.

The bus was trying to stay dry under the umbrella? Interesting mental picture, but try:

> At the bus stop, **Sam, *trying to stay dry under his umbrella,*** didn't see the bus.

The second and more important problem with misplaced modifiers occurs when a phrase introduced by a verbal, such as a participle, doesn't relate clearly to another word or phrase in the sentence. The problem is often the lack of a clear relationship between the subject of the sentence and the phrase.

In the following sentence, the true subject is missing.

> *Holding the umbrella sideways, the car* splashed him anyway.

What the writer meant to say was:

> ***Holding the umbrella sideways, Sam*** was splashed by the car anyway.

Who entered the bus in the following sentence?

> *On entering the bus, there* were no seats.

Clarify like this:

> ***On entering the bus, Sam saw*** there were no seats.

This sentence doesn't work well either:

> *Hot and tired, that* was the perfect end to a perfect day thought Sam ironically.

Rewrite the sentence like this instead:

> ***Hot and tired, Sam thought ironically that*** it was the perfect end to a perfect day.

The above examples are all simple so that you can easily see the problem and the correction. But the following example shows what can happen when a writer writes quickly to get thoughts down. See if you can spot the errors in this excerpt from an essay and then rework the excerpt to correct them.

> The arts make an important contribution to the economy of communities across the nation this is true. Even when the economy is in trouble. Governments should fund arts programs. When arts programs thrive, tax receipts flow into government coffers. It's not just the artists who make money. But people who work in allied businesses. For example, my small city has a live theater company that produces three plays a year plus has several concerts and dance programs. Having no other theater for a 75-mile radius, it brings in people from the region. These people go to dinner at local restaurants they park in a garage near the theater if they come early, they shop in local stores. All this brings in money to stores and restaurant that have to hire people to serve these theatergoers. Every sale means sales tax for the city and for the state, jobs and income taxes for the state and the federal government.

TIP

An easy way to recognize a participle is by the **-ing** ending. Not all participles end in **-ing** in English, but many do.

_____

_____

_____

_____

_____

_____

_____

_____

_____

_____

_____

A revised version might read like this:

> The arts make an important contribution to the economy of <u>communities. Across</u> the nation this is true. Even when the economy is in <u>trouble, governments</u> should fund arts programs. When arts programs thrive, tax receipts flow into government coffers. It's not just the artists who make <u>money, but </u>also people who work in allied businesses. For example, my small city has a live theater company that produces three plays a year plus has several concerts and dance programs. <u>Having no other theater for a 75-mile radius, people come to it from across the region.</u> These people go to dinner at local <u>restaurants and park </u>in a garage near the <u>theater. If</u> they come early, they shop in local stores. All this brings in money to stores and restaurant that have to hire people to serve these theatergoers. Every sale means sales tax for the city and for the <u>state and jobs </u>and income taxes for the state and the federal government.

As you can see from the examples in this rewritten excerpt, it is often necessary to rework sentences to establish the clear relationship between the misplaced word, phrase, or clause and the word it modifies. Keep this in mind as you revise your practice drafts so that on test day, you'll be able to spot problems quickly and know a range of options for correcting them.

SUBJECT-VERB AGREEMENT

The following are probably two rules that you've heard a thousand times:

- A singular subject takes a singular verb.
- A plural subject takes a plural verb.

However, the correct subject-verb agreement can still elude a writer when several words, phrases, or even a clause comes between the subject and the verb. This is especially true when the subject is singular, but a plural noun comes just before the verb, or vice versa. Such an error usually doesn't impede understanding and one or two won't hurt your score, but try for as few of these problems as possible. For example:

Sam's *umbrella* along with his briefcase and gym *shoes were* under his desk.

The correct version may sound odd to your ear, but the verb should be *was*.

Sam's **umbrella** along with his briefcase and gym shoes **was** under his desk.

In the following example, the comma after "color" should clue you in that "color" can't be the subject of the verb.

The *umbrellas*, which belonged to Sam and Jack and were a riot of color, *was* a welcome sight on the gray day.

The correct agreement is:

The **umbrellas**, which belonged to Sam and Jack and were a riot of color, **were** a welcome sight on the gray day.

Pronoun Problems

There are a variety of pronouns and a variety of problems you can get into when using them. The most common problems involve using incorrect forms, having unclear antecedents, and confusing pronouns with other words. One or two or even three mistakes with pronouns shouldn't be reflected in your score, but consistent mistakes throughout your response could. Unclear antecedents is a meaning issue; if the reader can't tell to whom or to what you're referring, it can affect the meaning of your sentences.

Unclear Antecedents for Pronouns

The antecedent is the word that the pronoun refers to, or stands in for, in the sentence. When you review your essays, check for any problems with telling to whom or to what pronouns refer.

Jack and Sam went back to their offices to get their umbrellas because it was starting to rain. They were gone for a few minutes because *theirs* were across the floor from the elevator.

A clearer version is:

Jack and Sam went back to their offices to get their umbrellas because it was starting to rain. They were gone for a few minutes because *their offices* were across the floor from the elevator.

Incorrect Forms

Is it *I* or *me, she* or *her, he* or *him, we* or *them?* Most people don't have trouble figuring out which pronoun to use when the subject of a sentence or clause is singular. The trouble comes when the subject is plural.

> *Her* and I went.
>
> *Him* and I went.
>
> We and *them* went. *Us* and *them* went.

The sentences should read:

> **She** and I went.
>
> **He** and I went.
>
> **We** and they went.

Objects of verbs and prepositions (*of, for, in, on,* etc.) are another problem area for pronoun forms.

> The umbrellas belong to him and *I*, to *he* and *I*.
>
> The umbrellas belong to her and *I*, to s*he* and *I*.
>
> The umbrellas belong to them and *I*, to *they* and *I*.

The correct forms are:

> The umbrellas belong to **him** and **me**.
>
> The umbrellas belong to **her** and **me**.
>
> The umbrellas belong to **them** and **me**.

Confusing Pronoun Forms with Other Words

You've probably heard these rules in every English/language arts class you've ever taken, but they're worth repeating because many writers still make these errors.

1. *it's* or *its*

    It's is a contraction that stands for *it is: **It's** raining. (**It is** raining.)

    Its is an adjective that modifies a noun: The dog got **its** coat wet because **it's** raining.

    An easy way to test which word you should use is to substitute *it is* in the sentence: The dog got *it is* coat wet because *it is* raining. "It is coat" doesn't make sense, so it must be "*its* coat."

2. *who's* or *whose*

    This pair of often confused words is similar to the problem—and the solution—with *it's* and *its*.

    Who's is a contraction that stands for *who is: **Who's** going to take an umbrella? (**Who is** going to take an umbrella?)

    Whose is an interrogative pronoun that shows possession: **Whose** umbrella will we take?

Like testing out *it's* and *its*, substitute *who* and *whose* into the sentence: **Who is** going to take **who is** umbrella? "Who is umbrella" doesn't make sense, so it must be "**whose** umbrella."

3.   *they're, their, or there*

They're is a contraction that stands for *they are*: **They're** going to take umbrellas. (**They are** going to take umbrellas.)

Their is an adjective that shows possession or ownership: Jack and Sam are taking **their** own umbrellas.

There is a pronoun that is used to introduce a clause or a sentence when the subject comes after the verb: **There** were no umbrellas in the closet.

Substitute *they are* in a sentence to see if the substitution makes sense: **They are** looking in **they are** desks for umbrellas. "They are desks" makes no sense, so it must be "**their** desks."

Knowing the difference between *there* and the other two forms is one that you must learn; there's no easy solution, which brings up the issue of *there's* and *theirs*.

Theirs is a personal pronoun that shows ownership: Those umbrellas are **theirs**. (The umbrellas belong to certain people.)

There's is a contraction that stands for *there is*: **There's** no umbrella in the closet. (**There is** no umbrella in the closet.)

To find the right word, substitute *there is* in the sentence. For example: **There is** one umbrella in the closet, but I doubt that it's either one of *there is*. "There is" at the end of the sentence doesn't make sense, so the missing word must be *theirs*, meaning something belonging to two or more.

A FEW ADDITIONAL WORDS OF ADVICE

The following advice belongs more to the category of good writing than grammar, usage, or mechanics, but keep these ideas in mind as you write and revise your responses:

- **Use dashes sparingly.** They often mark the work of writers who don't have a command of Standard Written English, don't know how to develop ideas clearly, or have little to say. Use dashes if you want to show a break in thought, or to emphasize an idea, for example, ". . . would be a sufficient reason—unless you are a dog owner."

- **Use active voice whenever possible.** Passive voice (the parts of the verb *to be*) can weaken your writing. Instead of "ticket sales were underwritten by a grant," try "a grant underwrote ticket sales."

- **Get rid of redundancies.** Avoid wordiness and redundancies just to fill up space. It's the quality of your thoughts that counts toward your score, not the length. Repetition and wordiness can mask a good analysis.

- **Don't use jargon and clichés.** Jargon and slang don't fit the tone and style appropriate for these essays, and clichés indicate that the writer is not a very original thinker or trying to fill up space.

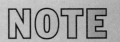

NOTE

A persuasive essay can use more than one type of rhetorical strategies.

RHETORICAL SKILLS

Once you know the basics of composing a mechanically sound sentence, it is imperative to understand how to make every sentence in your persuasive essay work toward getting your point across. After all, a persuasive essay must be thoroughly persuasive, and you can sharpen your powers of persuasion with a quick review of rhetorical skills.

Strategy

As you may recall from the Critical Reading chapter, rhetorical strategies are the methods an author uses to convince the reader of a particular position or belief. As we also discussed in that chapter, there are several basic rhetorical strategies. Here's a quick review of them along with some familiar examples:

An appeal to reason uses logic to persuade the reader.

Example: *If you go out in a storm without proper rain gear, you will get wet.*

  An emotional appeal attempts to manipulate the readers' feeling in order to win support.

Example: *You would feel terrible about yourself if you did not donate some of your pay to charity.*

  An ethical appeal affects the readers' sense of right and wrong.

Example: *It is simply unfair to gorge oneself during every meal when so many throughout the world are starving.*

  Anecdotes personalize an argument.

Example: *Only after I got cancer did I realize the absolute necessity of universal health coverage.*

  Quoting an expert can lend credence to a piece of rhetorical writing.

Example: *As renowned genius Albert Einstein said, "The world is a dangerous place to live not because of the people who are evil but because of the people who don't do anything about it."*

  Studies or other data also lend credence to a piece of rhetorical writing.

Example: *A recent study by Chicago University reveals that older people tend to be happier than those under 18.*

Organization

We discussed organization at length in the previous chapter in the section on the step-by-step process of composing an essay, so this review will be especially brief. Just remember that a well-written essay is also a well-structured one, and a well-organized essay must include the following components:

Introduction: the opening paragraph that introduces the problem and alludes to a solution or acknowledges that a solution is necessary.

Body: a minimum of three paragraphs that each focus on a different aspect of the problem or solution.

Conclusion: the final paragraph, which may provide a little new information but is mostly concerned with wrapping up the discussion and summarizing the essay's findings.

Style

There are many different kinds of writing, and although there is some flexibility, each kind of writing basically has its own style. You would not use the same friendly, informal style you'd probably use in an email to a sibling that you would use in a cover letter to a potential employer.

There are some stylistic conventions you will probably want to stick to when writing your persuasive essay on the PCAT Writing subtest.

- **Understand your audience**. In the case of the PCAT, your audience is the test scorers. The test scorers certainly do not wish you any ill will, but they are not exactly your friends either. Adopt a formal tone in your essay. Do not use slang.

- **Third person is safest**. Try to avoid the first and second person—in other words, do not refer to yourself as *I* or *me* or your reader as *you*. It lacks formality.

- **Stick to your guns**. Your argument will not be very persuasive if you can't stick to it. Do not undermine your own position by wavering on it or presenting evidence or arguments that contradict it. At the same time, make sure the evidence you use to make your point is well reasoned and logical.

- **Choose appropriate words**. Make sure that your wording is sufficiently sophisticated and that your vocabulary is not overly simplistic. However, if you choose advanced vocabulary words, be positive that you are using them correctly. If you are unsure of the meaning of a word, don't use it!

- **Select your evidence carefully**. Make sure that every sentence you write supports your main idea clearly and convincingly. The test scorers will know when you are merely padding your essay.

- **Keep the flow**. Each paragraph should have its own main idea, but it should also flow logically from the paragraph that followed it. Use transitional words and phrases such as *first of all*, *furthermore*, *next*, and *consequently* both at the beginning of paragraphs and between related ideas within paragraphs to aid the flow of your essay.

- **Mix it up**. Reusing the same words over and over or only using simple sentence not keys to composing a compelling essay. Vary your wording and your sentence structure. While revising your essay, look out for words you overuse and substitute them with fresh synonyms. If you overuse a particular sentence structure, reword your sentences for the sake of variety.

Structure

Because it has a unique job to do, persuasive writing also has particular structural elements. After all, you want to get your reader on your side and you want her or him to stay there. Try these structural techniques to build the strongest argument you can build.

- **Hook your readers**. Do not begin your essay with a blunt statement of intention. Hook your reader with an interesting anecdote, a provocative question, fascinating background details, or a thought-provoking quotation. This will make your readers want to read your essay.

- **Keep it clear**. If you are introducing a concept or term that may be unfamiliar to your readers, be sure to define it. On the same note, avoid any unnecessary technical jargon that may be unclear to your particular audience.

NOTE

Eliminate any unnecessary details from your essay during the revision phase.

- **Don't forget the thesis**. Your thesis clearly states the intention of your essay. Don't forget to include your thesis statement in your introductory paragraph.

- **Stay focused**. Each of your body paragraphs should focus on one particular idea or subtopic. If you are veering into new ideas, start a new paragraph.

- **Don't forget your topic sentences**. To help clarify the purposes of your body paragraphs, make sure each one includes a topic sentence that links back to the main thesis while also fleshing it out.

- **Don't forget the evidence**. Your own personal opinions will never be as convincing as evidence from an outside source. Be sure to support your argument with reliable, relevant evidence, and don't forget to ensure that your evidence links up with your thesis clearly.

- **End on a strong note**. The final sentence of your essay may be even more important than the first one. It is the sentence your reader will read last and remember most. End with a strong restatement of your position or even a provocative question the reader may ponder well after finishing your essay.

MODEL ESSAY PROMPT

Now let's take a look at one more sample essay to see how all of these mechanical, strategic, organizational, stylistic, and structural elements can work together to build a high-scoring essay.

In this bustling age, it can sometimes be difficult to always get a minimum of seven-hours of sleep, but it is crucial to one's health since sleep deprivation can lead to such health issues as heart disease, kidney disease, high blood pressure, diabetes, stroke, depression and risk of injury. Discuss a solution to the problem of sleep deprivation.

Work, school, eating, errands, chores, entertainment, socializing, and meetings—these are just some of the activities the modern person crams into her or his day every day. For some people, the old saying that "there just aren't enough hours in the day" really rings true. In fact, for some individuals, the daily schedule becomes so packed that there is barely time for one thing every human must do: sleep. Consequently, sleep deprivation is becoming more and more of a problem, and it can have serious repercussions on one's physical and mental health if time is not made to get proper rest.

For the exceptionally active person, sleep may seem like more of an annoyance than a necessity; it becomes a period of hours in which the things that need to get done are not being done. However, considering the very serious issues linked to sleep deprivation, sleep may be the day's most crucial activity. Sleep deprivation can lead to diseases of the heart or kidney, and it can increase blood pressure or risk of stroke or diabetes. At the most fundamental, sleep deprivation greatly increases the risk of injury for those operating machinery such as cars or power tools.

Personal health can never be lower priority than staying on task. After all, one cannot complete the day's tasks when working below his or her full physical powers. This is a key fact to impart to anyone who simply refuses to make time to get adequate rest.

It is also important to change popular attitudes regarding sleep. Too often it is stigmatized or viewed as a mark of laziness. Authority figures from bosses to teachers to parents regularly repeat tired lines such as "stop sleeping your life away" that perpetuate the stigma. Such people need to be reminded of the healthfulness of sleep as assuredly as the sleep-deprived do.

Furthermore, steps need to be made to promote a culture that truly values sleep. Managers need to shorten work hours or even make room for naps in the daily schedule. After all, science has proven that the siesta culture is actually very healthful, as a short nap after lunch is both refreshing and very good for the heart.

In the current cultural climate, it is hard to imagine an American work environment that would make room for daily naps in the schedule or even take the rest of employees seriously. That is why change must begin with education and a complete attitude about face. If everyone knew what was at stake, sleep deprivation would become a far less pervasive problem.

This essay earns it 5.0 score by:

- avoiding such common sentence problems as comma splices, run-ons, fragments, misplaced modifiers, pronoun problems, unclear antecedents, incorrect forms,

- maintaining subject-verb agreement

- appealing to reason (one cannot be sleep deprived and maintain a busy schedule since the health risks associated with sleep deprivation would prevent one from working at his or her peak powers)

- maintaining strong organization with a clear introductory paragraph, three body paragraphs, and a concluding paragraph

- maintaining a formal tone for the given audience of test scorers

- sticking to the third-person point of view

- using appropriate words and sophisticated vocabulary such as *repercussions*, *stigmatized*, and *pervasive*.

- avoiding unnecessary information

- using transitional words and phrases such as *consequently*, *however*, *at the most fundamental*, *furthermore*, and *after all*

- varying wording and sentence structure with simple (*Personal health can never be lower priority than staying on task.*), compound (*Consequently, sleep deprivation is becoming more and more of a problem, and it can have serious repercussions on one's physical and mental health if time is not made to get proper rest.*), and complex (*At the most fundamental, sleep deprivation greatly increases the risk of injury for those operating machinery such as cars or power tools.*) sentences all represented

- hooking readers with a strong and provocative opening statement (*Work, school, eating, errands, chores, entertainment, socializing, and meetings—these are just some of the activities the modern person crams into her or his day every day.*)

- presenting a clear thesis statement (*Consequently, sleep deprivation is becoming more and more of a problem, and it can have serious repercussions on one's physical and mental health if time is not made to get proper rest.*)

- focusing on a particular topic in each body paragraph: the health risks of sleep deprivation (paragraph 2), how sleep deprivation affects productivity (paragraph 3), how to change attitudes about sleep deprivation (paragraph 4), and promoting restfulness in our culture (paragraph 5)

- supporting each topic with evidence

- ending on a strong note with an urgent concluding statement (*If everyone knew what was at stake, sleep deprivation would become a far less pervasive problem.*)

Practice Prompt

OK, now it's your turn to get some practice by answering the following prompt. Be sure to respond to this prompt under test-like conditions. That means planning, writing, and revising it in 30 minutes.

Corporate culture tends to emphasize productivity above all else, but this attitude sometimes comes at the expense of employee's personal health. Discuss a solution to the problem of creating a more health-conscious environment in the work place.

Sample 5.0 response

By its very nature, corporate culture is built on the generation of revenue and the productivity of its employees. Thus long work hours, meals grabbed on the go, and constantly being on call are regular components of the corporate lifestyle. While this lifestyle may increase profits in the short run, it will inevitably have negative effects on the lives of those trapped in a culture that emphasizes financial gain over wellness and happiness in the long run. Fortunately, by being more tuned into the needs of those working in that culture, corporate life does not need to be so unhealthful.

Outings are a big part of corporate culture. Very often employees spend their hours outside of the office together and discussing work. Maybe instead of meeting up at a pub, employees can be encouraged to get together at a gym or health-food restaurant to encourage them to engage in physical fitness and well without shirking their duties.

However, there must be time for an out-of-office life that has nothing to do with work responsibilities. While it may seem antithetical to the entire corporate culture, it is valuable to encourage employees to spend their nights and weekends simply relaxing. Well-rested employees will ultimately be more productive than exhausted ones. A company-sponsored meditation retreat can also be a wonderful way to refresh employees in mind and body.

Such encouragements can find their way into an official company wellness plan. Corporations can actually offer incentives for healthful living. Paying for that outing to a healthy restaurant or gym can be an incentive in itself.

This is just a small selection of suggestions for making the work place a more healthful environment. Creative thinking and openness to employee suggestions will open up the possibilities even further. Upper management who remain skeptical of the necessities of promoting physical fitness, healthy eating, and restfulness among employees should ask themselves one key question: who will be a more productive asset to the company— the rundown employee or the physically fit one?

Sample 3.0 response

Corporations just want employees to be productive. They want employees to work all the time. Think about what this does to employee health! Without a doubt this is a very short sighted way to run a business. But there is a solution.

Corporations can start making their employees healthier by installing gyms in the office. Yes, it is a major initial expense, but think of the benefits! Employees who once went to the gym on their lunch breaks will now spend that time in the office probably talking with other employees about work business. So they will still productive during their break time while also being more physically fit than if they went to a fast food place.

Also the corporation can promote use of the gym by having official events. There can be weight lifting competitions or weight loss competitions or something. Events and competitions bring employees together and that builds strong team skills. Plus they would be in the office for these competitions and again work matters would probably get discussed.

Another reason an on-sight gym is great for an office is because sometimes people will leave work early or not want to stay late because they have to "get to the gym." With a gym actually in the office, they can never use that excuse again!

So in conclusion, the corporate environment can become a healthy environment with new gyms. It is a great solution to a serious problem.

Sample 1.0 response

These days people just work and work. It's all part of the corporate culture. This is not a culture at all it is just a way to keep people working all the time. They don't even have time to go to the gym and get some exercise. They don't even eat well. So this culture needs to be changed now. Only by altaring our lifestyles will we be better employees in the so called corporate culture in which so many of us are forced to work in.

PART VIII
TWO PRACTICE TESTS

PRACTICE TEST 2: ANSWER SHEETS

Biological Processes

1. Ⓐ Ⓑ Ⓒ Ⓓ	11. Ⓐ Ⓑ Ⓒ Ⓓ	21. Ⓐ Ⓑ Ⓒ Ⓓ	31. Ⓐ Ⓑ Ⓒ Ⓓ	40. Ⓐ Ⓑ Ⓒ Ⓓ
2. Ⓐ Ⓑ Ⓒ Ⓓ	12. Ⓐ Ⓑ Ⓒ Ⓓ	22. Ⓐ Ⓑ Ⓒ Ⓓ	32. Ⓐ Ⓑ Ⓒ Ⓓ	41. Ⓐ Ⓑ Ⓒ Ⓓ
3. Ⓐ Ⓑ Ⓒ Ⓓ	13. Ⓐ Ⓑ Ⓒ Ⓓ	23. Ⓐ Ⓑ Ⓒ Ⓓ	33. Ⓐ Ⓑ Ⓒ Ⓓ	42. Ⓐ Ⓑ Ⓒ Ⓓ
4. Ⓐ Ⓑ Ⓒ Ⓓ	14. Ⓐ Ⓑ Ⓒ Ⓓ	24. Ⓐ Ⓑ Ⓒ Ⓓ	34. Ⓐ Ⓑ Ⓒ Ⓓ	43. Ⓐ Ⓑ Ⓒ Ⓓ
5. Ⓐ Ⓑ Ⓒ Ⓓ	15. Ⓐ Ⓑ Ⓒ Ⓓ	25. Ⓐ Ⓑ Ⓒ Ⓓ	35. Ⓐ Ⓑ Ⓒ Ⓓ	44. Ⓐ Ⓑ Ⓒ Ⓓ
6. Ⓐ Ⓑ Ⓒ Ⓓ	16. Ⓐ Ⓑ Ⓒ Ⓓ	26. Ⓐ Ⓑ Ⓒ Ⓓ	36. Ⓐ Ⓑ Ⓒ Ⓓ	45. Ⓐ Ⓑ Ⓒ Ⓓ
7. Ⓐ Ⓑ Ⓒ Ⓓ	17. Ⓐ Ⓑ Ⓒ Ⓓ	27. Ⓐ Ⓑ Ⓒ Ⓓ	37. Ⓐ Ⓑ Ⓒ Ⓓ	46. Ⓐ Ⓑ Ⓒ Ⓓ
8. Ⓐ Ⓑ Ⓒ Ⓓ	18. Ⓐ Ⓑ Ⓒ Ⓓ	28. Ⓐ Ⓑ Ⓒ Ⓓ	38. Ⓐ Ⓑ Ⓒ Ⓓ	47. Ⓐ Ⓑ Ⓒ Ⓓ
9. Ⓐ Ⓑ Ⓒ Ⓓ	19. Ⓐ Ⓑ Ⓒ Ⓓ	29. Ⓐ Ⓑ Ⓒ Ⓓ	39. Ⓐ Ⓑ Ⓒ Ⓓ	48. Ⓐ Ⓑ Ⓒ Ⓓ
10. Ⓐ Ⓑ Ⓒ Ⓓ	20. Ⓐ Ⓑ Ⓒ Ⓓ	30. Ⓐ Ⓑ Ⓒ Ⓓ		

Chemical Processes

1. Ⓐ Ⓑ Ⓒ Ⓓ	11. Ⓐ Ⓑ Ⓒ Ⓓ	21. Ⓐ Ⓑ Ⓒ Ⓓ	31. Ⓐ Ⓑ Ⓒ Ⓓ	40. Ⓐ Ⓑ Ⓒ Ⓓ
2. Ⓐ Ⓑ Ⓒ Ⓓ	12. Ⓐ Ⓑ Ⓒ Ⓓ	22. Ⓐ Ⓑ Ⓒ Ⓓ	32. Ⓐ Ⓑ Ⓒ Ⓓ	41. Ⓐ Ⓑ Ⓒ Ⓓ
3. Ⓐ Ⓑ Ⓒ Ⓓ	13. Ⓐ Ⓑ Ⓒ Ⓓ	23. Ⓐ Ⓑ Ⓒ Ⓓ	33. Ⓐ Ⓑ Ⓒ Ⓓ	42. Ⓐ Ⓑ Ⓒ Ⓓ
4. Ⓐ Ⓑ Ⓒ Ⓓ	14. Ⓐ Ⓑ Ⓒ Ⓓ	24. Ⓐ Ⓑ Ⓒ Ⓓ	34. Ⓐ Ⓑ Ⓒ Ⓓ	43. Ⓐ Ⓑ Ⓒ Ⓓ
5. Ⓐ Ⓑ Ⓒ Ⓓ	15. Ⓐ Ⓑ Ⓒ Ⓓ	25. Ⓐ Ⓑ Ⓒ Ⓓ	35. Ⓐ Ⓑ Ⓒ Ⓓ	44. Ⓐ Ⓑ Ⓒ Ⓓ
6. Ⓐ Ⓑ Ⓒ Ⓓ	16. Ⓐ Ⓑ Ⓒ Ⓓ	26. Ⓐ Ⓑ Ⓒ Ⓓ	36. Ⓐ Ⓑ Ⓒ Ⓓ	45. Ⓐ Ⓑ Ⓒ Ⓓ
7. Ⓐ Ⓑ Ⓒ Ⓓ	17. Ⓐ Ⓑ Ⓒ Ⓓ	27. Ⓐ Ⓑ Ⓒ Ⓓ	37. Ⓐ Ⓑ Ⓒ Ⓓ	46. Ⓐ Ⓑ Ⓒ Ⓓ
8. Ⓐ Ⓑ Ⓒ Ⓓ	18. Ⓐ Ⓑ Ⓒ Ⓓ	28. Ⓐ Ⓑ Ⓒ Ⓓ	38. Ⓐ Ⓑ Ⓒ Ⓓ	47. Ⓐ Ⓑ Ⓒ Ⓓ
9. Ⓐ Ⓑ Ⓒ Ⓓ	19. Ⓐ Ⓑ Ⓒ Ⓓ	29. Ⓐ Ⓑ Ⓒ Ⓓ	39. Ⓐ Ⓑ Ⓒ Ⓓ	48. Ⓐ Ⓑ Ⓒ Ⓓ
10. Ⓐ Ⓑ Ⓒ Ⓓ	20. Ⓐ Ⓑ Ⓒ Ⓓ	30. Ⓐ Ⓑ Ⓒ Ⓓ		

Critical Reading

1. Ⓐ Ⓑ Ⓒ Ⓓ	11. Ⓐ Ⓑ Ⓒ Ⓓ	21. Ⓐ Ⓑ Ⓒ Ⓓ	31. Ⓐ Ⓑ Ⓒ Ⓓ	40. Ⓐ Ⓑ Ⓒ Ⓓ
2. Ⓐ Ⓑ Ⓒ Ⓓ	12. Ⓐ Ⓑ Ⓒ Ⓓ	22. Ⓐ Ⓑ Ⓒ Ⓓ	32. Ⓐ Ⓑ Ⓒ Ⓓ	41. Ⓐ Ⓑ Ⓒ Ⓓ
3. Ⓐ Ⓑ Ⓒ Ⓓ	13. Ⓐ Ⓑ Ⓒ Ⓓ	23. Ⓐ Ⓑ Ⓒ Ⓓ	33. Ⓐ Ⓑ Ⓒ Ⓓ	42. Ⓐ Ⓑ Ⓒ Ⓓ
4. Ⓐ Ⓑ Ⓒ Ⓓ	14. Ⓐ Ⓑ Ⓒ Ⓓ	24. Ⓐ Ⓑ Ⓒ Ⓓ	34. Ⓐ Ⓑ Ⓒ Ⓓ	43. Ⓐ Ⓑ Ⓒ Ⓓ
5. Ⓐ Ⓑ Ⓒ Ⓓ	15. Ⓐ Ⓑ Ⓒ Ⓓ	25. Ⓐ Ⓑ Ⓒ Ⓓ	35. Ⓐ Ⓑ Ⓒ Ⓓ	44. Ⓐ Ⓑ Ⓒ Ⓓ
6. Ⓐ Ⓑ Ⓒ Ⓓ	16. Ⓐ Ⓑ Ⓒ Ⓓ	26. Ⓐ Ⓑ Ⓒ Ⓓ	36. Ⓐ Ⓑ Ⓒ Ⓓ	45. Ⓐ Ⓑ Ⓒ Ⓓ
7. Ⓐ Ⓑ Ⓒ Ⓓ	17. Ⓐ Ⓑ Ⓒ Ⓓ	27. Ⓐ Ⓑ Ⓒ Ⓓ	37. Ⓐ Ⓑ Ⓒ Ⓓ	46. Ⓐ Ⓑ Ⓒ Ⓓ
8. Ⓐ Ⓑ Ⓒ Ⓓ	18. Ⓐ Ⓑ Ⓒ Ⓓ	28. Ⓐ Ⓑ Ⓒ Ⓓ	38. Ⓐ Ⓑ Ⓒ Ⓓ	47. Ⓐ Ⓑ Ⓒ Ⓓ
9. Ⓐ Ⓑ Ⓒ Ⓓ	19. Ⓐ Ⓑ Ⓒ Ⓓ	29. Ⓐ Ⓑ Ⓒ Ⓓ	39. Ⓐ Ⓑ Ⓒ Ⓓ	48. Ⓐ Ⓑ Ⓒ Ⓓ
10. Ⓐ Ⓑ Ⓒ Ⓓ	20. Ⓐ Ⓑ Ⓒ Ⓓ	30. Ⓐ Ⓑ Ⓒ Ⓓ		

answer sheet

Quantitative Reasoning

1. Ⓐ Ⓑ Ⓒ Ⓓ   11. Ⓐ Ⓑ Ⓒ Ⓓ   21. Ⓐ Ⓑ Ⓒ Ⓓ   31. Ⓐ Ⓑ Ⓒ Ⓓ   40. Ⓐ Ⓑ Ⓒ Ⓓ

2. Ⓐ Ⓑ Ⓒ Ⓓ   12. Ⓐ Ⓑ Ⓒ Ⓓ   22. Ⓐ Ⓑ Ⓒ Ⓓ   32. Ⓐ Ⓑ Ⓒ Ⓓ   41. Ⓐ Ⓑ Ⓒ Ⓓ

3. Ⓐ Ⓑ Ⓒ Ⓓ   13. Ⓐ Ⓑ Ⓒ Ⓓ   23. Ⓐ Ⓑ Ⓒ Ⓓ   33. Ⓐ Ⓑ Ⓒ Ⓓ   42. Ⓐ Ⓑ Ⓒ Ⓓ

4. Ⓐ Ⓑ Ⓒ Ⓓ   14. Ⓐ Ⓑ Ⓒ Ⓓ   24. Ⓐ Ⓑ Ⓒ Ⓓ   34. Ⓐ Ⓑ Ⓒ Ⓓ   43. Ⓐ Ⓑ Ⓒ Ⓓ

5. Ⓐ Ⓑ Ⓒ Ⓓ   15. Ⓐ Ⓑ Ⓒ Ⓓ   25. Ⓐ Ⓑ Ⓒ Ⓓ   35. Ⓐ Ⓑ Ⓒ Ⓓ   44. Ⓐ Ⓑ Ⓒ Ⓓ

6. Ⓐ Ⓑ Ⓒ Ⓓ   16. Ⓐ Ⓑ Ⓒ Ⓓ   26. Ⓐ Ⓑ Ⓒ Ⓓ   36. Ⓐ Ⓑ Ⓒ Ⓓ   45. Ⓐ Ⓑ Ⓒ Ⓓ

7. Ⓐ Ⓑ Ⓒ Ⓓ   17. Ⓐ Ⓑ Ⓒ Ⓓ   27. Ⓐ Ⓑ Ⓒ Ⓓ   37. Ⓐ Ⓑ Ⓒ Ⓓ   46. Ⓐ Ⓑ Ⓒ Ⓓ

8. Ⓐ Ⓑ Ⓒ Ⓓ   18. Ⓐ Ⓑ Ⓒ Ⓓ   28. Ⓐ Ⓑ Ⓒ Ⓓ   38. Ⓐ Ⓑ Ⓒ Ⓓ   47. Ⓐ Ⓑ Ⓒ Ⓓ

9. Ⓐ Ⓑ Ⓒ Ⓓ   19. Ⓐ Ⓑ Ⓒ Ⓓ   29. Ⓐ Ⓑ Ⓒ Ⓓ   39. Ⓐ Ⓑ Ⓒ Ⓓ   48. Ⓐ Ⓑ Ⓒ Ⓓ

10. Ⓐ Ⓑ Ⓒ Ⓓ   20. Ⓐ Ⓑ Ⓒ Ⓓ   30. Ⓐ Ⓑ Ⓒ Ⓓ

SECTION 1: WRITING

1 Essay • 30 Minutes

> **Directions:** Answer the following prompt in 30 minutes.

One out of every 4 children in developed countries is obese due to lack of exercise and poor diets, which can lead to health issues such as diabetes, heart disease, and asthma.

_____

_____

_____

_____

_____

_____

_____

_____

_____

_____

_____

_____

_____

_____

_____

_____

_____

_____

_____

_____

_____

practice test 2

SECTION 2: BIOLOGICAL PROCESSES

48 Items • 40 Minutes

> **Directions:** Choose the best answer for each question.

Refer to the following passage for Questions 1–7.

Proteins have a huge array of functions and are absolutely essential for the cell to function properly. They are found free or in the membrane, in cellular structures or as enzymes, and even in microbes like viruses.

1. Which of the following is a type of cellular transport that relies upon proteins in the lipid bilayer?
   A. Diffusion
   B. Osmosis
   C. Facilitated transport
   D. Protein transport

2. Through which of the following mechanisms are amino acids brought to the site of protein synthesis?
   A. Amino acids bind to the codons on a DNA strand to synthesize new proteins.
   B. mRNA delivers amino acids to the ribosomes for protein synthesis.
   C. tRNA attaches to amino acids in the cytoplasm and transports them to the ribosomes.
   D. Amino acids are stored in the ribosomes so they are ready for protein synthesis.

3. Which statement best describes what occurs after a substrate binds to an enzyme's active site?
   A. The active site remains rigid and loosely binds the substrate.
   B. The enzyme changes its shape and wraps around the substrate.
   C. The substrate changes shape to better fit in the active site.
   D. The enzyme remains bound to the substrate indefinitely.

4. On which side does a protein enter the Golgi apparatus for modification, transport, or storage?
   A. Cis face
   B. Trans face
   C. Proximal side
   D. Distal side

5. The function of a coenzyme is to transfer
   A. vitamins from one reaction to another.
   B. substrate from one reaction to another.
   C. enzymes from one reaction to another.
   D. the product from one reaction to another.

6. Antibodies recognize a small exposed portion of the antigen surface called the
   A. antigen-binding site.
   B. antibody-binding site.
   C. MHC.
   D. epitope.

7. Which portion of an mRNA strand becomes the ribosome binding site in translation?
   A. Leader region
   B. Promoter region
   C. Poly-A tail
   D. 5' cap

Refer to the following passage for Questions 8–12.

The synthesis stage of the cell cycle is absolutely essential for proper cell division because it is the stage during which all DNA in a somatic cell is replicated. The process of DNA replication occurs here via its typical mode. Accordingly, this is the stage during which sister chromatids, linked at the centromere, are generated in preparation for mitotic cell division.

8. Which is the longest phase of the cell cycle?
   A. G_1
   B. G_2
   C. S
   D. M

9. Okazaki fragments are joined together by which of the following enzymes?
   A. DNA helicase
   B. DNA primase
   C. DNA polymerase II
   D. DNA ligase

10. Which phase of the cell cycle is represented by the illustration below?

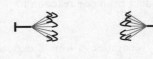

   A. Prophase
   B. Metaphase
   C. Anaphase
   D. Telophase

11. Which of the following statements best describes how viral DNA is replicated?
   A. Viruses have their own replication enzymes and proteins.
   B. Viral DNA takes over the nucleus and is replicated on its own.
   C. Viral DNA attaches to the host chromosome and is replicated with the host DNA.
   D. A virus kills the host cell and replicates on its own.

12. The regions of DNA that do not code for a specific gene are called
   A. exons.
   B. introns.
   C. promoters.
   D. initiation sites.

Refer to the following passage for Questions 13–17.

In biology, form directs function; that is, the shape and structure of organisms and their parts directly contribute to what they do. Natural selection is a well-studied example of this; structures in organisms that prove to be beneficial for organismal survival are passed along to future generations, while structures in organisms that are not beneficial disappear over time.

13. Which of the following best describes the viral shape of most plant viruses?
   A. Cylindrical or helical
   B. Complex
   C. Polyhedral
   D. Icosahedral

14. Which of the following is a good approximation of the shape and appearance of a staphylococcus?

A.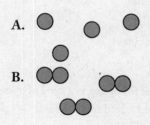

B.

C.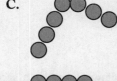

D.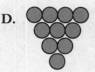

15. The tubular cell walls surrounded by plasma membrane in fungi are called
    A. mycelia.
    B. hyphae.
    C. septa.
    D. chitin.

16. Which of the following equations shows the dependence of ventilation on the pressure and volume of the thoracic cavity?
    A. $P_1V_1 = P_2V_2$
    B. $PV = nRT$
    C. $\dfrac{P_1}{V_1} = \dfrac{P_2}{V_2}$
    D. $\dfrac{P_1V_1}{T_1} = \dfrac{P_2V_2}{T_2}$

17. Two species that have similar structures with different functions are said to be
    A. homoplasies.
    B. homologies.
    C. genetically related.
    D. fossils.

Refer to the following passage for Questions 18–20.

Meiosis is the process by which haploid gametes are generated from diploid somatic cells in humans. Meiosis has two stages and produces four gametes from a single somatic cell, undergoing two nuclear divisions. With regard to zygote formation, the events of meiosis help to explain why offspring in sexual reproduction exhibit such genetic variety.

18. The idea that two alleles of a gene separate during gamete formation is expressed in the
    A. law of independent assortment.
    B. law of segregation.
    C. law of inheritance.
    D. laws of probability.

19. Which of the following describes an event that takes place during interkinesis?
    A. DNA is replicated.
    B. DNA is partially elongated.
    C. DNA is condensed.
    D. DNA chromosomes line up in the middle of the cell.

20. Recombination during meiosis occurs via crossing over, which takes places during
    A. prophase I.
    B. prophase II.
    C. metaphase I.
    D. metaphase II.

The following questions are standalone and not tied to a passage.

21. Which of the following statements about viruses is most accurate?
    A. Viruses initiate nonspecific infections.
    B. Viruses have receptors that bind to any type of cell in any type of host.
    C. Viruses have receptors that bind to any type of cell in a specific host.
    D. Viruses have receptors that recognize proteins on specific host cells.

practice test 2

22. Which of the following is the main input and output center for all sensory information?
    A. Thalamus
    B. Epithalamus
    C. Hypothalamus
    D. Midbrain

23. The two kingdoms into which the kingdom Monera has now been divided are
    A. Archaea and Fungi.
    B. Eukarya and Bacteria.
    C. Archaea and Bacteria.
    D. Bacteria and Animalia.

24. Bone flexibility is provided by which of the following components?
    A. Hydroxyapatites and calcium
    B. Bone marrow and collagen
    C. Calcium and glycoproteins
    D. Collagen and glycoproteins

25. Sexual reproduction in fungi relies upon the release of
    A. pheromones.
    B. signal transduction proteins.
    C. receptors.
    D. corticosteroids.

26. Bacteria that obtain energy from aerobic respiration in the presence of a low concentration of oxygen are called
    A. obligate aerobes.
    B. microaerophiles.
    C. aerotolerant anaerobes.
    D. facultative anaerobes.

27. Which layer of the heart is made up of contractile muscles necessary to pump blood?
    A. Myocardium
    B. Endocardium
    C. Septum
    D. Valves

28. Which type of white blood cells involved in the inflammatory response to an allergic reaction?
    A. Neutrophils
    B. Basophils
    C. Lymphocytes
    D. Eosinophils

29. Which of the following is a type of asexual reproduction carried out in yeast?
    A. Spore production
    B. Plasmogamy
    C. Budding
    D. Karyogamy

30. Which of the following acts as a second messenger in the release of the hormone gonadotropin?
    A. GTP
    B. GDP
    C. cAMP
    D. Protein kinase

31. Drastic changes in an environment that reduce the size of a population can lead to
    A. the founder effect.
    B. an increase in mutations.
    C. the bottleneck effect.
    D. Hardy-Weinberg equilibrium.

32. The observation that energy is lost to the environment in the form of thermal energy is stated in the
    A. first law of thermodynamics.
    B. second law of thermodynamics.
    C. third law of thermodynamics.
    D. zeroth law of thermodynamics.

33. Parasitic bacteria that can only survive within the cell of an animal host are called
    A. spirochetes.
    B. gram-positive bacteria.
    C. cyanobacteria.
    D. chlamydias.

34. What type of ions in the small intestine aid in the digestion of food?
    A. Sodium ions
    B. Calcium ions
    C. Magnesium ions
    D. Bicarbonate ions

35. In the urinary system, toxic substances are eliminated from the blood through the process of
    A. filtration.
    B. reabsorption.
    C. secretion.
    D. excretion.

36. Which of the following occurs during the follicular phase of the ovarian cycle?
    A. When the egg is not fertilized, the corpus luteum degenerates within about 10 days.
    B. If fertilization occurs, the corpus luteum grows, causing an increase in progesterone.
    C. LH transforms the vesicular follicle into the corpus luteum.
    D. Primary follicles with two or more layers are targeted by FSH.

37. *Streptococcus* belongs to which of the following taxonomic domains?
    A. Archaea
    B. Bacteria
    C. Eukarya
    D. Protista

38. Which of the following statements describes the function of chemiosmosis?
    A. Chemiosmosis is a phosphorylation reaction that generates ATP.
    B. Chemiosmosis is a method of transporting water across a cell membrane.
    C. Chemiosmosis transports H+ ions into the cell.
    D. Chemiosmosis is a way for cells to store ATP.

39. In which type of metabolic pathway is energy released by breaking down complex molecules into simpler molecules?
    A. Anabolic pathway
    B. Biosynthetic pathway
    C. Catabolic pathway
    D. Protein synthesis pathway

40. Which type of bonding holds together the two polynucleotide strands of a DNA molecule?
    A. Phosphodiester linkage
    B. Covalent bonds
    C. Ionic bonds
    D. Hydrogen bonds

41. Which of the following proteins in the transcription initiation complex first recognizes the TATA box on a DNA strand?
    A. RNA polymerase III
    B. TFIIA
    C. TFIIC
    D. TFIID

42. What two components are necessary for the start of the Krebs cycle?
    A. Oxygen and glucose
    B. Oxygen and pyruvate
    C. Carbon dioxide and pyruvate
    D. Oxygen and citric acid

43. Human blood types are an example of
    A. codominance.
    B. pleiotropy.
    C. epistasis.
    D. polygenic inheritance.

44. In which cellular organelle is the main function to break down fatty acids?
    A. Centrosome
    B. Golgi apparatus
    C. Peroxisomes
    D. Lysosomes

45. The order in which food passes through the digestive system is:
    A. small intestine, large intestine, and stomach.
    B. large intestine, small intestine, and stomach.
    C. stomach, large intestine, and small intestine.
    D. stomach, small intestine, and large intestine.

46. The function of alveoli is to:
    A. exchange CO2 and O2 in the lungs.
    B. filter waste products from the blood.
    C. carry oxygen-depleted blood toward the heart.
    D. connect the larynx to the lungs.

47. Which of the following organisms is a type of fungus?
    A. bacteriophage
    B. coral
    C. paramecium
    D. yeast

48. The region of a bacterium in which its genetic material can be found is called the
    A. capsule.
    B. nucleoid.
    C. nucleus.
    D. pilus.

SECTION 3: CHEMICAL PROCESSES

48 Items • 40 Minutes

Directions: Choose the best answer for each question.

Refer to the following passage for Questions 1–6.

Water is a very versatile and unique substance. Because water molecules form strong intermolecular forces called hydrogen bonds, water has a number of unique properties. Water is also polar and can dissolve many substances well. For this reason, water is widely known as the universal solvent.

1. What property of water molecules gives them their fluid property?
   A. Molecules are held close together.
   B. Molecules can move past one another.
   C. Liquid takes the shape of its container.
   D. Intermolecular forces keep the molecules in a fixed volume.

2. Which of the following is a TRUE statement about the surface tension of a liquid?
   A. Molecules on a liquid's surface do not interact with other molecules.
   B. Molecules on a liquid's surface are pushed upward by other molecules.
   C. Molecules on a liquid's surface are pulled in every direction by other molecules.
   D. Molecules on a liquid's surface are pulled downward and sideways by other molecules.

3. Which of the following statements describes what might happen if a single crystal is added to a supersaturated solution?
   A. The addition of a single crystal will increase the concentration of the dissolved solute.
   B. The addition of a single crystal of solute will cause the solute to form crystals.
   C. The addition of a single crystal will cause an exothermic reaction.
   D. The addition of a single crystal will have no effect.

4. If the specific heat of water is 4.184 J/g·°C, calculate the heat capacity of 50.0 g of water.
   A. 0.0836 J/°C
   B. 11.95 J/°C
   C. 209.2 J/°C
   D. 418.4 J/°C

5. When a weak acid and a strong base react, the overall pH of the reactant solution is
   A. 7.0.
   B. < 7.0.
   C. > 7.0.
   D. 0.

6. How much solvent must be added to 250 mL of a 0.72 M solution to get a 0.24 M solution?
   A. 250 mL
   B. 500 mL
   C. 750 mL
   D. 1,000 mL

Refer to the following passage for Questions 7–12.

One's ability to read the periodic table of elements can make for an easy and accessible understanding of chemical properties. Based on the periodic table, one can figure out the numbers of sub-atomic particles in atoms, ions, or isotopes. One can determine mass information, and based on periodic trends, one can even compare elements with one another based on physical properties. For example, comparing the electronegativities of atoms in a bond can help one to determine whether the bond is polar or nonpolar, and toward which atom electrons will tend within a bond.

7. What is the atomic mass of a mol of mercury atoms?

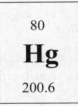

| 80 |
| **Hg** |
| 200.6 |

     A. 80 g/mol

     B. 200.6 g/mol

     C. 2.50 g/mol

     D. 120 g/mol

8. In an element with an atomic number Z = 9, how many protons and electrons does an ion with a +2 charge have?

     A. P = 9, E = 9

     B. P = 8, E = 8

     C. P = 9, E = 7

     D. P = 7, E = 9

9. In a bond between an S atom and an H atom, which statement describes the bond that forms?

     A. Polar bond with the electrons closer to the H atom

     B. Polar bond with the electrons closer to the S atom

     C. Nonpolar bond with electrons closer to the S atom

     D. Nonpolar bond with the electrons shared equally

10. Why do the noble gases have a low reactivity?

     A. They are all gases.

     B. They are nonflammable.

     C. They are in the last group of the Periodic Table.

     D. They have a full valence electron shell.

11. Which of the following statements is most accurate with respect to the energy of atomic orbitals?

     A. The energy of an orbital decreases as the distance from the nucleus increases.

     B. The energy of an orbital increases as the distance from the nucleus increases.

     C. The energy of an orbital increases as the distance from the nucleus decreases.

     D. The energy of each atomic orbital is equal.

12. Calculate the molecular mass of CO_2, given that the atomic mass of carbon is 12.01 g/mol and the atomic mass of oxygen is 16.00 g/mol.

     A. 18.01 g/mol

     B. 44.01 g/mol

     C. 3.99 g/mol

     D. 192.16 g/mol

Refer to the following passage for Questions 13–18.

The temperature at which a liquid is converted to a gas is called its boiling point. This conversion is called a phase change. Liquids have a distinct volume but not a distinct shape. In contrast, gases have neither a distinct volume nor a distinct shape.

13. Calculate the volume of 8.0 g of ammonia gas (NH_3) at standard temperature and pressure.
    A. 179.29 L
    B. 10.52 L
    C. 95.05 mL
    D. 181.67 mL

14. Which method is best used to determine the molecular formula of the gas $C_xH_yO_z$?
    A. Distillation
    B. Chromatography
    C. Combustion analysis
    D. Sublimation

15. Which of the following is the best explanation as to why alcohols have a higher boiling point than their corresponding hydrocarbons?
    A. The OH group can hydrogen bond to other molecules.
    B. The OH group binds to other hydrogen atoms on the alcohol.
    C. The OH bonds more strongly to the carbon atom.
    D. The OH group bonds weakly to carbon.

16. If a gas mixture contains 0.74 g of argon gas, 4.5 mol of neon gas, and 2.6 mol of xenon gas, and the total pressure of the mixture is 2.00 atm, what is the partial pressure of argon gas?
    A. 0.189 atm
    B. 0.74 atm
    C. 1.181 atm
    D. 2.00 atm

17. If a mixture of substances A, B, and C is separated by distillation, which substance can be isolated first if the boiling point of A is 100 °C, of B is 97 °C, and of C is 150°C?
    A. A
    B. B
    C. C
    D. They cannot be separated by distillation methods.

18. The temperature of a liquid at which its vapor pressure is equal to the external pressure is called the
    A. melting point.
    B. freezing point.
    C. boiling point.
    D. sublimation point.

The following questions are standalone and not tied to a passage.

19. In a carbonyl condensation reaction, which molecule acts like a nucleophile?
    A. Enolate ion
    B. Carbonyl group
    C. H_2O
    D. OH^-

20. The main difference between an electrolytic cell and a galvanic cell is that
    A. electrons migrate from the cathode to the anode.
    B. electrons migrate from the anode to the cathode.
    C. the redox reaction in an electrolytic cell is spontaneous.
    D. the redox reaction in an electrolytic cell is nonspontaneous.

21. In an E1 reaction, which of the following is the rate-limiting step?
    A. Loss of proton
    B. Breaking of C-H bond
    C. Nucleophilic attack
    D. Dissociation of leaving group

22. Which of the following best categorizes the compound below?

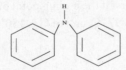

   A. Carbonyl
   B. Amine
   C. Aromatic
   D. Amide

23. Which of the following statements is TRUE according to the VSEPR model?
   A. Molecules with two electron pairs are linear.
   B. Molecules with three electron pairs form a bipyramidal structure.
   C. Molecules with four electron pairs form an octahedral.
   D. Molecules with five electron pairs form a tetrahedral.

24. A good tool for determining the functional groups of an unknown compound is
   A. UV-Vis spectroscopy.
   B. IR spectroscopy.
   C. mass spectroscopy.
   D. HPLC.

25. Which of the following is the correct classification of the molecule $CH_3COOH_2CH_3$?
   A. Aldehyde
   B. Ketone
   C. Ester
   D. Carboxylic acid

26. Which of the following is a factor that affects the rate of a reaction?
   A. An increase in temperature decreases the kinetic energy of the reactants.
   B. A reaction is independent of its medium.
   C. Catalysts inhibit reaction rates.
   D. An increase in reactant concentration increases the reaction rate.

27. Which of the following explains why a specific radio frequency is applied to molecules in NMR?
   A. The level of radio frequency depends on the size of the molecule.
   B. The level of radio frequency depends on the energy state of the atoms.
   C. The level of radio frequency depends on the type of nucleus being irradiated.
   D. The level of radio frequency depends on the magnetic moment of the instrument.

28. The last step in an esterification reaction involves
   A. the loss of a proton.
   B. the transfer of a proton from one O atom to another.
   C. activation of a carbonyl group.
   D. a nucleophilic addition reaction.

29. Which of the following is a temporary and weak intermolecular force?
   A. Dipole-dipole interaction
   B. Dispersion force
   C. Hydrogen bonding
   D. Covalent bonding

30. Which type of orbital hybridization results in the tetrahedral geometry seen in methane molecules?
   A. s
   B. sp
   C. sp^2
   D. sp^3

31. According to the rules of spin-spin splitting, how many peaks are given for a proton that has three equivalent neighboring protons?
   A. 1
   B. 2
   C. 3
   D. 4

32. On which two factors is the strength of an ionic bond dependent?
   A. Ionic radius and ionic charge
   B. Ionic radius and atomic number
   C. Ionic radius and lattice structure
   D. Ionic charge and lattice energy

33. Name the following oxacid: H_3PO_3.
   A. Phosphoric acid
   B. Phosphorous acid
   C. Hydrogen phosphate
   D. Hypophosphorous acid

34. Which of the following can be used as a mobile phase in gas chromatography?
   A. Silica gel
   B. Alumina
   C. Helium
   D. Sodium chloride

35. The release of usable energy from a chemical reaction indicates that
   A. $\Delta G = 0$
   B. $\Delta G < 0$
   C. $\Delta G > 0$
   D. ΔG is nonstandard.

36. Which of the following statements best describes the equivalence point of a titration reaction?
   A. The point at which the standard solution is first added
   B. The point at which the concentrations of unknown and standard solution are equal
   C. The point at which the acid has completely reacted with the base
   D. The point when the number of moles of H^+ is equal to 1.00

37. Which of the following statements about reaction order is TRUE?
   A. The reaction order is independent of the stoichiometric coefficient of the reactant.
   B. The reaction order can be determined by the concentration of the products.
   C. Reaction order is always defined in terms of the concentration of a given product.
   D. The rate constant is determined by the rate and the concentration of the products.

38. The link between a head group and a fatty acid in a lipid is called a(n)
   A. ester bond.
   B. glycosidic bond.
   C. peptide bond.
   D. phosphodiester bond.

39. The type of reaction that connects amino acids in a polypeptide chain is a(n)
   A. acid-base reaction.
   B. condensation reaction.
   C. hydrolysis reaction.
   D. single displacement reaction.

40. When a protein is stressed (e.g. by high temperatures), it can unfold and lose its function. Which of the following terms describes this behavior?
   A. catalysis
   B. denaturation
   C. hydrophobic effect
   D. spontaneous generation

41. Which of the following statements is true of cofactors?

    A. Cofactors are technically enzymes.

    B. Cofactors decrease the efficiency of enzymes.

    C. Cofactors change the shape of an enzyme's active site, but they bind somewhere away from the active site.

    D. The two types of cofactors are coenzymes and prosthetic groups.

42. The three parts of a nucleotide are:

    A. a glycerol, a polar head group, and a fatty acid tail.

    B. a pentose sugar, a phosphate group, and a nitrogenous base.

    C. the primary structure, the secondary structure, and the tertiary structure.

    D. mRNA, tRNA, and rRNA.

43. A double-stranded DNA molecule has a total of 100 nucleotides in its strands. Exactly 40 of those nucleotides are C. How many T nucleotides are there in the DNA molecule?

    A. 10

    B. 20

    C. 40

    D. 80

44. Examples of lipids include:

    A. fructose and sucrose.

    B. candle wax and vegetable oil.

    C. DNA polymerase and hemoglobin.

    D. DNA and RNA.

45. Enzymes are different from other catalysts because they

    A. are biomolecules.

    B. are small molecules.

    C. are not found in the human body.

    D. increase the rate of a chemical reaction.

46. A –CH2OH group is characteristic of a

    A. primary alcohol.

    B. secondary alcohol.

    C. tertiary alcohol.

    D. quaternary alcohol.

47. During DNA replication, ligase

    A. unwinds DNA.

    B. holds the separated DNA strands apart.

    C. initiates lagging strand replication.

    D. closes the gap between Okazaki fragments.

48. Organic compounds with the same chemical formula but different connectivities are

    A. stereoisomers.

    B. structural isomers.

    C. isotopes.

    D. enantiomers.

SECTION 4: CRITICAL READING

48 Items • 50 Minutes

> **Directions:** Choose the best answer for each question.

(1)   While Dmitri Mendeleev is routinely credited as the creator of the Periodic Table of the Elements, the knowledge that contributed to the construction of the table evolved over time and beautifully represents the famous words Newton penned in a letter to Robert Hooke: "If I have seen further, it is by standing on the shoulders of giants." So it was that the knowledge codified in the content and arrangement of the periodic table did not begin with Dmitri Mendeleev, nor did it end with him.

(2)   Perhaps the first contribution to the table was Aristotle's four element theory (even if his "elements," such as water, were misnamed). From that we must flash forward more than two thousand years to Antoine Lavoisier's first list of some thirty-three elements in which metals were distinguished from nonmetals. Just thirty or so years later, in 1828, Jons Jakob Berzelius developed a table of atomic weights and used letters to symbolize the elements. In 1829, Johann Dobereiner developed triads of elements, such as chlorine, bromine, and iodine; these triads were the forerunners of groups. By the 1860s, John Newlands arranged the elements in order of atomic weights and noticed similarities between the first and ninth, second and tenth, and so on. From these similarities, he developed the notion of octaves, another characteristic of the table we know today.

(3)   In 1868, both Dmitri Mendeleev and Lothar Meyer developed remarkably similar periodic tables independently of each other. Mendeleev's was published in 1869 and Meyer's in 1870. As Mendeleev wrote later, he understood that "the properties of elements are in periodic dependence upon their atomic weights." This enabled him to leave blanks for elements that had not yet been discovered, simultaneously predicting their discovery and their properties. Within less than two decades, some of Mendeleev's predictions were borne out when gallium, scandium, and germanium were all discovered between 1875 and 1886.

(4)   Progress went on after Mendeleev as, first, Lord Rayleigh discovered the element called argon and, shortly after, William Ramsay added all the noble gases to the table. By means of measurement with X-rays, Henry Moseley helped confirm earlier theories that an element's properties are more dependent on its atomic number than on its atomic weight, leading to changes in the arrangement of elements on the table. Glenn Seaborg discovered and added all the transuranic elements from 94 to 102. And, as we all know, 16 more elements have been added since.

1. Information in the passage suggests that the author views Dmitri Mendeleev as
   A. a consummate scientist.
   B. a person who did not deserve his fame.
   C. one of many people who helped develop the Periodic Table.
   D. the first person to understand John Newlands' work.

2. Which of these is NOT mentioned in the passage as a contribution to the Periodic Table?
   A. The addition of transuranic elements
   B. The shift in arrangement from atomic weight to atomic number
   C. The concept of octaves, or groups of eight
   D. The first geometric representation of the periodic law

3. The primary purpose of this passage is to
   A. bolster Dmitri Mendeleev's reputation.
   B. present a brief history of the Periodic Table.
   C. clarify misconceptions about the Periodic Table.
   D. contrast Mendeleev's contributions with those of other scientists.

4. Which word best describes the author's overall tone in the passage?
   A. Subjective
   B. Disapproving
   C. Confused
   D. Impartial

5. The first two sentences of paragraph 3 suggest that
   A. Lothar Meyer could easily have been credited as the creator of the Periodic Table.
   B. Mendeleev's contributions to the Periodic Table are overrated.
   C. Mendeleev added nothing original to the development of the Periodic Table.
   D. Meyer likely copied some of the work already developed by Mendeleev.

6. The statement about Moseley in the last paragraph suggests that Moseley
   A. originated the idea of arrangement by atomic number.
   B. did the definitive work that resulted in the table's current arrangement.
   C. was the first to understand arrangement by atomic weight.
   D. refined the ideas of periodicity by discovering new elements.

7. In paragraph 1, the author's main purpose in quoting Newton's letter to Hooke is to
   A. include two more important contributors to the Periodic Table.
   B. add support for the main thesis of the passage.
   C. introduce the idea of one scientist using the ideas of others to make progress.
   D. prepare the reader for the introduction of specific "giants" in the following paragraphs.

8. The information in the last paragraph helps to support the thesis by showing that
   A. work on the periodic table did not begin with Mendeleev.
   B. work on the periodic table did not end with Mendeleev.
   C. Mendeleev's assumption about atomic weight proved accurate.
   D. Henry Moseley deserves most of the credit for the Periodic Table in use today.

(1)   Some studies come up with findings that are hard to believe; a recent study conducted in Cork, Ireland, came up with findings that were rather difficult for me to digest. The work focused on microbes, and specifically on those tiny organisms that live in our gut and help us with digestion and the smooth functioning of our intestines. Findings from the study suggest that these microbes alter brain chemistry and could affect our state of mind.

(2)   Working with two groups of normal, healthy mice, one of which was fed a diet fortified with microbes (specifically *Lactobacillus rhamnosus,* a gut bacteria that may be found in yogurt and other dairy products) and the other group was fed an ordinary, unfortified diet, the Cork research team came up with some interesting results. When put in a maze with open and closed tunnels, the microbe munchers, or those juiced up on bacteria, tended to venture out into the open two times as often as those on the ordinary diet. It might not be reaching for me to interpret that they were more confident, willing, or adventurous than the other mice; the researchers saw such behavior as indicative of a positive mood.

(3)   In another part of the experiment, the mice were forced to swim in a container. The container was filled with water, and it was impossible for the mice to get out of the container on their own. Those with the microbe-enriched diets swam longer before they finally gave up and were rescued. (The paper's abstract says that researchers were looking at anxiety-related behavior; I guess they got it.) Researchers read these results in emotional terms, too, ascribing the behavior of the microbe eaters to a more positive <u>mood</u> than that of the mice on the ordinary diet.

(4)   Observational results were then combined with some direct measurements. One of the measurements showed that corticosterone, a stress hormone, was at a lower level in the mice with the microbe-enriched diets. Furthermore, the microbe-enriched mice had more GABA (a neurotransmitter that reduces the activity of neurons) receptors in the areas of the brain associated with emotions and memory. Other direct measurements seemed to confirm the role of bacteria in communication along what researchers call the "gut-brain axis."

(5)   Will the results in mice translate to people? Whatever your gut feelings on the matter, it may make you think twice about asking for antibiotics the next time you have an ailment that isn't necessarily bacterial. The probiotic organisms in our guts, it seems, like bacteria, and we may all end up feeling better for it. Or, minimally, should someone try to drown us, we'll perhaps swim longer before we give up.

9. Which word best describes the author's overall tone in this passage?
   A. Excited
   B. Doubtful
   C. Amused
   D. Serious

10. Which statement from the passage is an example of an opinion held by the author?
    A. "The work focused on microbes, and specifically on those tiny organisms that live in our gut and help us with digestion and the smooth functioning of our intestines."
    B. "It might not be reaching for me to say that they were more confident, willing, or adventurous than the other mice."
    C. "The container was filled with water, and it was impossible for the mice to get out of the container on their own."
    D. "Observational results were then combined with some direct measurements."

11. At the end of the passage, what does the author conclude?
    A. The results in mice are quite likely to translate to people.
    B. The findings are worthy of consideration.
    C. The findings will make us more eager to take antibiotics.
    D. The findings were elicited at too high a cost to the mice involved.

12. Which statement from the passage lends most credibility to the idea that microbes may alter brain chemistry?
    A. "Other direct measurements seemed to confirm the role of bacteria in communication along what researchers call the 'gut-brain axis.'"
    B. "One of them showed that corticosterone, a stress hormone, was at a lower level in the mice with the microbe-enriched diets."
    C. "Researchers read these results in emotional terms, too, ascribing the behavior of the microbe eaters to a more positive mood than that of the mice on the ordinary diet."
    D. "The probiotic organisms in our guts, it seems, like bacteria, and we may all end up feeling better for it."

13. What additional evidence could the author have included that would best support the main point?
    A. Examples of ways the mice were overstressed or mistreated
    B. The other direct measurements that led to the findings
    C. Specific details about the maze and its tunnels
    D. Prior research findings on the gut-brain axis

14. In paragraph 3, the word *mood* refers to a
    A. state of mind or feeling.
    B. category of verb use.
    C. state of sullenness.
    D. means of operation.

15. Which most likely states the author's opinion of the tests that the mice were subjected to?
    A. One of them appeared to be particularly cruel to the mice.
    B. Both of them elicited a persuasive amount of statistical data.
    C. The results were more persuasive than the direct measurements.
    D. One of them yielded more conclusive evidence than the other did.

16. In paragraph 2, the author suggests that labeling the mice as "confident, willing, or adventurous" on the basis of their performance in the maze may be
    A. a possibly unmerited value judgment.
    B. antithetical to the judgments made by the researchers.
    C. more accurate as a label for the behavior of the mice in the water-filled container.
    D. scientifically defensible on the basis of the experiment results.

(1)   In *The Emperor of All Maladies,* Siddhartha Mukherjee recounts several histories large and small, including the search for curative substances in general and cancer cures in specific. He begins this story with the early world of synthetic chemistry of the 1850s. According to Mukherjee, the laboratory synthesis of a dye called aniline mauve led to questions of whether synthesized chemicals could work in the treatment of disease in living organisms. Paul Ehrlich was the first to discover that not only could aniline dyes stain animal tissues, but they could do so selectively. They would bind to only some structures in the cells. As Ehrlich wondered if such discriminating binding could be the method of targeting diseased cells, the idea of chemotherapy was first conceived.

(2)   While Ehrlich was able to target specific bacteria with synthetic chemicals, the targeting of malignant human cells eluded him. Although Ehrlich had worked steadfastly for years with a vast array of synthetic chemicals, the next step in the development of chemotherapy, according to Mukherjee, occurred right after Ehrlich's death and more or less by accident when mustard gas was used as a chemical weapon during World War I. US pathologists who studied the long-term effects of nitrogen mustard found that it depleted the bone marrow; that is, it seemed to have a targeted effect on a particular kind of cell, the white blood cell. Soon, other scientists speculated on whether the properties of nitrogen mustard could be controlled and dosed to target malignant white cells. Some began specific research into chemicals that could block bacterial growth by inhibiting DNA. When researcher Gertrude Elion focused specifically on a single class of compounds called purines, 6-MP was eventually developed. When used in patients with ALL (acute lymphoblastic leukemia), it produced remissions, though they were short-lived.

(3)   Some researchers continued to seek and target synthetic chemicals, though many did so in an atmosphere of extremely negative public and private opinion. Temporary remission was initially thought to be cruel, giving hope to patients only to return them to grim reality all too soon. Moreover, any cure for cancer was widely believed impossible.

(4)   So it was that those who pioneered combination therapies did so in a general atmosphere of derision. In trial after trial beginning in the late 1950s, various combinations of cytotoxic drugs were tried on leukemia patients, many of whom were children. While the absence of regulation, particularly in human trials, helped this work go forward at a dizzying pace, it also elicited cries of inhumanity as researchers effectively used children as their petri dishes. In fact, some people at the National Cancer Institute, which was newly formed in 1937 and still in its relative institutional infancy, publicly mocked what they called the "poison of the month" approach as dedicated, dogged, and, according to some public opinion, demonic researchers scrambled to find the right combinations of chemicals in the right dosages and on the right schedule through repeated trial and error. To the considerable amazement of detractors, it was these combination therapies, and the unregulated atmosphere in which the correct chemicals, dosages, and chemicals were found, that led in 1963 to the cure for Hodgkin's lymphoma, a cancer of the immune system and, later, to effective adjuvant therapy for specific cancers.

practice test 2

17. The emperor referred to in the title of Mukherjee's book is most likely
    A. chemotherapy.
    B. cancer.
    C. nitrogen mustard.
    D. Paul Ehrlich.

18. Which of the following is the author's thesis statement?
    A. "In *The Emperor of All Maladies*, Siddhartha Mukherjee recounts several histories large and small, including the search for curative substances in general and cancer cures in specific."
    B. "According to Mukherjee, the laboratory synthesis of a dye called aniline mauve led to questions of whether synthesized chemicals could work in the treatment of disease in living organisms."
    C. "As Ehrlich wondered if such discriminating binding could be the method of targeting diseased cells, the idea of chemotherapy was first conceived."
    D. "While Ehrlich was able to target specific bacteria with synthetic chemicals, the targeting of malignant human cells eluded him."

19. The author suggests that the breakthroughs in combination therapies for cancer might not have occurred
    A. in an atmosphere of less criticism.
    B. in a time of greater regulation.
    C. in a laboratory using only synthetic chemicals.
    D. before the existence of the National Cancer Institute.

20. The author's attitude toward unregulated research often undertaken on children beginning in the late 1950s is largely
    A. critical.
    B. biased.
    C. objective.
    D. indignant.

21. How is information in paragraph 3 organized?
    A. In chronological order
    B. By main idea and details
    C. By comparison and contrast
    D. In order of cause and effect

22. According to the passage, the relationship between aniline mauve and nitrogen mustard is that
    A. both eventually were used in the development of combination therapies.
    B. both led to speculations on the use of synthetic chemicals for curing disease.
    C. the properties of aniline mauve led to the development of nitrogen mustard.
    D. the use of nitrogen mustard finally proved that chemical substances could bind selectively.

23. Which of the following is the best title for this passage?
    A. "Defeating the Emperor"
    B. "Demonic Researchers Triumph!"
    C. "The Cure for Hodgkin's Lymphoma"
    D. "Synthetic Chemicals Lead to a Cure"

24. In the context in which it appears, *derision* in paragraph 4 means
    A. scorn.
    B. contradiction.
    C. disease.
    D. hopefulness.

(1)   The bacteria *Borrelia burgdorferi* causes Lyme disease when vector ticks (*Ixodes scapularis* and *Ixodes pacificus*) that have bitten mice or deer with the disease in turn bite humans. The CDC calls Lyme disease the most commonly reported vectorborne disease in the United States, noting that 95% of all cases arise in just nine states, all of them on the East coast or in the Mid-Atlantic region except Wisconsin and Minnesota. Lyme disease is also one of the most insidious diseases as it is difficult to detect and treat.

(2)   Vector ticks in the western United States (*Ixodes pacificus*) have a much lower infection rate with *B. burgdorferi* than do vector ticks in the Northeast and Upper Midwest states with high endemicity. In "The Clinical Assessment, Treatment, and Prevention of Lyme Disease, Human Granulocytic Anaplasmosis, and Babesiosis: Clinical Practice Guidelines by the Infectious Disease Society of America," Dr. Gary P. Wormser et al. refer to research that explains this difference. The *Ixodes pacificus* ticks "feed on lizards, the blood of which is bactericidal to *B. burgdorferi*."

(3)   The most common clinical manifestation of early cutaneous infection in Lyme disease is erythema migrans. Because the bite of the *I. scapularis* may lead not only to Lyme disease, but also to HGA (human granulocytic anaplasmosis) and babesiosis, and extracutaneous manifestations can be undetectable in the early years of the disease, diagnostic laboratory testing is required for confirmation of extracutaneous Lyme disease, HGA, and babeosis. Because Lyme disease can be so challenging to detect and diagnose, those exhibiting symptoms of the disease would be foolish to fail to seek medical advice when exhibiting such symptoms.

(4)   Antimicrobial prophylaxis or serological testing after a tick bite are recommended only if the following conditions exist in concert: an adult or nymphal *I. scapularis* has been attached for more than 36 hours and that attachment is evident based either on the degree of tick engorgement or on the certainty of the time of the bite, prophylaxis begins within 72 hours of tick removal, local rates of infection with *B. burgdorferi* are greater than 20%, and there are no counterindications for doxycycline.

25. How is information in paragraph 2 organized?
    A. Order of importance
    B. Problem–solution
    C. Main idea–details
    D. Effect–cause

26. Which of the following is the author's thesis statement?
    A. "The bacteria *Borrelia burgdorferi* causes Lyme disease when vector ticks (*Ixodes scapularis* and *Ixodes pacificus*) that have bitten mice or deer with the disease in turn bite humans."
    B. "The CDC calls Lyme disease the most commonly reported vectorborne disease in the United States, noting that 95% of all cases arise in just nine states, all of them on the East coast or in the Mid-Atlantic region except Wisconsin and Minnesota."
    C. "Lyme disease is also one of the most insidious diseases as it is difficult to detect and treat."
    D. "Vector ticks in the western United States (*Ixodes pacificus*) have a much lower infection rate with *B. burgdorferi* than do vector ticks in the Northeast and Upper Midwest states with high endemicity."

27. In the last paragraph, *in concert* means
    A. while playing.
    B. together.
    C. sequentially.
    D. with certainty.

28. Which word or term from the passage reveals a connotation bias on the part of the author?
    A. Commonly (paragraph 1)
    B. Insidious (paragraph 1)
    C. High (paragraph 2)
    D. Greater (paragraph 4)

29. Which word or words from the passage reflect the author's opinion?
    A. Undetectable (paragraph 3)
    B. Foolish (paragraph 3)
    C. Recommended only (paragraph 4)
    D. Local rates (paragraph 4)

30. According to the passage, HGA and babesiosis are related to Lyme disease in that both HGA and babesiosis are
    A. caused by *Ixodes scapularis* and *Ixodes pacificus*.
    B. caused by *Ixodes scapularis*.
    C. serological tests.
    D. antimicrobial prophylaxes.

31. The author's primary purpose in this passage is to
    A. persuade readers to adopt more specific guidelines for treating Lyme disease.
    B. explain the basic causes and immediate treatments for Lyme disease.
    C. compare and contrast Lyme disease with HGA and babesiosis.
    D. present causes and effects of Lyme disease and related diseases.

32. The last paragraph suggests that doxycycline is
    A. an antimicrobial prophylaxis that is always indicated for a tick bite.
    B. a serological test that is always indicated for a tick bite.
    C. effective only if 72 or fewer hours have elapsed since the tick removal.
    D. warranted anytime a visibly engorged tick is present.

(1)   Methane, a chemical compound known as CH_4, is a colorless, odorless gas known principally today as one of the greenhouse gases. Emitted from sources both anthropogenic (such as natural gas and petroleum systems) and natural (such as wetlands), methane is best known for its role in trapping heat in the atmosphere. As if the rap sheet on methane weren't bad enough, paleoecologists are now suggesting that the rapid or explosive release of methane can trigger massive extinction events.

(2)   Such an eruption of methane is sometimes referred to as a clathrate gun. A link between methane and mass extinction is known as the clathrate gun hypothesis. (Methane is stored in structures called clathrates, crystalline solids that look like ice and may be found on seafloors.) Some believe that the Paleocene epoch came to an end because of a sudden release of methane.

(3)   Was such a rapid release of methane also responsible for the end-Triassic extinction? (This was the major extinction that left dinosaurs with little competition on land, as most vertebrate fauna were eliminated forever; thus, the rise of the dinosaurs became possible.) The preferred hypothesis for this event has until recently been that massive eruptions of volcanoes that lasted for some 600,000 years finally brought the Triassic period to an end.

(4)   Now, however, an analysis of chemical trace remains of dying plants from some 230 to 210 million years ago is showing a spike in the amount of nonbiological carbon released over a period of some 10,000 to 20,000 years. That is, of course, much shorter than the 600,000-year period that has generally been thought causative for the end-Triassic extinction. This has led to the speculation that the carbon came from a clathrate gun, which would have resulted in an exceptionally rapid warming of the climate. In fact, an analysis of sediment composition from the period yields corroborative evidence that such warming occurred.

(5)   It is quite possible that the release of methane could have been triggered by the volcanic eruptions of the period. Both the methane and volcanic theories might plausibly exist side by side. Whatever happened, the Earth warmed rapidly, if briefly, and some 70% of all land species were eliminated. If methane alone wiped out the species, a mass extinction may be substantially easier to trigger than has been previously believed.

33. According to the passage, the end-Triassic extinction
   A. was not caused by volcanoes after all.
   B. wiped out all the dinosaurs.
   C. was less devastating to species than the end of the Paleocene epoch.
   D. made the era of the dinosaurs possible.

34. Which statement from the passage is an example of an opinion held by the author?
   A. "Some believe that the Paleocene epoch came to an end because of a sudden release of methane."
   B. "Both the methane and volcanic theories might plausibly exist side by side."
   C. "Paleoecologists are now suggesting that the rapid or explosive release of methane can trigger massive extinction events."
   D. "In fact, an analysis of sediment composition from the period yields corroborative evidence that such warming occurred."

35. In the context of paragraph 1, the term *rap sheet* is used to mean
   A. list of negative effects.
   B. criminal history.
   C. syncopated evolution.
   D. chemical composition.

36. The main point of the passage is that
   A. the clathrate gun hypothesis has been proven.
   B. methane is more dangerous than people realize.
   C. methane emissions must be contained to prevent catastrophe.
   D. a sudden release of methane may have caused a mass extinction.

37. Which of these would add most credibility to the hypothesis presented in the passage?
   A. Evidence of sudden, brief change from plants and the fossil record
   B. Evidence of prolonged climate change from volcanic eruptions
   C. Evidence of methane involvement in the rise of the dinosaurs
   D. Evidence of clathrates or gas hydrates at the bottom of the ocean

38. Which of the following statements about methane is supported by the passage?

    A. Methane traps heat in the atmosphere more effectively than any other gas.

    B. The sudden eruption of methane in the atmosphere is caused by global warming.

    C. Methane triggered massive eruptions of volcanoes that caused the end-Triassic.

    D. Stores of methane are available for rapid and potentially cataclysmic release.

39. How does the term *clathrate gun* relate to the speculation that occurs in the last sentence of the final paragraph?

    A. This hypothesis would have to be disproved for the speculation to be plausible.

    B. This phenomenon would actually have to occur to make the speculation possible.

    C. This term explains the release of methane that forms a basis for the speculation.

    D. This speculation forms the basis of most mass extinction theories, of which the last line is one.

40. On the basis of paragraph 1 of the passage and the last sentence of the passage, it is possible to conclude that

    A. the sudden release theory will help to assuage worries about the impact of global warming.

    B. the sudden release theory is especially provocative in an era when people are already worried about global warming.

    C. methane is most likely relatively benign in relation to the total of all greenhouse gases.

    D. mass extinctions that are triggered by the sudden release of methane are unlikely to recur.

(1)   Enter your brain's medial temporal role and you will find a set of neurons known as the amygdala (from the Greek for "almond," the amygdala's shape). This subcortical brain structure is the seat of human (and animal) fear and pleasure responses. As such, it is often involved in self-preservation, as well as implicated in the worst of human behaviors, those unforgivable actions that can range from bad decisions in moments of stress to hurting ourselves and others. The amygdala turns on adrenaline and the adrenocorticotropic hormone (ACTH). It is linked to all responses to fear, including aggression.

(2)   The whole nervous system is responsible for the response to environmental stimuli associated with fear and stress, but the amygdala appears to be at the heart of the "flight or fight" reaction that is so often manifested in the increased rate and intensity of one's heartbeat; shakes, shivers, or tremors; sweaty palms on otherwise cold hands; and, in some cases, a feeling of being sick to one's stomach. In the presence of some of these reactions, some people simply freeze; others run; still others put up a fight.

(3)   What is it about the amygdala specifically, or the nervous system in general, that makes responses to fear so difficult to overcome or redirect? Why do they seem to overtake and control us, instead of the other way around? For one thing, such reactions may help to keep us alive. We have evolved to understand vicerally what threatens us and act in self-preserving accordance with that urgent information. That, however, is only part of the story.

(4)   According to an article published by the center for Neural Science at New York University, "[n]euroanatomists have shown that the pathways that connect the emotional processing system of fear, the amygdala,

with the thinking brain, the neocortex, are not symmetrical—the connections from the cortex to the amygdala are considerably weaker than those from the amygdala to the cortex." The article goes on to suggest that this is why, once an emotion is overtaking us, we can't seem to turn it off or get beyond it. The article adds, "The asymmetry of these connections may also help us understand why psychotherapy is often such a difficult and prolonged process—it relies on imperfect channels of communication between brain systems involved in cognition and emotion."

41. The main purpose of paragraph 3 is to
 A. answer questions related to "fight or flight."
 B. underscore our lack of knowledge about the amygdala.
 C. confirm the thesis.
 D. create a transition to current theories.

42. Which of the following statements about the amygdala is best supported by the passage?
 A. It is at the heart of the thinking brain.
 B. It will continue to play a vital role in our evolution as a species.
 C. It has an asymmetrical effect on our emotions.
 D. It is unfairly implicated in some of our worst actions.

43. In paragraph 1, the author mentions the Greek origins of the word *amygdala* in order to
 A. clarify the purpose of the passage.
 B. introduce a detail about the amygdala.
 C. introduce a main idea about the amygdala.
 D. suggest problems related to the amygdala.

44. Which of these adds the most credibility to the information presented in the passage?
 A. The Greek root explained in paragraph 1
 B. The quotation in paragraph 4
 C. The descriptions of "fight or flight" reactions in paragraph 2
 D. The questions posed in paragraph 3

45. Which word best describes the author's overall tone in the passage?
 A. Benevolent
 B. Earnest
 C. Mocking
 D. Informative

46. Which words from the passage reflect the author's opinion?
 A. *fear and pleasure* (paragraph 1)
 B. *worst* (paragraph 1)
 C. *unforgivable* (paragraph 1)
 D. *at the heart of* (paragraph 2)

47. As used in paragraph 1, the word *subcortical* means
 A. below the cortex.
 B. under the brain.
 C. throughout the brain.
 D. related to structure.

48. Which question did the neuroanatomists referred to in paragraph 4 most likely ask?
 A. What is the best type of psychotherapy for fearful people?
 B. Why are there asymmetrical connections in the human brain?
 C. How does the amygdala function in the "fight or flight" response?
 D. What is the anatomical explanation for the primacy of fear over reason?

practice test 2

SECTION 5: QUANTITATIVE REASONING

48 Items • 50 Minutes

> **Directions:** Choose the best answer for each question.

1. A financial advisor uses the function

   $$T = T(p) = \frac{5,000 - p}{0.04 p}, \quad 0 < p < 5,000,$$

   to determine the time (in years) it takes for an investment of p dollars to reach \$5,000. Which function below describes the inverse relationship, namely the amount an initial investment p should be to reach \$5,000 in T years?

   A. $p = \dfrac{0.04T}{5,000 - T}$

   B. $p = 5,000 - 0.04T$

   C. $p = \dfrac{5,000}{1 + 0.04T}$

   D. $p = \dfrac{5,000}{0.4T} + 1$

2. The distance, d, (in feet) a snow sled travels down a children's mountain slope in t seconds is described by the function $d(t) = \frac{7}{2}t + \frac{1}{2}t^2$. How long does it take the sled to travel 49 feet?

   A. 3.5 seconds

   B. 7 seconds

   C. 10.5 seconds

   D. 14 seconds

3. What is $\dfrac{\frac{1}{3} + 3}{3}$?

   A. $\dfrac{10}{9}$

   B. $\dfrac{8}{9}$

   C. $\dfrac{4}{9}$

   D. $\dfrac{1}{10}$

SHOW YOUR WORK HERE

4. What is $\lim_{x \to 1^+}\left(\dfrac{-1}{x-1}\right)$?

   A. $-\infty$

   B. -1

   C. 0

   D. ∞

5. The average age of a 17-member track-and-field team is 26 years. After one member leaves the team because of injury, the average age of the remaining members is 25.625. What is the age of the injured member of the team?

   A. 33

   B. 32

   C. 31

   D. 30

6. The average speed at which traffic moves along a highway during the morning of a typical workday is described by the following graph. Here, $t = 0$ corresponds to 6 a.m. and $t = 4$ corresponds to 10 a.m.

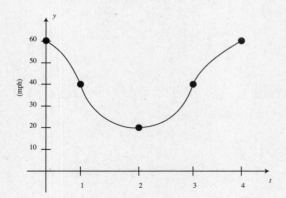

This graph represents a period of which function??

   A. $F(t) = 40\cos\left(\dfrac{\pi}{2}t\right)$

   B. $F(t) = 20\sin\left(\dfrac{\pi}{2}t\right) + 60$

   C. $F(t) = 40\sin(4t)$

   D. $F(t) = 20\cos\left(\dfrac{\pi}{2}t\right) + 40$

SHOW YOUR WORK HERE

practice test 2

7. A bookcase is comprised of 3 shelves, each of which is $2\frac{3}{4}$ feet long. You have a large collection of hard-bound classics, each of which is $1\frac{5}{8}$ inches wide. How many such books can fit into this bookcase?
   A. 20
   B. 33
   C. 60
   D. 99

8. The sponsors of the annual *Bark for Life* event are designing the route contestants and their dogs will follow through the city streets. They incorporate rest stations along the way. The distance between successive rest stations are $\frac{5}{8}$ mile, $1\frac{1}{3}$ miles, $\frac{3}{4}$ mile, and $1\frac{1}{4}$ miles. Contestants complete two laps through the course. How many miles, total, does each contestant walk?

   A. $3\frac{23}{24}$ miles

   B. $6\frac{1}{2}$ miles

   C. $7\frac{11}{12}$ miles

   D. $8\frac{1}{12}$ miles

9. Functions $f(x)$ and $g(x)$ are such that the graph of function $f(x)$ lies entirely above the x-axis and the graph of $(fg)(x)$ also lies entirely above the x-axis. Which of the following CANNOT be true?
   A. The graph of $g(x)$ lies entirely above the x-axis.
   B. The graph of $(f+g)(x)$ lies entirely above the x-axis.
   C. The graph of $\left(\frac{f}{g}\right)(x)$ lies entirely below the x-axis.
   D. The graph of $(f-g)(x)$ lies entirely below the x-axis.

SHOW YOUR WORK HERE

10. If $f(x) = \ln x$ and $g(x) = x^2$, what is the derivative of $f(g(x))$ at $x = 2$?

    A. -1

    B. $\ln 2$

    C. 1

    D. $4\ln 2 + 2$

11. Morgan needs to buy 0.6 liters of a certain liquid. If the liquid is sold in 30-milliliters vials, how many vials must he buy?

    A. 20

    B. 200

    C. 2,000

    D. 20,000

12. What is the value of $\int_{2\pi}^{2\pi} \csc x \cot x\, dx$?

    A. -1

    B. 0

    C. 1

    D. $\dfrac{\sqrt{2}}{2}$

13. The frequency table below shows the number of students who joined a particular arts club during the fall semester.

Arts Club	Frequency
Dance	6
Painting	5
Music	9
Theatre	7
Photography	8

    To the nearest integer, what percentage of the students who joined an arts club joined the painting club?

    A. 20%

    B. 17%

    C. 14%

    D. 13%

SHOW YOUR WORK HERE

SHOW YOUR WORK HERE

14. On a trip to the store, Martha bought tomatoes, cucumbers, and onions in the ratio 3:1:2. She bought nothing else on this trip. If she bought 2 cucumbers, how many items did she buy in total?
    A. 7
    B. 9
    C. 10
    D. 12

15. Which of the following is equivalent to $\log 72$?

    A. $\ln 72$
    B. $\log 144 - \log 2$
    C. $9 \log 8$
    D. $\log 12 - \log 6$

16. Carl is a collector of unique toys from the 1980s. Last year, his most valuable piece, a sealed in-box cartoon action figure, was worth $640. This year, it is now worth $720. What is the percent increase in its value?
    A. 11.1%
    B. 12.5%
    C. 40.4%
    D. 80.0%

17. A popular automobile parts vendor gathered data on the average life of 50 brands of car batteries. She summarized the data in the following box plot:

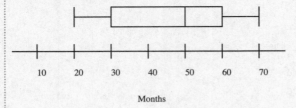

Months

Which of the following characteristics of the data set can be determined from this graph?
    A. Median only
    B. Mean and range
    C. Median and range
    D. Mean and standard deviation

18. What is the value of

$$\lim_{x\to\infty}\left(\frac{-3x^3+2x^2-x}{2}\right)?$$

A. $-\infty$

B. $-\dfrac{3}{2}$

C. 0

D. ∞

SHOW YOUR WORK HERE

19. The total resistance R_T (measured in ohms) in a circuit comprised of three parallel branches—1, 2, and 3—with resistance R_1, R_2, and R_3, respectively, is given by the formula

$$\frac{1}{R_T}=\frac{1}{R_1}+\frac{1}{R_2}+\frac{1}{R_3}.$$

If the total resistance is 25 ohms, the resistance emitted by branch 1 is 200 ohms, and the resistance emitted by branch 3 is 100 ohms, what is the resistance emitted by branch 2?

A. 30 ohms

B. 40 ohms

C. 50 ohms

D. 75 ohms

20. What is the slope of a line tangent to the function $f(x)=\cos(2x)$ at $x=\dfrac{\pi}{2}$?

A. -2

B. 0

C. 1

D. 2

21. Mary bought a figurine for $50.00. A few years later, she sold it to her cousin Michael for $40.00. Michael then sold the figurine to a collector friend for 50% more than he paid to buy it. What percentage of Mary's purchase price was the price for which Michael sold the figurine?

A. 120%

B. 60%

C. 40%

D. 20%

22. The mid-level difficulty slope at a ski lodge has a 35° slope and is $\frac{1}{2}$ mile high. The chair lift starts at the base of the mountain and travels to the peak along the slope. How many feet long is the cable along which the chairs on the chair lift move?

   A. $\dfrac{2,640}{\cos(35°)}$ feet

   B. $2,640\cos(35°)$ feet

   C. $\dfrac{2,640}{\cos(55°)}$ feet

   D. $\dfrac{2,640}{\sin(35°)}$ feet

23. A local kennel keeps track of the duration (in days) that a new rescue puppy is in their care prior to being adopted. A sample of these times (in days) from the most recent batch is as follows:

   1   4   4   8   2   1   1   5   4   6   10

   1   2   3   12   6   8

   What is the median number of days a puppy is in their care?

   A. 1
   B. 4
   C. 5
   D. 12

24. What is the value of $\int xe^x dx$ when integration by parts is used?

   A. $xe^x + c$

   B. $\dfrac{x^2}{2}e^x + xe^x + c$

   C. $xe^x - e^x + c$

   D. $xe^x + e^x + c$

SHOW YOUR WORK HERE

25. Melissa is a freelance consultant. In 2011, she had four clients in New York, two in New Jersey, and six in Pennsylvania. If *a* represents the average fee she earns in New York, *b* represents the average fee she earns in New Jersey, and *c* represents the average fee she earns in Pennsylvania, which of the following represents the average fee she earns in all three states?

   A. $\frac{1}{3}a + \frac{1}{6}b + \frac{1}{2}c$

   B. $\frac{1}{4}a + \frac{1}{6}b + \frac{1}{2}c$

   C. $\frac{2}{5}a + \frac{1}{5}b + \frac{3}{5}c$

   D. $4a + 2b + 6c$

26. During the testing phase at an aerospace company, engineers put a model of a helicopter rotor with 4 blades into a wind tunnel and rotate it at a rotational speed of 490 revolutions per minute. If 1 revolution = 2π radians, what is the speed in *radians per hour*?

   A. $(490 \times 2\pi)$ radians per hour

   B. $\dfrac{490 \times 2\pi}{60}$ radians per hour

   C. $\dfrac{490}{2\pi \times 60}$ radians per hour

   D. $(490 \times 60 \times 2\pi)$ radians per hour

27. A chemical solution consists of 1 part liquid A and 3 parts liquid B. If a third liquid is added, doubling the total volume of the solution, what percent of the new solution does liquid B represent?

   A. 12.5%

   B. 37.5%

   C. 45%

   D. 60%

SHOW YOUR WORK HERE

28. The thickness of an expansion joint on a massive bridge is a linear function of the temperature of the above paved roadway. When the temperature of the roadway is $100°F$, the thickness of the joint is 0.8 inch, and when the temperature is $20°F$, the thickness of the joint is 1.2 inches. What is the thickness of the joint when the temperature is $70°F$?

A. 0.85 inch

B. 0.90 inch

C. 0.95 inch

D. 1.05 inches

29. What is $\log_{1,000} 100$ equal to?

A. $\frac{2}{3}$

B. $\frac{3}{2}$

C. 2

D. 10

30. What is the approximate area bounded by the graph of the function $f(x) = 8 - x^3$ and the x-axis over the interval $[0,2]$, when the left Riemann sum with four subintervals is used?

A. 8

B. 9.75

C. 12

D. 13.75

31. Based on the box plot below, what is the range of the data set?

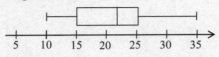

A. 10

B. 22

C. 25

D. 35

SHOW YOUR WORK HERE

32. The graph below shows the probabilities that it will rain in four cities on a given day. A company has offices in each of these four cities. If a job applicant who is asked to interview for the company on that particular day is equally likely to be asked to go to any of these cities for the interview, what is the probability that it will rain in the city in which she interviews?

SHOW YOUR WORK HERE

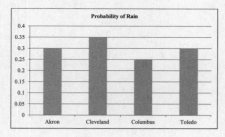

- **A.** 0.25
- **B.** 0.3
- **C.** 0.35
- **D.** 0.5

33. Tsunamis are a growing concern for coastal regions. Scientists can calculate the speed, s, at which a tsunami travels through the ocean based on the depth, d, of the ocean. In turn, this information can be used to predict when the wave will reach shore. The formula for the speed is $s = \sqrt{9.8\,d}$, where the speed is measured in meters per second and the depth d is measured in meters. For what range of ocean depths is the speed of the tsunami between 80 meters per second and 100 meters per second?

- **A.** 653 meters to 1,020 meters
- **B.** 67 meters to 104 meters
- **C.** 2,044 meters to 3,194 meters
- **D.** 6,400 meters to 10,000 meters

34. If $\log_2 x = y$, what is $\log_2 4x$?

    A. $2y$

    B. $4y$

    C. $2 + y$

    D. $2 - y$

35. Which of the following is equivalent to $\dfrac{6}{5,000}$?

    A. 0.0012

    B. 0.012

    C. 0.12

    D. 1.2

36. What is the value of y, if $-y + 3 = 2x$ and $x - 4 + y = 0$?

    A. -1

    B. $-\dfrac{1}{3}$

    C. $\dfrac{11}{3}$

    D. 5

37. The value of an account after t years in which \$5,000 is initially invested and for which interest is compounded continuously at a rate of 6% is given by the function $A(t) = 5,000e^{0.06t}$. After how many years will the account be worth \$11,000?

    A. $\ln\left(\dfrac{11}{5} \times \dfrac{50}{3}\right)$ years

    B. $\ln\left(\dfrac{11}{5}\right)^{\frac{50}{3}}$ years

    C. $\dfrac{3}{50} \times \ln\left(\dfrac{11}{5}\right)$ years

    D. $\ln\left(\dfrac{5}{11}\right) + \dfrac{50}{3}$ years

SHOW YOUR WORK HERE

38. Mark scored an 87 on his fourth chemistry test, raising his average to 83. If on his first two tests he received scores of 76 and 86, what was his score on the third test?

A. 81

B. 83

C. 85

D. 87

39. A pharmacist needs 120 liters of 40% alcohol solution. She has containers of 25% solution and of 70% solution in the storage cabinet. Which system below can be used to determine the number of liters of each solution she must use to produce 120 liters of 40% solution?

A. $\begin{cases} x + y = 40 \\ 0.25x + 0.70y = 144 \end{cases}$

B. $\begin{cases} x + y = 120 \\ 25x + 70y = 4,800 \end{cases}$

C. $\begin{cases} 25x + 70y = 120 \\ x + y = 48 \end{cases}$

D. $\begin{cases} x + y = 120 \\ 25x + 70y = 48 \end{cases}$

SHOW YOUR WORK HERE

practice test 2

40. Which of the following is the graph of $f(x)$ $= -x^2 + x + 3$?

SHOW YOUR WORK HERE

A.

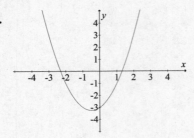

B.

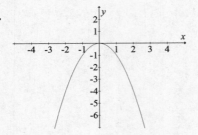

C.

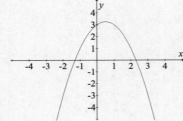

D.

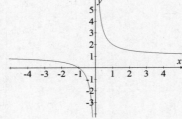

41. A family owns two doggie day care facilities. The profit (in thousands of dollars), $P1(t)$, of one facility is described by $P_1(t) = 290 - 3t - \frac{1}{2}t^2$, and the profit, $P_2(t)$, of the second facility is described by $P_2(t) = 381 - \frac{2}{5}t$. Both functions are defined for t = 0, 1, 2, 3, and 4, where t = 0 corresponds to 2013. Which function represents the total profit earned in year t by both facilities?

A. $\left(P_1 \cdot P_2\right)(t)$

B. $\left(P_1 + P_2\right)(t)$

C. $\left(P_2 \circ P_1\right)(t)$

D. $\left(P_2 - P_1\right)(t)$

42. What is the solution set of $\sqrt{2x+3} < 5$?

A. $x \geq -\frac{3}{2}$

B. $x < 11$

C. $x < -\frac{3}{2}$ or $x > 11$

D. $-\frac{3}{2} \leq x < 11$

43. The manufacturer's recommended tire pressure for your vehicle is 30 pounds per square inch (psi). What is the equivalent measurement in *ounces per square foot*?

A. $(30 \times 16 \times 144)$ ounces per square foot

B. $\dfrac{30}{16 \times 144}$ ounces per square foot

C. $\dfrac{30}{144}$ ounces per square foot

D. $\dfrac{30 \times 144}{16}$ ounces per square foot

SHOW YOUR WORK HERE

practice test 2

44. What is the solution set of the inequality $x^2 + 3x > -2$?

    A. $(-\infty, -2) \cup (-1, \infty)$

    B. $(-\infty, -2)$

    C. $(-1, \infty)$

    D. $(-2, -1)$

45. An online survey from a cable television provider asks customers to indicate the average number of hour-long prime-time television shows they regularly watch, in total, Monday through Friday. The data is summarized in the below table:

Number of television shows	Number of customers
0	1
1	8
2	15
3	40
4	21
5	15
6	30
7	18
8	2

What is the median and range of this data set?

    A. The median is 4 and range is 8.

    B. The median is 3 and range is 8.

    C. The median is 4 and range is 7.

    D. The median is 3 and range is 1.

46. What is $1.2 \times 10^{-2} + 1.2 \times 10^{-1} + 1.2$?

    A. 13.32

    B. 1.332

    C. 0.1332

    D. 0.01332

SHOW YOUR WORK HERE

47. What is the x-intercept of the function $f(x) = e^{5x} + 2$?

A. 0

B. $\dfrac{\ln 2}{5}$

C. 3

D. This function does not have an x-intercept.

48. The university administration is performing a 10-year self-study. As part of this study, they categorize faculty members based on gender and number of years of service to the university. This data is summarized in the below table:

Number of Years of Service	Female	Male
Less than 5	9	10
Less than 10 and at least 5	6	9
Less than 20 and at least 10	18	30
Less than 30 and at least 20	10	8
At least 30	3	7

What is the probability that a faculty member, chosen randomly from this group, has given at least 20 years of service to the university?

A. $\dfrac{9}{55}$

B. $\dfrac{38}{55}$

C. $\dfrac{3}{22}$

D. $\dfrac{14}{55}$

SHOW YOUR WORK HERE

practice test 2

ANSWER KEYS AND EXPLANATIONS

Section I: Writing

Sample of a Superior Response

The problem of childhood obesity not only diminishes the joy of childhood, but it also threatens the lives and safety of America's children and dramatically challenges our health-care system. To solve this problem, we must work through our schools to promote healthy lifestyles, reduce unhealthful food choices, and change attitudes.

To promote healthy lifestyles, schools have to teach the facts about, as well as incorporate, reward, and encourage, activity and exercise. Stretching, running in place, and other simple activities can be incorporated into any downtime during the school day: from unused homeroom minutes to times of day when some students are waiting for others to line up, fill an auditorium, or pass out of the cafeteria. Students need to learn why such exercise is fundamental to their health and need to be encouraged to incorporate it into their lives. They also need to learn to prefer active leisure, such as walking and playing a sport, to inactive leisure, such as television and social networking. Teachers need to model activity and participate in stretching, running in place, and so on. Teachers and administrators also need to introduce the concept to parents and encourage them to model the same.

Schools also need to teach and model the facts about high-calorie foods and empty calories. They can begin doing this by removing all high-fat, empty-calorie, and other unhealthful choices from their cafeteria menus, from school parties, from vending machines, and from snack time. This includes removing all sugary sweets, all white bread, all deep-fried foods, and all drinks with empty calories, including those that have labels that suggest that they are healthful when they are not. All sodas and high-fructose juice drinks should be replaced with a choice between water and low-fat milk. Birthdays can be celebrated with fun and games, not cake. Recess can be a time to drink water and to eat fruit, not pull out the supposedly healthy packaged "bar," which is filled with calories. Even fruit eating should be restricted to those actually feeling hunger; let's end the actions of eating just because it's time to eat, especially in those cases where it is known that children have come to school after eating breakfast.

We must also change attitudes. In much of the press today, there is an "it's okay" attitude about people who are overweight, even grossly overweight. The truth is, however, that it's not okay, and that obesity ruins lives both physically and socially. A gentle, careful, individual message must be sent to each student that overweight is not okay in terms of his or her future. Clearly, being overweight or obese does not make a person less valuable as a person, but it does create huge problems that the person himself or herself can work to avoid. We must also promote the attitudes that while losing or keeping off weight can be very hard work, it is truly not optional.

None of these solutions will be simple to put into action, and some may require changes on the parts of the educators who must teach and model them. Yet, if we want to protect our nation's children from the scourge of diabetes, other serious diseases, and premature death, is there really any choice? Let's work through our schools to end the problem of childhood obesity.

This essay earns a 5.0 score for the following reasons:

- In the introductory paragraph, the writer offers a solution to the problem (…*we must work through our schools to promote healthy lifestyles, reduce unhealthful food choices, and change attitudes.*) which will be fleshed out in the preceding paragraphs.

- Each of the first body paragraphs deals with a facet of the solution: education and rewards (paragraph 2), modeling facts about poor diets (paragraph 3), and changing attitudes (paragraph 4). That facet is made clear at the beginning of each paragraph in a clear topic sentence.

- The transitional words and phrases *To solve this problem*, *They can begin*, and *Clearly* guide the reader through the explanation in a clear, systematic way.

- Many details (such as the kinds of exercises students can perform in class and actions schools can take to improve student diets on site) make the writing cogent and work toward supporting the main idea. Nothing is repeated. There are no digressions.

- The reasoning throughout the essay is logical.

- The conclusion ends with an admission of the challenges facing the solution but a strong argument for it despite the challenges.

- There are no errors in sentence structure, and the sentences are varied and fluid.

- Words are used correctly and well.

- The essay is persuasive, the tone is appropriately serious, the voice of the writer is clear and engaged, and the first and second person are avoided.

- There are no mechanical errors.

Sample of a Weak Response

Look around the classrooms of America, you will see many ways in which the students there has changed in the last fifty years. One of the most biggest changes, size and shape, America's elementary and high school students have gotten bigger and bigger. In fact, they have pile on so much weight on average that we now have a obesity epidemic. Solving this problem being a number one priority for the country now.

These overweight and obese students are really in big trouble. Many of them already has diabetes, many of them will get it soon if they do not change there ways. Some of them are going to get too big to pass through some doorways, others are going to get too big to fit in their own bathtubs. Getting on an airplane is going to be super hard for them, in the future, they might even have to start paying for two seats. They are going to get diseases too like heart disease and maybe even cancers. Plus other kids are going to make fun of them and they will eventually have a lot of trouble getting dates and finding happiness.

Noone says the solution to this problem is easy but children have to be learned to eat right when they are really young. This has to start at home with families returning to the habit of having family dinner together. The reason being that at family dinner, someone puts healthful food on the table and kids have something like a balanced meal, including vegetables, instead of a cheap takeout meal, which might be loaded with carbohydrates and calories but have no vegetables at all, or only really high calorie vegetables like French fries, which have so much fat and salt that they aren't good for you anymore, just the opposite, in fact. Than the family can be sitting down together and talking about there day and enjoying a meal. All of which will help to solve the terrible problem of childhood obesity in our nation.

This essay earns a 1.0 score for the following reasons:

- This essay is inadequate in terms of supporting details and problem solving. The writer introduces only one idea to support his or her solution and does not explain it in a cogent way.

- The solution of eliminating obesity through family dinners simplistic.

- The essay lacks organization. The second paragraph is a listing of somewhat absurd consequences of obesity.

- There are enough errors in sentence construction to make much of the essay unintelligible.

- There are a number of instances in which the subject and verb do not agree.

- There are numerous mechanical and usage errors.

Section 2: Biological Processes

1. C	**11.** C	**21.** D	**31.** C	**41.** D
2. C	**12.** B	**22.** A	**32.** B	**42.** B
3. B	**13.** A	**23.** C	**33.** D	**43.** A
4. A	**14.** D	**24.** D	**34.** D	**44.** C
5. D	**15.** B	**25.** A	**35.** C	**45.** D
6. D	**16.** A	**26.** B	**36.** D	**46.** A
7. A	**17.** B	**27.** A	**37.** B	**47.** B
8. C	**18.** B	**28.** B	**38.** A	**48.** B
9. D	**19.** B	**29.** C	**39.** C	
10. C	**20.** A	**30.** C	**40.** D	

1. **The correct answer is C.** Facilitated transport is a third form of passive transport that relies upon the concentration gradient. Certain proteins within the cell membrane can assist in transporting molecules across the membrane. Some proteins act as channels and are, therefore, called *channel proteins*, whereas others act as transporters and are called *carrier proteins*. Choice A is incorrect because diffusion describes a gradual change in concentration of a molecule either with, or along, a concentration gradient. Choice B is incorrect because osmosis is defined as the diffusion of water across the membrane. There is an aqueous solution on either side of the membrane, and the net movement of the water is determined by what biologists call *tonicity*. Choice D is incorrect because there is no specific type of transport defined as protein transport. Proteins can move across the gradient via facilitated or active transport.

2. **The correct answer is C.** Transfer RNA, tRNA, attaches to amino acids in the cytoplasm and transports them to the ribosomes for protein synthesis. Choice A is incorrect because although the codon sequence is found in the DNA sequence, tRNA recognizes the codon on an mRNA strand for protein synthesis to occur. Amino acids are brought to the mRNA on ribosomes via tRNA. Choice B is incorrect because tRNA, not mRNA, delivers the amino acids to the ribosomes for protein synthesis. The mRNA acts as a template for the growing amino acid chain. Choice D is incorrect because amino acids are found in the cytoplasm of cells and are brought to the ribosomes by tRNA.

3. **The correct answer is B.** Once the substrate recognizes and binds to the active site, the enzyme changes its shape and is able to wrap around, or embrace, the substrate. This is known as an *induced* fit and allows the enzyme to be in the best position to catalyze a given reaction. Choice A is incorrect because the active site changes shape to embrace the substrate. Choice C is incorrect because the enzyme changes shape to more tightly hold the substrate, but the substrate does not change shape. Choice D is incorrect because once bound together, the active site of the enzyme catalyzes the conversion of reactant into product, and the

product is then released from the enzyme, leaving it free to bind another substrate molecule. This cycle occurs so quickly that a single enzyme molecule can bind at least a thousand substrate molecules per second.

4. **The correct answer is A.** A protein enters the Golgi from its cis face and exits the Golgi from the other side known as the trans face. Choice B is incorrect because proteins leave the Golgi from the trans face. Choices C and D are incorrect because a protein enters a golgi from its cis face.

5. **The correct answer is D.** Most vitamins are either coenzymes or the starting material from which coenzymes are made. Coenzymes function to transfer the product from one reaction to another. In this way, they can link together two unrelated molecules. Choice A is incorrect because most vitamins are coenzymes, but it is the vitamin that transfers a product from one reaction to another. Choice B is incorrect because it is the product that is transferred by coenzymes. Choice C is incorrect because a coenzyme transfers reaction product, not enzymes from one reaction to another.

6. **The correct answer is D.** Antigenic determinants, also known as *epitopes*, are the small surface-exposed regions of an antigen that are recognized by antibodies. An antigen-binding site on the antibody recognizes an antigenic determinant because the binding site on the antibody and the antigenic determinant have complementary shapes, much like an enzyme and a substrate. An antigen may have several different determinants so that different antibodies can bind to the same antigen. Choice A is incorrect because the antigen-binding site is on the surface of the antibody, not the antigen. Choice B is incorrect because the correct name for site of antibody binding is *the antigenic determinant of epitope.* Choice C is incorrect

because MHC coats all cells as a mechanism of self-recognition.

7. **The correct answer is A.** The first region of DNA after the promoter to be transcribed is called the *leader region*. This is the portion of mRNA that will become the ribosome binding site for each mRNA. Choice B is incorrect because the promoter region is a portion of the DNA sequence that is not transcribed. It is the site where the transcription initiation complex binds to DNA. Choice C is incorrect because the poly-A tail is at the 3' end of newly transcribed mRNA, and is thought to help promote the export of mRNA from the nucleus to the ribosomes. Choice D is incorrect because the 5' cap may also help to promote the export of mRNA to ribosomes.

8. **The correct answer is C.** The S phase is the longest part of interphase and the longest phase of the cell cycle. It last about 10 to 12 hours. This is the phase in which the DNA of the cell is replicated. Choice A is incorrect because the G_1 phase lasts about 5 to 6 hours and is the time in which cellular content (except for the chromosomes) is duplicated. Choice B is incorrect because the G_2 phase lasts about 4 to 6 hours and is the phase in which the cell checks for mistakes in the newly replicated DNA. Choice D is incorrect because the M phase, during which mitosis occurs, is a relatively quick phase lasting only about one hour.

9. **The correct answer is D.** DNA ligase functions on the 3' lagging strand of DNA to join together the newly synthesized Okazaki fragments. Choice A is incorrect because helicase acts to unwind the parent double helix at the replication fork. Choice B is incorrect because DNA primase synthesizes a primer on the end of each Okazaki fragment, but does not join the fragments together. Choice C is incorrect because

DNA polymerase II elongates each Okazaki primer by adding new nucleotides to its primer.

10. **The correct answer is C.** Anaphase begins when the sister chromatids in each pair separate. In order for this to happen, the spindle fibers that are attached to the kinetochore of each chromatid begin to shorten. Each chromatid thus becomes a chromosome, and the two liberated chromosomes move toward opposite poles (ends) of the cell. Because the microtubules are attached to the centromeres, the chromosomes move from the centromere, first in a "V" shape, toward opposite sides. Choice A is incorrect because during prophase, each chromosome that has been duplicated during the S phase joins together with its sister chromatid and attaches to the center of the centromere. Choice B is incorrect because during metaphase, the chromosomes align in the middle of the cell. Choice D is incorrect because during telophase, the microtubules disappear, and the cell begins to divide into two cells.

11. **The correct answer is C.** Viral DNA is transported into the cell nucleus. In the nucleus, it is attached to the end of a host cell chromosome. The cell then is under the control of the virus. The host cell is partially shut down and taken over by viral DNA. Choice A is incorrect because viruses do not have their own replication machinery. They rely on their host cell for replication. Choice B is incorrect because viral DNA attaches to the host DNA and is replicated with the host. Choice D is incorrect because the virus needs the host cell to function so that it can be replicated along with the host. The host cell continues to function for the benefit of the virus.

12. **The correct answer is B.** In higher-order eukaryotic organisms, there are some regions of DNA that do not code for genes as they are transcribed into mRNA. These regions are called *introns*, and in humans, they comprise 98% of our chromosomal DNA. Choice A is incorrect because exons are the regions between introns that do contain genetic information. Choice C is incorrect because a promoter is the sequence at the start of a gene onto which the transcription machinery binds. Choice D is incorrect because an initiation site is the site on the DNA strand at which transcription of a gene begins.

13. **The correct answer is A.** Most plant viruses are cylindrical in shape. Choice B is incorrect because the most complex capsid shapes are found among viruses that infect bacteria. These viruses are called *bacteriophages* and *mycophages*. These phages generally have a polyhedral hollow head that contains DNA and a tail apparatus. Choice C is incorrect because most animal viruses are icosahedral or another polyhedral shape. The viral head is made of protein and is hollow. The inside of the head contains DNA or RNA. The protein head, or capsid, is built from protein subunits called *capsomeres*. Choice D is incorrect because most animal viruses are icosahedral, which is a category of polyhedral shapes.

14. **The correct answer is D.** Staphylococus bacteria form irregular bunches of cocci (spherical-shaped bacteria). Choice A is incorrect because this image represents a single coccus. Choice B is incorrect because this image represents a diplococcus which is two bacteria cells (cocci) linked together. Choice C is incorrect because a chain of cocci is representative of the streptococci bacteria.

15. **The correct answer is B.** The bodies of multicellular fungi typically form a network of tiny filaments called *hyphae*. Hyphae are

made of tubular cell walls that are surrounded by plasma membrane. Choice A is incorrect because mycelia are the mass formed by the interwoven hyphae. Choice C is incorrect because the septa are the crosswalls that divide the hyphae into cells. Choice D is incorrect because chitin is a strong and flexible nitrogen-containing polysaccharide that makes up the cell walls of fungi.

16. **The correct answer is A.** Ventilation is dependent upon change in volume in the thoracic cavity, and the pressure and volume in the thoracic cavity is dependent upon Boyle's gas law ($P_1V_1 = P_2V_2$). Choice B is incorrect because the ideal gas law does not show the dependence of the thoracic cavity of changes in pressure and volume. Choice C is incorrect because pressure and volume are not inversely proportional. Choice D is incorrect because temperature is not a factor because internal body temperature is relatively constant.

17. **The correct answer is B.** Structures that are anatomically alike, but differ functionally are *homologies*. These species have shared ancestry. DNA sequence homology can indicate common ancestry and function. Choice A is incorrect because homoplasies are structures that are similar, but have a different origin. Homoplasies give evidence of convergent evolution. Choice C is incorrect because species that are genetically related would most likely have similar structures with similar functions. Choice D is incorrect because fossils give physical evidence of differences that emerge among species, but don't prove that a similar structure has a different function.

18. **The correct answer is B.** The law of segregation states that two alleles for a specific inheritable character, or trait, separate (segregate) during gamete formation and end up in two different gametes (during meiosis). Choice A is incorrect because the law of independent assortment states that each pair of alleles for a specific gene segregates independently of the alleles for another gene during gamete formation. Choice C is incorrect because the laws of inheritance are the law of segregation and the law of independent assortment. Choice D is incorrect because the laws of probability are used to determine the likelihood of certain inheritance patterns.

19. **The correct answer is B.** Interkinesis is the period in meiosis between the two cell divisions in which partial elongation of DNA takes place. The DNA does not replicate again during interkinesis. Choice A is incorrect because DNA does not replicate a second time during the interkinesis phase of meiosis. Choice C is incorrect because DNA condenses during prophase II. Choice D is incorrect because chromosomes are positioned on the metaphase plate (middle of the cell) during metaphase, not during interkinesis.

20. **The correct answer is A.** Synapsis is the process by which homologous chromosomes come together during early prophase I, and crossing over takes place once the homologous chromosomes have formed tetrads. Choice B is incorrect because crossing over occurs during prophase I, not prophase II; homologous chromosomes are only paired up during meiosis I, which is a requirement for crossing over. This is also why Choice D is incorrect, as homologous chromosomes at this point are in separate haploid cells. Choice C is incorrect because crossing over has already taken place by the time the cells reach metaphase I.

21. **The correct answer is D.** Most viruses are specific to the organism that they infect, and the particular tissue type they infect. On the head of the virus, there are receptor proteins

that recognize a specific protein on specific cells of a host. Choice A is incorrect because most viruses are very specific as to their host. Choice B is incorrect because viruses have receptors that recognize a specific cell type in a specific host. Choice C is incorrect because viruses have receptors that are specific to a particular cell type in a specific host.

22. **The correct answer is A.** The thalamus is the main input center for sensory information coming from all regions of the body going into the cerebrum and the main output center for motor information leaving the cerebrum to all regions of the body. In the thalamus, sensory information is sorted and sent to the correct region of the cerebrum, and motor information is also sorted and sent to the correct region of the body. Choice B is incorrect because the epithalamus is important for regulating sleep-wake cycles. Choice C is incorrect because the hypothalamus is important for homeostatic regulation. It is the autonomic control center for blood pressure, heart rate regulation, respiration rate, and digestive tract function, and overlaps in function with the medulla oblongata. It also contains the body's thermostat, as well as centers for regulating hunger, thirst, and other basic survival mechanisms. The hypothalamus also plays a role in sexual and mating behaviors and is part of the limbic system that controls emotional responses. Choice D is incorrect because the midbrain contains centers for the receipt of different types of sensory information. It also sends sensory information to specific regions of the forebrain.

23. **The correct answer is C.** In the past, Archaea and Bacteria were classified as one kingdom known as Monera. Choice A is incorrect because the kingdom Fungi is not similar enough to Archaea for them to have been classified as one kingdom. Choice B is incorrect because Eukarya is a domain

classification, not a kingdom. Choice D is incorrect because the kingdoms Animalia and Bacteria are too divergent to have been classified as one kingdom.

24. **The correct answer is D.** Osteoid is composed of collagen and glycoproteins, both of which provide flexibility to bones. Collagen also provides strength to the bone structure. Choice A is incorrect because hydroxyapatites and calcium are minerals that impart hardness to bones. Choice B is incorrect because bone marrow contains stem cells and stores fat. Choice C is incorrect because calcium imparts hardness, not flexibility, to bones.

25. **The correct answer is A.** Generally, sexual reproduction in fungi begins when hyphae, which have haploid nuclei from two distinct mycelia, release sexually signaling molecules called *pheromones*. Choice B is incorrect because sexual reproduction requires the release of pheromones. Choice C is incorrect because sexual reproduction requires the release of pheromones, which bind to the surface receptors of other mycelia. Choice D is incorrect because corticosteroids do not play a role in sexual reproduction of fungi.

26. **The correct answer is B.** Microaerophile bacteria require only a low concentration of oxygen. Energy comes from aerobic respiration. Choice A is incorrect because an obligate aerobe grows in the presence of oxygen, but bacteria that grow only in a low concentration of oxygen are more specifically categorized as a microaerophile. Choice C is incorrect because an aerotolerant anaerobe does not require oxygen for growth. Energy for these bacteria cells comes from anaerobic respiration. Choice D is incorrect because facultative anaerobe grows best in an oxygenated environment with energy supplied through anaerobic respiration.

27. **The correct answer is A.** The myocardium is the bulk of the heart. It is the contractile muscle tissue of the organ. The left ventricle of the heart pumps blood out of the heart to the body. Choice B is incorrect because the endocardium layer of the heart is the innermost layer that lines the chambers of the heart, covers the valves, and is continuous with the blood vessels. The endocardium is made up of epithelial cells and connective tissue. Choice C is incorrect because the septum acts to divide the chambers of the heart and is not made of contractile muscles. Choice D is incorrect because the valves are heart structures that allow blood to flow only in one direction.

28. **The correct answer is B.** Basophils are the least abundant of all white blood cells. They are involved in the inflammatory response to an allergic reaction. Basophils also attract more WBCs to infected areas, to help reduce infection. Choice A is incorrect because neutrophils are recruited to sites of injury and are the hallmark of inflammation at the site of a wound or injury. Choice C is incorrect because lymphocytes reside in lymphatic tissue. They destroy foreign cells, respond to virus-infected cells and tumor cells, and produce antibodies. Choice D is incorrect because eosinophils contain digestive enzymes and are part of the immune system that combats multicellular parasites and certain other infections.

29. **The correct answer is C.** Budding is the process of asexual reproduction carried out in yeast. DNA is first replicated in the nucleus. The nucleus then splits and forms a daughter nucleus, which migrates to the edge of the cell. The daughter nucleus is then surrounded by cytoplasm. Cell wall material is then laid between the parent and the daughter nuclei (bud). The small bud continues to grow until it separates from the parent cell. Once it separates, it is fully mature and the same size as the parent. Choice A is incorrect because spore production is a method of asexual reproduction in molds and fungi, not yeast. Choice B is incorrect because plasmogamy is a step in the sexual reproduction process of fungi. Choice D is incorrect because karyogamy is a step in the sexual reproduction process of fungi.

30. **The correct answer is C.** Adenylate cyclase generates the second messenger, cyclic AMP (cAMP) from an ATP molecule. cAMP diffuses through the cell, triggering a cascade of chemical reactions. The first protein activated in the cascade is protein kinase. Choice A is incorrect because GTP activates the G-protein that, in turn, activates the effector enzyme. Choice B is incorrect because GDP turns off the G-protein. Choice D is incorrect because protein kinase phosphorylates various proteins and is responsible for mediating the cellular response to hormones.

31. **The correct answer is C.** The bottleneck effect is due to a drastic change in environment that greatly reduces the size of a population (forest fire, flood, human activity). After a drastic reduction in populations there are a few survivors, and the gene pool is no longer representative of the original population. These few survivors are said to have passed through a hypothetical "bottleneck." Choice A is incorrect because the founder effect is seen when a few individuals become isolated from a larger population. This smaller population may develop a gene pool that is less variable than that of the larger population. Choice B is incorrect because an increase in mutations may lead to a decrease in population, but it is not a direct effect of a decrease. Choice D is incorrect because the Hardy-Weinberg equilibrium refers to a population that has a steady frequency of alleles from one

generation to the next. This is not an effect of reduced population size.

32. **The correct answer is B.** The second law of thermodynamics states that during every energy conversion or transfer, some energy becomes unavailable to do work. This energy is lost to the surrounding environment as heat. Heat is thermal energy, but it is unusable in that it cannot perform work on a system. Another way of stating this law is to say that the entropy of the universe increases in a spontaneous process and remains unchanged in an equilibrium process. Choice A is incorrect because the first law of thermodynamics states that energy cannot be created or destroyed. Choice C is incorrect because the third law of thermodynamics states that the entropy of a perfect crystalline substance at absolute zero temperature is zero. Choice D is incorrect because the zeroth law of thermodynamics states that if two systems are at equilibrium with a third system, they are also in equilibrium with each other.

33. **The correct answer is D.** Chlamydias are parasitic bacteria that can only survive within an animal cell. (*Only* is the operative word in this question.) These types of bacteria depend on their host for resources such as ATP. Choice A is incorrect because spirochetes are helical heterotrophs that can live either independently or in a host. Choice B is incorrect because gram-positive bacteria do not require a host for survival. Choice C is incorrect because cyanobacteria are photoautotrophs with the plant-like ability to carry out oxygen-generating photosynthesis.

34. **The correct answer is D.** Chemical digestion in the small intestine is accomplished by digestive enzymes, bile, and bicarbonate ions. Choice A is incorrect because sodium ions do not aid in chemical digestion of food; they help in regulating the electric potential of cells. Choice B is incorrect because calcium ions help to develop hardness in bones. They do not play a role in digestion. Choice C is incorrect because magnesium ions do not play a role in digestion of food.

35. **The correct answer is C.** The secretion process in the urinary system eliminates drugs and toxic substances from the blood. In both secretion and reabsorption, water and solutes pass through interstitial fluid between tubules and capillaries. During secretion, the second process to refine filtrate, substances in the blood are transported into the filtrate. For example, excess H^+ ions are secreted into filtrate to keep blood at the proper pH level. Choice A is incorrect because during the filtration process in the urinary system, water and small molecules are forced through capillary walls and enter the nephron tubules from the glomerulus. Choice B is incorrect because in the reabsorption process, the first steps of refining the filtrate occur. Water and all valuable solutes are returned to the blood. Choice D is incorrect because excretion is the process of eliminating urine from the body.

36. **The correct answer is D.** During the follicular phase of the ovarian cycle, primary follicles with two or more layers are targeted by FSH. This phase follows the development of the follicle until ovulation. Choice A is incorrect because degeneration occurs in the luteal phase if fertilization does not occur. Choice B is incorrect because if fertilization occurs, the corpus luteum grows, causing an increase in progesterone production during the luteal phase. Choice C is incorrect because LH transforms the vesicular follicle into the corpus luteum during the luteal phase.

37. **The correct answer is B.** The Bacteria domain includes almost all of the common prokaryotes such as the pathogenic species

that cause strep (*streptococcus*) and staph infections, and other diseases such as pneumococcal infections. Choice A is incorrect because *streptococcus* is classified in the domain Bacteria. Choice C is incorrect because the domain Eukarya consists of all eukaryotic species, and *streptococcus* is a prokaryotic organism. Choice D is incorrect because Protista is one of the six kingdoms, and it is not a domain.

38. **The correct answer is A.** Chemiosmosis is a type of phosphorylation reaction that generates ATP. In chemiosmosis, energy stored in the form of an H⁺ ion gradient across a membrane is used to drive cellular work such as the synthesis of ATP. Chemiosmosis is part of oxidative phosphorylation, a more complex method than substrate-level phosphorylation. It depends on osmotic pressure, so a concentration gradient across a membrane is essential. This method generally results in a high yield of ATP. Choice B is incorrect because osmosis is a way of transporting water into and out of a cell, but chemiosmosis is a phosphorylation reaction that generates ATP. Choice C is incorrect because chemiosmosis does not transport H⁺ ions into the cell. It acts as a method for generating ATP. Choice D is incorrect because chemiosmosis is a method of ATP production, not a way to store it.

39. **The correct answer is C.** Catabolic pathways are metabolic pathways that release energy by breaking down complex molecules into simpler molecules. Cellular respiration is a major catabolic pathway in cells. Choice A is incorrect because an anabolic pathway is one in which an energy input is required to build complicated molecules from simpler ones. Choice B is incorrect because a biosynthetic pathway is simply an anabolic pathway. Choice D is incorrect because a pathway that builds up proteins would be a type of protein synthesis pathway, but a catabolic

pathway breaks down large molecules into smaller ones.

40. **The correct answer is D.** The two polynucleotide chains are held together by hydrogen bonds between the paired bases and van der Waals interactions between the stacked bases. Even though hydrogen bonds are generally weak bonds, the huge number of hydrogen bonds in a DNA double helix makes the molecule very stable. Choice A is incorrect because phosphodiester linkages hold together the nucleotides in each polynucleotide strand, creating the sugar-phosphate backbone of the DNA double helix. Choice B is incorrect because hydrogen bonds, not strong covalent bonds, hold the two polynucleotide strands of DNA together. Choice C is incorrect because the strands are held together by hydrogen bonding, not ionic bonding.

41. **The correct answer is D.** The name TATA is given because of the sequence of DNA in this region: TATAAAA. The TATA box is significant because the first protein of the transcription initiation complex, TFIID (transcription factor IID), recognizes the TATA sequence and binds to DNA. This triggers the formation of the initiation complex and the start of transcription. Choices A, B, and C are, therefore, incorrect. Choice B, TFIIA, can join the initiation complex after the binding of TFIID, and TFIIA acts to stabilize the transcription complex. Choice C is incorrect because TFIIC is not a type of transcription factor in eukaryotic cells; it is a transcription factor involved in transcription by RNA polymerase III, choice A.

42. **The correct answer is B.** If there is oxygen present in the cell, the pyruvate molecules, which are the product of glycolysis, enter the mitochondrion and the enzymes involved in the Krebs cycle, or citric acid cycle,

complete the oxidation process and release the stored energy. The goal of the Krebs cycle is to completely oxidize the remnants of the original glucose molecule. Choice A is incorrect because glucose is broken down into two pyruvate molecules during glycolysis. These pyruvate molecules enter into the Krebs cycle or citric acid cycle. Choice C is incorrect because carbon dioxide is given off by reactions in the Krebs cycle, but oxygen is required to begin the cycle. Choice D is incorrect because citric acid is formed in one of the steps of the Krebs cycle.

43. **The correct answer is A.** In the case of codominance, two different alleles of a gene are expressed phenotypically. A good example of codominance is blood type in humans. The codominant blood type is AB. Choice B is incorrect because pleiotropy refers to the property of a gene in which it affects multiple phenotypes. Choice C is incorrect because epistasis involves a gene at one locus on the chromosome altering the phenotypic expression of a gene at a different locus. Choice D is incorrect because polygenic inheritance refers to variations of a single trait due to a gene at one locus on the chromosome that alters the phenotypic expression of a gene at a different locus.

44. **The correct answer is C.** Peroxisomes use oxygen molecules to oxidize organic molecules. Hydrogen peroxide is given off as a product of these oxidation reactions. The main function of peroxisomes is to break down fatty acids. Choice A is incorrect because the main function of the centrosome is to act as a microtubule organizing center. Choice B is incorrect because the main

function of the Golgi apparatus is to modify, store, and transport proteins leaving the ER. Choice D is incorrect because the main function of the lysosomes is to rid the cell of debris.

45. **The correct answer is D.** Food passes from the mouth to the esophagus, and into the stomach. After stomach acids break down the food into chyme, the digested food is passed through the small and large intestines for nutrient absorption. Choice A incorrectly places the stomach after the intestines. Choice B is incorrect because it reverses the proper organ order. Choice C is incorrect because it swaps the positions of the small and large intestines.

46. **The correct answer is A.** Alveoli are the tiny air sacs in the lungs that allow for rapid gas exchange. Choice B is incorrect. This is the function of the glomerulus of the kidney. Choice C is incorrect because this is the function of veins. Choice D is incorrect because this is the function of the trachea.

47. **The correct answer is D.** Yeast are fungi. Choice A is incorrect because it is a virus. Choice B is incorrect because it is an invertebrate animal. Choice C is incorrect because it is a protist.

48. **The correct answer is B.** The nucleoid is the region of genetic material concentration within a prokaryote. Choice A is incorrect because the capsule is the outer envelope of a bacterial cell. Choice C is incorrect because bacteria do not have nuclei. Choice D is incorrect because the pilus is the structure bacteria use for conjugation, a mode of horizontal gene transfer.

Section 3: Chemical Procesess

1. B	11. B	21. D	31. D	40. B
2. D	12. B	22. B	32. A	41. D
3. B	13. B	23. A	33. B	42. B
4. C	14. C	24. B	34. C	43. A
5. C	15. A	25. C	35. B	44. B
6. B	16. A	26. D	36. C	45. A
7. B	17. B	27. C	37. A	46. A
8. C	18. C	28. A	38. A	47. D
9. B	19. A	29. B	39. B	48. B
10. D	20. D	30. D		

1. **The correct answer is B.** The molecules in a liquid are held close together, but they are not held as rigidly as in a solid. Molecules in a liquid can move past one another, which gives liquids the property of fluidity. Choice A is incorrect because the closeness of molecules in a liquid is not what gives them their fluid property. Choice C is incorrect because although liquids take the shape of their container, the property that gives them their fluidity is their ability to move past one another. Choice D is incorrect because it is the fact that liquid molecules can move past one another that gives them fluidity.

2. **The correct answer is D.** Molecules at the surface of a liquid are pulled downward and sideways by other liquid molecules. This causes the surface of liquids to tighten like an elastic film, thus creating surface tension. Choice A is incorrect because surface molecules in a liquid do interact with other molecules in the liquid. Choice B is incorrect because molecules are pushed downward, not upward, and sideways by other molecules. Choice C is incorrect because molecules in a liquid are pulled in every direction by intermolecular forces, but at the surface of a liquid are pulled downward and sideways by other liquid molecules.

3. **The correct answer is B.** A supersaturated solution contains more solute than is present in a saturated solution. This is a very unstable solution, and the addition of a single crystal of solute will cause the solute to come out of solution and form crystals (crystallization). Choices A and C are incorrect because the addition of a crystal to a supersaturated solution will cause some solute to come out of solution and form crystals. Neither of these answers apply to this effect. Choice D is incorrect because the addition of a single crystal does have an effect on a supersaturated solution in that other crystals form as the solid comes out of solution.

4. **The correct answer is C.** Since the heat capacity is defined as $C = ms$, the value of C can be calculated to be 209.2 J/°C. Choice A is incorrect because the formula for heat capacity is $C = ms$. Choice B is incorrect because the value of C is 209.2, according to the equation $C = ms$. Choice D is incorrect because the value of C is calculated by the equation $C = ms$.

5. **The correct answer is C.** When a weak acid reacts with a strong base, the salt that forms hydrolyzes to reform the acid. Hydroxide ions form due to the hydrolysis of water, and, therefore, the overall solution is basic. Therefore, the pH of the reaction solution is greater than 7.0. Thus, choice A is incorrect. Choice B is incorrect because a pH of less than 7.0 would indicate an acidic environment. Choice D is incorrect because the pH of the solution will be basic (> 7.0), not 0.

6. **The correct answer is B.** Using the dilution equation $M_1V_1 = M_2V_2$ to determine the unknown volume gives a value of 750 mL. Since there are already 250 mL of solvent in the 0.72 M solution, 500 mL of solvent must be added to get a concentration of 0.24 M. Choice A is incorrect because adding 250 mL would give a final concentration of 0.36 M. Choice C is incorrect because 750 mL is the final volume of solution, but since there is already 250 mL of solvent, only 500 mL need to be added. Choice D is incorrect because adding 1,000 mL would give a solution with a final concentration of 0.18 M.

7. **The correct answer is B.** The average atomic mass of an atom is found under the element symbol on the Periodic Table. Therefore, the atomic mass of mercury is 200.6 g/mol. Choice A is incorrect because 80 is the atomic number, which is equivalent of the number of protons in the nucleus. Choices C and D are incorrect because the atomic mass of mercury is shown under the element symbol on the Periodic Table.

8. **The correct answer is C.** An element's atomic number, Z, is defined as the number of protons the element has. The number of protons in an atom does not vary. Electrons can be added or removed from an atom in a process called ionization. Ionization leads to an overall positive (loss of electrons) or negative (gain of electrons) charge of the atom. Therefore, an ion with a +2 charge has a proton number equal to the atomic number and two fewer electrons than protons. Choice A is incorrect because an ion with a +2 charge has lost two of its electrons. Choice B is incorrect because the number of protons in an ion does not vary. Choice D is incorrect because the number of protons in an ion does not vary.

9. **The correct answer is B.** S is more electronegative that H, so the electrons in the bond will be pulled more closely toward the sulfur atom than toward the hydrogen atom. Therefore, the bond that forms will be a polar bond. Choice A is incorrect because sulfur atoms are more electronegative than hydrogen atoms, so the electrons would be pulled toward the S atom. Choice C is incorrect because the atoms differ in electronegativity, so the bond would be polar. Also, a nonpolar bond would have the electrons shared equally, so this choice cannot be accurate. Choice D is incorrect because since the atoms differ in electronegativity, the bond would be polar.

10. **The correct answer is D.** Because their outer shells are completely filled, noble gases have a low chemical reactivity. These gases have been called inert gases, and very few compounds exist with noble gases, and for the most part, those are unreactive. Choice A is incorrect because simply being a gas does not make them inert. Choice B is incorrect because the fact that they are nonflammable does not make them inert. Choice C is incorrect because the fact that they have a full valence electron shell makes them unable to react well with other elements regardless of their place on the Periodic Table.

11. **The correct answer is B.** The energy of an electron in an atom is lower than the energy

of a free electron, which is infinitely far from a nucleus. Thus, the energy of an electron in an orbital increases as the orbital increases in distance from the atomic nucleus. Choice A is incorrect because the energy of an electron increases as it gets farther from the nucleus. Choice C is incorrect because the energy level of an orbital is lower as it approaches the nucleus. Choice D is incorrect because the energy varies depending on the distance of the orbital from the nucleus.

12. **The correct answer is B.** The molecular mass of a compound is equal to the sum of the atomic masses of its elements in the correct stoichiometric ratio. Therefore, the molecular mass of carbon dioxide is 44.01 g/mol. Choice A is incorrect because there are two oxygen atoms in a molecule of CO_2, so the molecular mass is 44.01 g/mol. Choices C and D are incorrect because the molecular mass is equal to the sum of the atomic mass of each element.

13. **The correct answer is B.** The volume of gas can be calculated using the ideal gas law $PV = nRT$ under standard temperature and pressure. 8.0 g of ammonia gas are equal to 0.47 mol. The gas constant is 0.08205 L·atm/K·mol. Standard pressure is 1 atm, and standard temperature is 273.15K (0°C). The volume of gas is 10.52 L. Choice A is incorrect because using the correct values for the moles of gas (not the mass) and the ideal gas equation the volume of gas is equal to 10.52 L. Choices C and D are incorrect because the correct calculations result in a volume of 10.52 L.

14. **The correct answer is C.** Empirical and molecular formulas of organic compounds can be determined through the process of combustion analysis. The mass of the product to be analyzed is determined, and then the product is burned completely. If a product only contains one or some of the following atoms: carbon, hydrogen, and oxygen atoms, as is the case in many organic compounds, then the only products of combustion (burning) are carbon dioxide and water. Carbon dioxide and water that result from combustion are collected in separate tubes that contain materials specific to adsorbing either water or CO_2. The mass of carbon and hydrogen can be determined by the samples collected, and the mass of oxygen can be determined by subtracting the calculated mass of carbon and hydrogen from the mass of the original sample. All of this data collected can be used to calculate the empirical and molecular formulas of the starting compound. Choice A is incorrect because the molecular formula cannot be determined through distillation methods, and distillation is used to separate volatile liquids. Choice B is incorrect because chromatography separates compounds, not individual elements of the compound. Choice D is incorrect because sublimation is a process of separating a volatile solid from another substance.

15. **The correct answer is A.** Oxygen atoms have a strong electronegativity, and, therefore, the hydrogen atom in the OH group can hydrogen bond to other molecules. The hydrogen bonding that alcohols can participate in typically gives an alcohol derivative a higher boiling point than its corresponding hydrocarbon. Choice B is incorrect because hydrogen bonding does not occur between the OH and the hydrogen atoms on the same molecule. Choice C is incorrect because the carbon atom does not play a role in the high boiling point. Choice D is incorrect because the carbon and the oxygen form a strong bond because O is a strongly electronegative atom.

16. **The correct answer is A.** The partial pressure of each gas component is represented by the equation $P_i = X_i P_{\text{total}}$ and the mole fraction

of argon can be calculated by dividing the moles of argon over the sum of the moles of all three gases. Using these equations, the partial pressure of argon is determined to be 0.189 atm. Choices B, C, and D are incorrect because the correct computation gives the value of 0.189 atm.

17. **The correct answer is B.** In a crude mixture of two or more volatile liquids with different boiling points, a process of fractional distillation can separate the liquids. The more volatile liquid with the lower boiling point distills first, and the higher boiling point liquid is distilled next. Because B has the lowest boiling point, it will be isolated first. Choice A is incorrect because the boiling point of B is the lowest of the three substances. Choice C is incorrect because C has the highest boiling point so it should distill last. Choice D is incorrect because all three substances can be separated from each other because they have different boiling points.

18. **The correct answer is C.** The boiling point of a liquid is the temperature at which the vapor pressure of the liquid is equal to the external pressure. Bubbles of gas form within a liquid as it reaches its boiling point. The pressure inside the bubble is due solely to the vapor pressure of the liquid. When the vapor pressure inside the bubble becomes equal to the external pressure, the bubble rises to the surface of the liquid and bursts. Choices A and B are incorrect because the melting point is the temperature at which a solid changes to a liquid, and the freezing point is the temperature at which a liquid changes to a solid. Choice D is incorrect because sublimation refers to the phase change from a solid to a vapor.

19. **The correct answer is A.** The carbonyl condensation reaction is a combination between a nucleophilic addition reaction and a substitution reaction. In a carbonyl condensation reaction, a carbonyl with a hydrogen atom in its alpha position is converted by base (OH^-) into its enolate anion. The enolate ion acts as a nucleophile electron donor and donates an electron pair to the electrophilic carbonyl group. Choice B is incorrect because the carbonyl group acts as an electrophilic acceptor. Choice C is incorrect because water is required for protonation of the final product. Choice D is incorrect because the OH^- ion converts the reactant to an enolate ion.

20. **The correct answer is D.** A redox reaction that occurs in an electrolytic cell is a nonspontaneous reaction, and a redox reaction in a galvanic cell is spontaneous. Choices A and B are incorrect because electrons migrate from the anode to the cathode in both types of cells. Choice C is incorrect because the redox reaction in a galvanic cell is spontaneous, and it is nonspontaneous in an electrolytic cell.

21. **The correct answer is D.** All E1 elimination reactions occur by spontaneous dissociation of the leaving group and the loss of a proton from an intermediate carbocation. The loss of the proton occurs after the dissociation of the leaving group, which is the rate-limiting step. Choice A is incorrect because the loss of the proton is a fast step in an E1 reaction. Choice B is incorrect because the breaking of the C-H bond occurs as the H^+ ion is lost, and it is a rapid step. Choice C is incorrect because a nucleophilic attack does not occur in an E1 reaction.

22. **The correct answer is B.** Amines are organic molecules with properties of a base. They have the general formula, R_3N, where R is an H atom or a hydrocarbon group. The name of the compound shown is diphenylamine. Choice A is incorrect because a carbonyl has the basic structure RCOR. Choice C is incorrect because although this

compound has two aromatic groups, it is best categorized as an amine (R_3N). Choice D is incorrect because an amide has the basic structure CONHC.

23. **The correct answer is A.** According to the VSEPR (valence-shell electron-pair repulsion) model, certain geometric arrangements of electron pairs around a central atom can be determined. The VSEPR model indicates that molecules with two electron pairs are linear. Choice B is incorrect because covalent compounds with three electron pairs form a triagonal planar structure. Choice C is incorrect because compounds with a central atom containing four electron pairs form a tetrahedral shape. Choice D is incorrect because a covalent compound with central atoms containing five electron pairs forms a triagonal bipyramidal shape.

24. **The correct answer is B.** Molecules are in constant motion, and when a molecule absorbs infrared radiation, the molecular motion of the molecule increases in intensity. Since each radiation frequency corresponds to a different motion, IR spectroscopy reveals the different types of motion within a given molecular sample. Interpreting the IR spectra can help to determine what kinds of functional groups are in the molecule. Choice A is incorrect because UV-Vis spectroscopy is best used to identify compounds based on color. Choice C is incorrect because the mass of a molecule or compound is determined by mass spectroscopy. Choice D is incorrect because HPLC is a sensitive method of chromatography that separates substances from one another.

25. **The correct answer is C.** Esters have the general formula R'COOR. R' can be either an H or a hydrocarbon, and R is a hydrocarbon group. The formula shown is for ethyl acetate, a common ester molecule. Choice A is incorrect because an aldehyde is formed when at least one of the R groups attached to the carbon atom is an H atom. It has the general formula RCOH. Choice B is incorrect because a ketone has the general structure RCOR. Choice D is incorrect because a carboxylic acid compound contains a carboxyl group, COOH.

26. **The correct answer is D.** The greater the concentration of the reactants, the greater number of collisions between molecules per unit of time will occur. Thus, an increase in concentration of reactants greater than zero order to a determined maximum level will increase the reaction rate. Choice A is incorrect because in almost all reactions, an increase in temperature will increase the reaction rate. Choice B is incorrect because the rate of a reaction may be affected by the medium in which it takes place. Choice C is incorrect because a catalyst is a substance that increases the rate of a chemical reaction without being consumed in the reaction.

27. **The correct answer is C.** The amount of radio-frequency energy required depends on the strength of the external magnetic field and the type of nucleus being irradiated. Radio-frequency energy in the 60 MHz range is required to bring an ^1H nucleus into resonance, and 15 MHz is required to bring a ^{13}C nucleus into resonance. Choice A is incorrect because the radio frequency depends on the strength of the external magnetic field and the type of nuclei that is being detected. Choice B is incorrect because the energy state of the atom "flips" to the higher-energy state once the radio wave is applied. Choice D is incorrect because the magnetic moment is proportional to the spin, but does not determine the amount of radio frequency applied to a sample molecule.

28. **The correct answer is A.** In the last step of an esterification reaction, a proton is lost, leaving a free ester product. The loss of the

proton also serves to regenerate the acid catalyst for further use. Choice B is incorrect because the transfer of a proton from one oxygen atom to another occurs after the nucleophilic attack, or in the third step of the 5-step reaction. Choice C is incorrect because activation of the carbonyl group is the first step in an esterification reaction. Choice D is incorrect because the second step of the reaction is a nucleophilic addition reaction.

29. **The correct answer is B.** Dispersion, or London, forces are the attractive forces that are the result of a temporary dipole induced in a nonpolar atom or molecule by a surrounding molecule. Dispersion forces are temporary forces, and they are generally weaker than other intermolecular forces. Choice A is incorrect because dipole-dipole interaction is attractive forces between polar molecules. Polar molecules are arranged such that the partially positive end of one molecule is in close proximity to the partially negative end of another molecule. This forms a dipole-dipole interaction between the molecules, since the opposite ends of each molecule are attracted to each other. Dipole-dipole interactions are stronger than dispersion forces. Choice C is incorrect because hydrogen bonding is the strongest type of intermolecular force, and it is not a temporary interaction between molecules. Choice D is incorrect because covalent bonds are intramolecular forces, not intermolecular forces.

30. **The correct answer is D.** A molecule with a central carbon atom can form four bonds with hydrogen to form methane (CH_4). The geometry of this structure is tetrahedral because the carbon atom in its excited state forms four sp^3 hybridized orbitals. Choice A is incorrect because an s orbital is not a hybridized orbital. Choice B is incorrect because a carbon atom in its excited state has four unpaired electrons that form sp^3 hybridized orbitals. Choice C is incorrect because carbon forms four sp^3 hybridized orbitals due to four unpaired electrons in the valence shell of carbon in its excited state.

31. **The correct answer is D.** According to the rules of spin-spin splitting, in ^1H NMR, a proton with n equivalent neighboring protons gives a signal that is split into $n + 1$ peaks with a coupling constant, J. A proton with three equivalent neighboring protons will have $3 + 1$, or four, peaks. For this reason, choices B and C are incorrect. Choice A is incorrect because the peak is split if there are neighboring equivalent protons.

32. **The correct answer is A.** Lattice energy is the measure of bond strength of a particular ionic compound in its solid state. It is defined as the amount of energy required to completely separate one mole of solid ionic compound into individual ions in their gaseous state. The bond strength depends on two factors: ionic radius and ionic charge. Choice B is incorrect because the bond strength is dependent on the radius of the ion and the charge of the ion, not the atomic number. Choice C is incorrect because the lattice structure is determined by the lattice energy, or bond strength, of the ions forming the compound. Choice D is incorrect because lattice energy is the measure of bond strength of a particular ionic compound.

33. **The correct answer is B.** The removal of an oxygen atom from H_3PO_3, phosphoric acid, changes the name of the compound to phosphorous acid. Choice A is incorrect because phosphoric acid would have the formula H_3PO_4. Choice C is incorrect because hydrogen phosphate would have the formula HPO_4^{2-}. Choice D is incorrect because the formula for hypophosphorous acid is H_3PO_2.

34. The correct answer is C. Gas chromatography employs a carrier gas such as nitrogen as the mobile phase solvent. Helium, another gas, can also be used as a mobile phase in gas chromatography. Choice A is incorrect because alumina is used as a solid mobile phase in chromatography. Choice B is incorrect because silica gel is used as a solid mobile phase in chromatography. Choice D is incorrect because sodium chloride is not a compound used as a mobile phase in chromatography.

35. The correct answer is B. A negative ΔG value indicates the release of usable energy during a reaction. This type of reaction is spontaneous. Choice A is incorrect because a ΔG value of zero indicates that the system is at equilibrium. Choice C is incorrect because a positive ΔG value indicates that additional energy is required for a reaction to proceed, and the reaction is nonspontaneous. Choice D is incorrect because the release of energy indicates a spontaneous reaction and a negative ΔG value.

36. The correct answer is C. The point at which the acid has completely reacted with the base is called the *equivalence point*. It is measured in terms of pH, and it indicates that the number of moles of H^+ ions that have reacted is equivalent to the number of moles of OH^- ions that have reacted. Choice A is incorrect because the equivalence point concerns the point at which there are the same number of moles of H^+ and moles of OH^-. Choice B is incorrect because the equivalence point at which the acid has completely reacted with the base and the number of moles of H^+ ions that have reacted is equivalent to the number of moles of OH^- ions that have reacted. Choice D is incorrect because the equivalence point is the point at which the number of moles of H^+ ions that have reacted is equivalent to the number of moles of OH^- ions that have reacted.

37. The correct answer is A. Reaction order enables one to understand how the reaction is dependent on the concentration of a given reactant. In the reaction $aA + bB \rightarrow cC + dD$ where the rate is $k[A][B]^2$, the reaction orders are $x = 1$ and $y = 2$. The reaction order is independent of the stoichiometric coefficient of the reactant. Choice B is incorrect because the reaction order can be determined by the concentration of the reactants. Choice C is incorrect because the reaction order is always defined in terms of the concentration of a given reactant. Choice D is incorrect because the rate constant is determined by the rate and the concentration of the reactants.

38. The correct answer is A. An ester bond links fatty acids to a head group. Choice B is incorrect because glycosidic bonds connect monosaccharides in carbohydrates. Choice C is incorrect because peptide bonds connect amino acids in proteins. Choice D is incorrect because phosphodiester bonds link nucleotides in nucleic acids.

39. The correct answer is B. A condensation reaction connects amino acids, releasing a water in the process. Choice A and D are incorrect because they are other reaction types that are not relevant to polymerization of amino acids. Choice C is incorrect because a hydrolysis reaction is the reaction that can disrupt a peptide bond and separate amino acids, with an input of water.

40. The correct answer is B. The unfolding of a protein due to high temperature or some other stress is called *denaturation*. Choice A is incorrect because catalysis describes the increased reaction rate due to a catalyst, like an enzyme. Choice C is incorrect because the hydrophobic effect describes the way a protein folds so that its hydrophilic residues interact with water and its hydrophobic residues do not. Choice D is incorrect because spontaneous generation describes the now-debunked theory that life can arise from non-life.

41. **The correct answer is D.** Coenzymes and prosthetic groups are subcategories of cofactors. Choice A is incorrect because cofactors do not catalyze reactions without enzymes. Choice B is incorrect because cofactors are needed to increase the efficiency, or provide the functionality, of enzymes. Choice C is incorrect because this choice describes allosteric regulators.

42. **The correct answer is B.** Each of these three parts can be found in each of A, C, G, T, and U. Choice A is incorrect because these are various parts of a lipid. Choice C is incorrect because these are three levels of protein structure. Choice D is incorrect because these are the three main types of RNA.

43. **The correct answer is A.** If there are 40 C's, there are 40 G's, 10 A's, and 10 T's. Choice B is incorrect because this is the total number of A's and T's combined. Choice C is incorrect because this is the number of C's or G's. Choice D is incorrect because this is the total number of C's and G's combined.

44. **The correct answer is B.** Waxes and oils are types of lipids. Choice A is incorrect because these are types of carbohydrates. Choice C is incorrect because these are types of proteins. Choice D is incorrect because these are types of nucleic acids.

45. **The correct answer is A.** Non-enzymatic catalysts are not biomolecules, but all enzymes are biomolecules. Choice B is incorrect. Catalysts can be small molecules, but enzymes are not small molecules. Choice C is incorrect because enzymes are found in the human body. Choice D is incorrect because enzymes and other catalysts alike increase the rate of a chemical reaction.

46. **The correct answer is A.** A primary alcohol possesses a hydroxyl group on a primary carbon, like that in $-CH_2OH$. Choice B is incorrect because a secondary alcohol has a hydroxyl group on a secondary carbon. Choice C is incorrect because a tertiary alcohol has a hydroxyl group on a tertiary carbon. Choice D is incorrect because a quaternary alcohol cannot exist; it would break the octet rule.

47. **The correct answer is D.** Ligase connects Okazaki fragments into a continuous DNA strand. Choice A is incorrect because helicase unwinds DNA. Choice B is incorrect because single-stranded binding proteins hold the separated DNA strands apart. Choice C is incorrect because this describes the role of primase in DNA replication.

48. **The correct answer is B.** Structural, or constitutional, isomers have the same chemical formula but are bonded differently. Choice A is incorrect because stereoisomers differ in three-dimensional orientation. Choice C is incorrect because isotopes are atoms that differ in number of neutrons. Choice D is incorrect because enantiomers are non-identical molecules that are non-superimposable mirror images of each other and have at least one chiral center.

Section 4: Critical Reading

1. C	**11.** B	**21.** B	**31.** B	**40.** B
2. D	**12.** B	**22.** B	**32.** C	**41.** D
3. B	**13.** B	**23.** D	**33.** D	**42.** B
4. D	**14.** A	**24.** A	**34.** B	**43.** B
5. A	**15.** A	**25.** D	**35.** A	**44.** B
6. B	**16.** A	**26.** C	**36.** D	**45.** D
7. C	**17.** B	**27.** B	**37.** A	**46.** C
8. B	**18.** C	**28.** B	**38.** D	**47.** A
9. C	**19.** B	**29.** B	**39.** C	**48.** D
10. B	**20.** C	**30.** B		

1. **The correct answer is C.** Choice C is correct because the passage credits many others, beginning with Aristotle and continuing through Glenn Seaborg. Choices A, B, and D are incorrect because the passage neither states nor implies any of these negative or positive opinions. Rather, it suggests that Mendeleev was one scientist among many who developed the Periodic Table.

2. **The correct answer is D.** Choice D is correct because the passage does not mention a geometric representation. Choice A is incorrect because the addition of transuranic elements is mentioned in the last paragraph. Choice B should be eliminated because the shift in arrangement from atomic weight to atomic number is also mentioned in the final paragraph. Choice C must be ruled out because the concept of octaves is mentioned in paragraph 2.

3. **The correct answer is B.** Although the passage begins with Mendeleev, it is in fact a history of the development of the Periodic Table. Choice A must be ruled out because the passage does not bolster Mendeleev's reputation; if anything, it diminishes his reputation as creator of the Periodic Table, noting that he is only one of the important contributors to the development of Periodic Table. Choice C is not the best choice because the passage does not clarify misconceptions about the table itself; rather, it clarifies misconceptions about Mendeleev's role in its development. Choice D is nearly correct but must be eliminated because, while the passage does effectively provide some contrast, its main purpose is to provide a history that shows that many people contributed to the development of the Periodic Table.

4. **The correct answer is D.** Choice D is correct because this is an objective history, based on fact. Choice A is incorrect; there are no personal pronouns or other suggestions that the facts have been gathered to further a strictly personal agenda. Choice B is incorrect. Little, if any, attitude can be heard in the author's voice, and certainly disapproval is not present. Choice C is incorrect because the author presents the facts confidently and without any backpedaling or other signs of confusion about chronology or the authorship of additions to the table.

5. **The correct answer is A.** Choice A is the correct answer because, in the matter of two apparently remarkably similar tables, credit went to the one published first. Choice B must be ruled out because the author credits Mendeleev with important contributions to the development of the Periodic Table. Choice C must be ruled out because the author credits Mendeleev not only with development of a table, but also predicting elements that would eventually fill it. Choice D is incorrect because the passage clearly states that Mendeleev and Meyer worked independently of each other.

6. **The correct answer is B.** Choice B is the correct answer because the final paragraph states that Moseley's work led to the arrangement of the table as we know it today. Choice A must be ruled out because the passage says that Moseley confirmed earlier ideas about this. Choice C is not correct because Mendeleev had arranged the table by atomic weight. Choice D must be ruled out because the passage does not credit Moseley with discovering new elements.

7. **The correct answer is C.** Choice C is correct because the letter penned by Newton to Hooke summarizes an idea about the sequential development of a breakthrough that the passage supports. Choice A should be ruled out because the author does not include Newton and Hooke as developers of the table. Choice B is incorrect because the main thesis of the passage is that Mendeleev deserves only some of the credit for the creation of the Periodic Table. Choice D must be ruled out. "Giants" are, indeed, discussed, but the purpose of the quotation is not to cause the reader to think about giants, but rather to cause the reader to think about how one important thinker or creator uses the work of a previous one to further develop a concept.

8. **The correct answer is B.** Choice B is correct because the last paragraph discusses ways the Periodic Table changed (and became more accurate) after Mendeleev published his version of it. Choice A must be ruled out because the last paragraph makes no mention of work that occurred before Mendeleev's time. Choice C, while tempting, is incorrect because the thesis is not about Mendeleev's being incorrect or only partially correct; it is about his role in an entire sequence of development. Choice D is incorrect because the passage does not say on who deserves most or even more credit; rather, its main thesis is that the table was the result of the work of many thinkers.

9. **The correct answer is C.** Choice C is correct because the tone is perhaps most evident in the final sentence, but earlier clues to the author's amusement include the puns about information that was "difficult to digest" and the reference to the reader's "gut feelings." The statement in parentheses in the third paragraph is also certainly droll. Choice A is incorrect because the author does not convey excitement. The author is clearly interested in the findings, but also finds them entertaining. Choice B is incorrect because the author does not convey doubt. Instead, the author regards the findings as both interesting and amusing. Choice D must be ruled out because details about information that was "difficult to digest" and the reference to the reader's "gut feelings," as well as the statement in parentheses in the third paragraph, all show attempts at humor and a decidedly less than completely serious attitude toward the study and its findings.

10. **The correct answer is B.** Choice B is the correct answer; the use of the first person is the best clue. In addition, the author is interpreting the findings or offering his or her own opinion here. Choices A, C, and

D are incorrect because each is a statement of fact, not opinion.

11. **The correct answer is B.** Choice B is correct because everything the author says in the final paragraph suggests that the author is thinking through the implications of the study's findings. Choice A is incorrect because the author never concludes this; rather, the author does a little speculation on what the findings might imply. Choice C is incorrect; the final paragraph suggests just the opposite. Choice D is incorrect; although the author's sympathy for the mice is clear, this is not what the author concludes, nor is it the topic of the end of the passage.

12. **The correct answer is B.** Choice B is correct because the first paragraph links brain chemistry with an altered state of mind. A lower level of stress suggests an altered state of mind. Choice A is incorrect because the statement focuses on communication between gut and brain rather than on the alteration of brain chemistry or any effect of such alteration. Choice C is a good answer, but not the best one, because, while its content about a positive mood seems to refer to the alteration of brain chemistry, the statement is interpretive ("researchers read these results as ...") and, therefore, more speculative than clearly supportive. Choice D is incorrect; it is very general and does not speak specifically to the alteration of brain chemistry.

13. **The correct answer is B.** Choice B is correct because the author's purpose is mainly to inform and the author's main points have to do with how the experiment shows how microbes affect brain activity; therefore, more data would be more informative. Choice A is incorrect because the writer's main point is not about the treatment of the mice. Choice C is incorrect because the maze and tunnels made up just one part of the experimental data. Choice D should

be eliminated. While the gut-brain axis is indeed at the heart of this informative piece, the focus is nevertheless on what the Cork researchers did and found, and the best answer is related to their research.

14. **The correct answer is A.** Choice A is correct because the context for the word *mood* refers to a state of mind. Choice B is incorrect because there is no context related to grammar. Choice C is incorrect because there is no context related to sullenness. Choice D is incorrect; this answer choice is closer to a definition of *mode* than a definition of *mood*.

15. **The correct answer is A.** Choice A is the correct answer because the author makes it clear more than once that the experiment that nearly drowned the mice seemed excessive. Choice B must be ruled out because the author neither states nor implies this. Choice C is not correct because the author makes no such claim; if anything, the reference to "direct measurements" seems to suggest validation for less quantifiable evidence. Choice D is tempting but incorrect, as nowhere does the author really suggest that anything is conclusive about these experiments.

16. **The correct answer is A.** Choice A is the correct answer because the author prefaces such comments with "it might not be reaching," which suggests that the comments could very well be a reach. Choice B should be ruled out because the author doesn't suggest that the statement is antithetical. Instead, the author suggests that such labels simply take the researchers' labels one step further. Choice C is incorrect. There is no specific application of the label; furthermore, the description of that part of the experiment comes after the relevant text. Choice D is incorrect because the author neither makes nor implies any such claim.

17. **The correct answer is B.** While the passage is about chemotherapy, the malady being treated is cancer. For this reason, choice A is incorrect. Choice C should be eliminated because nitrogen mustard is a minor detail in this passage about chemotherapy, and chemotherapy is used to treat the malady called cancer. Choice D is incorrect because the answer must name a malady, or illness, not a person.

18. **The correct answer is C.** In this passage, the author works to prove that Ehrlich's consideration of how discriminating binding could be the method of targeting diseased cells gave birth to the idea of chemotherapy, and choice C captures that goal in a clear statement. While the thesis statement of a passage is often presented in the first sentence, that is not the case in this particular passage, since the opening sentence focuses on Siddhartha Mukherjee rather than Paul Ehrlich. Therefore, choice A is incorrect. Choice B can be eliminated because it similarly focuses on Mukherjee rather than Ehrlich. Choice D is the topic sentence of the second paragraph; not the thesis statement that captures the author's purpose in writing the passage as a whole.

19. **The correct answer is B.** Choice B is correct because paragraph 4 says directly that "the absence of regulation . . . helped this work go forward at a dizzying pace." Choice A is incorrect because the work went on and led to results despite great criticism. Choice C is incorrect because the passage is mainly about synthetic chemicals and combination therapies using synthetic chemicals. Choice D must be ruled out because the National Cancer Institute actually mocked the work, so it did more to stand in its way than promote it.

20. **The correct answer is C.** Even though the passage documents the criticisms of others, it also makes clear that a cure for one kind of cancer resulted from the unregulated research. There is no attitude of criticism or indignation, choices A and D, so eliminate them. Choice B should be eliminated because the passage contains no evidence of bias, or prejudice, in favor of or against the history it retells.

21. **The correct answer is B.** Choice B is correct because the main idea of paragraph 3 is that researchers went forward despite very negative criticism. Supporting ideas include the idea that temporary remission (which the researchers brought about with their chemicals) was thought cruel and that people didn't believe cancer could be cured (and, therefore, the reader may infer, did not respect the researchers' work). Choice A is incorrect. There is no series of events related in time order. Choice C should be eliminated. The paragraph does not compare or contrast. Choice D is incorrect because, even though the passage documents the criticisms of others, it also makes clear that a cure for one kind of cancer resulted from the unregulated research.

22. **The correct answer is B.** The discovery of aniline mauve caused Ehrlich to consider the targeting of diseased cells, which is what happens in chemotherapy. The study of nitrogen mustard revealed a similar targeted effect, just as the goal of chemotherapy is to target diseased cells without killing normal cells. Choice A must be ruled out because nothing suggests that either aniline mauve or nitrogen gas were ever used in chemotherapy or combination therapies. Choice C is not the best choice because nothing in the passage suggests this. Choice D is incorrect because nothing in the passage suggests this.

23. **The correct answer is D.** Choice D is correct because the passage focuses on synthetic chemicals and how they eventually

led to a cure. Choice A must be ruled out because just one form of cancer, Hodgkin's lymphoma, was defeated. Choice B is not the best choice because the author's attitude toward the researchers is fairly objective, even though it is clear that others thought them demonic. Also, the triumph described in the passage was hardly total—it was a beginning. Choice C is incorrect because even though the passage ends with this victory, most of the passage is about how synthetic chemicals were used and targeted to create the first successful chemotherapy.

24. **The correct answer is A.** Choice A is correct because researchers were regarded with scorn for their attempts to find chemical cures. Choice B is incorrect. The context does not suggest that the atmosphere was one of contradiction. Choice C is incorrect. Researchers may have worked to combat disease, but it makes no sense to say that they were regarded with an "attitude of disease." Choice D is incorrect. The passage suggests that the general atmosphere was more likely to be characterized as hopelessness.

25. **The correct answer is D.** Choice D is correct because paragraph 2 is organized in an effect–cause order. It begins with the lower infection rate and explains the cause, ticks' diet. Choice A must be ruled out because the focus of the paragraph is on why there is a lower infection rate from vector ticks in the western United States. There is no order of importance to the information. Choice B is incorrect because this would not be seen as a problem, but as a positive. Choice C is incorrect because main ideas and supporting details is not an organizational structure.

26. **The correct answer is C.** The thesis statement sums up the author's main goal, and in the case of this passage, the author is mainly concerned with proving that Lyme disease is difficult to detect (the topic of

paragraph 3) and treat (the topic of paragraph 4). Therefore, choice C is the best answer. Choice A may be the first sentence of the passage, but it is not a strong thesis statement because it does not capture the author's main goal in writing this passage. Choice B simply provides some statistics about Lyme disease; it does not capture the author's main goal. Choice D is the topic sentence of paragraph 2, not the thesis statement of the entire passage.

27. **The correct answer is B.** Choice B is correct because the paragraph details a number of conditions and implies, mainly by means of the conjunction *and* in the last sentence, that they must exist together. Choice A must be ruled out, though it may be tempting if you think of "while playing" as a definition of *interplay* or *interact*. Choice C is not correct because "in concert" never means "sequentially." Choice D must be eliminated because "in concert" never means "with certainty"; furthermore, the conjunction *and* that relates to all the conditions, suggests another meaning and answer choice.

28. **The correct answer is B.** The author's bias is revealed in descriptive words reflecting the author's opinion, and as it is used in paragraph 1, *insidious* is one such word, so choice B is the best answer. Choice A, *commonly*, choice C, *high*, and choice D, *greater*, are all descriptive words, but none of them reflect the author's opinion in their respective contexts.

29. **The correct answer is B.** The author categorizing potential Lyme disease sufferers as foolish in paragraph 3 is a reflection of a personal opinion that everyone might not share, so choice B is the best answer. As they are used in their respective contexts, choice A, *undetectable*, choice C, *recommended only*, and choice D, *local rates*, are used factually because they cannot be disputed.

30. **The correct answer is B.** Choice B is the correct answer because the second sentence of paragraph 3 directly states that "the bite of the *I. scapularis* may lead not only to Lyme disease but also to HGA . . . and babesiosis." Choice A must be ruled out because the passage never says this. Furthermore, a specific statement in the third paragraph suggests a better answer. Choices C and D must be ruled out because HGA and babesiosis are diseases.

31. **The correct answer is B.** Choice B is the correct answer because the passage presents the causes (vector tick bites) and some treatments. Choice A must be ruled out because the passage is informational, not persuasive. Choice C is not correct because the focus of the passage is clearly on Lyme disease; mentions of HGA and babesiosis are included to illuminate that main topic. Choice D must be ruled out because the focus of the passage is on Lyme disease, not related diseases; furthermore, while causes of the disease are discussed, few effects are noted.

32. **The correct answer is C.** This is stated in the final paragraph. Choice A is incorrect. Doxycycline is an antimicrobial prophylaxis, but the last paragraph clearly states that its use is not always indicated. Choice B is incorrect because doxycycline is an antimicrobial prophylaxis, not a serological test. Choice D must be ruled out; paragraph 4 makes it clear that the use of doxycycline is warranted only in some cases.

33. **The correct answer is D.** Choice D is correct because paragraph 3 states this directly. Choice A must be ruled out because the final paragraph concedes that volcanoes may have caused the release of methane. Choice B is incorrect because the extinction promoted the rise of the dinosaurs. Choice

C is incorrect; the passage makes no comparison of the amount of devastation.

34. **The correct answer is B.** This opinion, not fact, is stated in the fifth paragraph. Choice A is incorrect because it quotes an opinion held by others, not necessarily by the author. Choices C and D are incorrect because they are statements of fact.

35. **The correct answer is A.** Choice A is the correct answer because the term refers back to one negative effect, trapping greenhouse gases, and ahead to another negative effect, causing mass extinctions. Choice B must be ruled because methane is inanimate and cannot have a criminal history—except metaphorically. Choice C is not correct because the passage makes no mention of syncopated evolution. Choice D is incorrect because it does not make sense.

36. **The correct answer is D.** Choice D is correct because this informative, not persuasive, passage focuses on new evidence for the possibility that methane caused the end-Triassic. Choice A should be ruled out because the passage never credits the clathrate gun idea with being anything more than a hypothesis. Choice B is tempting but incorrect; choice D is a far better answer that more adequately reflects the focus of the passage. Choice C is incorrect because, first, the passage is informative and not persuasive, and second, the implied need for the control of methane is not a main idea.

37. **The correct answer is A.** Choice A is correct because the new study focuses on sudden and relatively brief change, and studying plants and the fossil record could show this. Choice B should be eliminated; it would discredit the hypothesis presented in the passage. Choice C is incorrect because the hypothesis is not about the rise of the dinosaurs, which is a fact. Choice D is irrelevant because the

passage states directly that clathrates are found on seafloors.

38. **The correct answer is D.** Choice D is correct because the passage says that the clathrates are on the seafloors, and the entire passage is about the kind of cataclysm such stores could cause. Choice A is incorrect; the passage does say methane traps heat but does not compare it with other gases. Choice B is incorrect; the passage does not mention global warming (even if the reader's mind does, naturally, go there). Choice C should be eliminated; the passage says the opposite: that the eruption of volcanoes might have triggered a release of methane.

39. **The correct answer is C.** Choice C is correct because the last line of the passage speculates that mass extinctions are relatively easy to trigger if all it takes is a sudden release of methane, or a clathrate gun. Choice A is incorrect because the clathrate gun hypothesis is the basis of the final speculation. Choice B makes no sense because the last sentence of the last paragraph is a speculation; the phenomenon does not make the speculation possible. Choice D is incorrect because the passage does not mention a number of mass extinction theories or draw conclusions about most of them.

40. **The correct answer is B.** Choice B is the correct answer because the information in paragraph 1 is specifically relevant to global warming: greenhouse gases, trapping heat in the atmosphere, and the final statement that suggests a sudden, mass release of that greenhouse gas. Choice A must be ruled out; the passage suggests just the opposite. Choice C is not correct because the passage neither implies nor makes any such claim. Choice D is incorrect; the final sentence of the passage suggests the opposite.

41. **The correct answer is D.** Choice D is the correct answer; the third paragraph asks questions that lead up to, and effectively provide background for, the research described in paragraph 4. Choice A should be ruled out because the second paragraph focuses more specifically on this topic. Choice B is tempting because the paragraph does ask questions; if there were no paragraph 4, or if the fourth paragraph contained different information, it would be the best choice. Choice C makes no sense; a paragraph that mainly asks questions confirms nothing.

42. **The correct answer is B.** Paragraph 3 suggests this continuing role of the evolution of the species. Choice A is incorrect because the passage makes a distinction between the amygdala and the thinking brain, or neocortex. Choice C should be eliminated because the passage suggests that the communication between the amygdala and the neocortex is asymmetrical, not what the effect on emotions is. Choice D is incorrect because the passage states clearly that the amygdala is linked to aggression.

43. **The correct answer is B.** Choice B is correct because the detail is that the amygdala is shaped like an almond. Choice A must be ruled out. The purpose of the passage is to explain the amygdala and a theory about why it is so difficult to overcome, counterbalance, or act in a way that is contrary to its signals. Choice C is incorrect because the shape of the amygdala is a detail, not a main idea. Choice D is incorrect because the shape of the amygdala is in no way related to problems.

44. **The correct answer is B.** Writers use quotations from credible sources such as academic leaders from respected institutions such as New York University to lend credibility to their assertions, so choice B is the best answer. Choices A and C may help clarify

information in the passage, but they do not necessarily make the passage more credible. Choice D sets up an explanation, which is a strategy for getting the reader to think about a problem before its solution is offered, but it is not a rhetorical strategy for strengthening the credibility of a piece of writing.

45. **The correct answer is choice D.** The author of the passage is mostly concerned with imparting information about the amygdala in a straightforward manner, so *informative* is the best description of its tone. Choice D is the best answer. Choice A, *benevolent*, suggests that the author is trying to improve the reader's life in some way, but that does not seem to be the express purpose of this particular passage. *Earnest*, choice B, suggests an intense sincerity, which would apply to a passage with a more emotional tone than this one. Choice C, *mocking*, suggests an author making fun of someone or something, and nothing like that is happening in this particular passage.

46. **The correct answer is choice C.** Different people have different ideas about what is and isn't forgivable, so a term such as *unforgivable* is generally used to reflect an opinion rather than a fact. So choice C is the best answer. As it is used in paragraph 1, *fear and pleasure* relates to the undisputable function of the amygdala, and not the author's personal opinion about anything, so choice A is incorrect. While in certain contexts *worst* can certainly be reflective of an opinion, that is not how it is used in the context of paragraph 1, so choice B is also wrong. *At the heart of* is an idiom, not a reflection of an opinion, so choice D is incorrect.

47. **The correct answer is A.** Choice A is the only possible correct choice because *sub-* can mean "beneath" or "below;" the relationship to the cortex is made clear later. Choices B, C, and D must be ruled out because there is no structural evidence within the word itself or the passage to support any of these choices.

48. **The correct answer is D.** Choice D is correct because paragraph 3, which leads up to the presentation of this information, effectively asks this question, and the quoted information from the research is a stab at answering it. Choice A must be ruled out because there is no mention of specific therapies. Choice B is incorrect because the point made by the neuroanatomists was the discovery of the asymmetry and what it might explain, not the reasons for it. Choice C is incorrect because the neuroanatomists were looking at a more specific question about why the amygdala can seem to overrule the thinking brain.

Section 5: Quantitative Reasoning

1. C	11. A	21. A	31. C	40. C
2. B	12. B	22. A	32. B	41. B
3. A	13. C	23. B	33. A	42. D
4. A	14. D	24. C	34. C	43. A
5. B	15. B	25. A	35. A	44. A
6. D	16. B	26. D	36. D	45. A
7. C	17. C	27. B	37. B	46. B
8. C	18. A	28. C	38. B	47. D
9. C	19. B	29. A	39. B	48. D
10. C	20. B	30. D		

1. **The correct answer is C.** Compute the inverse function of $T = \dfrac{5,000 - p}{0.04\,p}$ by solving for p:

$$T = \frac{5,000 - p}{0.04\,p}$$
$$0.04T \cdot p = 5,000 - p$$
$$p + 0.04T \cdot p = 5,000$$
$$p(1 + 0.04T) = 5,000$$
$$p = \frac{5,000}{1 + 0.04T}$$

2. **The correct answer is B.**

Solve the equation $\frac{7}{2}t + \frac{1}{2}t^2 = 49$:

$$\frac{7}{2}t + \frac{1}{2}t^2 = 49$$
$$7t + t^2 = 98$$
$$t^2 + 7t - 98 = 0$$
$$(t + 14)(t - 7) = 0$$
$$t = \cancel{-14},\ 7$$

So, it takes 7 seconds for the sleigh to move 49 feet.

3. **The correct answer is A.** First, simplify the numerator by changing 3 into the fraction $\frac{9}{3}$ and adding it to $\frac{1}{3}$. Then simplify the complex fraction by multiplying the numerator by the reciprocal of the denominator:

$$\frac{\frac{1}{3} + 3}{3} = \frac{\frac{1}{3} + \frac{9}{3}}{3} = \frac{\frac{10}{3}}{3} = \frac{\frac{10}{3}}{\frac{3}{1}} = \frac{10}{3} \times \frac{1}{3} = \frac{10}{9}$$

4. **The correct answer is A.** Leave the negative sign on the numerator aside for starters. As x approaches 1 from the right, that is, as it takes successively the values 4, 3, 2, 1.5, and so on, the denominator is positive, but diminishing toward 0. That means that the fraction (ignoring the negative sign, still) keeps increasing toward infinity. Now, taking into account the negative sign, you have a negative number whose absolute value keeps increasing toward infinity. Thus, the right-hand limit equals negative infinity.

5. **The correct answer is B.** The combined age of the 17 team members was $17 \times 26 = 442$ years. The combined age of the remaining 16 team members is $16 \times 25.625 = 410$ years. Thus, the age of the injured team member is $442 - 410 = 32$ years.

6. **The correct answer is D.** Extract the essential characteristics from the graph. First, the minimum occurs at $t = 2$, and the maximum occurs when $t = 0$ and 4. As such, look for a function of the form $y = A\cos(Bt) + C$. The period is 4; so, $\frac{2\pi}{B} = 4$, so that $B = \frac{\pi}{2}$. Next, the midline is $y = 40$, and the minimum and maximum values are 20 and 60, respectively. So, the amplitude A must be 20 (the average of the minimum and maximum values). Finally, since the midline is $y = 40$, the graph $y = 20\cos\left(\frac{\pi}{2}t\right)$ is translated up 40 units to get the final function $f(t) = 20\cos\left(\frac{\pi}{2}t\right) + 40$.

7. **The correct answer is C.** First, make certain all measurements are expressed using the same units. Using $2\frac{3}{4}$ feet $= \frac{11}{4}$ feet with the fact that 1 foot = 12 inches yields

$$\frac{\frac{11}{4} \text{ feet}}{} \times \frac{12 \text{ inches}}{1 \text{ foot}} = 33 \text{ inches}$$

This is the width of the shelf. For each shelf, you can fit $\frac{33 \text{ inches}}{1\frac{5}{8} \text{ inches}} = \frac{33}{\frac{13}{8}} = \frac{264}{13} = 20.31\ldots$.

So, 20 books can be fit on a single shelf. Thus, 60 such books can be fit into the bookcase.

8. **The correct answer is C.** Add the four distances to get the length of one full lap:

$$\frac{5}{8} + 1\frac{1}{3} + \frac{3}{4} + 1\frac{1}{4} = \frac{5}{8} + \frac{4}{3} + \frac{3}{4} + \frac{5}{4}$$
$$= \frac{15}{24} + \frac{32}{24} + \frac{18}{24} + \frac{30}{24}$$
$$= \frac{95}{24}$$

Since they are walking two laps, the total distance being walked is $2 \times \frac{95}{24} = \frac{95}{12} = 7\frac{11}{12}$ miles.

9. **The correct answer is C.** If the graph of function $f(x)$ lies entirely above the x-axis, then all values of $f(x)$ are positive, regardless of what x is. If the graph of $(fg)(x)$ also lies entirely above the x-axis, then all values of $g(x)$ must also be positive because $f(x)$ is always positive—and only if you multiply a positive number by another positive number will you get a positive result. Thus, the statement in choice A is correct, and choice A is not the right answer. Similarly, the statement in choice B is correct (the sum of two positive numbers is also positive), so choice B is not the right answer. However, the statement in choice D cannot be correct because the quotient of a positive number by another positive number can never be negative. Thus, choice C is the correct answer. For the record, the statement in choice D can be true—if, for instance, $f(x) = x^2 + 1$ and $g(x) = x^2 + 3$, in which case $f(x) - g(x) = -2$.

10. **The correct answer is C.** You're asked to find the derivative of $\ln x^2$. You can use the chain rule here, but you don't have to. Recall that $\ln x^2 = 2 \ln x$. Thus: $\frac{d}{dx}\left(\ln x^2\right) = \frac{d}{dx}\left(2 \ln x\right) = \frac{2}{x}$. When $x = 2$, the derivative equals 1.

11. **The correct answer is A.** One liter equals 1,000 milliliters, so 0.6 liters equals 600 milliliters. If x is the number of vials Morgan has to buy, then:

$$30x = 600 \Rightarrow x = 20$$

12. **The correct answer is B.** You may recall that $\int \csc x \cot x\, dx = -\csc x + c$, and that an angle's cosecant is the reciprocal of its sine. However, you do not need to worry about all this for this problem. Rather, note that the limits of the definite integral are equal to each other. Since $\int_a^b f(x)dx = F(b) - F(a)$, and in this case a

$= b$, then the definite integral you are looking for becomes $F(b) - F(a) = F(a) - F(a) = 0$.

13. **The correct answer is C.** The total number of students who joined an arts club is 6 + 5 + 9 + 7 + 8, that is, 35. Of them, 5 joined the painting club. In order to find what percentage of 35 that is, set up and solve a proportion:

$$\frac{5}{35} = \frac{x}{100}$$

$$\frac{1}{7} = \frac{x}{100}$$

$$7x = 100$$

$$x = \frac{100}{7}$$

$$x \approx 14.29$$

To the nearest integer, the answer is 14%.

14. **The correct answer is D.** Martha bought 3 tomatoes for every 1 cucumber. Since she bought 2 cucumbers, she bought 2 × 3, that is, 6 tomatoes. Likewise, she bought 2 onions for every 1 cucumber, so she bought 2 × 2, that is, 4 onions. In total, she bought 6 + 2 + 4 = 12 items.

15. **The correct answer is B.** Choice A is incorrect; the logarithm of the same number (other than 1) varies depending on the base of the logarithm. Since log and ln are logarithms in different bases, the logarithm of 72 in one base will be different from the logarithm of 72 in another base. The other three choices play (correctly or incorrectly) with the following three properties of logarithms:

$$\log_a (xy) = \log_a x + \log_a y$$

$$\log_a \left(\frac{x}{y}\right) = \log_a x - \log_a y$$

$$\log_a x^r = r \log_a x$$

The only answer choice that uses one of these properties correctly is choice B:

$$\log 72 = \log \frac{144}{2} = \log 144 - \log 2$$

16. **The correct answer is B.** To compute percent increase, subtract the two values, divide the difference by the original value, and then multiply by 100%. Doing so yields $\frac{720 - 640}{640} \times 100\% = 12.5\%$.

17. **The correct answer is C.** In a boxplot, the median is the middle vertical segment contained within the box portion of the plot (which here is 50), and the range is the difference between the maximum and minimum values, which are the extreme ends of the plot (which here are 20 and 70).

18. **The correct answer is A.** Do not substitute directly into the fraction because you'll get the indeterminate form $-\infty + \infty - \infty$. Rather, begin by factoring x^3 out of the numerator:

$$\lim_{x \to \infty} \left(\frac{-3x^3 + 2x^2 - x}{2} \right)$$

$$= \lim_{x \to \infty} \frac{1}{2} \left[x^3 \left(-3 + \frac{2}{x} - \frac{1}{x^2} \right) \right]$$

$$= \frac{1}{2} \times \infty \left(-3 + 0 - 0 \right)$$

$$= -\infty$$

19. The correct answer is B. Substitute the following values into the formula: $R_T = 25$, $R_1 = 200$, and $R_3 = 100$; then, solve for $R2$:

$$\frac{1}{25} = \frac{1}{200} + \frac{1}{R_2} + \frac{1}{100}$$

$$\frac{1}{25} - \frac{1}{200} - \frac{1}{100} = \frac{1}{R_2}$$

$$\frac{8 - 1 - 2}{200} = \frac{1}{R_2}$$

$$\frac{5}{200} = \frac{1}{R_2}$$

$$\frac{1}{40} = \frac{1}{R_2}$$

$$40 = R_2$$

20. The correct answer is B. The slope is equal to the derivative of the function at that point. Use the chain rule in order to differentiate:

$$\frac{d}{dx}\cos 2x = \frac{d}{du}(\cos u)\frac{d}{dx}u$$

$$= -2\sin u$$

$$= -2\sin(2x)$$

When $x = \frac{\pi}{2}$, the sine you are looking for is that of π, which is 0. Thus, the derivative at that point is also 0.

21. The correct answer is A. Michael sold the figurine for 50% more than the $40 he paid. So, the price for which he sold it is: $\$40 + \frac{1}{2}\$40 = \$60$. You need to find out what percent of $50 (Mary's purchase price) the sale price of $60 is. Set up and solve a proportion:

$$\frac{60}{50} = \frac{x}{100}$$

$$\frac{6}{5} = \frac{x}{100}$$

$$\frac{6}{1} = \frac{x}{20}$$

$$x = 120$$

Therefore, the price for which Michael sold the figurine was 120% of Mary's purchase price.

22. The correct answer is A. Note that half a mile equals $\frac{1}{2}(5,280) = 2,640$ feet. Let y be the hypotenuse, which is the length of the chair lift cable. Model the scenario using the following diagram:

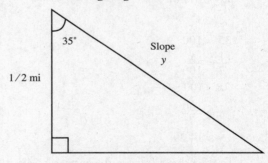

Then, $\cos(35°) = \dfrac{2,640}{y}$, so that

$$y = \frac{2,640}{\cos(35°)}\text{ feet.}$$

23. The correct answer is B. First, arrange the data in increasing order, as follows:

1 1 1 1 2 2 3

4 $\boxed{4}$ 5 6 6 8 8

10 12

The median is the value in the 9th position because there are 17 data values. This value is 4.

24. The correct answer is C. The integration by parts formula is $\int f(x)g'(x)dx = f(x)g(x) - \int f'(x)g(x)dx$. For the integral in question, since $(e^x)' = e^x$, let $g(x) = e^x$. Then:

$$\int xe^x dx = \int x\left(e^x\right)' dx$$
$$= xe^x - \int x'e^x dx$$
$$= xe^x - \int e^x dx$$
$$= xe^x - e^x + c$$

25. The correct answer is A. Melissa had a total of 12 clients (4 plus 2 plus 6) from which she earned a total fee of $4a + 2b + 6c$. Thus, the average fee she earned equals $\frac{4a + 2b + 6c}{12}$, which can be broken into $\frac{4}{12}a + \frac{2}{12}b + \frac{6}{12}c$, or $\frac{1}{3}a + \frac{1}{6}b + \frac{1}{2}c$.

26. The correct answer is D. Use the facts that 1 hour = 60 minutes and 1 revolution = 2π radians to convert the units as follows:

$$\frac{490 \text{ revolutions}}{1 \text{ minute}} \times \frac{60 \text{ minutes}}{1 \text{ hour}}$$
$$\times \frac{2\pi \text{ radians}}{1 \text{ revolution}} = (490 \times 60 \times 2\pi)$$

radians per hour

27. The correct answer is B. If there are 1 part liquid A and 3 parts liquid B in the original solution, then there are 4 parts in total, 3 of which are liquid B. Thus, liquid B is $\frac{3}{4}$ of the original solution. In problems such as this one, in which you are not given specific numbers for the quantities involved, it's wise to pick the number 100 to represent the original total. So, let 100 be the original volume of the solution. Then, the volume of liquid B is three quarters of 100, that is, 75. When the third liquid is added, the new volume of the solution is 200. What percent of 200 is 75?

$$\frac{75}{200} = \frac{x}{100}$$
$$\frac{75}{2} = \frac{x}{1}$$
$$x = 37.5$$

So, liquid B is 37.5% of the new solution.

28. The correct answer is C. Let x represent the temperature of the roadway and y the thickness of the joint. Find the equation of the line using the points (100, 0.8) and (20, 1.2). The slope is $m = \frac{0.8 - 1.2}{100 - 20} = -0.005$. Using point-slope form $y - y_1 = m(x - x_1)$ with $m = -0.005$ and (20, 1.2) as the point (x_1, y_1) gives the equation $y - 1.2 = -0.005(x - 20)$, which simplifies to $y = -0.005x + 1.3$. Next, compute $y(70)$: $y(70) = -0.005(70) + 1.3 = 0.95$ inch.

29. The correct answer is A. Calculate the logarithm:

$$\log_{1,000} 100 = y$$
$$1,000^y = 100$$
$$10^{3y} = 10^2$$
$$3y = 2$$
$$y = \frac{2}{3}$$

30. The correct answer is D. The approximate area will be equal to the sum of the areas of four rectangles, each with width $\frac{2-0}{4} = \frac{1}{2}$. In the left Riemann sum, the height of each rectangle will be the value of the function at the left endpoint of the subinterval to which the rectangle corresponds. For the left-most subinterval, that endpoint is 0; for the second subinterval from the left, the left endpoint is $0 + \frac{1}{2}$; in general, for each subinterval the left endpoint is $\frac{1}{2}i$, where i = 0, 1, 2, 3. Thus, the height of each rectangle equals $8 - \left(\frac{1}{2}i\right)^3$ and the Riemann sum becomes:

$$\sum_{i=0}^{3}\left[\frac{1}{2}\left(8 - \left(\frac{1}{2}\right)^3\right)\right] = \frac{1}{2}\left[8 - \left(\frac{1}{2} \times 0\right)^3 + 8 - \left(\frac{1}{2} \times 1\right)^3 + 8 - \left(\frac{1}{2} \times 2\right)^3 + 8 - \left(\frac{1}{2} \times 3\right)^3\right]$$

$$= \frac{1}{2}\left[8 - 0 + 8 - \left(\frac{1}{2}\right)^3 + 8 - 1^3 + 8 - \left(\frac{3}{2}\right)^3\right]$$

$$= \frac{1}{2}\left(31 - \frac{1}{8} - \frac{27}{8}\right)$$

$$= \frac{1}{2}\left(31 - \frac{28}{8}\right)$$

$$= \frac{1}{2}\left(31 - \frac{7}{2}\right)$$

$$= \frac{1}{2} \times \frac{55}{2}$$

$$= 13.75$$

31. The correct answer is C. The endpoints of the whiskers indicate the range of the data set. In this case, the range is 35 minus 10, that is, 25.

32. The correct answer is B. The applicant is equally likely to have to go to any of these four cities, so the probability she will have to go to any of them is 0.25. To find the probability that the applicant will be in each city and it will rain in that city, multiply the probability she will have to go to that particular city by the probability it will rain in that city.

The probability she will go, for example, to Akron and it will be raining there is 0.25 × 0.3.

Finally, to find the probability that it will rain in the city in which she interviews, add the four probabilities you calculated in the previous step:

$$P = 0.25 \times 0.3 + 0.25 \times 0.35 + 0.25 \times 0.25 + 0.25 \times 0.3$$

$$= 0.25 \times (0.3 + 0.35 + 0.25 + 0.3)$$

$$= 0.25 \times 1.2$$

$$= 0.3$$

33. The correct answer is A. Substitute $s = 80$ and $s = 100$ into the formula $s = \sqrt{9.8 \times d}$ and solve for d in each case:

$$80 = \sqrt{9.8 \times d}$$
$$6,400 = 9.8 \times d$$
$$d = \frac{6,400}{9.8} \approx 653 \text{ meters}$$
$$100 = \sqrt{9.8 \times d}$$
$$10,000 = 9.8 \times d$$
$$d = \frac{10,000}{9.8} \approx 1,020 \text{ meters}$$

So, the range is 653 meters to 1,020 meters.

34. The correct answer is C. Start by noting that $\log_2 4x = \log_2 4 + \log_2 x$. Now, evaluate $\log_2 4$:

$$\log_2 4 = n \Rightarrow 2^n = 4 \Rightarrow n = 2$$

Therefore, $\log_2 4x$ equals $2 + y$.

35. The correct answer is A. You could divide the numerator by the denominator, but this would be unnecessarily complicated. Take a look at the answer choices: all of them are of the form "12 times a negative power of 10." This should give you a clue: If possible, you should manipulate the fraction so that you get the number 12 somewhere. You can achieve this by multiplying both numerator and denominator by 2. Then, $\frac{6}{5,000}$ becomes $\frac{12}{10,000}$. This division is much easier: Simply add a decimal point four spots to the left of the "2" in 12:

$$\frac{6}{5,000} = \frac{12}{10,000} = 0.0012$$

36. The correct answer is D. Solve the second equation for x:

$$x - 4 + y = 0 \Rightarrow x = 4 - y$$

Now substitute this expression for x into the first equation:

$$-y + 3 = 2x$$
$$-y + 3 = 2(4 - y)$$
$$-y + 3 = 8 - 2y$$
$$y = 5$$

37. The correct answer is B. Solve the equation $11,000 = 5,000\, e^{0.06t}$ for t:

$$11,000 = 5,000\, e^{0.06t}$$
$$\frac{11}{5} = e^{0.06t}$$
$$\ln\left(\frac{11}{5}\right) = 0.06t$$
$$\frac{1}{0.06} \ln\left(\frac{11}{5}\right) = t$$
$$\frac{50}{3} \ln\left(\frac{11}{5}\right) = t$$
$$\ln\left(\frac{11}{5}\right)^{50/3} = t$$

38. The correct answer is B. Let x be Mark's score on the third test. Now you can set up and solve the following equation for the average of his four test scores:

$$\frac{76 + 86 + x + 87}{4} = 83$$
$$\frac{249 + x}{4} = 83$$
$$249 + x = 332$$
$$x = 83$$

39. The correct answer is B. Let x be the number of liters of 25% solution and y the number of liters of 70% solution. The sum of these two quantities must be 120, giving the equation $x + y = 120$. The amount of alcohol in x liters of 25% solution is $0.25x$, and the amount of alcohol in y liters of 70% solution is $0.70y$. The sum of these two quantities must be the amount of alcohol in 120 liters of 40% solution, namely $0.40(120) = 48$. This leads to the equation $0.25x + 0.70y = 48$. Taking these equations together results in the system in choice B.

40. The correct answer is C. Look at the answer choices. First, $f(x)$ is a parabola with a negative coefficient of the x-squared term. This means it must open downward. Only the graphs in choices B and C do, so you can eliminate the other two choices. Further, $f(x)$ does not pass through the origin: when x equals 0, y equals 3. So, you can eliminate choice B, leaving you with the correct choice C.

41. The correct answer is B. Combined profit from both facilities is the sum of the profits. This is precisely the function $(P_1 + P_2)(t)$.

42. The correct answer is D. You need to solve the inequality, but also make sure that the radical is a real number. For that to be the case, the quantity under the radical must be greater than or equal to 0:

$$2x + 3 \geq 0 \Rightarrow x \geq -\frac{3}{2}$$

Now solve the inequality:

$$\sqrt{2x + 3} < 5$$
$$\left(\sqrt{2x + 3}\right)^2 < 5^2$$
$$2x + 3 < 25$$
$$2x < 22$$
$$x < 11$$

So, the solution of the inequality is the union between $x \geq -\frac{3}{2}$ and $x < 11$, which is

$$-\frac{3}{2} \leq x < 11.$$

43. The correct answer is A. Use the facts that 1 pound = 16 ounces and 1 foot = 12 inches, so that 1 square foot = 12^2 inches = 144 inches to convert the units, as follows:

$$\frac{30 \text{ pounds}}{1 \text{ square inch}} \times \frac{16 \text{ ounces}}{1 \text{ pound}} \times$$

$$\frac{144 \text{ square inches}}{1 \text{ square foot}} =$$

$$= (30 \times 16 \times 144) \text{ ounces per square foot}$$

44. The correct answer is A. Begin by factoring the quadratic:

$$x^2 + 3x > -2$$
$$x^2 + 3x + 2 > 0$$
$$x^2 + 2x + x + 2 > 0$$
$$x(x + 2) + x + 2 > 0$$
$$(x + 2)(x + 1) > 0$$

The two factors on the left are 0 when x equals -1 and -2, respectively. Set up a table and see how each factor behaves for values of x to the left and right of these two values:

	$x < -2$	$-2 < x < -1$	$x > -1$
$(x + 1)$	Negative	Negative	Positive
$(x + 2)$	Negative	Positive	Positive
$(x + 2)(x + 1)$	**Positive**	Negative	**Positive**

The expression is positive when both factors are positive—that is, when x is less than -2 or greater than -1.

45. The correct answer is A. The median is the average of the 75th and 76th data values because there are 150 data values in this sample. Here, this value is $\frac{4 + 4}{2} = 4$. The range is the difference between the maximum and minimum data values, namely $8 - 0 = 8$.

46. The correct answer is B. Convert the second and third terms as products of a number and 10^{-2} in order to make the operations easier:

$$1.2 \times 10^{-2} + 1.2 \times 10^{-1} + 1.2$$
$$= 1.2 \times 10^{-2} + 12 \times 10^{-2} + 120 \times 10^{-2}$$
$$= 10^{-2} \times (1.2 + 12 + 120)$$
$$= 10^{-2} \times 133.2$$
$$= 1.332$$

47. The correct answer is D. A function's x-intercept occurs at the point at which the function crosses the x-axis. The function e^x lies entirely above the x-axis—it consists of all the powers of a positive number. The function $e^x + 2$ also lies entirely above the x-axis, since it is the sum of two positive numbers. Thus, this function does not have an x-intercept.

48. The correct answer is D. Sum the values in the cells in the last two rows: $10 + 8 + 3 + 7 = 28$. Divide this by 110, the sum of all the cells in the table (which corresponds to the number of data points all told). Doing so yields a probability of $\frac{28}{110} = \frac{14}{55}$.

PRACTICE TEST 3: ANSWER SHEETS

Biological Processes

1. Ⓐ Ⓑ Ⓒ Ⓓ	11. Ⓐ Ⓑ Ⓒ Ⓓ	21. Ⓐ Ⓑ Ⓒ Ⓓ	31. Ⓐ Ⓑ Ⓒ Ⓓ	40. Ⓐ Ⓑ Ⓒ Ⓓ
2. Ⓐ Ⓑ Ⓒ Ⓓ	12. Ⓐ Ⓑ Ⓒ Ⓓ	22. Ⓐ Ⓑ Ⓒ Ⓓ	32. Ⓐ Ⓑ Ⓒ Ⓓ	41. Ⓐ Ⓑ Ⓒ Ⓓ
3. Ⓐ Ⓑ Ⓒ Ⓓ	13. Ⓐ Ⓑ Ⓒ Ⓓ	23. Ⓐ Ⓑ Ⓒ Ⓓ	33. Ⓐ Ⓑ Ⓒ Ⓓ	42. Ⓐ Ⓑ Ⓒ Ⓓ
4. Ⓐ Ⓑ Ⓒ Ⓓ	14. Ⓐ Ⓑ Ⓒ Ⓓ	24. Ⓐ Ⓑ Ⓒ Ⓓ	34. Ⓐ Ⓑ Ⓒ Ⓓ	43. Ⓐ Ⓑ Ⓒ Ⓓ
5. Ⓐ Ⓑ Ⓒ Ⓓ	15. Ⓐ Ⓑ Ⓒ Ⓓ	25. Ⓐ Ⓑ Ⓒ Ⓓ	35. Ⓐ Ⓑ Ⓒ Ⓓ	44. Ⓐ Ⓑ Ⓒ Ⓓ
6. Ⓐ Ⓑ Ⓒ Ⓓ	16. Ⓐ Ⓑ Ⓒ Ⓓ	26. Ⓐ Ⓑ Ⓒ Ⓓ	36. Ⓐ Ⓑ Ⓒ Ⓓ	45. Ⓐ Ⓑ Ⓒ Ⓓ
7. Ⓐ Ⓑ Ⓒ Ⓓ	17. Ⓐ Ⓑ Ⓒ Ⓓ	27. Ⓐ Ⓑ Ⓒ Ⓓ	37. Ⓐ Ⓑ Ⓒ Ⓓ	46. Ⓐ Ⓑ Ⓒ Ⓓ
8. Ⓐ Ⓑ Ⓒ Ⓓ	18. Ⓐ Ⓑ Ⓒ Ⓓ	28. Ⓐ Ⓑ Ⓒ Ⓓ	38. Ⓐ Ⓑ Ⓒ Ⓓ	47. Ⓐ Ⓑ Ⓒ Ⓓ
9. Ⓐ Ⓑ Ⓒ Ⓓ	19. Ⓐ Ⓑ Ⓒ Ⓓ	29. Ⓐ Ⓑ Ⓒ Ⓓ	39. Ⓐ Ⓑ Ⓒ Ⓓ	48. Ⓐ Ⓑ Ⓒ Ⓓ
10. Ⓐ Ⓑ Ⓒ Ⓓ	20. Ⓐ Ⓑ Ⓒ Ⓓ	30. Ⓐ Ⓑ Ⓒ Ⓓ		

Chemical Processes

1. Ⓐ Ⓑ Ⓒ Ⓓ	11. Ⓐ Ⓑ Ⓒ Ⓓ	21. Ⓐ Ⓑ Ⓒ Ⓓ	31. Ⓐ Ⓑ Ⓒ Ⓓ	40. Ⓐ Ⓑ Ⓒ Ⓓ
2. Ⓐ Ⓑ Ⓒ Ⓓ	12. Ⓐ Ⓑ Ⓒ Ⓓ	22. Ⓐ Ⓑ Ⓒ Ⓓ	32. Ⓐ Ⓑ Ⓒ Ⓓ	41. Ⓐ Ⓑ Ⓒ Ⓓ
3. Ⓐ Ⓑ Ⓒ Ⓓ	13. Ⓐ Ⓑ Ⓒ Ⓓ	23. Ⓐ Ⓑ Ⓒ Ⓓ	33. Ⓐ Ⓑ Ⓒ Ⓓ	42. Ⓐ Ⓑ Ⓒ Ⓓ
4. Ⓐ Ⓑ Ⓒ Ⓓ	14. Ⓐ Ⓑ Ⓒ Ⓓ	24. Ⓐ Ⓑ Ⓒ Ⓓ	34. Ⓐ Ⓑ Ⓒ Ⓓ	43. Ⓐ Ⓑ Ⓒ Ⓓ
5. Ⓐ Ⓑ Ⓒ Ⓓ	15. Ⓐ Ⓑ Ⓒ Ⓓ	25. Ⓐ Ⓑ Ⓒ Ⓓ	35. Ⓐ Ⓑ Ⓒ Ⓓ	44. Ⓐ Ⓑ Ⓒ Ⓓ
6. Ⓐ Ⓑ Ⓒ Ⓓ	16. Ⓐ Ⓑ Ⓒ Ⓓ	26. Ⓐ Ⓑ Ⓒ Ⓓ	36. Ⓐ Ⓑ Ⓒ Ⓓ	45. Ⓐ Ⓑ Ⓒ Ⓓ
7. Ⓐ Ⓑ Ⓒ Ⓓ	17. Ⓐ Ⓑ Ⓒ Ⓓ	27. Ⓐ Ⓑ Ⓒ Ⓓ	37. Ⓐ Ⓑ Ⓒ Ⓓ	46. Ⓐ Ⓑ Ⓒ Ⓓ
8. Ⓐ Ⓑ Ⓒ Ⓓ	18. Ⓐ Ⓑ Ⓒ Ⓓ	28. Ⓐ Ⓑ Ⓒ Ⓓ	38. Ⓐ Ⓑ Ⓒ Ⓓ	47. Ⓐ Ⓑ Ⓒ Ⓓ
9. Ⓐ Ⓑ Ⓒ Ⓓ	19. Ⓐ Ⓑ Ⓒ Ⓓ	29. Ⓐ Ⓑ Ⓒ Ⓓ	39. Ⓐ Ⓑ Ⓒ Ⓓ	48. Ⓐ Ⓑ Ⓒ Ⓓ
10. Ⓐ Ⓑ Ⓒ Ⓓ	20. Ⓐ Ⓑ Ⓒ Ⓓ	30. Ⓐ Ⓑ Ⓒ Ⓓ		

Critical Reading

1. Ⓐ Ⓑ Ⓒ Ⓓ	11. Ⓐ Ⓑ Ⓒ Ⓓ	21. Ⓐ Ⓑ Ⓒ Ⓓ	31. Ⓐ Ⓑ Ⓒ Ⓓ	40. Ⓐ Ⓑ Ⓒ Ⓓ
2. Ⓐ Ⓑ Ⓒ Ⓓ	12. Ⓐ Ⓑ Ⓒ Ⓓ	22. Ⓐ Ⓑ Ⓒ Ⓓ	32. Ⓐ Ⓑ Ⓒ Ⓓ	41. Ⓐ Ⓑ Ⓒ Ⓓ
3. Ⓐ Ⓑ Ⓒ Ⓓ	13. Ⓐ Ⓑ Ⓒ Ⓓ	23. Ⓐ Ⓑ Ⓒ Ⓓ	33. Ⓐ Ⓑ Ⓒ Ⓓ	42. Ⓐ Ⓑ Ⓒ Ⓓ
4. Ⓐ Ⓑ Ⓒ Ⓓ	14. Ⓐ Ⓑ Ⓒ Ⓓ	24. Ⓐ Ⓑ Ⓒ Ⓓ	34. Ⓐ Ⓑ Ⓒ Ⓓ	43. Ⓐ Ⓑ Ⓒ Ⓓ
5. Ⓐ Ⓑ Ⓒ Ⓓ	15. Ⓐ Ⓑ Ⓒ Ⓓ	25. Ⓐ Ⓑ Ⓒ Ⓓ	35. Ⓐ Ⓑ Ⓒ Ⓓ	44. Ⓐ Ⓑ Ⓒ Ⓓ
6. Ⓐ Ⓑ Ⓒ Ⓓ	16. Ⓐ Ⓑ Ⓒ Ⓓ	26. Ⓐ Ⓑ Ⓒ Ⓓ	36. Ⓐ Ⓑ Ⓒ Ⓓ	45. Ⓐ Ⓑ Ⓒ Ⓓ
7. Ⓐ Ⓑ Ⓒ Ⓓ	17. Ⓐ Ⓑ Ⓒ Ⓓ	27. Ⓐ Ⓑ Ⓒ Ⓓ	37. Ⓐ Ⓑ Ⓒ Ⓓ	46. Ⓐ Ⓑ Ⓒ Ⓓ
8. Ⓐ Ⓑ Ⓒ Ⓓ	18. Ⓐ Ⓑ Ⓒ Ⓓ	28. Ⓐ Ⓑ Ⓒ Ⓓ	38. Ⓐ Ⓑ Ⓒ Ⓓ	47. Ⓐ Ⓑ Ⓒ Ⓓ
9. Ⓐ Ⓑ Ⓒ Ⓓ	19. Ⓐ Ⓑ Ⓒ Ⓓ	29. Ⓐ Ⓑ Ⓒ Ⓓ	39. Ⓐ Ⓑ Ⓒ Ⓓ	48. Ⓐ Ⓑ Ⓒ Ⓓ
10. Ⓐ Ⓑ Ⓒ Ⓓ	20. Ⓐ Ⓑ Ⓒ Ⓓ	30. Ⓐ Ⓑ Ⓒ Ⓓ		

answer sheet

Quantitative Reasoning

1. Ⓐ Ⓑ Ⓒ Ⓓ   11. Ⓐ Ⓑ Ⓒ Ⓓ   21. Ⓐ Ⓑ Ⓒ Ⓓ   31. Ⓐ Ⓑ Ⓒ Ⓓ   40. Ⓐ Ⓑ Ⓒ Ⓓ

2. Ⓐ Ⓑ Ⓒ Ⓓ   12. Ⓐ Ⓑ Ⓒ Ⓓ   22. Ⓐ Ⓑ Ⓒ Ⓓ   32. Ⓐ Ⓑ Ⓒ Ⓓ   41. Ⓐ Ⓑ Ⓒ Ⓓ

3. Ⓐ Ⓑ Ⓒ Ⓓ   13. Ⓐ Ⓑ Ⓒ Ⓓ   23. Ⓐ Ⓑ Ⓒ Ⓓ   33. Ⓐ Ⓑ Ⓒ Ⓓ   42. Ⓐ Ⓑ Ⓒ Ⓓ

4. Ⓐ Ⓑ Ⓒ Ⓓ   14. Ⓐ Ⓑ Ⓒ Ⓓ   24. Ⓐ Ⓑ Ⓒ Ⓓ   34. Ⓐ Ⓑ Ⓒ Ⓓ   43. Ⓐ Ⓑ Ⓒ Ⓓ

5. Ⓐ Ⓑ Ⓒ Ⓓ   15. Ⓐ Ⓑ Ⓒ Ⓓ   25. Ⓐ Ⓑ Ⓒ Ⓓ   35. Ⓐ Ⓑ Ⓒ Ⓓ   44. Ⓐ Ⓑ Ⓒ Ⓓ

6. Ⓐ Ⓑ Ⓒ Ⓓ   16. Ⓐ Ⓑ Ⓒ Ⓓ   26. Ⓐ Ⓑ Ⓒ Ⓓ   36. Ⓐ Ⓑ Ⓒ Ⓓ   45. Ⓐ Ⓑ Ⓒ Ⓓ

7. Ⓐ Ⓑ Ⓒ Ⓓ   17. Ⓐ Ⓑ Ⓒ Ⓓ   27. Ⓐ Ⓑ Ⓒ Ⓓ   37. Ⓐ Ⓑ Ⓒ Ⓓ   46. Ⓐ Ⓑ Ⓒ Ⓓ

8. Ⓐ Ⓑ Ⓒ Ⓓ   18. Ⓐ Ⓑ Ⓒ Ⓓ   28. Ⓐ Ⓑ Ⓒ Ⓓ   38. Ⓐ Ⓑ Ⓒ Ⓓ   47. Ⓐ Ⓑ Ⓒ Ⓓ

9. Ⓐ Ⓑ Ⓒ Ⓓ   19. Ⓐ Ⓑ Ⓒ Ⓓ   29. Ⓐ Ⓑ Ⓒ Ⓓ   39. Ⓐ Ⓑ Ⓒ Ⓓ   48. Ⓐ Ⓑ Ⓒ Ⓓ

10. Ⓐ Ⓑ Ⓒ Ⓓ   20. Ⓐ Ⓑ Ⓒ Ⓓ   30. Ⓐ Ⓑ Ⓒ Ⓓ

SECTION 1: WRITING

1 Essay • 30 Minutes

> **Directions:** Answer the following prompt in 30 minutes.

Healthcare costs in the United States are spiraling out of control due to such factors as the high costs of doctors and hospitals and the practices of private health insurance companies. Discuss a solution to the problem of spiraling healthcare costs.

_____

_____

_____

_____

_____

_____

_____

_____

_____

_____

_____

_____

_____

_____

_____

_____

_____

_____

_____

practice test 3

SECTION 2: BIOLOGICAL PROCESSES

48 Items • 30 Minutes

Directions: Choose the best answer for each question.

Refer to the following passage for Questions 1–4.

Aerobic cellular respiration is a highly efficient pathway for ATP production. However, when oxygen is unavailable, cells must revert to alternative pathways that allow for energy production in an oxygen-independent, albeit inefficient, manner. Muscle cells and many bacteria undergo lactic acid fermentation, producing lactate after glycolysis for minimal ATP production. Yeast cells, in contrast, undergo alcohol fermentation, during which ethanol is produced after glycolysis for minimal ATP production.

1. Which of the following statements about ATP synthesis is TRUE?
   A. ATP production increases as cells become more active.
   B. ATP production decreases as cells become more active.
   C. ATP is transferred from one area of the body to another, as needed.
   D. ATP synthesis is an exothermic process.

2. Which of the following is the location of glycolysis in the cell?
   A. Plasma membrane
   B. Mitochondrial matrix
   C. Nucleus
   D. Cytoplasm

3. During alcohol fermentation, which of the following processes regenerates a supply of NAD+?
   A. Pyruvate is converted to acetylaldehyde.
   B. Acetylaldehyde is reduced.
   C. CO_2 is released from pyruvate.
   D. Phosphoenolpyruvate is converted to pyruvate.

4. Energy for ATP synthesis is supplied by which of the following?
   A. Phosphorylation
   B. Other ATP molecules
   C. Electron transport chain
   D. Proton gradient

Refer to the following passage for Questions 5–12.

DNA is essential for providing the genetic blueprint for cellular function. As organisms grow, DNA must replicate prior to cell division so that each newly produced cell contains the full genome for the organism. Without this DNA, new cells will not be able to produce the essential protein products at the ribosomes for functionality. In prokaryotes, transcription and translation produce mRNA and then proteins based on a DNA sequence, while in eukaryotes, there is an RNA processing step in between transcription and translation.

5. Which nonmembraneous organelle is involved in the synthesis of ribosomes?
   A. Nucleus
   B. Nucleolus
   C. Endoplasmic reticulum
   D. Lysosome

6. What is the antiparallel sequence for the DNA segment 5'GGCTACATC3'
   A. 5'CCGAUGUAG3'
   B. 3'GGCTACATC5'
   C. 5'CCGATGTAG3'
   D. 3'CCGATGTAG5'

7. Which of the following occurs during RNA processing?
   A. The transcription initiation complex forms.
   B. Nucleotides are joined together.
   C. Introns are spliced out of RNA.
   D. Exons are spliced out of RNA.

8. Which of the following lists the correct order of enzymes acting in the DNA replication process?
   A. Helicase, topoisomerase, primase, DNA polymerase III
   B. Primase, DNA polymerase III, helicase, topoisomerase
   C. DNA polymerase III, primase, topoisomerase, helicase
   D. Topoisomerase, helicase, DNA polymerase III, primase

9. If a particular protein is 100 amino acids long, how many nucleotides are necessary to code for this protein?
   A. 100
   B. 200
   C. 300
   D. 400

10. If a chemical is added to cells to prevent DNA synthesis, at which part of the cell cycle would cells stop growing?
    A. G_1
    B. G_2
    C. M
    D. S

11. In which position on the deoxyribose sugar does the nucleotide base bind?
    A. C1'
    B. C2'
    C. C3'
    D. C4'

12. Which of the following steps occurs after $tRNA_{met}$ attaches to the P site of the ribosome?
    A. $tRNA_{met}$ moves to the A site to make room for another tRNA.
    B. Another tRNA molecule displaces the $tRNA_{met}$ at the P site.
    C. Another tRNA molecule binds to the methionine at the P site.
    D. Another tRNA molecule recognizes the A site.

Refer to the following passage for Questions 13–16.

Enzymes are biomolecules, primarily proteins, that lower the activation energy of a chemical reaction to allow the reaction to proceed at a more rapid rate. Enzymes, however, do not always act alone. Input reactants for an enzyme-catalyzed reaction are substrates, with products produced. Inhibitors can slow enzyme activity, while activators can promote enzyme activity. Allosteric regulators can fall under either of these categories. Additionally, some enzymes require cofactors or coenzymes in order to function properly and efficiently.

13. Which of the following statements best describes allosteric regulation?
    A. A product of the reaction pathway blocks substrate binding.
    B. The binding of a protein stabilizes a favorable or unfavorable enzyme conformation.
    C. A protein binds to the active site, blocking the substrate.
    D. Substrate concentration is increased to overcome inhibition.

14. Which point on this graph represents a temperature at which the enzyme degrades and loses efficiency?

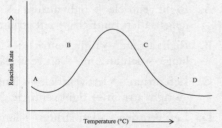

A. A
B. B
C. C
D. D

15. Which of the following is an enzyme cofactor that contains an iron atom which loses and gains an electron via alternating oxidation and reduction reactions?

A. NAD^+
B. FAD
C. Cytochrome C
D. Coenzyme A

16. Which type of energy best describes the energy released as a chemical reaction moves forward?

A. Mechanical energy
B. Kinetic energy
C. Potential energy
D. Electrical energy

Refer to the following passage for Questions 17–20.

Changes in genotypes and phenotypes of a group of organisms over time can be tracked via a number of different biological analyses. Some of these analyses are based on visual evidence from current organisms or organisms past, while others are based on DNA, relying on genetics to analyze the relatedness of individual organisms or groups of organisms.

17. Chemical similarities in species can be observed through genetic analysis, and physical similarities can be studied through

A. adaptations.
B. behavioral analysis.
C. fossil records.
D. genetic variation.

18. Changes that occur in the gene frequency of a population are referred to as

A. macroevolution.
B. microevolution.
C. natural selection.
D. adaptation.

19. Which of the following statements reveals the usefulness of a pedigree analysis?

A. A pedigree can only show a history of genetic disorder.
B. A pedigree can help to manipulate human mating patterns.
C. A pedigree can help to predict the likelihood of genetic disorders in future generations.
D. A pedigree can help to predict the sex of offspring.

20. What is the chemical basis for having one source as the originator of all life?

A. Gene flow
B. Fossil records
C. Similarities in DNA across species
D. The presence of mutations in DNA

The following questions are standalone and not tied to a passage.

21. The presence of human stomach bacteria, *E. coli*, contributes to good overall health. This bacteria is considered to be a(n)

A. pathogen.
B. opportunistic pathogen.
C. nonpathogen.
D. microaerophile.

22. Which of the following statements is TRUE of all viruses?
    A. All viruses contain DNA.
    B. Penetration of the virus into the host cell causes an attack by the immune system.
    C. A virus has its own mechanism of DNA replication.
    D. A virus cannot survive and reproduce outside a host cell.

23. In which phase of fungal reproduction do fungi have two nuclei?
    A. Heterokaryotic phase
    B. Karyogamy
    C. Plasmogamy
    D. Spore-producing phase

24. Which type of cells form multi-layered coiled wrappings around the axons of motor neurons in the PNS?
    A. Astrocytes
    B. Radial glia
    C. Schwann cells
    D. Oligodendrocytes

25. Which of the following requires the assistance of a transport protein to cross the cell membrane?
    A. H_2O
    B. O_2
    C. CO_2
    D. Na^+

26. Which of the following is a specialized fibrous joint that holds together teeth, mandible, and maxima?
    A. Gomphoses
    B. Sutures
    C. Syndesmoses
    D. Diarthroses

27. Which of the following shows the correct direction of blood flow through the heart and lungs?
    A. Right ventricle → right atrium → lungs → left ventricle → left atrium
    B. Right atrium → right ventricle → lungs → left atrium → left ventricle
    C. Left atrium → left ventricle → lungs → right atrium → right ventricle
    D. Left ventricle → left atrium → lungs → right ventricle → right atrium

28. Lymph reenters the circulatory system via the
    A. lymph nodes.
    B. lymphatic vessels.
    C. thoracic duct.
    D. lymphatic capillaries.

29. Insulin and human growth hormone help to promote bone growth. When these two hormones work together to produce positive effects that are greater than the sum of the individual effects of both hormones, it is an example of
    A. permissiveness.
    B. antagonism.
    C. synergism.
    D. inhibition.

30. Which of the following time periods in bacterial growth is marked by equal rates of reproduction and cell death?
    A. Stationary period
    B. Logarithmic growth period
    C. Lag time
    D. Decline period

31. Which of the following is a correct statement about the respiratory system?

    A. Cells produce a continuous supply of oxygen for cellular respiration.

    B. The oropharynx is the place where the paths for air and food cross each other.

    C. Cells take up CO_2 and release O_2 into the bloodstream.

    D. The O_2 that diffused into the bloodstream attaches to hemoglobin in the red blood cells.

32. Which of the following is an accurate statement about the structure of the heart?

    A. The myocardium is the innermost layer of the heart.

    B. The left ventricle receives oxygen-rich blood.

    C. The tricuspid valve is located between the left atrium and left ventricle.

    D. The aortic valve allows blood flow in both directions between the left ventricle and the aorta.

33. Which of the following statements explains why HIV is considered a retrovirus?

    A. HIV synthesizes RNA from its DNA genome.

    B. HIV synthesizes DNA from its RNA genome.

    C. HIV RNA synthesizes complementary RNA strands.

    D. HIV is an enveloped virus.

34. A bacterial species that looks like a rod-shaped chain of cells and has flagella can be classified as

    A. streptococcus.

    B. streptobacilli.

    C. vibrio.

    D. spirillum.

35. Which of the following statements about the kidneys is accurate?

    A. The corticoid nephron is found mostly in the loop of Henle.

    B. The peritubular capillary beds pick up filtered solutes and remove them.

    C. The juxtamedullary capillary beds help to concentrate urine.

    D. Vasa recta are veins in the kidneys that are perpendicular to the loop of Henle.

36. Sperm get nourishment from

    A. a thin, watery fluid secreted by the seminal vesicles.

    B. a thin fluid secreted by the prostate gland.

    C. a thick, clear alkaline mucous secreted from the bulbourethral glands.

    D. nutrients in the bloodstream.

37. Which two forms of chemical energy are produced by the light reactions of photosynthesis?

    A. ATP and ADP

    B. ATP and $NADP^+$

    C. ATP and NADPH

    D. ATP and photons

38. Antiviral proteins that are made by an infected cell and prevent viral replication in other cells are

    A. memory B cells.

    B. antigens.

    C. antibodies.

    D. interferons.

practice test 3

39. Which of the following is the function of microvilli in the small intestine?
    A. The microvilli help to move nutrients along the small intestines.
    B. The microvilli increase the surface area available for the absorption of nutrients.
    C. Microvilli help to dispose of waste material in the intestine.
    D. Microvilli aid in chemical digestion of nutrients.

40. Inhaling soil dust contaminated by certain bird droppings can lead to which type of yeast infection?
    A. *Saccharomyces cerevisiae*
    B. *Pneumocystis jirovecii*
    C. *Candida*
    D. *Cryptococcus neoformans*

41. Follicle-stimulating hormone (FSH) and luteinizing hormone (LH) are secreted by the
    A. adrenal glands.
    B. pituitary gland.
    C. thymus gland.
    D. thyroid gland.

42. Which of the following suggests conditions under which asexual reproduction is favorable?
    A. Consistent, adverse conditions
    B. Extreme environmental conditions
    C. Consistent, favorable environment
    D. Changing environmental conditions

43. Peristalsis refers to
    A. the process of discharging waste from the body.
    B. metabolic equilibrium maintained by numerous body systems to stabilize conditions.
    C. the wave-like muscle contractions that move food through the digestive tract.
    D. the ability of a liquid to flow in narrow spaces without the assistance of gravity.

44. An antidiuretic drug is administered in order to
    A. loosen stools and increase bowel movements.
    B. neutralize the acid produced by your stomach.
    C. relax muscles in the airways to increase airflow to the lungs.
    D. control water balance by reducing urine production.

45. The main cells that compose the hypodermis, or subcutaneous layer, of the skin are
    A. adipocytes.
    B. melanocytes.
    C. phagocytes.
    D. thymocytes.

46. Cilia remove foreign particles and mucus from the surface of the
    A. circulatory system.
    B. digestive system.
    C. integumentary system.
    D. respiratory system.

47. Competent cells can
    A. take up DNA from the environment.
    B. halt the cell cycle and stop cell division.
    C. undergo conjugation.
    D. prevent integration of viral DNA into their genome.

48. The benefits of most antiviral drugs are limited because
    A. mutation rates can be very high in viruses.
    B. viruses produce proteins that detoxify the drugs.
    C. host cells resist the activity of the drugs.
    D. bacteria develop resistance to antibiotics.

SECTION 3: CHEMICAL PROCESSES

48 Items • 30 Minutes

Directions: Choose the best answer for each question.

Refer to the following passage for Questions 1–7.

Research in both general and organic chemistry relies on a number of techniques to, first of all, purify organic compounds of interest, either from a mixture or as products of a chemical reaction, and then secondly, to analyze those compounds to confirm their identity or purity. An extraction is a technique used to separate a desired substance that is mixed with others.

1. Which type of laboratory equipment is best used to extract one liquid from another?
   A. Separatory funnel
   B. Column
   C. Filter paper
   D. Graduated cylinder

2. A cation radical is formed in which type of spectroscopy?
   A. Infrared spectroscopy
   B. Mass spectroscopy
   C. NMR
   D. UV-Vis spectroscopy

3. Which of the following would be the best technique for purifying the solid sulfanilamide from ethanol?
   A. Liquid chromatography
   B. Distillation
   C. Sublimation
   D. Crystallization

4. The least efficient method of chromatography is
   A. liquid chromatography.
   B. gas chromatography.
   C. high-pressure liquid chromatography.
   D. paper chromatography.

5. The analysis of a compound before and after combustion would reveal information about the compound's
   A. physical properties.
   B. chemical properties.
   C. boiling point.
   D. color.

6. In a combustion analysis, 3.6 g of H_2O and 4.4 g of CO_2 are collected. Which of the following is most likely the starting compound?
   A. CH_3
   B. C_2H_4
   C. CH_4
   D. C_2H_6

7. Which of the following statements about 1 H NMR is TRUE?
   A. Two groups of protons coupled to each other can have different coupling constants.
   B. Protons closer than four carbons in a molecule exhibit coupling.
   C. A proton with equivalent neighbors gives a signal split into $n + 2$ peaks.
   D. Chemically equivalent protons do not exhibit spin-spin splitting.

Refer to the following passage for Questions 8–11.

Sulfuric acid, H2SO4, is a strong acid. Sulfate, on the other hand, is a very weak base. This pattern is observed in strong acids and their complementary bases; accordingly, the pH of H2SO4 is very low. Sulfuric acid is a diprotic acid, which means it has two hydrogens to donate.

8. If the pH and pOH of a solution must add up to 14, what is the H_3O^+ concentration of a solution with a pOH of 6?

    A. 1×10^{-14}M

    B. 1×10^{-10}M

    C. 1×10^{-6}M

    D. 1×10^{-8}M

9. Calculate the molecular mass in g/mol of H_2SO_4 (H = 1.008 amu, S = 32.07 amu, O = 16.00 amu).

    A. 49.08 g/mol

    B. 65.08 g/mol

    C. 82.026 g/mol

    D. 98.09 g/mol

10. Which of the following are the atoms found in an oxacid molecule?

    A. Carbon, hydrogen, oxygen, and another element

    B. Carbon, hydrogen, and another element

    C. Carbon, oxygen, and another element

    D. Hydrogen, oxygen, and another element

11. Which of the following is a TRUE statement about buffers?

    A. A buffer changes in pH when a small amount of acid or base is added to it.

    B. The acid and base components of a buffer must not undergo a neutralization reaction.

    C. A buffer solution is a solution of a weak acid and base.

    D. Buffers contain a strong acid and a salt.

Refer to the following passage for Questions 12–15.

Real gases deviate from ideal gases in several ways. Particles of real gases have volumes, which the principles of ideal gases assume is not the case. Real gases also have attractive and repulsive forces; ideal gas particles are assumed to have no interactive forces, resulting in perfectly elastic collisions. The van der Waals equation helps to account for these deviations in behavior of real gases from ideal gases. However, for the sake of straightforward calculations, ideal gas principles do a solid job of explaining the behaviors of gases, and ideal gas laws are generally used for analysis of gases and their properties. Common gases at room temperature include oxygen, O2, and methane, CH4.

12. The temperature of gas A is 51°C, and the temperature of gas B is 27°C. Calculate the ratio of the volume of 1 mole of gas A to 1 mole of gas B at 1 atm.

    A. 51:27

    B. 27:25

    C. 9:7

    D. 3:2

13. Which of the following statements is accurate with respect to the reaction below?

    $2CO_{2 (g)} \rightarrow 2CO_{(g)} + O_{2 (g)}$, at 25°C $\Delta H = 566$ kJ/mol and $\Delta S = 0.174221$ kJ/K·mol

    A. ΔG is negative and the reaction is spontaneous.

    B. ΔG is negative and the reaction is nonspontaneous.

    C. ΔG is positive and the reaction is nonspontaneous.

    D. ΔG is positive and the reaction is spontaneous.

14. Which gas law states that the volume of a gas is directly proportional to the number of moles of gas at constant temperature and pressure?

    A. Avogadro's law

    B. Boyle's law

    C. Charles's law

    D. Dalton's law

15. What is the correct bond angle in a methane molecule CH_4?

    A. 90°

    B. 109°

    C. 120°

    D. 180°

Refer to the following passage for Questions 16–19.

The mole has become a regular unit of quantity used in chemistry. In particular, the mole has been useful in stoichiometry as a means of relating quantities of chemicals that are not necessarily present initially in the same type of units (e.g., various components of a solution). Moles provide a means of standardizing quantities within a system or chemical reaction so that they can be related to each other in a meaningful way.

16. Which of the following examples are representative of Avogadro's number?

    A. The number of protons in a 1-liter sample of 1 M HCl

    B. The number of molecules it takes to fill a 1-liter beaker

    C. The number of atoms in 1 g $_{12}C$

    D. The number of O atoms in 500 mL 1 M H_2SO_4

17. What is the percent yield of the product CO_2 in the neutralization reaction below if the approximate atomic masses of the elements are as follows: H = 1, Cl = 35, Na = 23, O = 16, and C = 12; 24 g of HCl are mixed with an excess amount of sodium carbonate at STP; and 12.71 g of CO_2 are produced?

    $2HCl + Na_2CO_3 \rightarrow 2NaCl + H_2O + CO_2$

    A. 43.4%

    B. 50.0%

    C. 87.5%

    D. 97.9%

18. Which of the following would be the equation for the formation of aluminum oxide, Al_2O_3?

    A. $Al_2 + O_3 \rightarrow Al_2O_3$

    B. $2Al_2 + 3O_2 \rightarrow 2Al_2O_3$

    C. $2Al + 3O \rightarrow Al_2O_3$

    D. $4Al + 3O_2 \rightarrow 2Al_2O_3$

19. 26.3 g of NaCl is added to 100 mL of water and mixed until completely dissolved. This solution is then added to a beaker of water such that the final volume in the beaker is 750 mL. Which of the following is the final concentration of the solution?

    A. 4.50 M

    B. 6×10^{-6} M

    C. 0.60 M

    D. 0.34 M

The following questions are standalone and not tied to a passage.

20. Which of the following hydrocarbon compounds has four carbon atoms and one carbon-carbon double bond?

    A. Butene

    B. Propene

    C. Butane

    D. Ethane

21. What is the name of the following compound?

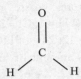

A. Acetone
B. Carboxylic acid
C. Methyl butyrate
D. Formaldehyde

22. The two structures below are an example of

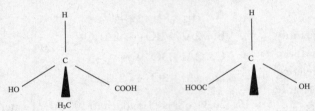

A. achiral.
B. diastereomers.
C. enantiomers.
D. polarization.

23. Which DNA nucleotides are purines?
A. adenine and guanine
B. adenine and thymine
C. cytosine and guanine
D. cytosine and thymine

24. If the molecule below undergoes an S_N2 reaction in which the nucleophile attacks the H functional group, which of the following is the leaving group?

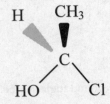

A. H
B. OH
C. Cl
D. CH_3

25. Which type of enzyme facilitates a dehydration reaction?

   A. Acid catalyst

   B. Hydroxylase

   C. Dehydrogenase

   D. Base catalyst

26. Which of the following is the resulting product of the reaction below?

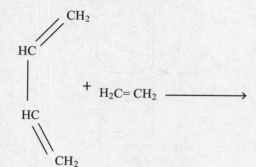

$+$ $H_2C = CH_2$ $\longrightarrow$

   A.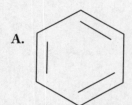

   B.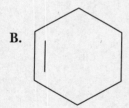

   C. $CH_3CH_2CH_2CH_2CH_2CH_2$

   D.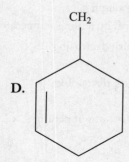

27. An amino acid is characterized by the presence of

   A. a central carbon surrounded by a hydrogen, amino group, carboxyl group, and variable R group.

   B. a pentose sugar, a nitrogenous base, and a phosphate group.

   C. a hydrocarbon chain, with or without double bonds, with a carboxylic acid at the end.

   D. a carbon ring or chain with hydrogens and hydroxyl groups on them.

28. The only known enzyme that is not a protein is

   A. a carbohydrate.

   B. a DNA molecule.

   C. a lipid.

   D. an RNA molecule.

29. The following reaction forms an iodine ion and which type of product?

$CH_3CH_2CH_2O^-$ $+$ CH_3I $\rightarrow$ $CH_3CH_2CH_2OCH_3 + I^-$

   A. Carbonyl

   B. Ether

   C. Ester

   D. Alcohol

30. Which of the following lists the elements in the correct order from largest atomic radius to smallest?

   A. He, Li, N, F

   B. He, F, N, Li

   C. Li, N, F, He

   D. F, N, Li, He

31. Which of the following is a TRUE statement about elimination reactions?
    A. An E2 reaction forms a carbocation intermediate.
    B. In an E1 reaction, the nucleophile attacks and a double bond forms in the same step.
    C. The transition state of an E2 reaction is very stable.
    D. The dissociation of the leaving group is the rate limiting step in an E1 reaction.

32. Which property of electrons was still puzzling to physicists after Bohr introduced his atomic theory?
    A. Electrons move from one orbital to another.
    B. Electrons behave like wave particles.
    C. Electrons orbit around the nucleus of an atom.
    D. The energies of electrons can be quantized in a hydrogen atom.

33. In which group(s) on the Periodic Table are the elements called the transition metals?
    A. Group 1
    B. Group 2
    C. Groups 3–12
    D. Group 17

34. Which of the following chemical formulas represents the molecule magnesium sulfate heptahydrate?
    A. $H_{14}MgSO_{11}$
    B. $MgSO_4 \cdot 7H_2O$
    C. $MgSO_4 \cdot 6H_2O$
    D. $H_{12}MgSO_{10}$

35. Which of the following compounds has the carbon-carbon bond with the shortest bond length?
    A. Butane
    B. Butene
    C. Butyne
    D. Ethane

36. What is the overall order of a reaction in which rate = $k[A]^0[B]^2$?
    A. 0
    B. 1
    C. 2
    D. 3

37. The below diagrams which type of hybridized orbital?

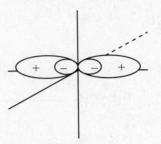

overlapping *sp*
hybrid orbitals

    A. *sp*
    B. sp^2
    C. sp^3
    D. *p*

38. The following compound is classified as an

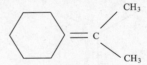

    A. alkane.
    B. alkyne.
    C. alkene.
    D. aromatic.

39. The viscosity of a liquid
    A. increases with increasing temperature.
    B. decreases with decreasing temperature.
    C. increases with decreasing temperature.
    D. is independent of temperature.

40. Which of the following compounds is held together by covalent bonding only?
- **A.** LiCl
- **B.** MgO
- **C.** CH$_2$O
- **D.** B$_2$O$_3$

41. To form a triglyceride from glycerol and fatty acids, what is released in the process as a byproduct?
- **A.** An ester group
- **B.** 3CO2 and 3O2
- **C.** 3H2O
- **D.** Three hydrocarbon chains

42. The order in which nucleotides are moved along the ribosomal binding sites is:
- **A.** A, P, E.
- **B.** P, E, A.
- **C.** E, P, A.
- **D.** E, A, P.

43. The direct result of translation is
- **A.** a protein.
- **B.** an mRNA molecule.
- **C.** a cDNA molecule.
- **D.** a tRNA molecule bound to an amino acid.

44. Which of the following jobs is performed by DNA polymerase?
- **A.** Adding new nucleotides to the leading strand during DNA replication
- **B.** Closing gaps by forming phospho-diester bonds between Okazaki fragments on the lagging strand during DNA replication
- **C.** Generating an RNA primer on the lagging strand during DNA replication
- **D.** Adding new nucleotides to the growing nucleic acid during transcription

45. Alpha helices and beta sheets are characteristic features of which level of protein structure?
- **A.** Primary
- **B.** Secondary
- **C.** Tertiary
- **D.** Quaternary

46. "Kinks" in fatty acid chains, as opposed to straight chains, are caused by
- **A.** the presence of oxygen within the chains.
- **B.** the presence of double bonds within the chains.
- **C.** the presence of methyl groups on carbons in the chains.
- **D.** intramolecular dispersion forces between separate chains within one molecule.

47. During fatty acid synthesis, which molecule is sued as an energy source to polymerize fatty acid chains?
- **A.** NADPH
- **B.** NADH
- **C.** FADH2
- **D.** CO2

48. Which of the following statements is accurate about the formation of molecular bonds?
- **A.** One electron occupies the bonding orbital and a second electron occupies the antibonding orbital.
- **B.** Two electrons occupy the bonding orbital.
- **C.** Two electrons occupy the antibonding orbital.
- **D.** The bonding orbital is higher in energy than the antibonding orbital.

practice test 3

SECTION 4: CRITICAL READING

48 Items • 50 Minutes

> **Directions:** Choose the best answer for each question.

(1)   Because treatment options abound for the asthma sufferer, the medical professional must always evaluate the strengths and weaknesses of various treatment options through the lens of the patient's age, as well as specific and individual symptoms, with a special focus on their duration and severity. First and foremost, asthma sufferers should avoid known triggers of their attacks and remove all such triggers from their environment. For those with repeated attacks in the moderate to severe range, carrying and using a peak flow meter can aid in the management of asthma medications by alerting the patient to changes that may signal an attack before it occurs.

(2)   Quick relief options include short-acting beta agonists (bronchodilators) as well as oral and intravenous corticosteroids. They are intended for rapid relief during an asthma attack and not for long-term use. Quick relief options may be used before exercise for those with exercise-induced asthma.

(3)   For people with allergic asthma, specific immunotherapy, or desensitization, can prove beneficial. For other asthma sufferers seeking long-term control of their symptoms, inhaled corticosteroids, which prevent the swelling of airways, are often prescribed. This daily and ongoing treatment may not become maximally beneficial until several days or weeks after the beginning of treatment, but it does offer the benefit of relatively few side effects. In some cases, combined medications with both an inhaled steroid and a beta-2 agonist are prescribed.

Oral corticosteroids and oral beta-2 agonists that are not long-acting may also be used.

(4)   More controversy surrounds the use of leukotriene modifiers, which help to prevent asthma symptoms for up to twenty-four hours, because of psychological side effects that include hallucinations, aggression, agitation, and even the triggering of suicidal thoughts or impulses. Without question, this "treatment" should be avoided at all costs. Bronchial thermoplasty, which is reserved for asthmatics who do not respond to other treatments, is also controversial. This procedure involves using a electrode to heat the airways in the lungs, thereby limiting the ability of the airways to tighten.

(5)   While advocacy for training in specific breathing techniques appears to be on the rise, the effects are uncertain. Such techniques, which include, but are not limited to so called "yoga breathing" or pranayama, will probably help people to relax, but they have not yet been proven to relieve asthma attacks. Other dubious alternative approaches to the treatment of asthma run the gamut from herbal remedies such as gingko extract to higher ingestion rates of Omega-3 fatty acids.

1. Paragraph 3 suggests that desensitization is a treatment for those

   A. who have allergic triggers.

   B. with especially sensitive nasal passages.

   C. with exercise-induced asthma.

   D. who carry peak flow meters.

2. Which of the following would be the best title for the passage?
   A. "Asthma: The Search for the Cure"
   B. "Asthma Treatments"
   C. "Long-Term Treatments for Asthma"
   D. "Getting Relief from Allergic Asthma"

3. The ideas in paragraphs 4 and 5 are mainly related by
   A. main idea.
   B. sequence.
   C. cause and effect.
   D. problem and solution.

4. According to the passage, the asthma sufferer with repeated moderate-to-severe attacks should
   A. use long-term medications such as inhaled corticosteroids.
   B. consider controversial therapies such as leukotriene modifiers.
   C. find relief from the worst attacks through ingestion of gingko extract.
   D. get the most relief from specific immunotherapy.

5. Which statement from the passage best shows the author's attitude toward leukotriene modifiers?
   A. "More controversy surrounds the use of leukotriene modifiers, which help to prevent asthma symptoms for up to twenty-four hours…"
   B. "…because psychological side effects that include hallucinations, aggression, agitation, and even the triggering of suicidal thoughts or impulses."
   C. "Without question, this "treatment" should be avoided at all costs."
   D. "Bronchial thermoplasty, which is reserved for asthmatics who do not respond to other treatments, is also controversial."

6. Which of the following conclusions is most effectively supported by information in the passage?
   A. Ginko extract will ultimately prove to be the most effective treatment for asthma.
   B. There is not yet any relief for those who suffer from asthma.
   C. Inhaled corticosteroids are a more effective treatment for asthma than pranayama is.
   D. Avoiding triggers will prevent asthma sufferers from ever having an asthma attack.

7. Information in the passage suggests that the author views Omega-3 fatty acids as
   A. ridiculously ineffectual.
   B. an ineffective treatment.
   C. highly effective for some people.
   D. damaging to one's health.

8. What can be concluded from the passage about the use of bronchodilators for the treatment of asthma?
   A. Athletes with asthma should use them after each exercise session.
   B. Athletes with asthma should never use them.
   C. They are always administered orally.
   D. They may constitute the entire treatment plan for some asthma sufferers.

(1)   While the unofficial history of the generic drug is long and complicated and probably stretches as far back as the first drugs ever sold, the official history of the generic drug could be said to have begun in this nation in 1888 when the American Pharmaceutical Association published the National Formulary, a document intended to prevent the counterfeiting of branded drugs. In the ensuing years, much government effort was spent not only on ensuring the safety and efficacy of pharmaceutical products, but also on preventing low-quality or mis-leading substitutions for them. Landmark legislation was passed in 1906, during Theodore Roosevelt's administration, that not only required product labeling, but also marked the true beginning of government regulation. This regulation was effectively enlarged and expanded by the Food, Drug, and Cosmetic Act of 1938.

(2)   One of the most significant dates in the official history of the generic drug was 1962. In that year, the federal government first required a long and expensive drug testing process, including large-scale human trials, to prove a drug was safe and effective before it hit the market. Because this law applied to both new and generic drugs, the production of the latter slowed considerably. In fact, between 1962 and 1984, the FDA approved only sixteen generic drugs.

(3)   Beginning in the second half of the 1960s, however, and in the decades following, the Medicare and Medicaid Amendment to the Social Security Act in 1967 drove home to lawmakers the need for generic drugs. Specifically, it was acknowledged that a flood of generics could create healthy competition in the pharmaceutical market and, therefore, help keep prices low. It would take time before the government fully responded to this realization with effective legislation, but once it did, the floodgates for generics opened.

(4)   By 1984, the Hatch-Waxman Act made it possible for the FDA to approve applications to market generic versions of brand-name drugs released after 1962 without repeating efficacy and safety research. That is, the generic maker did not have to submit an ANDA, or Abbreviated New Drug Application. The thinking was that the research had already been done on the active ingredient by the pharmaceutical company that first patented it. The generic maker did not have to re-invent that pharmaceutical wheel. Instead, it had only to prove <u>bioequivalence</u> to the pioneer drug. The generic maker also had to prove that the active ingredient in its drug was absorbed into the body at a rate that was within 20% of the rate of absorption speed of the reference drug.

(5)   On its Web site, the Generic Pharma-ceutical Association quotes President Ronald Reagan crediting the Hatch-Waxman Act with "regulatory relief, increased competition, economy on government, and best of all, the American people will save money, and yet receive the best medicine that pharmaceutical science can provide." Indeed, in 1983, only about 35% of the bestselling drugs that had gone off patent had any generic competition at all. Today, it is generally the case that all of them do. Furthermore, in a little more than two decades following the passage of the Hatch-Waxman Act, the generic drug industry grew into a $63 billion dollar business. According to one source, an estimated 69% of all prescriptions today are filled with generic drugs, yet generic drug spending accounts for, by some estimates, only 16 cents of every drug dollar spent. This translates into billions of dollars a year in savings for consumers, managed care organizations, and the U.S. government. Few changes in government spending have been more welcome than this one.

9. Paragraph 4 suggests that a pioneer drug is also called a(n)
   A. generic drug.
   B. reference drug.
   C. off-patent drug.
   D. managed care drug.

10. By *bioequivalence* (paragraph 4), the author most likely means the same
    A. active ingredient and effect.
    B. dosage rate.
    C. drug manufacturing practices.
    D. fillers, flavors, and dyes.

11. The passage suggests that there were no laws requiring that drugs be tried out on humans until
    A. 1938.
    B. 1962.
    C. 1967.
    D. 1984.

12. According to the passage, the fewest new generic drugs were likely produced between
    A. 1906 and 1938.
    B. 1938 and 1962.
    C. 1962 and 1984.
    D. 1984 and the date the author wrote it.

13. Which of these statements from the passage expresses a personal opinion?
    A. "Because this law applied to both new and generic drugs, the production of the latter slowed considerably."
    B. "It would take time before the government responded to this need with effective legislation, but once it did, the floodgates for generics opened."
    C. "According to one source, an estimated 69% of all prescriptions today are filled with generic drugs, yet generic drug spending accounts for, by some estimates, only 16 cents of every drug dollar spent."
    D. "Few changes in government spending have been more welcome than this one."

14. At the end of the passage, what does the author conclude?
    A. The government has a history of wasting money.
    B. The government finally made a smart decision in passing the Hatch-Waxman Act.
    C. The Hatch-Waxman Act has been very beneficial to the public.
    D. Generic drugs are destroying the branded drugs industry.

15. The tone of the quoted information in paragraph 5 is
    A. celebratory.
    B. ambivalent.
    C. disapproving.
    D. objective.

16. Paragraph 1 suggests that the National Formulary most likely
    A. outlawed "counterfeit" or generic drugs.
    B. listed drugs approved by the American Pharmaceutical Association.
    C. provided formulas for making drugs approved by the National Pharmaceutical Association.
    D. effectively ended the manufacture of generic drugs until 1906.

practice test 3

(1)   Today, we tend to identify Antoine Lavoisier as the man who, among other things, developed an oxygen theory. In Lavoisier's own time, however, he was the man who disproved the phlogiston theory. Before Lavoisier proved otherwise, the theory of combustion stated that everything that could be burned contained phlogiston. When a substance was burned, the phlogiston was liberated in the process. In 1669, Johann Joachim Becher had called this substance combustible earth. The name *phlogiston* was coined a few decades later by Georg Ernst Stahl. (*Phlog* is the Greek root for "flame.") At any rate, the theory that was given credence before Lavoisier's breakthrough was that things burned because they contained phlogiston, which was released into the air during the process of burning. So it was that what remained after combustion came to be described, by no less than Joseph Priestley, as <u>dephlogisticated</u>.

(2)   Not only did the phlogiston theory help to explain combustion, but it also gave a consistent explanation for other processes that were not understood at the time. These processes included respiration. After all, something was released into and absorbed by the air during that process, too, but what was it? The obvious problem with the theory, however, was that whatever was going into the air, and many thought it was phlogiston, was not measurable. Scientists could hypothesize about, not prove, its presence or its properties. Still, they thought they could answer questions such as, "Why would a human die after being placed for some time in a small, closed space?" (The air was became saturated with phlogiston.) "Why does fire stop burning in a small, closed space?" (The burning saturates the air with phlogiston.)

(3)   The problem with the theory that most disturbed—and probably, therefore, most motivated—Lavoisier related to calcination. When a metal was heated by an intense flame, it left a residue called calx, which weighed more than the original metal. Maybe it was not the thing subjected to the flame, Lavoisier posited, but the air itself that contained both something vital and something suffocating.

(4)   Lavoisier endeavored to prove his theory by using a specially designed flask and pure mercury—an element that was already known to have unique properties related to heat. He was able to calculate depletion of the vital air when the mercury was burned. He was also able to determine that the process of burning released suffocating air. He called the vital air oxygen; today we know the suffocating air as carbon dioxide.

17. Based on this article, a person could most reasonably speculate that the term *oxidation*

   A. was introduced after Lavoisier disproved the phlogiston theory.

   B. is a misnomer for the liberation of phlogiston.

   C. could be said to help validate the phlogiston theory.

   D. is only partially accurate when applied to the process of combustion.

18. According to the passage, before Lavoisier, phlogiston was believed to be
    A. anything that could be subjected to a flame.
    B. the reason for respiration.
    C. part of a residue called calx.
    D. a by-product of combustion and other processes.

19. What evidence could the author have included that would best support the main point?
    A. The implications of the fact that heated metal leaves calx
    B. An example of a process not understood before the phlogiston theory
    C. The scientific name of the flask Lavoisier designed
    D. Answers to the questions in paragraph 2

20. Which strategy does the author use to support the overall thesis?
    A. References to studies
    B. Emotional appeals
    C. Ethical appeals
    D. Personal anecdotes

21. In paragraph 1, the author mentions the Greek origins of the word *phlogiston* in order to
    A. show its relationship to the process of burning.
    B. relate its meaning to liberation, or freeing.
    C. explain how earth may be combustible.
    D. describe the flame created by phlogiston.

22. In the overall context of the passage, the questions at the end of paragraph 2 serve mainly to show
    A. the main components of air.
    B. the problems with phlogiston theory.
    C. why scientists before Lavoisier accepted the theory of phlogiston.
    D. how scientists before Lavoisier arrived at the theory of phlogiston.

23. According to the passage, how does the process of calcination relate to the evolution of the scientific understanding of air?
    A. Like air itself, calcination leaves behind a residue.
    B. Like the process of respiration, calcination is vital to life.
    C. The earlier phlogiston theory did not completely explain this process.
    D. Calcination took place in the most dephlogisticated air.

24. The topic of the passage relates mainly to Lavoisier's thinking processes related to
    A. understanding why phlogiston was liberated during burning.
    B. identifying the nature of suffocating air.
    C. identifying the nature of vital air.
    D. debunking a theory marred by an observable illogic.

(1)   Not everyone has heard of transposons, but they are crucial to our understanding of multicellular organisms. Transposons are specific DNA sequences; another way to refer to transposons is to call them jumping genes. The name *transposon* comes from the two Latin word parts, the prefix *trans-*, meaning "across" and the root *pos*, meaning "position" or "place." The far less lofty and Latinate term *jumping genes* may sound like the name of a musical band, a denim brand, or even a playground game, but the understanding of jumping genes could have possibilities as big and as grand as the understanding of Mendelian genetics or the structure of DNA.

(2)   The word *jumping* in the term *jumping genes* refers to the ability of a transposon to jump, or move to or between chromosomes and to different positions on a chromosome. Once in the new position, a transposon often "turns off," or prevents the expression of a gene. In some cases, a transposon can also "turn on" a gene. A transposon acts as a regulator. More broadly, the existence and movement of transposons can cause mutations, and mutations can result in observable changes to an organism, such as changes in color to the kernels of an ear of corn.

(3)   How were jumping genes discovered? A scientist named Barbara McClintock spent a lifetime of work on corn genetics. A starting point for her work was the fact that the numbers of variegated grains on cobs of Indian corn did not conform to the principle, or, more specifically, the ratios set forth by Mendel. Something had to account for a nonconforming ratio of corn kernel colors.

(4)   McClintock proposed that transposons were responsible for the speckled or striped patterns in some kernels of Indian corn.

Unfortunately, when McClintock first published her results in the 1950s, many scientists did not comprehend the significance of her discovery. They were apparently too busy to turn momentarily off their own avenues of endeavor or to think about the lowly corn plant. In fact, it wasn't until 1983 that McClintock was awarded the Nobel Prize in Physiology or Medicine for her groundbreaking discovery.

(5)   In those intervening years, and since, research in molecular genetics has confirmed or logically suggested the enormous significance of McClintock's work. For example, scientists now know that transposons can block transcription (transcription is the synthesis of RNA from a DNA template) and can leave copies of themselves behind before they jump. Therefore, they can contribute both to duplication, as well as to deletions and other genome modifications. Some researchers are also currently suggesting that transposons may have played an important role in significant evolutionary changes in species. Who knew that such massive implications could grow out of a humble ear of Indian corn?

25. According to the passage, jumping genes can
   A. transcribe RNA.
   B. regulate genes.
   C. enable transcription.
   D. copy a DNA template.

26. Which of the following would be the best title for this passage?
   A. "Barbara McClintock Discovers Corn Genetics"
   B. "Secrets in an Ear of Corn"
   C. "Transpositions and Transcriptions"
   D. "Jumping Genes"

27. The third and fourth sentences in paragraph 3 relate to each other by
   A. contrasting two different understandings.
   B. showing how one discovery led to another.
   C. narrowing down the problem.
   D. supporting the overall claim of the passage.

28. Which of the following statements expresses a personal opinion?
   A. "The far less lofty and Latinate term *jumping genes* may sound like the name of a musical band, a denim brand, or even a playground game, but the understanding of jumping genes could have possibilities as big and as grand as the understanding of Mendelian genetics or the structure of DNA."
   B. "More broadly, the existence and movement of transposons can cause mutations, and mutations can result in observable changes to an organism, such as changes in color to the kernels of an ear of corn."
   C. "In fact, it wasn't until 1983 that McClintock was awarded the Nobel Prize in Physiology or Medicine for her groundbreaking discovery."
   D. "Some researchers are also currently suggesting that transposons may have played an important role in significant evolutionary changes in species."

29. In paragraph 1, the author mentions the Latin origins of the word *transposon* in order to
   A. compare the term with its familiar substitute, *jumping genes*.
   B. contrast the term with its familiar substitute, *jumping genes*.
   C. help explain the meaning of the term.
   D. provide background information for details about genes.

30. In paragraph 3, the author mentions non-conforming corn kernel colors in order to
   A. introduce the observable evidence that led McClintock to her theory.
   B. explain how variation in nature can result in mutations.
   C. provide evidence of significant evolutionary changes in species.
   D. explain how transposons can block transcription and leave copies of themselves.

31. The author of this passage ties together the introduction and conclusion by
   A. explaining claims about the implications of knowledge of jumping genes.
   B. making clear what precisely happens when jumping genes "jump."
   C. explaining how researchers today are overturning the principles of Mendelian genetics.
   D. second-guessing the implications of Barbara McClintock's discovery.

32. The author of the passage would agree that the best explanation of a transposon is
   A. a jumping gene.
   B. a specific DNA sequence that can regulate genes.
   C. the key to understanding multicellular organisms.
   D. the basis for evolutionary changes.

(1)   I tend to page through our local hospital's monthly *Health & Wellness* magazine with very casual interest at best, but this month my eye landed on a new lung cancer-screening program. What my hospital was promising was the use of low-dose-radiation CT scans to detect lung cancer early—and, by early, I mean early enough to cure.

(2)   The screening is not yet recommended by the American Cancer Society, and therefore not paid for by most insurance companies. Nevertheless, I immediately called my uncle and aunt and encouraged them to make an appointment. There was nothing frivolous about this. The findings that had led my local hospital to invest in this program came from a large study called the National Lung Screening Trial (NLST) that was sponsored by the National Cancer Institute; the results had been published by the *New England Journal of Medicine*. What the study specifically found was that the odds of tumor detection increase dramatically when a CT scan is used instead of a chest X-ray. While chest X-rays can detect cancers, there is no known effect on death rate by means of such detection. In contrast, CT scans not only pick up information about lung tumors at earlier stages, but they may also detect other illnesses and save lives that way.

(3)   The study, which was conducted with 53,000 current or former smokers, found that one cancer death could be prevented in every 300 to 320 people screened. Those odds may not sound that promising—unless, of course, you happen to be the one. To me, however, they seemed like the chance of a lifetime for potentially helping my aunt and uncle who each had smoked well over a pack a day for some twenty-five years before quitting just about a decade ago.

(4)   Indeed, my aunt and uncle fit the profile for those who were eligible for screening. To be eligible, a person had to be at least 55 years of age or older and a current or past smoker with at least a 30-pack per year smoking history (that's over a half pack per day). If the prospective participant had quit smoking, she or he had to have done that less than fifteen years ago. The illuminating study was carried out on a similar population: participants were 55 to 74 years of age, and had either smoked a pack a day for 30 years or two packs a day for fifteen years. Those who had quit less than 15 years ago were eligible to take part in the study.

(5)   A history of heavy smoking makes a lot of people nervous, and for good reason. It is estimated that lung cancer will claim the lives of some 157,000 people this year. That's more than from breast, colorectal, prostate, and pancreatic cancers combined. More convincing are these stark numbers: one in ten. Those are said to be the chances that an older smoker will get lung cancer.

33. Which word best describes the author's overall tone in this passage?
   A. Concerned
   B. Alarmed
   C. Skeptical
   D. Optimistic

34. Which statement from the passage best shows the author's attitude toward the research?
   A. "The findings that had led my local hospital to invest in this program came from a large study called the National Lung Screening Trial (NLST) that was sponsored by the National Cancer Institute; the results had been published by the *New England Journal of Medicine*."

B. "What the study specifically found was that the odds of tumor detection increase dramatically when a CT scan is used instead of a chest X-ray."

C. "The study, which was conducted with 53,000 current or former smokers, found that one cancer death could be prevented in every 300 to 320 people screened."

D. "To me, however, they seemed like the chance of a lifetime for potentially helping my aunt and uncle who each had smoked well over a pack a day for some twenty-five years before quitting just about a decade ago."

35. As used in paragraph 4, the word *profile* means
    A. side view.
    B. data set.
    C. outline.
    D. genome.

36. Which of the following statements from the passage provides the least support for the author's attitude toward the new screening method?
    A. "What my hospital was promising was the use of low-dose-radiation CT scans to detect lung cancer early—and by early, I mean early enough to cure."
    B. "The screening is not yet recommended by the American Cancer Society, and, therefore, not paid for by most insurance companies."
    C. "The study, which was conducted with 53,000 current or former smokers, found that one cancer death could be prevented in every 300 to 320 people screened."
    D. "In contrast, CT scans not only pick up information about lung tumors at earlier stages, but they may also detect other illnesses and save lives that way."

37. Information in the passage suggests that
    A. lung cancer progresses rapidly.
    B. lung cancer is among the most curable cancers.
    C. chest X-rays do not detect lung cancer.
    D. chest X-rays do not improve odds for those with lung cancer.

38. Which word or phrase from the passage best reveals the author's bias?
    A. Frivolous (paragraph 2)
    B. Promising (paragraph 3)
    C. Chance of a lifetime (paragraph 3)
    D. For good reason (paragraph 5)

39. Which word from the passage reflects the author's opinion?
    A. eligible (paragraph 4)
    B. prospective (paragraph 4)
    C. illuminating (paragraph 4)
    D. similar (paragraph 4)

40. Which of these adds most credibility to the information presented in the passage?
    A. The author's tendency to read *Health & Wellness* magazine.
    B. The reference to the American Cancer Society.
    C. The author's experiences with her aunt and uncle.
    D. The results of the study the *New England Journal of Medicine* conducted.

(1) Few people bothered to unglue their eyes from their computer or television screens when part of Earth came within metaphorical inches of annihilation on November 8, 2011. That's when the asteroid 2005 YU55 careened by us at 29,000 miles per hour and at a perilously close 200,000 miles or so. This is the closest that 2005 YU55 has ever come to Earth. A little closer, and at least some people would have begun associating the city-block sized asteroid with the kind of dirty work done by the giant asteroid—or other gigantic, hurtling object—that cratered the Yucatan and led to the disappearance of dinosaurs.

(2) At 1,300 feet wide, 2005 YU55 is not the largest of the asteroids, several of which are more than 3,300 feet wide. But then again most asteroids, which may appear to be like stars, but are more like planets in their movement, whirl predictably around between Mars and Jupiter. Others stay at a safe distance closer to the sun than to Earth. Some, however, can cross planet orbits within the inner solar system.

(3) Because of the information-gathering potential, the illustrious scientists at NASA's Jet Propulsion Laboratory regarded the event as an astronomical field day. Prior to the asteroid's near collision with Earth, however, one of the JPL groups issued this sober warning: "Due to its size and proximity to Earth, the Minor Planet Center has designated 2005 YU55 as a 'Potentially Hazardous Asteroid.'" Simultaneously, the group reassured the potentially hazardously nervous public with this analysis: "Despite this designation, this object cannot hit Earth during the entire interval over which its motion can be computed reliably." That interval happens to be only several hundred years.

(4) Hundreds of telescopes worldwide, including NASA's own sophisticated Arecibo radio-telescope in Puerto Rico, were trained on the asteroid, which was not visible to the naked eye and presented some challenges for viewing by the amateur astronomer with a telescope. Few astronomers, however, and certainly none with an interest in asteroids, wanted to miss the chance for viewing an asteroid temporarily at closer range than the moon.

(5) As predicted, the asteroid's impact turned out to be far more emotional than physical. Not only was there no jarring jolt or slamming strike, but 2005 YU55's gravity was too weak to have any effect on earthquake activity or tides. It's currently uncalculated, but the greatest impact will most likely reveal itself slowly as scientists unpack and analyze data gathered from the closest visit of an asteroid to Earth since 1976. And, as impingement goes, most of us prefer the intellectual variety.

41. The author's main purpose in this passage is to
   A. issue a warning about the potential hazards of 2005 YU55.
   B. detail the possible damage from the asteroid's close encounter with Earth.
   C. persuade viewers not to miss the great opportunity to see 2005 YU55.
   D. explain the asteroid, scientific response to it, and its probable effect.

42. Which best characterizes the organization of information in paragraph 3?
   A. Problems and solution
   B. Chronological order
   C. Cause and effect
   D. Main idea and details

43. Which of the following statements from the passage provides least support for the author's claim that "at least part of Earth came within metaphorical inches of annihilation on November 8, 2011"?

   A. "Some, however, can cross planet orbits within the inner solar system."

   B. "At 1,300 feet wide, 2005 YU55 is not the largest of the asteroids, several of which are more than 3,300 feet wide."

   C. "Due to its size and proximity to Earth, the Minor Planet Center has designated 2005 YU55 as a 'Potentially Hazardous Asteroid.'"

   D. "Few astronomers, however, and certainly none with an interest in asteroids, wanted to miss the chance for viewing an asteroid at closer range than the moon."

44. The statement that "That interval happens to be only several hundred years" in paragraph 3 shows that the author

   A. discounts the idea of potential peril.

   B. creates a new interpretation of JPL's data.

   C. misinterprets JPL's statement.

   D. makes JPL's statement more threatening than JPL does.

45. According to the passage, 2005 YU55's greatest impact will be

   A. new scientific knowledge.

   B. cratering of the land.

   C. possible extinction of species.

   D. a slight, temporary change in the tides.

46. Which word from the passage best reveals the author's bias?

   A. Bothered (paragraph 1)

   B. Perilously (paragraph 1)

   C. Largest (paragraph 2)

   D. Illustrious (paragraph 3)

47. The details in paragraphs 2 through 5 help show that many details in paragraph 1 are

   A. inaccurate.

   B. hyperbolic.

   C. unverifiable.

   D. apocryphal.

48. Which of the following conclusions is best supported by the information in the passage?

   A. Little or nothing has been known about 2005 YU55 until now.

   B. 2005 YU55 is likely among the top five asteroids of scientific interest.

   C. 2005 YU55 is among the largest threats to our planet.

   D. 2005 YU55 presented scientists with a unique opportunity for gathering data.

SECTION 5: QUANTITATIVE REASONING

48 Items • 50 Minutes

> **Directions:** Choose the best answer for each question.

1. Before the stock market opened on April 20, an electronics company announced better than expected quarterly results. Consequently, its stock price increased by 20% that day. On April 21, news came out of a class action lawsuit against the company, causing the stock price to drop 10% that day. If, before the quarterly results announcement, the company's stock sold for $30 per share, what was the stock's closing price on April 21?

   A. $31.00
   B. $32.40
   C. $33.00
   D. $39.60

2. Melanie is selling her collection of antique plates using an online vendor. Initially, she planned to sell each plate for $22. Doing so would earn $1,430 before any fees were applied. If her goal is to earn $2,080 prior to fees, by approximately what percent should she increase the price she charges for a single plate?

   A. 10%
   B. 31%
   C. 32%
   D. 45%

SHOW YOUR WORK HERE

3. If a rock is tossed into a calm pond, ripples in the form of concentric circles emanate outward from the point of impact. The radius (in feet) of the outermost ripple is given by $r(t) = \frac{4}{5}t$, where t is the number of seconds following the time at which the rock hits the pond. The area of a ripple with radius r is $A(r) = \pi r^2$. Which of the following is an accurate interpretation of the function $(A \circ r)(t)$?

A. The area of the outermost ripple at the time of impact

B. The maximum area that ripples will reach before they dissipate

C. The area of the outermost ripple t seconds after the rock hit the pond

D. The radius that corresponds to the area of the ripple at time t

4. What is $\dfrac{\frac{1}{3}}{\frac{2}{5}+1}$?

A. $4\frac{1}{5}$

B. $\frac{5}{9}$

C. $\frac{7}{15}$

D. $\frac{5}{21}$

5. A contestant on a television show has scored 13, 18, 9, and 15 points over the first four challenges. If she needs an average score of at least 15 over the first five challenges in order to qualify for the next round, what is the lowest score she may receive on the fifth challenge and still qualify?

A. 21

B. 20

C. 18

D. 15

SHOW YOUR WORK HERE

practice test 3

6. If David bought 3 cans of soda at s cents each and four sticks of gum at g cents each, how much money did he spend, in cents?

   A. $3g + 4s$

   B. $7s + 7g$

   C. $3s + 4g$

   D. $3s - 4g$

7. A baseball game will definitely take place if there is no rain, while there is a 40% chance that the game will take place if there is rain. If the chance of rain is 80%, what is the overall chance that the game will take place?

   A. 0.064

   B. 0.4

   C. 0.52

   D. 0.92

8. If $f(x) = 3x$ and $g(x) = \log_5 x$, what is $(g - f)$ (25)?

   A. 73

   B. 50

   C. −70

   D. −73

9. What is $\lim\limits_{x \to -\infty} \left(\dfrac{1 - x^3}{x + 2} \right)$?

   A. $-\infty$

   B. 0

   C. $\dfrac{1}{2}$

   D. ∞

10. A bed frame is 2 meters long and 1.5 meter wide. What is its surface area?

   A. 30,000 squared centimeters

   B. 3,000 squared centimeters

   C. 300 squared centimeters

   D. 30 squared centimeters

SHOW YOUR WORK HERE

11. The figure below shows the box plots for two data sets. Which of the following is equal for the two data sets?

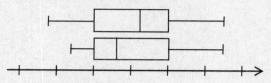

A. Average

B. Median

C. Range

D. Interquartile range

12. A state-of-the-art decorative fountain display that is the highlight of a nightly show at a local botanical gardens pumps water at a rate of 20,000 cubic feet per minute. What is the equivalent rate in *cubic yards per second*?

A. $\dfrac{20,000}{27 \times 60}$ cubic yards per second

B. $\dfrac{20,000}{9 \times 60}$ cubic yards per second

C. $\dfrac{20,000 \times 9}{60}$ cubic yards per second

D. $(20,000 \times 27 \times 60)$ cubic yards per second

13. A newly opened Internet café is selling shirts emblazoned with the company logo. The owner sells t-shirts for $10 each and collared shirts for $18 each. The total proceeds from the first weekend of sales is $566. If 43 shirts were sold, how many collared shirts were sold?

A. 17

B. 22

C. 26

D. 70

14. The diminishing population of Mexican red wolves in a national park t years after 2010 is described by the function $P(t) = \dfrac{350}{1 + 80\,e^{-0.2t}}$. After how many years will there be 50 Mexican red wolves in the park?

A. $5\left(\ln 3 + \ln 40\right)$ years

B. $\dfrac{\ln 3 - \ln 40}{5}$ years

C. $\ln\left(\dfrac{40}{3}\right)^5$ years

D. $\dfrac{1}{5}\ln\left(\dfrac{3}{40}\right)$ years

15. Two candidates ran for election for county coroner. Candidate A received 5,290 votes and candidate B received 7,406 votes. What is the approximate difference between the percentages of votes these two candidates each received?

A. 16.6%

B. 21.2%

C. 41.7%

D. 58.3%

16. On which of the following intervals is the function $f(x) = \dfrac{1}{3}x^3 - 3x^2 + 5x - 1$ increasing?

A. $(-\infty, -1) \cup (5, \infty)$

B. $(-\infty, 1) \cup (5, \infty)$

C. $(-1, 5)$

D. $(1, 5)$

17. Graham has mixed a cocktail that is 3 parts whiskey and 2 parts soda. If he mixed a total of 30 ounces of the cocktail, how many ounces of whiskey did he use?

A. 12

B. 18

C. 20

D. 24

SHOW YOUR WORK HERE

18. The graph below shows the number of tournaments a certain tennis player won between 2000 and 2010.

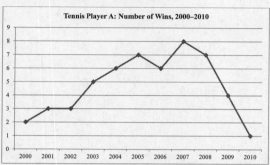

Rounded to the nearest tenth, what was the average number of tournaments this player won between 2003 and 2009, inclusive?

A. 6.8

B. 6.3

C. 6.1

D. 4.7

19. Two fighter jets, initially 1,800 miles apart, fly directly toward each other. Their speeds differ by 75 miles per hour. If they pass each other after 4 hours, what is the average of their speeds?

A. 187.5 miles per hour

B. 225 miles per hour

C. 262.5 miles per hour

D. 450 miles per hour

20. What is the reciprocal of $\dfrac{\frac{3}{4}}{\frac{5}{6}}$?

A. $-\dfrac{1}{12}$

B. $\dfrac{5}{8}$

C. $\dfrac{9}{10}$

D. $\dfrac{10}{9}$

21. Three friends workout at a local gym to-gether. There is a 20-station circuit involving a variety of nautilus machines, each of which has a fixed number of repetitions that must be completed before the athlete moves to the next station. The time it takes each of the three friends to complete the circuit are: 15 minutes 20 seconds, 14 minutes, and 16 minutes 52 seconds. What is the average number of seconds it takes this group to complete the circuit?

   A. 800 seconds

   B. 824 seconds

   C. 900 seconds

   D. 924 seconds

22. A food truck specializing in vegan food has worked at a local university during lunchtime for the past month. The owner analyzes the sales to determine the most profitable special to offer next month. Here is the data:

	Sweetened herbal tea	Vitamin water	No drink
Veggie wrap	40	65	25
Quinoa salad	15	30	10
Bean chili	65	45	15

If a customer is chosen randomly, how likely is it for him to purchase a quinoa salad given that he bought a vitamin water?

   A. $\frac{3}{31}$

   B. $\frac{11}{62}$

   C. $\frac{3}{14}$

   D. $\frac{6}{11}$

SHOW YOUR WORK HERE

23. If $\ln 12^x = \ln 48$, which of the following is incorrect?

   A. $\log 12^x = \log 48$

   B. $12^x = 48$

   C. $x \ln 12 = (\ln 6)(\ln 8)$

   D. $(\ln 12)(x - 1) = \ln 4$

24. A one-stop shop for automobile preventative maintenance boasts a quick time for standard oil changes. The times it took to complete an oil change for the last 10 customers, in minutes, are as follows:

18 21 20 19 20
16 24 18 18 16

What is the mean completion time?

   A. 18 minutes

   B. 18 minutes 30 seconds

   C. 19 minutes

   D. 24 minutes

25. A book is currently selling for $20. This price reflects a 20% discount compared to its original price. What was the book's original price?

   A. $15

   B. $16

   C. $24

   D. $25

SHOW YOUR WORK HERE

26. Concert venue owners are interested in knowing the number of concerts given by the top 25 rock band tours this year. This information is tabulated in the following stem-and-leaf plot:

Stem	Leaves
2	1 9
3	3 3 4 5
4	0 1 1 2 4 8
5	0 2 6 6 6 6 9 9
6	0 1
7	5
8	4 7

What is the range of this data set?

A. 48

B. 50

C. 56

D. 66

27. A decorative mulch bed is formed in the shape of a square with a side length of $4\frac{7}{8}$ feet. What is the perimeter of the mulch bed?

A. $9\frac{3}{4}$ feet

B. $16\frac{7}{8}$ feet

C. $19\frac{1}{2}$ feet

D. $23\frac{13}{16}$ feet

28. What is the second derivative of $f(x) = 2\cos x$?

A. $2\sin x$

B. $-2\sin x$

C. $2\cos x$

D. $-2\cos x$

SHOW YOUR WORK HERE

29. The average temperature in July in Serengeti is 61°F. The actual temperature can be 8 degrees warmer or colder. Which equation can be used to determine the minimum and maximum temperatures during July in this region?

A. $|x - 61| = 8$

B. $|x - 8| = 61$

C. $x - 61 = \pm 8$

D. $|x + 61| = 8$

30. The function $p(x) = x^2 - 40x$ describes the monthly profit, in dollars, that Ellen earns weekly by selling x dozen homemade miniature cupcakes. What is the least number of dozen cupcakes Ellen must sell to earn at least $500?

A. 10

B. 20

C. 40

D. 50

31. What is the value of $\int_0^\pi \sec^2 x\, dx$?

A. −1

B. 0

C. 1

D. π

32. What is 0.2% of $\frac{1}{5}$?

A. 0.0004

B. 0.004

C. 0.04

D. 0.4

33. If the average of a and b is 26 and the average of a and c is 18, what is $b - c$?

A. −16

B. 8

C. 16

D. 88

SHOW YOUR WORK HERE

practice test 3

SHOW YOUR WORK HERE

34. What is the solution of the inequality $3(2 - p) < 3 - 2(2p + 1)$?
    - A. $p > 5$
    - B. $p > -5$
    - C. $p < 5$
    - D. $p < -5$

35. What is the solution set of the inequality $|3x - 18| > -1$?
    - A. $(-\infty, -1) \cup (1, \infty)$
    - B. $(-\infty, \infty)$
    - C. $(-1, \infty)$
    - D. $(1, \infty)$

36. If $\ln e^7 = 1 - x$, what is x?
    - A. -6
    - B. $1 - \ln 7$
    - C. $\ln 7 - 1$
    - D. 6

37. What is $\dfrac{d}{dw}\left(\dfrac{w - 3}{2w + 1}\right)$ when $w = 3$?
    - A. $\dfrac{1}{7}$
    - B. $\dfrac{1}{2}$
    - C. 1
    - D. 7

38. The party planner in charge of coordinating Tom's parents' 50th wedding anniversary celebration ordered 250 flowers to decorate the hall. Specifically, she ordered white roses costing $4.25 each, long stem red roses costing $8.40 each, and tulips costing $3.75 each. She ordered 35 more tulips than white roses, and the total for the entire order, before sales tax and delivery, was $1,673.25. How many long stem red roses did she purchase?
    - A. 30
    - B. 65
    - C. 95
    - D. 155

39. The graphs of functions $f(x)$ and $g(x)$ are shown on the figure below. If $g(x)$ is perpendicular to $f(x)$, which of the following is the equation of $g(x)$?

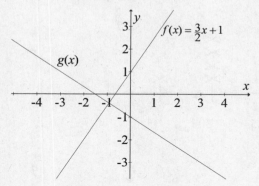

A. $g(x) = -\dfrac{2}{3}x - 1$

B. $g(x) = -\dfrac{2}{3}x + 1$

C. $g(x) = -\dfrac{3}{2}x + 1$

D. $g(x) = \dfrac{3}{2}x - 1$

40. Which of the following is equivalent to the vector w?

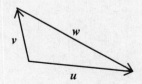

A. $v + u$

B. $2v + u$

C. $v - u$

D. $u - v$

practice test 3

41. A custodian has been tasked with counting the number of desks that are broken in each of 20 lecture halls in the science building. The results are illustrated in the following dot plot:

SHOW YOUR WORK HERE

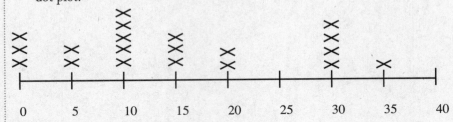

What is the median number of desks broken?

A. 10

B. 12.5

C. 15

D. 40

42. The table below shows the number of students at a particular college who are majoring in engineering.

Subject	Frequency
Chemical Engineering	10
Civil Engineering	15
Electrical Engineering	30
Mechanical Engineering	60

All students majoring in civil, electrical, or mechanical engineering are equally likely to be class president, while a student majoring in chemical engineering is twice as likely to be class president as a student majoring in civil engineering is. If it is certain that the class president will major in one of these four engineering disciplines, what is the probability that Kathy, a civil engineering major, will be class president?

A. $\frac{1}{75}$

B. $\frac{1}{25}$

C. $\frac{2}{23}$

D. $\frac{1}{5}$

43. The volume of a conical pile of gravel is 6,500 cubic feet. If the pile is 30 feet high, what is the radius of its base? (The volume of a cone with base radius r and height h is $V = \frac{1}{3}\pi r^2 h$.)

A. $\frac{650}{\pi}$ feet

B. $\sqrt{650\pi}$ feet

C. $\pi\sqrt{650}$ feet

D. $\sqrt{\frac{650}{\pi}}$ feet

SHOW YOUR WORK HERE

practice test 3

44. pH is often used to quantify the acidity level in a chemical solution. The definition is as follows: $pH = -\log[Z]$. If pH is 7.1, what is $[Z]$?

A. $e^{-7.1}$

B. $10^{-7.1}$

C. $-e^{7.1}$

D. $-10^{7.1}$

45. What is the value of $\int \dfrac{\ln 2x}{x}\,dx$?

A. $2\ln|x| + c$

B. $\dfrac{\ln 2x}{x} + c$

C. $\dfrac{\ln 2x}{2} + c$

D. $\dfrac{(\ln 2x)^2}{2} + c$

46. A summer camp focused on providing an enrichment experience to middle school children interested in space exploration keeps track of the number of female and male children attending the camp each year. Let $m(t)$ represent the number of males attending the camp in year t and $f(t)$ the number of females attending the camp in year t. Here, $t = 0$ corresponds to 2010. Which of these functions represents the portion of the total enrollment each year that is female?

A. $\dfrac{f(t)}{m(t)}$

B. $f(t) - m(t)$

C. $\big(f(t) + m(t)\big) \cdot \dfrac{1}{f(t)}$

D. $\dfrac{f(t)}{f(t) + m(t)}$

SHOW YOUR WORK HERE

47. Which of the following is the graph of $f(x) = 2 \sin x$?

SHOW YOUR WORK HERE

A.

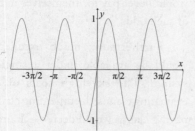

B.

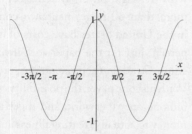

C.

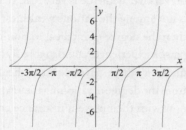

D.

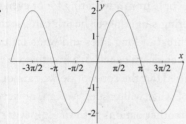

48. If $f(x)$ is a third-degree polynomial such that $f'(1) = 11, f''(1) = 10,$ and $f'''(1) = 12,$ which of the following could be $f(x)$?

A. $2x^3 - x^2 + 7x - 1$

B. $12x^3 + 10x^2 + 11x$

C. $x^3 + 2x^2 + 4x + 3$

D. $2x^3 - x^2 + 7$

ANSWER KEYS AND EXPLANATIONS

Section I: Writing

Sample of a Superior Response

The United States spends more on health care than any other nation in the world and, yet, by any number of measures that range from public opinion to life expectancy to rates of death from certain diseases, does not get the best results. To truly solve the problem of spiraling health-care costs, we must dramatically reduce our costs without compromising care. The best and fairest solution to this problem lies in adopting a single payer system.

At the first mention of single-payer health care, many people leap immediately to the assumption that care will be rationed. The truth of the matter is that care is rationed now by socioeconomic level and ability to pay as well as by private health insurance companies. There are now limits on what is available for most sick people. There are new treatments and possibilities only for those with the best insurance plans and the ability to pay their own way if absolutely necessary. Rationing is not by itself a dirty word, either. In a single-payer system, there is more fairness because what truly makes sense will be the standard for all, not just for the nation's poor or least demanding patients. Thus, a prostate screening test that costs more than $5 million for each prostate cancer life saved would be abandoned for all, not just for 90% of us. Similarly screenings, adjuvant therapies, and end-of-life care would also be evaluated through the lens of greatest good for the greatest number, or old-fashioned practicality. A much-needed end would come to the costly phenomenon of everybody wanting to take the 1 in 10,000 chance for a health treatment they would never pay for themselves in the face of such odds.

Furthermore, much excellent care would be available under a single-payer system. The sky-high costs of claims, evaluating claims, documenting claims, and paying claims would decrease dramatically with a single-payer system. Right now, more than 30 large insurance companies in the United States have costs of up to 30 percent just for the paperwork involved in administrating their insurance programs. With just one payer, the possibility of saving billions on paperwork, and diverting that money to actually treating illness and doing preventive medicine is very real. If a person is not among the nation's wealthiest people, then the degree of medical "rationing" that person experiences could markedly decrease under a single-payer form of health care from the degree of rationing they experience now with their current insurance company.

Many scare tactics are used to dissuade people from advocating for or even considering single-payer health care, such as the threat of long lines and waits for care and even death panels. It's true that we've never tried out the concept, so we cannot be sure of what will ensue. We can, however, look to other nations with single-payer systems, such as France, where the cost-to-benefits ratio for health care is far better and the cost to the nation as a whole is much lower. We might also notice that there are no death panels and no exaggerated or egregious waits there. We might further notice that there aren't 30 or more large health insurance corporations reaping enormous profits from the processing of, and often the denial of, claims, let alone the tragic tales of the uninsured.

While there remains much skepticism regarding the single-payer system, the fact is that it remains a viable solution to a dreadfully serious ongoing problem. Regardless of whether or not one agrees with this particular solution, there is little questioning that the current system is not working and needs to be fixed. As the single-payer system offers such benefits as fairness through standardization and the focus of funds on treatment rather than administration, and its effectiveness elsewhere in the world proves it viability, is it not worth trying here in the United States?

This essay earns a 5.0 score for the following reasons:

- In the introductory paragraph, the writer offers a solution to the problem (*adopting a single-payer system*), beginning the essay with a summary of that solution that will be fleshed out in the proceeding paragraphs.

- Each of the first body paragraphs deals with a facet of the solution: the truth about rationing (paragraph 2), the benefits of a single-payer system on the quality of care, and evidence of the effectiveness of the single-payer system (paragraph 3). That facet is made clear at the beginning of each paragraph in a clear topic sentence.

- The transitional words and phrases *Of course*, *Therefore*, and *To the argument* guide the reader through the explanation in a clear, systematic way.

- Many details (such as a scenario involving prostate cancer treatment to exemplify the fairness of the single-payer system and statistics regarding cost-draining issues affecting insurance companies) make the writing cogent and work toward supporting the main idea. Nothing is repeated. There are no digressions.

- The reasoning throughout the essay is logical.

- The conclusion ends a tidy summation of the passage's most important ideas as well as a provocative question to offer the reader some food for thought.

- There are no errors in sentence structure, and the sentences are varied and fluid.

- Words are used correctly and well.

- The essay is persuasive; the tone is appropriately serious; the voice of the writer is clear and engaged; and the first and second person are avoided.

- There are no mechanical errors.

Sample of a Weak Response

The United Sates does not have that many options when it comes to the problem of spiraling healthcare costs. We cannot sacrafice our high standerd of care and start bringing in death panels that tell you, no, you can't get anymore care and you have no options left. This is not what any American wants. Therefore, there is only one good way to really bring down the cost of healthcare. Ending entitlement programs, including those for healthcare, as soon as possible. We can all see the trouble that a nation like Greece is in now for having entitlement programs, those entitlement programs are way too big for any nation to handle and are going to bring it down sooner or later just like Greece got brung down. Entitlement programs are just not realistic. If we did not have these giant entitlements, we would not even have a deficit. Our economy would be better off, there would be jobs for every able body citizen who wanted to work. If you keep up a program like medicare, then you are going to see that deficit grow and grow as the healthcare costs go up. Also, as our population gets older and older, there are going to be more and more people putting in for their medicare claims and expecting the goverment to pay for everything they need. No matter how expensive those costs get. No one in this nation wants to take responsibility for theirselves any more. They just want other people to foot their bill.

In summary, the best thing to do is to end entitlement programs, especially healthcare entitlements, as soon as possible. This being the only real solution to the problem of spiraling healthcare costs.

This essay earns a 1.0 score for the following reasons:

- This essay is inadequate in terms of supporting details and problem solving. The writer introduces only one idea to support his or her solution and does not explain it in a cogent way.

- While the writer shows some insight in the idea selected for analysis, the idea is not explained and developed.

- The solution of ending entitlement programs to combat spiraling health care costs is overly simplistic.

- The essay lacks organization. It consists of only two paragraphs with the main idea and all supporting details crammed in the first paragraph and a weak conclusion in the second paragraph.

- There are enough errors in sentence construction to make much of the essay unintelligible.

- There are numerous errors in sentence construction. There are both run ons and fragments.

- There are numerous mechanical and usage errors.

Section 2: Biological Processes

1. A	11. A	21. C	31. D	41. B
2. D	12. D	22. D	32. B	42. C
3. B	13. B	23. A	33. B	43. C
4. D	14. C	24. C	34. B	44. D
5. B	15. C	25. D	35. C	45. A
6. D	16. C	26. A	36. B	46. D
7. C	17. C	27. B	37. C	47. A
8. A	18. B	28. C	38. D	48. A
9. C	19. C	29. C	39. B	
10. A	20. C	30. A	40. D	

1. **The correct answer is A.** Each cell produces its own supply of ATP as it is needed. As a cell becomes more active, ATP production increases, and as a cell becomes inactive, ATP production decreases. Choice B is incorrect because as a cell becomes more active it requires more ATP, and so the production of ATP increases. Choice C is incorrect because ATP is not transferred from one area of the body to another; therefore, its production depends upon the recycling of its components within a given cell. ATP is used continuously by cells in all organisms, but it is also a renewable resource within cells. Choice D is incorrect because ATP synthesis requires an input of energy; therefore, it is an endothermic reaction. ATP is synthesized from ADP and P_i.

2. **The correct answer is D.** Glycolysis occurs in the cytoplasm of the cell. Choice A is incorrect because glycolysis does not take place in the plasma membrane. Protein transport into and out of the cell occurs in the plasma membrane. Choice B is incorrect because the Krebs cycle occurs in the mitochondrial matrix, but glycolysis occurs in the cytoplasm. Choice C is incorrect because

the nucleus is the site of DNA replication, RNA transcription, and ribosome synthesis.

3. **The correct answer is B.** In alcohol fermentation, pyruvate is converted to ethanol in a two-step process. The first step releases CO_2 from the pyruvate, and the pyruvate is converted to acetaldehyde. In the second step, acetaldehyde is reduced by NADH to ethanol (ethyl alcohol). This step also regenerates the supply of NAD^+ needed for glycolysis. Choice A is incorrect because in the first step of alcohol fermentation, when pyruvate is converted to acetylaldehyde, NADH is not reduced. Therefore, NAD^+ does not form in this step. Choice C is incorrect because CO_2 is released from pyruvate in the first step of fermentation. Choice D is incorrect because the conversion of phosphoenolpyruvate to pyruvate occurs before formation in the process of glycolysis.

4. **The correct answer is D.** Chemiosmosis is a type of phosphorylation reaction that generates ATP for a cell. In this method, energy stored in the form of an H^+ ion (proton) gradient across a membrane is used to drive cellular work, such as the synthesis of ATP. Choice A is incorrect because a

phosphorylation reaction is the mechanism of ATP synthesis, but the energy to drive the reaction is supplied from a proton gradient. Choice B is incorrect because other ATP molecules do not provide energy for ATP synthesis. ATP hydrolysis that releases energy is used to power cellular functions. Choice C is incorrect because the electron transport chain is not the mechanism that supplies energy for protein synthesis. The electron transport chain is essential for oxidative phosphorylation.

5. **The correct answer is B.** A prominent structure within the nucleus of a cell is the nucleolus, which is a nonmembranous organelle involved in the production of ribosomes. A ribosome is made up of ribosomal RNA and proteins. Choice A is incorrect because the nucleus is a membrane-bound organelle. It contains the nucleolus, which is the site of ribosome synthesis. Choice C is incorrect because the endoplasm reticulum, ER, is the site of importance for protein and lipid synthesis. All transmembrane proteins are synthesized in the ER. Choice D is incorrect because the lysosome is a membrane-bound sac responsible for getting rid of cellular debris.

6. **The correct answer is D.** In a double helix of DNA, one strand runs 5' to 3' and the antiparallel strand runs 3' to 5'. The sequence of the antiparallel strand is complementary to the other strand. G nucleotides always pair with C, and A always pairs with T. Therefore, the antiparallel strand for the sequence shown is 3'CCGATGTAG5'. Choice A is incorrect because the strand shown is not in the antiparallel direction, and the sequence contains the base uracil, U, in place of thymine, T. Choice B is incorrect because although this strand is running 3' to 5' in the correct antiparallel direction, the sequence is not complementary to the one shown. Therefore, the two strands would

not form base pairs between each other. Choice C is incorrect because although this is a complementary base pair sequence, the strand is running parallel (5' to 3') to the given sequence instead of antiparallel (3' to 5').

7. **The correct answer is C.** RNA processing occurs in order to transform the precursor RNA into a mature mRNA strand. Introns are spliced out of the RNA sequence, and exons are joined together. These actions are performed by a protein complex called a spliceosome. The mature mRNA strand, therefore, has a continuous coding sequence. This process of preparing a mature mRNA molecule is called RNA splicing. Choice A is incorrect because the initiation complex binds to DNA before the start of transcription. Choice B is incorrect because the nucleotides are joined together during the transcription process. Choice D is incorrect because exons contain the genes, and, therefore, they are not spliced out of mature mRNA.

8. **The correct answer is A.** In DNA replication, the DNA helicase enzyme catalyses the unwinding of the double-stranded DNA. The next enzyme that is involved is DNA topoisomerase that acts to correct the overwinding of DNA just ahead of the replication fork. DNA primase then synthesizes a single RNA primer at the 5' end of the leading strand and primers at the end of each Okazaki fragment on the lagging strand. The final enzyme to act in the replication process is DNA polymerase III, which continually synthesizes new DNA on the leading strand and elongates the Okazaki fragments on the lagging strand. Choice B is incorrect because primase and DNA polymerase III cannot act on the DNA strands until the helicase and topoisomerase play their role in the unwinding. Choice C is incorrect because the enzymes work in the

opposite order than what is listed in choice C. Choice D is incorrect because helicase must unwind the DNA before topoisomerase is needed, and primase adds primers to the DNA before DNA polymerase III elongates the new strands.

9. **The correct answer is C.** Each amino acid codon is composed of three RNA nucleotides. Therefore, to make an amino acid chain that is 100 amino acids in length, 300 RNA nucleotides are needed in the RNA. Choice A is incorrect because three nucleotides are required for the addition of one amino acid to an amino acid chain. Choice B is incorrect because three nucleotides are required for each amino acid. Choice D is incorrect because three nucleotides are required for each amino acid.

10. **The correct answer is A.** Since DNA synthesis would not occur, the cells would be arrested at the G_1 phase, which is the phase immediately before the S phase. Choice B is incorrect because if cells could not replicate their DNA, they would not move past G_1. G_2 occurs after the S phase, so they would never reach this phase. Choice C is incorrect because the cells would move through the M phase and into G_1, and then not progress into the S phase. Choice D is incorrect because if DNA synthesis is prevented, cells would not enter the S phase.

11. **The correct answer is A.** The nucleotide base attaches to the C1' on the deoxyribose sugar. Choices B, C, and D are incorrect because the base binds to the C1' on the deoxyribose ring.

12. **The correct answer is D.** Since the initiator met-tRNA is in the P site, the A site is available to bind the next tRNA and amino acid. The two amino acids become joined together on the A site and the tRNA molecule dissociates from the P site. The ribosome then moves down to the next codon on the mRNA, and the tRNA-amino acid complex moves from the A site to the P site, leaving the A site free to receive the next tRNA and amino acid. Choice A is incorrect because the tRNA $_{met}$ remains on the P site until another tRNA binds to the A site. It dissociates when the methionine molecule binds to the amino acid at the A site. Choice B is incorrect because a second tRNA molecule joins the ribosome complex at the A site. Choice C is incorrect because another tRNA molecule binds to the A site, and then the methionine molecule binds to that amino acid.

13. **The correct answer is B.** Allosteric regulation is the term used to describe any case in which the function of a protein at one site is affected by the binding of a regulatory molecule at a different site. This regulatory molecule may serve either to activate or inhibit an enzyme's activity. An activating or inhibiting molecule binds to an allosteric site on the enzyme. The binding of an activator molecule stabilizes the enzyme in a conformation that is favorable to binding substrate to the active site. Conversely, the binding of an inhibitory molecule to an allosteric site will stabilize an inactive conformation of the enzyme so that the active site of the enzyme is not accessible to its substrate. Choice A is incorrect because a product acts to block substrate binding in the mechanism of feedback inhibition. Choice C is incorrect because a protein that binds to and blocks the active site is an example of competitive inhibition. Choice D is incorrect. Increasing substrate concentration is effective in overcoming the competitive inhibition because it increases the ratio of substrate to inhibitor molecules.

14. **The correct answer is C.** In general, an increase in temperature up to a maximum causes an increase in enzyme activity. Above this optimal temperature the enzyme begins to degrade and does not function as

efficiently as at the optimal temperature. Different enzymes have a different optimal temperature at which they catalyze a reaction most efficiently. Eventually, the enzyme becomes completely degraded and loses all functional activity. Choice A is incorrect because this point on the graph represents a temperature that is too low for optimal enzyme acidity. Choice B is incorrect because this point on the graph represents a temperature which is approaching the optimal temperature for enzyme activity. Choice D is incorrect because this point on the graph represents a temperature at which the enzyme is fully degraded and has lost all ability to catalyze the reaction.

15. **The correct answer is C.** Cytochromes are coenzymes that have a heme group, which is a ring structure surrounding an iron atom. Cytochromes transfer electrons to other molecules by alternating between oxidation and reduction reactions. In this process, the iron atom either gains or loses an electron. Choice A is incorrect because NAD$^+$ is a hydrogen carrier coenzyme and does not contain an iron atom. Choice B is incorrect because FAD is also a hydrogen carrier and does not contain an iron atom. Choice D is incorrect because coenzyme A does not contain an iron atom; it is a coenzyme that carries a small organic acid that is required for cellular respiration.

16. **The correct answer is C.** In a chemical reaction, chemical energy is referred to as the amount of potential energy available, which is the amount of energy released as the reaction moves forward. Choice A is incorrect because mechanical energy is the sum of an object's kinetic and potential energy and is required for motion. Mechanical energy is required for muscle movement and within the cell for movement of molecules around the cytoplasm. Choice B is incorrect because kinetic energy is the

energy of motion. Moving objects perform work by transferring motion from one object to another. Potential energy is the energy that matter possesses. Choice D is incorrect because electrical energy, a type of potential energy, is utilized when electrons move from one orbital to another or from one molecule to another.

17. **The correct answer is C.** Fossils are traces of previously existing organisms that give evidence that changes have occurred within a particular type of organism or species. Differences have emerged over long periods of time and have been documented. Fossils also reveal similarities in species. Choice A is incorrect because adaptation to an environment can cause changes in a species over time, but does not necessarily show physical similarities in species. Choice B is incorrect because behavioral analysis does not give physical evidence of the interrelatedness of species. Choice D is incorrect because genetic variation gives evidence of variation in a population, but does not provide physical evidence of species similarity.

18. **The correct answer is B.** Throughout evolution, mutations in genes are a method of change and modification in a species. Microevolution refers to a change in gene frequency within the population of a given organism in a given location. It can take only one generation for microevolution to occur, or it may take several generations. Choice A is incorrect because macroevolution refers to changes that occur in the family, order, and class of an organism. Fossil records can be used to study the history of macroevolution. Choice C is incorrect because natural selection is a process that can lead to evolution and a decrease in genetic variation in a population, but microevolution is more accurately described by the given statement. Choice D is incorrect because adaptation

refers to changes that individuals make to better survive in their environment.

19. **The correct answer is C.** Pedigrees are useful in families with a history of a genetic disorder. The pedigree can help predict the outcome of future generations with respect to disease. Choice A is incorrect because a pedigree can also help to predict the ratio of offspring likely to inherit a particular trait. Choice B is incorrect because it is unethical to manipulate human mating patterns. A pedigree can only help to predict what disorders or traits the offspring of two mates might inherit. Choice D is incorrect because a pedigree cannot help to predict the sex of offspring, only their inheritance patterns.

20. **The correct answer is C.** The fact that many species have a high percentage of similarities in their DNA gives strong chemical evidence to support the fact that all life originated from a single source. Choice A is incorrect because gene flow refers to the migration of individuals of one population to another. This does not provide a chemical basis for life originating from one source. Choice B is incorrect because fossil records can be used to study the history of macroevolution, but they do not provide chemical evidence. Choice D is incorrect because the presence of mutations in DNA does not indicate that all life originated from one source; it can only support the concept that species evolve over time.

21. **The correct answer is C.** A nonpathogen is a microorganism that almost never causes harm to a host. However, under the correct conditions, even these microorganisms can harm their hosts. *E. coli* are beneficial in maintaining the correct conditions in the gut, but *E. coli* can become an opportunistic pathogen under certain conditions. Choice A is incorrect because a pathogen is a microorganism that causes harm to host

organisms. The amount of harm or damage a pathogen can cause to humans depends on the ability of the immune system to respond to and attack the pathogen. Choice B is incorrect because opportunistic pathogens are those that cause harm to a host under ideal conditions. In cases of a host that has a suppressed immune system, opportunistic pathogens thrive. They also can thrive in certain areas of the body where they can exist in ideal conditions or in a symbiotic relationship with another organism. Choice D is incorrect because a microaerophile refers to bacteria that require only a low concentration of O_2 to thrive.

22. **The correct answer is D.** A virus requires a host cell to survive. A virus takes over the host cell in order to replicate and grow. The death of a virus only occurs outside its host. Choice A is incorrect because retroviruses contain RNA, not DNA. Choice B is incorrect because penetration of the virus into the host cell prevents it from being attacked by the immune system. Choice C is incorrect because a virus uses the host cell's replication machinery by attaching to the end of the host cell DNA and replicating with the host DNA.

23. **The correct answer is A.** If the haploid nuclei from each parent mycelium do not fuse immediately, the two genetically different nuclei can coexist in the mycelium. This type of mycelium is called a heterokaryon. In some species, heterokaryon can become mosaics. Choice B is incorrect because during karyogamy, the haploid nuclei from each parent fuse together to produce a diploid cell. Karyogamy is the only stage at which diploid cells exist in most fungi. Meiosis restores the cells to the haploid state. Choice C is incorrect, because during plasmogamy, the cytoplasm of two cells join together. Choice D is incorrect because two nuclei exist as a heterokaryon.

24. The correct answer is C. Schwann cells myelinate the axons of motor neurons in the PNS. Both Schwann cells and oligodendrocytes grow around axons in multi-layered coil wrappings. Since the layers are mostly composed of lipids, the myelin sheath is also a good form of insulation for the axons. Choice A is incorrect because astrocytes provide structural support for neurons and also regulate the extracellular concentration of ions (Na^+ and K^+) and recycle neurotransmitters. They have many projections that attach to the dendrites of neurons. Choice B is incorrect because radial glia form tracts along which newly formed neurons can migrate from the neural tube (pre-CNS in a developing embryo) to other positions in the body during embryonic development. Choice D is incorrect because although oligodendrocytes form a myelin sheath around the axons of neurons in the CNS, it is Schwann cells that form a myelin sheath around the axons of motor neurons in the PNS.

25. The correct answer is D. During active transport, energy in the form of ATP (adenosine triphosphate) is required to move molecules across the cell membrane and across the concentration gradient. In this type of transport, carrier or transport proteins are necessary. When these proteins interact with ATP, there is a change in the transport protein's conformation so that they bind specific ions such as Na^+, K^+, Ca^{2+}, and H^+ and carry them across the membrane either into or out of the cell. Choice A is incorrect because water can cross the cell membrane through the process of osmosis. Choice B is incorrect because oxygen is a gas and it can diffuse across the membrane. Choice C is incorrect because carbon dioxide can diffuse across the membrane in a similar manner to oxygen.

26. The correct answer is A. Gomphoses are specialized fibrous peg-in-socket joints between the teeth and the mandible and maxilla. These joints are secured with periodontal ligament and are immovable. Choice B is incorrect because sutures are fibrous joints that are found only in the skull. Choice C is incorrect because syndesmoses are fibrous joints held together by ligaments. These types of joints have minimal movement and are amphiarthroses. Choice D is incorrect because diarthroses are freely movable joints, whereas the joints connecting teeth to the mandible and maxima are immovable.

27. The correct answer is B. Oxygen-poor blood flows from the body via the superior and inferior vena cave into the right atrium of the heart. From the right atrium, it flows into the right ventricle and then to the lungs. From the lungs, oxygen-rich blood flows into the left atrium of the heart. Then oxygen-rich blood flows into the left ventricle of the heart. Choices A, C, and D are incorrect because they do not illustrate the correct flow of blood through the heart and lungs.

28. The correct answer is C. Lymph drains from lymphatic capillaries into larger lymphatic vessels. The thoracic duct and the right lymphatic duct are vessels through which lymph reenters the circulatory system. Choice A is incorrect because lymph flows back to the circulatory system via the thoracic duct and the right lymphatic duct. The two functions of lymph nodes are filtering and helping to activate the immune response mechanisms. Choices B and D are incorrect because lymph drains from the lymphatic capillaries into the lymphatic vessels. From the vessels, it flows into the ducts and then into the circulatory system.

29. **The correct answer is C.** Synergism involves two hormones working together to produce one outcome. Two hormones may also work together to produce a combined effect that is greater than the effect of one hormone acting alone. Growth hormone, insulin, insulin-like growth factor, calcitonin, and estrogen (female) or testosterone (male) all work together to promote bone growth. Choice A is incorrect because permissiveness involves the requirement of one hormone in order to bring about the full effect of a second hormone. In the case of bone growth, the hormones are working together to produce one result. Choice B is incorrect because antagonism is the effect observed when two hormones produce opposite effects from each other. Choice D is incorrect because the hormones work together in this example and are not inhibitory to one another.

30. **The correct answer is A.** The stationary period of bacterial growth is a 24- to 48-hour period in which there is an equal rate of growth and death. During this time, the bacterial population remains constant. Choice B is incorrect because the logarithmic growth period is a 12- to 24-hour period in which there is active doubling of bacteria through binary fission. Choice C is incorrect because the lag time of bacterial growth is a 20- to 30-minute period when a new colony is establishing itself and getting ready to reproduce. Choice D is incorrect because the decline period, which lasts 48 to 96 hours, is marked by rapid cell death by lysis. There is no new bacterial growth in this period.

31. **The correct answer is D.** The O_2 that is diffused into the bloodstream attaches to hemoglobin in the red blood cells, and hemoglobin also helps to transport CO_2 back out of the bloodstream. Choice A is incorrect because cells require a continuous supply of O_2 from outside the body for cellular respiration. Choice B is incorrect because the laryngopharynx is where the paths for air and food cross each other. Choice C is incorrect because cells take up O_2 and release CO_2 into the bloodstream so it can be exhaled out of the body.

32. **The correct answer is B.** The left ventricle receives oxygen-rich blood from the left atrium of the heart. The left atrium receives the blood through the four pulmonary veins extending from the lungs. The left ventricle pumps the blood to the aorta, the largest blood vessel of the body, and the aorta carries and distributes oxygen-rich blood to the rest of the body. Choice A is incorrect because the myocardium is the bulk of the heart consisting of the contractile muscle tissue; the endocardium is the innermost layer of the heart. Choice C is incorrect because the tricuspid valve is located between the right atrium and the right ventricle. Choice D is incorrect because the aortic valve is located between the left ventricle and the aorta and prevents backflow into the aorta as blood is pumped into the aorta. Heart valves are flap-like structures that allow blood to flow in one direction only. They prevent the backflow of blood as it is pumped from the atrium to the ventricle.

33. **The correct answer is B.** Retroviruses have an enzyme called reverse transcriptase rhat synthesizes DNA from RNA. This is the opposite of the DNA-to-RNA information flow of normal cells. HIV (human immunodeficiency virus) is a retrovirus that causes AIDS (acquired immunodeficiency syndrome). HIV is an enveloped virus that contains two identical RNA strands and two molecules of reverse transcriptase. Choice A is incorrect because retroviruses including HIV do not have a DNA genome. Their genome consists of RNA, and DNA is synthesized through reverse transcriptase. Choice C is incorrect because the RNA

in HIV and other retroviruses synthesizes DNA strands. Choice D is incorrect because the fact that HIV is an enveloped virus does not make it a retrovirus.

34. **The correct answer is B.** Rod-shaped bacteria that have flagella are bacilli. The average size of bacilli is 0.5 μm wide and 1 to 5 μm long. Bacilli are also named according to how many cells are linked together. Streptobacilli consist of a chain of cells in a rod-shaped configuration with a flagellum. Choice A is incorrect because a streptococcus bacteria would consist of a chain of round-shaped bacteria. Choice C is incorrect because vibrio are incomplete spirals that have a half-moon shape. Choice D is incorrect because a spirillum is a multi-bending spiral-shaped bacteria.

35. **The correct answer is C.** The juxtamedullary capillary beds help to concentrate urine. They are capillary beds that have vasa recta, which are straight arteries, not veins, in the kidneys that are ordered and perpendicular to the loop of Henle. Choice A is incorrect because the corticoid nephron is found mostly in the cortex of the kidney (although some are in the loop of Henle), and about 85% of all nephrons are corticoid nephrons. Choice B is incorrect because the peritubular capillary beds pick up solutes that have been filtered out in the glomerular bed and reabsorb them. Choice D is incorrect because the juxtamedullary capillary beds have vasa recta, which are straight arteries, not veins, in the kidneys, but are perpendicular to the loop of Henle.

36. **The correct answer is B.** The prostate gland secretes a thin fluid that further nourishes sperm. This milky, acidic fluid contains citrate, enzymes, and prostate-specific antigen (PSA). Choice A is incorrect because the seminal vesicles secrete a thick fluid that contains fructose, ascorbic acid, prostaglandins, and other substances that promote motility. The fructose provides most of the energy used by sperm to propel themselves through the female reproductive tract. Choice C is incorrect because the two small bulbourethral glands secrete a clear, thick, alkaline mucous that may act to neutralize the acidity of urine. It also lubricates the glans penis. Choice D is incorrect because the nutrients in the bloodstream do not supply nourishment to sperm; their nutrients come from the fluids of the prostate gland and seminal vesicles.

37. **The correct answer is C.** Light reactions reduce $NADP^+$ to NADPH, and they also generate ATP using chemiosmosis to drive the addition of a phosphate group to ADP. This process in plants is called photophosphorylation. The light reactions result in the production of chemical energy in the form of NADPH and ATP in the reaction: Light (photon) + H_2O + ADP + P_i + NADP → O_2 + ATP + NADPH. Choice A is incorrect because ADP is a breakdown product of ATP and is not considered an energy source for cells. Choice B is incorrect because $NADP^+$ is reduced to NADPH in light reactions, and NADPH is the energy source produced by the light reaction. $NADP^+$ is a reactant in the process. Choice D is incorrect because photons are another reactant in the light reaction, not an energy source produced by the reaction.

38. **The correct answer is D.** Interferons, or interleukins, are antiviral proteins made by cells infected with a virus. Interferons prevent viral replication in other cells. When interferons are made by an infected cell, they enter other cells preventing viral infection over a given time period in those cells. Interferons are not specific to a particular virus, and they are only produced in cells that are undergoing active infection. Choice A is incorrect because memory B cells are

made in the immune system to give antibody protections against future infection by the same virus. Choice B is incorrect because antigens do not prevent viral replication in other cells. Choice C is incorrect because antibodies prevent viral attachment to host cells.

39. **The correct answer is B.** Epithelial cells line the inner wall of the small intestine with small finger-like projections called villi, and a villus has many even smaller projections called microvilli. The microvilli extend into the lumen of the intestine and greatly increase the surface area available for the absorption of nutrients. Choice A is incorrect because microvilli help to increase the surface area for nutrient absorption. Choice C is incorrect because ridding the body of waste is a process that occurs in the large intestine. Choice D is incorrect because microvilli aid in abruption, but not chemical digestion.

40. **The correct answer is D.** The *Cryptococcus neoformans* strain of yeast is pathogenic and causes an infection called cryptococcosis. It is found in soil contaminated with certain types of bird droppings, like pigeon droppings. If humans inhale dust containing *C. neoformans*, they develop flu-like symptoms that can progress to pneumonia and lung scarring. Choice A is incorrect because *Saccharomyces cerevisiae* poses no health risk. Common examples of *Saccharomyces cerevisiae* are baker's yeast and brewer's yeast. Choice B is incorrect because *P. jiroveccii* affects the lungs and causes the formation of cysts. In immunosuppressed individuals, it causes pneumonia. However, it is not caused by inhaling infected bird droppings. Choice C is incorrect because *Candida* are the most common and most important type of yeast. There are many species of *Candida*. Candidiasis infections are commonly seen in humans as vaginitis, thrush, onchomycosis,

and dermatitis, but none come from bird droppings.

41. **The correct answer is B.** The pituitary gland additionally secretes growth hormone (GH) and thyroid-stimulating hormone (TSH). Choice A is incorrect because the adrenal glands produce hormones that include adrenaline and cortisol. Choice C is incorrect because the thymus gland is primarily involved in the immune system, developing T cells. Choice D is incorrect because the thyroid gland produces thyroxine and triiodothyronine.

42. **The correct answer is C.** In asexual reproduction, a consistent genotype can be propagated in order to take advantage of consistent ideal conditions. Choice A is incorrect because adverse conditions would lend themselves to sexual reproduction such that the fungus can adapt to its environment with genetic modifications. Choice B is incorrect because extreme environmental conditions would cause sexual reproduction to be favored, so that the optimal genotype is selected for survival. Choice D is incorrect because sexual reproduction is an advantage when environmental conditions are changing.

43. **The correct answer is C.** Peristalsis occurs in digestive organs like the small intestine to move digested food through. Choice A is incorrect because it describes excretion. Choice B is incorrect because it describes homeostasis. Choice D is incorrect because it describes capillary action.

44. **The correct answer is D.** Antidiuretics affect the kidneys in decreasing the production of urine. Choice A is incorrect because this describes a laxative drug. Choice B is incorrect because neutralization of stomach acid would disturb one's digestive processes. Choice C is incorrect because it describes an inhaler.

45. **The correct answer is A.** Adipocytes are specialized in fat accumulation and storage. Choice B is incorrect because melanocytes are found primarily in the epidermis, as well as in the inner ear and the uvea of the eye. Choice C is incorrect because phagocytes are white blood cells that play critical immune roles in the human body. Choice D is incorrect because thymocytes are found in the thymus and differentiate into mature T lymphocytes.

46. **The correct answer is D.** Cilia line the respiratory tract. Choices A, B, and C are incorrect because they do not reference the respiratory system.

47. **The correct answer is A.** Cells that are competent can undergo transformation and take up genetic material from the environment. Choice B is incorrect because certain proteins can do this, but not competent cells. Choice C is incorrect because cells that can undergo conjugation would be donor cells and recipient cells, with donors needing a fertility factor. Choice D is incorrect because cell competence is unrelated to viral resistance.

48. **The correct answer is A.** Because viruses can evolve, mutation rates tend to be high in viruses, which is why we need the flu shot annually. Choice B is incorrect because viruses lack the machinery to produce proteins themselves. Choice C is incorrect because it is not a generally true statement, even though viruses may use host cells for protection. Choice D is incorrect because antiviral drugs and antibiotics are not the same thing.

Section 3: Chemical Procesess

1. A	11. B	21. D	31. D	41. C
2. B	12. B	22. C	32. D	42. A
3. D	13. C	23. A	33. C	43. A
4. D	14. A	24. C	34. B	44. A
5. B	15. B	25. A	35. C	45. B
6. C	16. A	26. B	36. C	46. B
7. D	17. C	27. A	37. A	47. A
8. D	18. D	28. D	38. C	48. B
9. D	19. C	29. B	39. C	
10. A	20. A	30. C	40. C	

1. **The correct answer is A.** Liquid-liquid extraction is commonly performed in organic chemical reactions and is carried out in a separatory funnel. The liquid to be extracted and the extraction solvent are both added to the separatory funnel. A stopper is used to block off the opening of the funnel, and the mixture is shaken. The buildup of pressure from the shaken mixture is released by opening a stopcock at the end of the funnel. After a given time, layers of liquid are distinguishable, and the bottom layer can be removed via the stopcock on the end of the funnel. In some instances, multiple extractions are necessary to completely remove a liquid from its solvent. Choice B is incorrect because a column is used in chromatography techniques, not in an extraction experiment. Choice C is incorrect because filter paper can be used to dry crystals precipitated from a solution. Choice D is incorrect because a graduated cylinder is used to measure volume.

2. **The correct answer is B.** In mass spectroscopy a sample is placed into the spectrometer and bombarded by a stream of high-energy electrons. When a high-energy electron hits an organic molecule, it dislodges a valence electron from the sample molecule. This produces what is called a cation radical (positively charged, odd number of electrons). The process of electron bombardment also transfers a large quantity of energy to the molecules of the sample. This causes the cation radicals to fly apart (fragment). Some of the fragments retain a positive charge, and other fragments become neutral. The small fragments are passed through a magnetic field and only the positively charged fragments are deflected based on their charge-to-mass ratio. These positively charged fragments are sorted by the mass spectrometer and each group of a certain charge-to-mass ratio is recorded as a peak. Choice A is incorrect because wavelength is measured in IR spectroscopy. Cation radicals do not form. Choice C is incorrect because NMR does not rely on cation radicals. Instead, it relies on the generation of a magnetic field through the spinning of nuclei in a molecule. Choice D is incorrect because UV-Vis relies upon the absorbance of the substance at a specific wavelength.

3. **The correct answer is D.** Crystallization is a straightforward and effective way of purifying a solid. A crude sample of the reaction product is dissolved in a minimal amount of liquid solvent and heated to boiling. Once all the product has dissolved in the solvent, the solution is slowly cooled. As the solution cools, pure crystals form and precipitate out of the solution. The formation of crystals can be brought about by the addition of a seed crystal, or by scratching the side of the vessel containing the solution. The impurities are left behind in the solution, and the pure crystals are isolated through a process of filtration. Solid sulfanilamide can be isolated from an ethanol solution via crystallography. Choice A is incorrect because liquid chromatography is used to separate two liquids, not a solid and a liquid. Choice B is incorrect because distillation is a process for purifying a volatile liquid. Choice C is incorrect because sublimation is the process of separating a volatile solid from nonvolatile substances.

4. **The correct answer is D.** If the stationary phase is composed of very small, uniformly sized spherical particles, the efficiency of chromatography is improved. Small-sized spheres create a greater surface area for the adsorption of compounds, and the uniform size allows for the particles of the column to be tightly packed. Liquid chromatography, choice A; gas chromatography, choice B; and high-pressure liquid chromatography (HPLC), choice C, are very efficient forms due to this property. Paper chromatography has the least amount of surface area for the molecules to adsorb onto and so the correct answer is choice D.

5. **The correct answer is B.** Chemical properties of a substance are those observed when a chemical change of the substance takes place. Flammability, heat of combustion, and the ionization energy of an element are all examples of chemical properties. Choice A is incorrect because combustion of a material is a chemical property, not a physical property. Choice C is incorrect because the boiling point is not determined by a combustion analysis. Choice D is incorrect because color is a physical property and is not analyzed by combustion.

6. **The correct answer is C.** Converting grams of H_2O and CO_2 obtained to moles yields a molar ratio of 4 hydrogens per 1 carbon; therefore, the correct chemical formula of the analyzed compound is CH_4. All other choices have the wrong molar ratios.

7. **The correct answer is D.** Chemically equivalent protons do not exhibit spin-spin splitting. The equivalent protons can be on the same or different carbon atoms. They do not couple, and their signal appears as a singlet. Choice A is incorrect because two groups of protons coupled to each other have the same coupling constant. Choice B is incorrect because protons farther than two carbon atoms apart do not couple. Choice C is incorrect because a proton with n equivalent neighboring protons gives a signal that is split into $n + 1$ peaks with a coupling constant, J.

8. **The correct answer is D.** Since the sum of the pH and pOH of a solution must add up to 14, the pH of the given solution must be 8. The equation for the pH of a solution is $pH = -\log_{10} [H_3O^+]$. So to calculate the concentration of H_3O^+ ions, it is necessary to determine the antilog of the pH. In this case, it would be the antilog of $^-8$, since $^-8 = \log_{10} [H_3O^+]$. The antilog is 10^{-8}, and thus the concentration of H_3O^+ ions in the solution is 1×10^{-8}M. Choice A is incorrect because this would be the concentration if the pH was equal to 14. Choice B is incorrect because this would be the value if the pH of the solution were 10. Choice C is incorrect

because this would be the concentration of OH^- ions in the solution since the pOH is 6.

9. **The correct answer is D.** In a given molecule, if the atomic masses of each type of atom are known, it is possible to calculate the mass of the entire molecule. The molecular mass (also called the molecular weight) is the sum of all the atomic masses (or molar masses) in a molecule. Thus, the molecular mass can be calculated by multiplying the atomic mass of each element by the number of atoms of that element present in each molecule and adding all the values for each specific element. For H_2SO_4, there are 2 atoms of hydrogen (atomic mass of H = 1.008 amu), one atom of S (atomic mass of S = 32.07 amu), and four atoms of oxygen (atomic mass of O = 16.0 amu). Therefore, the total molecular mass of H_2SO_4 is 98.09 g/mol. Choices A, B, and C are incorrect because according to the atomic mass units and the correct number of atoms of each element, the molecular mass of H_2SO_4 is 98.09 g/mol.

10. **The correct answer is A.** Oxacids are those that contain oxygen, hydrogen, and another element (sulfuric acid, H_2SO_4; nitric acid, HNO_3; carbonic acid H_2CO_3). Choice B is incorrect because oxacids contain oxygen atoms. Choices C and D are incorrect because oxacids contain carbon, oxygen, hydrogen, and another element.

11. **The correct answer is B.** A buffer is a chemical solution of a weak acid or base and its salt. The buffer solution has the ability to resist changes in pH when small amounts of an acid or a base are added. Buffers play an important role in maintaining proper pH levels, especially in biological systems. Choice A is incorrect because a buffer does not change when small amounts of acid and base are added to the solution. Choice C is incorrect because a buffer solution contains a chemical solution of a weak acid or base and its salt. Choice D is incorrect because a buffer solution contains a weak acid or base and its salt.

12. **The correct answer is B.** Using the ideal gas law, $V_A = \dfrac{n_A R T_A}{P_A}$ and $V_B = \dfrac{n_B R T_B}{P_B}$.

Therefore, the ratio of $\dfrac{V_A}{V_B} = \dfrac{\dfrac{n_A R T_A}{P_A}}{\dfrac{n_B R T_B}{P_B}}$. Since each gas is a 1 mole sample, the pressure for each gas is 1 atm, and the gas constant, R, is in both equations. This ratio can be sim-

$$f(x) = 3\cos x$$

plified into $f'(x) = -3\sin x$, which is Charles's

$$f''(x) = -3\cos x$$

law. The temperature of each gas must be converted into degrees Kelvin so that $TA = 324$ K and $TB = 300$ K. The ratio of V_A to V_B then becomes $\dfrac{324}{300}$, or 324:300. This ratio can be simplified to 27:25. Therefore, the correct answer is Choice B Choice A is incorrect because 51:27 would be the ratio of the temperature in degrees Celsius, and it is always necessary to convert temperatures into degrees Kelvin in chemistry calculations. Choices C and D are incorrect because neither is an accurate ratio.

13. **The correct answer is C.** The change in free energy, ΔG, is calculated by the equation $\Delta G = \Delta H - T\Delta S$. Therefore, for the given reaction, $\Delta G = (566 \text{ kJ/mol}) - [(298 \text{ K})(0.17 \text{ kJ/K.mol})] = 515.34 \text{ kJ/mol}$. The positive value of ΔG indicates that the reaction is nonspontaneous. Choice A is incorrect because a negative ΔG value implies that the reaction is spontaneous. Choice B is incorrect because if the value of ΔG is negative, then the reaction is spontaneous. Choice D is incorrect because the value of ΔG is positive, which implies that the reaction is nonspontaneous.

14. **The correct answer is A.** Avogadro's law states that at constant pressure and temperature, the volume of a gas is directly proportional to the number of moles of the gas. This law can be represented by the equation $V = k_4 n$, where k_4 is the proportionality constant equal to RT/P. This equation shows that under constant temperature and pressure, equal volumes of gases have an equal number of particles, $\frac{V_1}{n_1} = \frac{V_2}{n_2}$. Choice B is incorrect because Boyle's law states that the pressure of a fixed amount of gas at a constant temperature is inversely proportional to the volume of the gas. The mathematical expression of Boyle's law is $P = k_1 \times \frac{1}{V}$, where k_1 is a proportionality constant, and the temperature and number of moles of gas remain constant. The proportionality constant k_1 is equal to the product of the number of moles (n), the temperature (T) and the gas constant ($R = 8.314$ J/K·mol). Choice C is incorrect because Charles's law states that the volume, V, of a constant amount of gas maintained at a constant pressure is directly proportional to temperature of the gas, T (in degrees Kelvin). This relationship is shown in the following equation: $V = k_2 T$, where k_2 is a proportionality constant. The value of k_2 is dependent upon the number of moles of gas (n), the gas constant ($R = 8/134$ J/K·mol) and the pressure of the gas, P. Similarly to Boyle's law this equation can be used to compare two sets of volume and temperature of a gas at a constant pressure: $\frac{V_1}{T_1} = \frac{V_2}{T_2}$. Choice D is incorrect because Dalton's law of partial pressures simply states that the total pressure of a mixture of gases is equal to the sum of the pressure that would be exerted by each individual gas if it occupied the space on its own. Mathematically, Dalton's law of partial

pressures is represented by the equation $P_{\text{total}} = P_1 + P_2 + P_3 \ldots$

15. **The correct answer is B.** Molecules with a central atom that has no lone pairs adopt certain geometrical structures. Molecules with two electron pairs are linear. Those with three electron pairs form a triagonal planar structure. Molecules with four electron pairs form a tetrahedral shape. Molecules with five electron pairs in the valence shell form a triagonal bipyramid, and those with six electron pairs form an octahedral. The bond angles are such that the molecules are placed as far apart as possible. In the case of methane, the hydrogen atoms arrange themselves around the central carbon atom at 109° angles. Choice A is incorrect because placing the H atoms as far apart as possible results in the maximum bond angle of 109°. Choice C is incorrect because the four H atoms cannot distribute themselves around the C atom at angles of 120°. Choice D is incorrect because it is impossible for four hydrogen atoms to arrange themselves at 180° angles around a single carbon atom.

16. **The correct answer is A.** A mole is the amount of a substance that contains as many atoms (or molecules or particles) as there are atoms in exactly 12 grams (g) of ^{12}C. The actual number of atoms in 12 g of ^{12}C has been determined experimentally, and this value is known as Avogadro's number (N_A). The accepted value for Avogadro's number is $N_A = 6.0221367 \times 10^{23}$. In Choice A, a 1-liter solution of 1 M HCl will contain 1 mole of HCl molecules. One mole of HCl contains exactly 6.02×10^{23} molecules of HCl, or Avogadro's number. Choice B is incorrect because the number of molecules it takes to fill a 1-liter beaker depends on the type of atoms filling the beaker. Choice C is incorrect because one mole corresponds to 12 g of ^{12}C, and one mole is representative of 6.02×10^{23} molecules. Choice D is incorrect

because in the case of 1 M H_2SO_4, 6.02 × 10^{23}, molecules of oxygen would be found in 250 mL of 1 M solution because there are four oxygen atoms per mole of H_2SO_4.

17. **The correct answer is C.** In a chemical reaction, the reaction yield is a theoretical yield that represents the maximum amount of product that can result if the entire limiting reagent is used up. The actual yield in a reaction is the amount of product that is actually obtained from a chemical reaction. The actual yield is almost always less than the theoretical yield. The reasons for the difference in yield vary. In this reaction, 24 g of HCl react with an excess of sodium carbonate. 24 g of HCl is equivalent to 0.66 mol HCl. Since the stoichiometric molar ratio of HCl to CO_2 is 2:1, 0.33 mol of CO_2 can form (theoretical yield). This molar value corresponds to 14.52 g of CO_2. Since we know the actual yield is 12.71, we can calculate the percent yield by dividing the actual yield by the theoretical yield and multiplying by 100. The percent yield is 87.5%. Choice A is incorrect because this is the percent yield calculated without taking into account the stoichiometric ratio of HCl to CO_2. Choices B and D are incorrect because the calculated percent yield is 87.5%.

18. **The correct answer is D.** The formation of aluminum oxide involves oxygen and the element aluminum, Al. Therefore, the reactant side of the equation should have the two reactants, Al and O_2. Since the product is Al_2O_3, this reaction must be balanced in order to determine the chemical equation. The proper balanced equation is choice D. Choice A is incorrect because the reactants are incorrect. Choice B is incorrect because the starting substance is Al, not Al_2. Choice C is incorrect because the reactant is O_2, not O.

19. **The correct answer is C.** Molarity is

$$\frac{\text{number of moles}}{\text{liters solution}} =$$

$$\frac{\text{grams NaCL}}{\text{molecular weight of NaCL}} \times \frac{1}{100} \text{ mL}$$

that is then multiplied by 1,000 mL, which equals moles of NaCl per liter. Therefore, the molarity of the prepared NaCl solution is $\frac{26.3 \text{ g NaCl}}{58.44 \text{ g/mole NaCl}} \times \frac{1}{100} \text{ mL} \times 1,000$ mL of water is 4.5 M. The solution is then diluted further by the addition of water to a final volume of 750 mL. Therefore, the concentration in terms of molarity decreases, which is called a dilution of the original solution. The concentration in terms of molarity can be determined for the dilute solution by using the equation $M_1V_1 = M_2V_2$. Thus, the final concentration of the NaCl solution is $\frac{(4.5 \text{ M})(0.1 \text{ L})}{(0.75 \text{ L})}$, or 0.6 M. Choice A is incorrect because the concentration of the initial solution is 4.5 M, and once it is diluted, the concentration becomes 0.6 M. Choice B is incorrect because the volume of each dilution of NaCl must be converted to liters for an accurate calculation. Choice D is incorrect because the correct concentration as calculated by the equations for molarity and dilution is not 0.34 M.

20. **The correct answer is A.** A hydrocarbon compound with four carbon atoms has the prefix *but-*. The presence of a carbon-carbon double bond changes the suffix of the hydrocarbon to *-ene*. A molecule of butene has the formula $CH_3CH = CHCH_3$. Choice B is incorrect because propene has three carbon atoms and a carbon-carbon double bond. Choice C is incorrect because butane has four carbon atoms, but only carbon-carbon single bonds. Choice D is incorrect because ethane is a hydrocarbon with two carbon atoms and no double bonds.

21. **The correct answer is D.** An aldehyde is formed when at least one of the *R* groups attached to the carbon atom is an H atom. If both *R* groups are H atoms, the compound formed is formaldehyde. Choice A is incorrect because acetone is a ketone molecule with the formula $CH_3C = OCH_3$. Choice B is incorrect because a carboxylic acid contains a carbonyl group, COOH. Choice C is incorrect because methyl butyrate is an ester molecule with the formula $CH_3CH_2CH_2COOCH_3$.

22. **The correct answer is C.** The two molecules shown are mirror images of each other. They are both forms of lactic acid and behave identically in a chemical reaction. The two compounds are called enantiomers. Choice A is incorrect because achiral compounds are superimposable on each other and have planes of symmetry. Choice B is incorrect because diastereomers are stereoisomers that are not mirror images of each other. Choice D is incorrect because these two compounds are not polarized.

23. **The correct answer is A.** Adenine and guanine have double rings and are therefore purines. Choices B and C are incorrect; purines are complementary to pyrimidines, so bases that pair up on opposite DNA strands cannot both be purines. Choice D is incorrect because these are the pyrimidines of DNA.

24. **The correct answer is C.** In an S_N2 reaction, the entering nucleophile attacks the substrate (electrophile) from a position that is 180° from the leaving group on the electrophile, and the reaction takes place all in one step without any intermediates formed. In the reaction process, as the leaving group departs from the electrophile, the remaining three groups change their orientation around the carbon atom. Therefore, if the H atom on the molecule is attacked by the nucleophile, then the leaving group would be the Cl^- atom since it is positioned 180° from the nucleophilic attack. Choice A is incorrect because the nucleophile is attacking the molecule at the H group. Therefore, it is not the leaving group. Choice B is incorrect because the OH group is not positioned at a 180° angle from the nucleophilic attack. Choice D is incorrect because the CH_3 group is not positioned 180° from the nucleophilic attack.

25. **The correct answer is A.** In most cases, an enzyme called an acid catalyst is present to facilitate the dehydration reaction. The lone pair of electrons on the hydroxyl group attracts a proton from a strong acid. OH^- is a poor leaving group, but the addition of the H^+ ion transforms it into a good leaving group by eliminating the negative charge. Choice B is incorrect because the enzyme that helps in a dehydration reaction is an acid catalyst. Choice C is incorrect because an acid catalyst, not a dehydrogenase, assists in the reaction. Choice D is incorrect because there is no such enzyme as a base catalyst.

26. **The correct answer is B.** The two reactants undergo a pericyclic reaction in which a six-carbon ring containing one carbon-carbon double bond forms. The double bond in the molecules breaks and reforms two single carbon-carbon bonds and a carbon-carbon double bond. The reaction results in a cyclical product:

Choice A is incorrect because the three double bonds break to form C – C bonds and one new C = C bond, so the resulting ring structure only has one double bond. Choice C is incorrect because the reaction forms a cyclical compound, not a linear compound. Choice D is incorrect because there are only six carbon atoms in the product, not seven.

27. **The correct answer is A.** This is the basic structure of an amino acid. Choice B is incorrect because it describes a nucleotide. Choice C is incorrect because it describes a fatty acid. Choice D is incorrect because it describes a monosaccharide.

28. **The correct answer is D.** Ribozyme is the only known enzyme that is not a protein, and it is catalytic RNA. Choice A is incorrect because no carbohydrates are known to be enzymes; the same goes for choice C, which is incorrect because no lipids are known to be enzymes. Choice B is incorrect because DNA is not currently known to act as an enzyme.

29. **The correct answer is B.** Ethers are organic compounds containing the general formula R-O-R', where R is a functional group. Ethers are formed by a reaction between an alkoxide (with an OR^- ion) and an alkyl halide. The reaction in the example shows the formation of *tert*-butyl methyl ether from a *tert*-butoxide ion and idomethane. Choice A is incorrect because a carbonyl has the general formula RC = OR. Choice C is incorrect because an ester is a carbonyl, and it has the general formula RCOOR. Choice D is incorrect because all alcohols have an OH functional group.

30. **The correct answer is C.** The atomic radius is half the distance between the nuclei of two touching atoms of an element. As the nuclear charge across a period increases, the electrons are drawn closer to the nucleus, which causes a decrease in the atomic radius of elements from left to right across the period. Moving down a group adds electron shells and increases the atomic radius. Therefore, in the list of elements in the question, Li has the largest atomic radius, N the next largest, and then F. He has the smallest atomic radius in the list. Choice A is incorrect because He has the smallest atomic radius because its electrons are pulled closest to the nucleus; the other elements are in the correct order. Choice B is incorrect because the order of this list is reversed; He has the smallest atomic radius, F the next smallest, then N, and finally Li. Choice D is incorrect because F has a smaller atomic radius the N, which has a smaller atomic radius than Li.

31. **The correct answer is D.** All E1 elimination reactions occur by spontaneous dissociation of the leaving group and the loss of a proton from an intermediate carbocation. As in the case of an S_N1 reaction, the loss of the proton (breaking of a C-H bond) occurs after the rate-limiting step of the dissociation of the

leaving group. Choice A is incorrect because a carbocation intermediate forms in an E1 reaction. No intermediate is formed in an E2 reaction. Choice B is incorrect because the transition state of an E2 reaction is a very short-lived and unstable state. Choice C is incorrect because it is an E2 reaction in which a nucleophile attacks and a double bond can form in the same step. This is because there is no intermediate in an E2 reaction.

32. **The correct answer is D.** Physicists were puzzled by Bohr's theory, and they questioned why the energies of a hydrogen electron would be quantized. Louis de Broglie reasoned that if light waves can behave like a stream of particles (photons), then perhaps particles such as electrons can behave as waves, and this helped to explain the phenomenon of quantized electron energies. Choice A is incorrect because it was understood and accepted that electrons could move from one energy orbital to another. Choice B is incorrect because de Broglie introduced the idea of electrons behaving like wave particles about 10 years after Bohr's atomic theory was proposed. Choice C is incorrect because it was well understood that the electrons orbited around the nucleus of an atom. What was puzzling was why they did so in quantized levels.

33. **The correct answer is C.** The elements in Groups 3 through 12 make up what are known as the transition elements. These elements are also called transition metals and are very hard, but malleable elements. These elements all have valence electrons in the *d* orbitals. The five *d* orbitals hold their electrons very loosely, and most of these elements are characterized by high melting points, high electrical conductivity, low ionization energies, and many oxidation states. Choice A is incorrect because the Group 1 elements are known as the alkali metals. Choice B is incorrect because the Group 2 elements on the Periodic Table are the Alkaline Earth metals. Choice D is incorrect because Group 17 elements on the Periodic Table are classified as halogens.

34. **The correct answer is B.** Hydrates are compounds that have a specific number of water molecules attached to them. These water molecules can be removed by heating the molecule. The resulting compound after heating is referred to as an anhydrous compound, meaning that the compound no longer has water molecules associated with it. A hydrate compound is written with the general formula $A \cdot X\mathrm{H_2O}$, where A is the chemical formula of a compound and X is the number of moles of water added. Therefore, the correct formula from the list shown is choice B, $\mathrm{MgSO_4 \cdot 7H_2O}$ because the prefix *hepta-* refers to seven. Choice A is incorrect because the water molecules are written separately from the chemical formula of the compound. The water molecules can easily be removed by heating the molecule without changing the chemical composition of the rest of the compound. Choice C is incorrect because *hepta-* refers to seven water molecules, not six. Choice D is incorrect because the water molecules are written separately from the rest of the molecule, and heptahydrate refers to seven water molecules.

35. **The correct answer is C.** Bond length is defined as the distance between the two nuclei of covalently bound atoms in a molecule. Multiple bonds are shorter than single bonds because the atoms are more strongly pulled toward one another. Triple bonds are shorter than double bonds, which are shorter than single bonds. Since butyne contains a triple bond, it is the molecule with the shortest bond length. Choice A is incorrect because a butane molecule contains only single carbon-carbon bonds. Choice B is incorrect because although this compound butane contains a double carbon-carbon bond, a triple bond is shorter than a double bond. Choice D is incorrect because ethane contains only a single carbon-carbon bond.

36. **The correct answer is C.** For the general reaction $aA + bB \rightarrow cC + dD$, the rate law is expressed by the equation rate = $k[A]^x[B]^y$, where the exponents of each reactant concentration correspond to the order of the reaction with respect to each reactant. Reaction order enables us to understand how the reaction is dependent on the concentration of a given reactant. In this reaction, the reaction is zero order for A, which means it is independent of the concentration of A and second order for B. The overall reaction order is the sum of the reaction order of each reactant, or $0 + 2 = 2$. Therefore, the overall reaction is second order. Choice A is incorrect because although the reaction order is zero order for A, the overall reaction order is 2. Choice B is incorrect because the reaction order is 2. Choice D is incorrect because the overall reaction order is $0 + 2$, or 2.

37. **The correct answer is A.** In addition to forming single and double bonds, carbon can also form triple bonds. In order to form a triple bond, carbon forms a third type of hybridization orbital called an sp hybrid. In an sp hybrid orbital, two of the p orbitals are used to form a triple bond between two carbon atoms ($C \equiv C$). The remaining p orbital hybridizes with the s orbital forming two sp hybrid orbitals. If the sp hybrid orbitals are close enough, they overlap head to head to form an sp-sp σ bond. The p_z and p_y orbitals overlap to form a p_z-p_z and p_y-p_y π bond. The σ and two π bonds form the carbon triple bond. The p_x and s orbitals form a hybrid orbital that has a straight 180° angle, giving a linear structure to the molecule. Choice B is incorrect because the sp^2 hybridized orbitals orient themselves in a triagonal shape. Choice C is incorrect because the sp^3 hybridized orbitals arrange themselves in a tetrahedral shape. Choice D is incorrect because a p orbital is not a hybridized electron orbital.

38. **The correct answer is C.** Alkenes are hydrocarbons that contain at least one carbon-carbon double bond. The general molecular formula for alkenes is C_nH_{2n}. The molecule shown has a carbon-carbon double bond, and, therefore, it is an alkene. Choice A is incorrect because an alkane only has carbon-carbon single bond. Choice B is incorrect because an alkyne molecule contains at least one carbon-carbon triple bond. Choice D is incorrect because an aromatic has a benzene ring as the parent compound. A benzene ring is a six-ring compound containing alternating single and double bonds.

39. **The correct answer is C.** Viscosity is the measure of a liquid's resistance to flow (fluidity). The greater the viscosity of a liquid, the more slowly it will flow. In general, the viscosity of a liquid increases with decreasing temperature. Liquids that have strong intermolecular forces have a higher viscosity than those that have weak intermolecular forces. Choice A is incorrect because the fluidity of a liquid will increase with increasing temperature. This is because there is an increase in the kinetic energy of the liquid molecules at higher temperatures such that they move past one another more frequently and faster. Choice B is incorrect because as temperature decreases, the viscosity increases. Choice D is incorrect because temperature does influence the viscosity of a liquid.

40. **The correct answer is C.** Ionic bonds typically form between a meta (cation) and a nonmetal (anion) ion. Covalent bonds form between molecules regardless of their properties. Most bonds between carbon and another element are covalent bonds. Therefore, the molecule CH_2O, formaldehyde, is held together by covalent bonds. Choice A is incorrect because the metal ion lithium forms an ionic bond with Cl. Choice B is incorrect because the metal ion Mg forms an ionic bond with O. Choice D

is incorrect because the metal atom boron forms ionic bonds with oxygen.

41. **The correct answer is C.** The described reaction is a condensation reaction, or dehydration synthesis, so water is produced during the reaction. Three ester bonds form, one between glycerol and each of the three fatty acids. Choice A is incorrect because even though an ester bond forms, an ester group is not released in the process. Choice B is incorrect because these are typical products of a combustion reaction of a hydrocarbon. Choice D is incorrect; hydrocarbon chains are added to a glycerol, not released as a byproduct.

42. **The correct answer is A.** mRNA enters the ribosome at A, moves through P, and finally passes through E. tRNA enters the ribosome and then exit in the same order. Choices B and D are incorrect because the ribosomal binding sites are listed out of order relative to one another. Choice C is incorrect because even though the sites are listed in the appropriate order relative to one another, the order is reversed with regard to mRNA interaction with the ribosome.

43. **The correct answer is A.** Translation occurs at the ribosome and produces proteins. Choice B is incorrect because this is the direct result of transcription. Choice C is incorrect because this is the direct result of reverse transcription, usually performed by reverse transcriptase of viruses. Choice D is incorrect because after translation, the tRNA dissociates from the amino acid as the amino acid is added to the growing chain, so free tRNA is directly produced during translation.

44. **The correct answer is A.** DNA polymerase adds new nucleotides to grow the copied leading strand during DNA replication. Choice B is incorrect because it describes the role of ligase during DNA replication. Choice C is incorrect because it describes

the role of primase during DNA replication. Choice D is incorrect because it describes the role of RNA polymerase during transcription.

45. **The correct answer is B.** Alpha helices and beta sheets are localized structures that are the main components of secondary structure. Choice A is incorrect because it refers to the amino acid sequence. Choice C is incorrect because it refers to the overall 3D structure of the protein. Choice D is incorrect because it refers to a complex of multiple polypeptide chains coming together to form a protein.

46. **The correct answer is B.** "Kinks" in unsaturated fatty acids are caused by double bonds in the hydrocarbon chains. Choice A is incorrect because oxygens are not present in hydrocarbon chains, and they would not cause these "kinks." Choice C is incorrect because methylation should not cause "kinks" in the backbone of the chain. Choice D is incorrect because dispersion forces are weak and would not cause "kinks" in the backbone of the chain.

47. **The correct answer is A.** NADPH is used as an energy source to polymerize fatty acid chains during fatty acid synthesis. Choices B, C, and D are incorrect because these molecules do not play this role.

48. **The correct answer is B.** When the atoms combine, a pair of molecular orbitals forms. One molecular orbital is lower in energy than the original atomic orbital, and the other is higher in energy than the original atomic orbitals. The two electrons from an atom occupy the bonding molecular orbital (lowest energy state), and the antibonding molecular orbital remains unoccupied. Choices A and C are incorrect because the antibonding orbital generally remains unoccupied. Choice D is incorrect because the lowest energy orbital is the bonding orbital and the higher energy orbital is the antibonding orbital.

Section 4: Critical Reading

1. A	11. B	21. A	31. A	41. D
2. B	12. C	22. C	32. B	42. D
3. A	13. D	23. C	33. D	43. B
4. A	14. C	24. D	34. D	44. D
5. C	15. A	25. B	35. B	45. A
6. C	16. B	26. D	36. B	46. D
7. B	17. A	27. C	37. D	47. B
8. D	18. D	28. A	38. C	48. D
9. B	19. A	29. C	39. C	
10. A	20. A	30. A	40. D	

1. **The correct answer is A.** Choice A is correct because the first sentence of the paragraph says that desensitization is for people with allergic asthma. Choice B is incorrect because the passage makes no mention of sensitive nasal passages. Choice C is incorrect because the paragraph does not mention exercise-induced asthma. Choice D is incorrect because the passage makes no connection between desensitization and peak flow meters.

2. **The correct answer is B.** Choice B is correct because the passage is not about curing asthma, but about treating it—getting relief from various forms of asthma, including exercise-induced asthma. While long-term treatments are discussed, so are quick relief and other controversial treatments. Choice A is incorrect because the passage is not about curing asthma, but treating it. Choice C should be eliminated because, while long-term treatments are discussed, so are quick relief and other controversial treatments. Choice D is incorrect because the passage is about getting relief from various forms of asthma, including exercise-induced asthma.

3. **The correct answer is A.** The main idea of the passage is treatments for asthma and paragraphs 4 and 5 are about different types of treatments. Choice B is incorrect because the fourth paragraph does not lead to the next in time or logical step order. Choice C is incorrect because both paragraphs present main ideas and details, not causes and effects. Choice D is incorrect because both paragraphs present main ideas and details, not problems and solutions.

4. **The correct answer is A.** Choice A is correct because the passage makes clear that sufferers with repeated moderate-to-severe attacks do not rely on quick relief options. Choice B is incorrect because the passage discusses these treatments, but does not suggest their use. Choice C is incorrect because the passage makes it clear that such a remedy is unproven. Choice D is incorrect because, while those with allergic asthma may benefit from specific immunotherapy, others will not.

5. **The correct answer is C.** The author makes his or her rather negative attitude toward leukotriene modifiers known by both subtle (placing the term *treatment* in quotation marks to indicate that they should not really

be considered a treatment) and explicit (stating that they should be "avoided at all costs") means. Choice A implies an attitude about leukotriene modifiers because of the word *controversy*, yet the word is used to reflect a general attitude about leukotriene modifiers rather than the author's personal attitude. Choice B explains the controversy without indicating anyone's attitude about anything. Choice D moves on to a completely different topic from leukotriene modifiers.

6. **The correct answer is C.** In paragraph 3, the author explains some proven benefits of treating asthma with inhaled corticosteroids (it prevents swelling of the airways and has few side effects) but indicates that pranayama only helps the sufferer to relax in paragraph 5, so there is reasonable support for the conclusion in choice C. The author provides virtually no details about using ginko extract as a treatment for asthma, so there is no support for the conclusion in choice A. The author describes more than one treatment that may provide some relief to the asthma sufferer, which contradicts the conclusion in choice B. Avoiding triggers may help the asthma sufferer from having attacks, but choice D reaches an extreme conclusion never suggested in the passage.

7. **The correct answer is B.** The author categorizes Omega-3 fatty acids as a "dubious" treatment, which supports the conclusion in choice B. Choice A is similarly negative, but it is too negative; *dubious* implies skepticism rather than the belief that something is anything as extreme as ridiculous. The author's use of the term *dubious* contradicts the conclusion in choice C. Like choice C, choice D is too extreme. The author merely implies that Omega-3 fatty acids are not effective treatments for asthma; she or he does not imply they are actually damaging to one's health.

8. **The correct answer is D.** Choice D is correct because the passage mainly notes options for those with frequent, moderate to severe attacks. Therefore, it stands to reason that quick-relief options may be enough for those with infrequent, mild attacks. Choices A and B must be ruled out because the passage says bronchodilators should be used before exercise. Choice C is incorrect because the passage does not discuss the method of administration.

9. **The correct answer is B.** Choice B is correct because the last sentence of paragraph 4 uses *reference drug* in the same way that the previous sentence uses *pioneer drug*. Choice A is incorrect because the pioneer drug comes before the generic drug and forms the standard on which the generic drug is based. Choice C is incorrect. The passage does not mention off-patent drugs. Choice D is incorrect because the passage does not mention managed care drugs, nor is the concept an entirely logical one.

10. **The correct answer is A.** Choice A is the correct answer because the word *bioequivalence* suggests "same life" or same effects on life. For that to be the case, of all the answers, the same active ingredient and effect is most logical. Choice B must be ruled out because the passage offers no details about dosage rate. Choice C is not correct because bioequivalence suggests something well beyond mere manufacturing processes. Choice D is incorrect because the important equivalent elements are the active ingredient and effect, not the coloring, flavoring, and fillers.

11. **The correct answer is B.** Choice B is correct because the passage states this fact directly in paragraph 2. Choices A, C, and D are incorrect because the passage directly states something to the contrary in paragraph 2.

12. **The correct answer is C.** Choice C is correct because the passage states, at the

end of paragraph 2, that "between 1962 and 1984, the FDA approved only sixteen generic drugs." Choices A, B, and D are incorrect because the passage states, at the end of paragraph 2, that "between 1962 and 1984, the FDA approved only sixteen generic drugs."

13. **The correct answer is D.** Choice D is correct because the author is not stating a fact or any information that the reader can verify. Choice A is incorrect: this is a statement of fact. Choice B is tempting and might be considered to have elements of an opinion, but there is a better choice. Despite the connotative language in this choice, terms and phrases such as "floodgates opened" can actually be backed up by fact. Choice C should be eliminated; it marshals only facts.

14. **The correct answer is C.** The author ends the passage with a very positive statement related to passage of the Hatch-Waxman Act, describing it as welcome, after describing all of the savings it has stimulated. Choice C is the best answer. Choices A and B are somewhat extreme interpretations of the concluding statement of the passage, and extreme statements should generally be avoided if they lack specific passage support, as these statements do. Since the author's concluding statement applies to generic drugs without any implications about branded drugs, choice D is not the most logical answer.

15. **The correct answer is A.** Choice A is the correct answer because Reagan's words are full of positives, such as "best medicine" and "economy" (in the sense of careful expenditure and saving money); the word *best* is used twice. Choice B must be ruled out because Reagan is not the least bit ambivalent; he clearly sees the change as auguring benefits. Choice C is not correct because Reagan is the opposite of disapproving,

rather he praises the change. Choice D is incorrect because Reagan is not objective at all; he clearly sees the change as extremely beneficial.

16. **The correct answer is B.** Choice B is the correct answer because, while the reader must infer the answer, the paragraph states the intent of protecting brand name drugs. Choice A should be ruled out because the paragraph does not state or imply this; in the absence of direct evidence, one must assume the National Formulary did something less radical to protect brand name drugs. Choice C is incorrect because it is illogical. The paragraph states the intent of protecting brand name drugs, thus ruling out this choice. Choice D is incorrect because the paragraph does not state or imply this; in the absence of direct evidence, one must assume the National Formulary did something less radical to protect brand name drugs.

17. **The correct answer is A.** Choice A is correct because the last sentence says that Lavoisier called the vital air oxygen; it seems likely that the term *oxidation* followed for naming processes involving oxygen. Choice B is incorrect because the last sentence says that Lavoisier called the vital air oxygen; this occurred as a result of his proving that it was not phlogiston that was liberated in the process of burning. Choice C should be eliminated because the reverse is nearly true: understanding oxygen, and therefore, most likely oxidation, was a result of debunking the phlogiston theory. Choice D is incorrect; nothing in the passage could be said to support or imply this idea.

18. **The correct answer is D.** Choice D is correct because the writer states this fact about combustion in paragraph 1. The second and third paragraphs name the other processes: respiration and calcination. Choices A, B, and C are incorrect. The passage gives details

to the contrary for each item; also, none of these answers make sense.

19. **The correct answer is A.** In paragraph 3, the author describes the understanding that heated metal leaves a residue called calx. This was a turning point in Lavoisier's oxygen theories but does not explain why. Such information would certainly help support the main idea, so choice A is the best answer. Choice B is incorrect because an example of a process not understood before the phlogiston theory (respiration) is given in paragraph 2. Choice C would not be irrelevant in this passage, but it would not do very much to support the main idea of the passage. Choice D is incorrect because the answers to the questions in paragraph 2 are answered in parenthetical statements.

20. **The correct answer is A.** The author supports the overall thesis with descriptions of experiments, so choice A is the best answer. There is nothing particularly emotional about this informative passage, so choice B does not make much sense. The author never tries to appeal to the reader's sense of right and wrong, so choice C is not correct. The author never includes any anecdotes about his or her own experiences either, so choice D is wrong.

21. **The correct answer is A.** Choice A is correct because the passage states that the word *phlogiston* comes from a Greek word for "flame." For this reason, choice B can be ruled out. Choice C should be eliminated because earlier information in the passage about combustible earth is not related to the etymology of *phlogiston*. Choice D, while tempting, is incorrect. The etymology is, in fact, related to flame, but nothing suggests a descriptive component in the word's history.

22. **The correct answer is C.** Choice C is correct because the questions and their answers show that the theory did logically explain common

phenomena. Choice A should be ruled out because there is a better choice. Also, the passage makes clear that those who accepted the phlogiston theory did not understand the main components of air. Choice B is incorrect because the questions and their answers do show that the theory did logically explain common phenomena. Choice D is tempting but incorrect; it could be correct, but the passage contains no information to verify that.

23. **The correct answer is C.** Choice C is correct because paragraph 3 explains that the phlogiston theory was illogical in relation to the process of calcination. Choice A must be ruled out because it does not make sense; respiration does not leave behind a residue. Choice B is not correct; calcination is not vital to life. Choice D is incorrect because nothing in the passage suggests this process is so.

24. **The correct answer is D.** Choice D is correct because the topic of the passage is stated in the second sentence; the entire passage is devoted to how Lavoisier debunked the theory, which had found support because there was much logic to it, but, at the same time, an observable illogic in the process of calcination. Choice A is incorrect. The topic of the passage is stated in the second sentence: through disproving the phlogiston theory, Lavoisier identified vital air, or oxygen. Choice B is incorrect. Lavoisier did not identify the nature of suffocating air, as the last paragraph makes clear. Choice C is a cautionary tale in reading all the answer choices carefully and completely. Indeed, Lavoisier did identify the nature of vital air, as the last paragraph explains. Nevertheless, the topic of the passage is stated in the second sentence, and the passage is devoted to developing that topic.

25. The correct answer is B. Choice B is correct; this is directly stated in paragraph 2. Choice A must be ruled out because the passage says that transposons can block transcription, not that they can perform it. Choice C is not correct because the passage says that transposons can block transcription, not that they can enable it. Choice D is incorrect because the passage does not make the claim that transposons can copy a DNA template.

26. The correct answer is D. Choice D is the best answer because the passage is generally about jumping genes, how they were discovered, what they do, and what their implications are. Choice A is incorrect because the passage focuses on Barbara McClintock's work for only two of its five paragraphs. Choice B is incorrect because the passage is not about ears of corn, even if it mentions the variegated kernels on an ear of corn in order to explain a concept. Choice C is tempting, but there is actually very little indeed about transcription in the passage, so this title does not adequately reflect the main idea of the passage.

27. The correct answer is C. Choice C is correct because sentence 3 states the problem of nonconformance; sentence 4 specifies "a nonconforming ratio of corn kernel colors." Choice A is incorrect because the two sentences do not offer a contrast. Choice B should be eliminated because the sentences are not about two separate discoveries, but rather about specifying the nature of a scientific problem. Choice D should be ruled out. This is an expository, not persuasive, passage; it does not make a claim.

28. The correct answer is A. Choice A is correct because the author states an opinion about the possibilities for the understanding of jumping genes. Choices B, C, and D must be eliminated because each states a fact.

29. The correct answer is C. Choice C is correct because the roots do, in this case, illuminate the word's meaning. Choice A is incorrect. The terms *transposon* and *jumping genes* are more contrasted than compared. Choice B is incorrect. The terms *transposon* and *jumping genes* are contrasted, but not specifically by means of the etymology of *transposon*. Choice D is incorrect because the etymology does not really provide background information; furthermore, there is a better answer choice.

30. The correct answer is A. Choice A is the correct answer because the passage clearly states that this phenomenon led to McClintock's hypothesis. Choices B, C, and D must be ruled out because the passage suggests a different link between the nonconforming colors and McClintock's work than any of these offer.

31. The correct answer is A. Choice A is the correct answer because the final paragraph does substantiate claims about the implications of the discovery of transposons. Choice B is a good answer, and very enticing, but not the best one. Paragraph 2 has already fulfilled some of this purpose, and the final paragraph provides more detail in service of a larger conclusion, which is the significance of the discovery of jumping genes. That same idea appears at the end of paragraph 1. Choice C is tempting, but the final paragraph has a larger purpose, which is to validate the idea proposed in paragraph 1 that transposons have enormous significance. Choice D must be ruled out because the final paragraph does not second-guess McClintock or criticize her in hindsight.

32. The correct answer is B. Choice B is correct because the author directly states both parts of this explanation in different parts of the passage. The author makes it clear that the regulation of genes, and not just the jumping, is what makes jumping genes significant. Choice A is tempting; *jumping gene* is indeed a synonym for *transposon*. Nevertheless, there is a better explanation among the choices. Choice C is somewhat correct, but it rather overstates the point that transposons are crucial (they are not the entire key) to our understanding of multicellular organisms. Choice D must be ruled out; the author does suggest that transposons are a basis for evolutionary changes, but choice B offers a better explanation of what a transposon is.

33. **The correct answer is D.** Choice D is correct because the author shows optimism in the first paragraph with the phrase "early enough to cure," as well as in the act of calling his or her own aunt and uncle and feeling as if the test were a "chance of a lifetime for them." The author also takes long odds and views them with a lottery-player's eyes by emphasizing the one who "wins," not the 300 plus who lose. Choices A and B must be ruled out because, while the author is clearly concerned about lung cancer, he or she greets the central topic, the new screening method, with enthusiasm and action. They are also incorrect because, while the author is clearly concerned or even alarmed about lung cancer and its deadly statistics, he or she greets the central topic, the new screening method, with enthusiasm and action. Choice C is incorrect because the author is not skeptical at all. Instead, the author also views the long odds with a lottery-player's eyes by emphasizing the one who "wins," not the 300 plus who lose.

34. **The correct answer is D.** Choice D is the best answer because it shows the author's personal involvement. Not only does he or she like the information, but takes action based on it. Choice A is not the best answer because even though it shows an attitude (that the study was not frivolous), there is an answer choice that shows an even more

personal and serious response to what was read. Choice B is incorrect because, despite the use of the word *dramatically*, it does not really reflect the author's attitude, and there is a far better answer. Choice C is not correct because it simply recounts the data without reflecting the author's attitude.

35. **The correct answer is B.** Choice B is the correct answer because the profile consists of data such as age and smoking history. Choices A, C, and D must be ruled out because there is no context to support any of these answers.

36. **The correct answer is B.** Choice B is correct because the author is optimistic about the new screening option, but this statement shows a good reason not to be so optimistic: the American Cancer Society does not yet recommend it. Choice A should be ruled out because this statement provides support for the author's optimism: the screening reveals tumors at a stage when cancer is curable. Choice C should be ruled out because, while it does not provide much support for the author's optimism, choice B provides even less support. Choice D should be ruled out because this statement provides support for the author's optimism: the screening detects information that can save lives.

37. **The correct answer is D.** Choice D is correct because the passage says that chest X-rays have no known effect on death rate. Choice A should be eliminated; the passage neither states nor implies that lung cancer progresses rapidly. Choice B is incorrect: the final paragraph suggests much the opposite. Choice C must be eliminated because the passage says that X-rays do detect cancers.

38. **The correct answer is C.** Choice C is correct because the phrase "chance of a lifetime" and the context in which it appears best reveal the author's optimism and enthusiasm, as well as, perhaps, some naiveté. Choice A is incorrect;

while *frivolous* is full of connotations, its use appears in the phrase "not frivolous." The author uses the word to validate the importance of the study she or he cites. Choice B is a worthy choice, because *promising* shows the author's positive attitude, but there is a better choice that shows the author's rather irrational enthusiasm. Choice D should be eliminated because, while the phrase "for good reason" does reflect the author's attitude, its use is less justified— borne out by the passage facts—than choice C.

39. **The correct answer is C.** Not everyone may find the same things to be illuminating, so choice C is a reflection of the author's personal opinion rather than an indisputable fact. Choices A and B are used to reflect a fact in paragraph 4—the specific requirements to participate in the study—rather than the author's personal opinions. While what is or isn't similar could be a matter of opinion, the author includes details indicating the indisputable similarity of the populations in question, so choice D is not the best answer.

40. **The correct answer is D.** Scientific studies are generally used to lend reliable credibility to a piece of writing, so choice D is a strong answer. A tendency to read a particular magazine, even if it is a science-related one, is not really a mark of credibility, so choice A is not the best answer. Merely referring to a particular group is not as convincing as referring to the findings of a scientific study, so choice B is another weak answer. Choice C is also weak since the author does not even mention whether or not the aunt and uncle participated in the screening; this is a minor aside rather than a credible supporting detail.

41. **The correct answer is D.** Choice D is the correct answer; the passage does explain the asteroid by giving details about its speed, size, and orbit; it does detail some scientific

response to it by including JPL statements and information about the telescope viewing; and it does suggest that the probable effect will be increased information. Choice A should be ruled out even though paragraph 1 does sound an exaggerated alarm; the rest of the passage does not follow along the same interest-grabbing and hyperbolic path. Choice B is incorrect because only paragraph 1 details possible physical damage, and the final paragraph repudiates that. Choice C is incorrect because most people could not see this event, which was not visible to the naked eye; furthermore, most of the information is expository in nature.

42. **The correct answer is D.** Choice D is the best answer because the paragraph is primarily about NASA's JPL and its assessment of the risk posed by 2005 YU55. This could be said to be the main idea, which all the other details in the paragraph support or lead up to. Choice A is incorrect because no real problem, and especially no solution, is presented. Choice B should be eliminated because, while there is some reference to time, there is no arrangement by chronology. Choice C is not correct; the paragraph is primarily about NASA's JPL and its assessment of the risk posed by 2005 YU55, which is neither a cause nor an effect.

43. **The correct answer is B.** Choice B is correct because the width of 2005 YU55 clearly categorizes it as relatively small; therefore, it is unlikely indeed to result in or cause annihilation, or, put another way, of all the factors cited, this seems least threatening. Choice A must be ruled out. The crossing of orbits suggests the reason 2005 YU55 can come so dangerously close to Earth. Choice C is incorrect because this statement generally supports the author's claim. Choice D is incorrect because an asteroid at closer range than Earth's own moon does suggest something to worry about.

44. **The correct answer is D.** Choice D is correct because it most accurately describes what the author does through the insertion of the word *only* in his description of the interval. In that way, the author makes the information more threatening than JPL does. Choice A is incorrect because the opposite is true; the author plays up the idea of potential peril. Choice B is incorrect because the author does not recreate the data or its meaning, but rather puts a more threatening spin on it. Choice C is incorrect because the author does not reinterpret the several-hundred-years interval; rather, the author chooses to make that interval sound threatening through the insertion of the word *only*.

45. **The correct answer is A.** Choice A is the correct answer because this information is stated in the final paragraph. Choice B is incorrect. Nowhere does the passage claim that the asteroid will crater the land, even if it does allude to what is probably the most fantastic cratering of all time. Choice C should be eliminated. Nowhere does the passage claim that the asteroid will cause species extinction, even if it does allude to a past mass extinction. Choice D is incorrect because the last paragraph clearly states that the asteroid had no effect on tides.

46. **The correct answer is D.** The glowing term *illustrious* reveals a very strong preference for the scientists at NASA, so choice D is the best answer. *Bothered* could be used to indicate a bias, but it does not perform that particular function as it is used in the context of paragraph 1. The word *perilously* may be used to indicate the author's opinion in paragraph 1, but it does not really reveal a bias, so choice B is not the best answer. The word *largest* is used objectively in paragraph 2 to indicate the fact that there are indisputably bigger asteroids than 2005 YU55, so it indicates no bias on the part of the author.

47. **The correct answer is B.** Choice B is correct because the first paragraph wildly exaggerates the asteroid's potential danger first by alluding to annihilation and second by suggesting a comparison with the impact that led to the extinction of the dinosaurs. The remainder of the paragraphs are much more reasonable and logical and less like television news in content and tone. Choice A should be ruled out because the first paragraph is accurate insofar as the facts reported. Choices C and D are incorrect because most information in paragraph 1, such as the small amount of attention received, the speed, the distance, and the statement about closeness to Earth, are all verifiable.

48. **The correct answer is D.** Choice D is correct because the final paragraph, as well as the first sentence of paragraph 3, makes this clear. Choice A must be ruled out because the answer is improbable. After all, JPL could predict the approach of the asteroid and knew its speed and size. Choice B is also improbable because there are many far larger asteroids. In addition, nothing in the passage actually suggests that this asteroid is of more interest than other asteroids. Choice C should be eliminated because the passage's facts do not imply anything about this asteroid being the largest threat to the planet; furthermore, the existence of many asteroids more than twice as large as 2005 YU55 seems to suggest otherwise.

Section 5: Quantitative Reasoning

1. B	11. D	21. D	31. B	40. D
2. D	12. A	22. C	32. A	41. B
3. C	13. A	23. C	33. C	42. A
4. D	14. C	24. C	34. D	43. D
5. B	15. A	25. D	35. B	44. B
6. C	16. B	26. D	36. A	45. D
7. C	17. B	27. C	37. A	46. D
8. D	18. C	28. D	38. D	47. D
9. A	19. B	29. A	39. A	48. A
10. A	20. D	30. D		

1. **The correct answer is B.** Twenty percent of the starting price of $30 is $6, so at closing on April 20, the stock's price was $30 + $6 = $36. Ten percent of $36 is $3.6, so at closing on April 21 the stock's price was $36 − $3.6 = $32.40.

2. **The correct answer is D.** First, determine the number of plates: $\frac{\$1,430}{\$22} = 65$. So, the new cost per plate using the goal profit of $2,080 is $\frac{\$2,080}{65} = \$32$. Thus, the percent increase in cost per plate is $\frac{32-22}{22} \times 100\% = \frac{10}{22} \times 100\% = 45\%$.

3. **The correct answer is C.** $(A \circ r)(t) = A(r(t)) = \pi(r(t))^2$. Since $r(t)$ is the radius of the outermost ripple t seconds after the rock hits the pond, this function represents the area of that ripple at time t.

4. **The correct answer is D.** First, simplify the denominator by changing 1 into the fraction $\frac{5}{5}$ and adding it to $\frac{2}{5}$. Then simplify the complex fraction by multiplying the numerator by the reciprocal of the denominator:

$$\frac{\frac{1}{3}}{\frac{2}{5}+1} = \frac{\frac{1}{3}}{\frac{2}{5}+\frac{5}{5}} = \frac{\frac{1}{3}}{\frac{7}{5}} = \frac{1}{3} \times \frac{5}{7} = \frac{5}{21}$$

5. **The correct answer is B.** Let x be the contestant's score on the fifth challenge. If she is to qualify for the next round, the average of her five scores must satisfy the following equation:

$$\frac{13+18+9+15+x}{5} \geq 15$$
$$\frac{55+x}{5} \geq 15$$
$$55+x \geq 75$$
$$x \geq 20$$

Alternatively, you can work backwards from the answer choices, calculating the average of 13, 18, 9, 15, and a particular answer choice. Choice D is unlikely to be the right answer because, based on the four scores the contestant has received so far, it looks like she needs a score higher than 15 in order to achieve an average of 15. Try choice C: the average of the contestant's four scores and 18 is 14.6, which is too low. Move on to choice B: the average of the contestant's four scores and 20 is 15, which is exactly what she needs.

6. **The correct answer is C.** David bought 3 cans of soda at s cents each, so he spent $3s$ cents on soda. He also bought 4 sticks of gum at g cents each, so he spent $4g$ cents on gum. Together, he spent $3s + 4g$ cents.

7. **The correct answer is C.** There are two cases to consider: One that it rains and the game takes place, and the other, that it does not rain and the game takes place. These two cases are mutually exclusive, since it cannot rain and not rain at the same time. Thus, you should add their probabilities in order to find the overall probability that the game will take place.

   $P = P\,(\text{rain+game}) + P\,(\text{no rain+game})$

   $= (80\%)(40\%) + (20\%) \times 1$

   $= 0.8 \times 0.4 + 0.2$

   $= 0.32 + 0.2$

   $= 0.52$

8. **The correct answer is D.** Subtracting f from g, you get: $(g - f)\,(x) = \log_5 x - 3x$. When $x = 25$, this becomes: $(g - f)\,(25) = \log_5 25 - 3 \times 25 = 2 - 75 = -73$.

9. **The correct answer is A.** Recall that the limit of a quotient of two polynomials as the variable approaches ∞ (or $-\infty$) equals the limit of the quotient of the highest degree terms in each polynomial. In this case:

   $$\lim_{x \to -\infty} \left(\frac{1 - x^3}{x + 2} \right) = \lim_{x \to -\infty} \left(\frac{-x^3}{x} \right)$$

   $$= \lim_{x \to -\infty} \left(-x^2 \right)$$

   $$= -\left(-\infty \right)^2$$

   $$= -\infty$$

   If you did not remember this fact, then you could factor x out of both numerator and denominator and simplify:

   $$\lim_{x \to -\infty} \left(\frac{1 - x^3}{x + 2} \right) = \lim_{x \to -\infty} \left(\frac{x\left(\frac{1}{x} - x^2 \right)}{x\left(1 + \frac{2}{x} \right)} \right)$$

   $$= \lim_{x \to -\infty} \left(\frac{\frac{1}{x} - x^2}{1 + \frac{2}{x}} \right)$$

   $$= \frac{0 - \left(-\infty \right)^2}{1 + 0}$$

   $$= \frac{0 - \infty}{1 + 0}$$

   $$= -\infty$$

10. **The correct answer is A.** One meter equals 100 centimeters. Therefore, the bed is 200 centimeters long and 150 centimeters wide. Multiply these two dimensions to find the surface area: $200 \times 150 = 30{,}000$ squared centimeters.

11. **The correct answer is D.** The interquartile range, which contains the middle 50% of the data, is shown by the rectangular box. The figure shows this to be the same for the two data sets. The median (marked by the vertical line inside the box) and the range (marked by the distance between the left and right endpoints of the "whiskers" of the plot) are different for the two data sets. As for the averages, this plot does not tell you anything about them, so you cannot draw any conclusions.

12. **The correct answer is A.** Since 1 yard = 3 feet, it follows that 1 cubic yard = 3^3 = 27 cubic feet. Using this with the fact that 1 minute = 60 seconds, convert the units as follows:

$$\frac{20,000 \text{ cubic feet}}{1 \text{ minute}} \times \frac{1 \text{ cubic yard}}{27 \text{ cubic feet}} \times$$

$$\frac{1 \text{ minute}}{60 \text{ seconds}} = \frac{20,000}{27 \times 60}$$

cubic yards per second

13. **The correct answer is A.** Let x be the number of collared shirts. Then, the number of t-shirts is $43 - x$. The amount earned by selling x collared shirts is $18x$ dollars, and the amount earned by selling $43 - x$ t-shirts is $10(43 - x)$ dollars. The sum of these two amounts must be $566. This gives the equation $10(43 - x) + 18x = 566$. Solve for x, as follows:

$$10(43 - x) + 18x = 566$$

$$430 - 10x + 18x = 566$$

$$8x = 136$$

$$x = 17$$

So, the owner sold 17 collared shirts.

14. **The correct answer is C.** Solve the equation $50 = \dfrac{350}{1 + 80e^{-0.2t}}$ for t:

$$50 = \frac{350}{1 + 80e^{-0.2t}}$$

$$50 + 4,000\,e^{-0.2t} = 350$$

$$4,000\,e^{-0.2t} = 300$$

$$e^{-0.2t} = \frac{300}{4,000}$$

$$-0.2t = \ln\left(\frac{3}{40}\right)$$

$$t = -\frac{1}{0.2}\ln\left(\frac{3}{40}\right)$$

$$t = -5\ln\left(\frac{3}{40}\right)$$

Using the log properties enables us to further simplify this as

$$t = -5\ln\left(\frac{3}{40}\right) = \ln\left(\frac{3}{40}\right)^{-5} = \ln\left(\frac{40}{3}\right)^{5}$$

years.

15. **The correct answer is A.** The total number of votes cast is 5,290 + 7,406 = 12,696. Now, compute the percentage of votes each candidate received:

$$\frac{5,290}{12,696} \times 100\% \approx 41.7\%$$

$$\frac{7,406}{12,696} \times 100\% \approx 58.3\%$$

So, the difference between these percentages is 58.3% − 41.7% = 16.6%.

16. **The correct answer is B.** Find the function's derivative: $f'(x) = x^2 - 6x + 5 = (x - 5)(x - 1)$. The function is increasing when $f'(x) > 0$, that is, when $(x - 5)$ and $(x - 1)$ have the same sign:

	$x < 1$	$1 < x < 5$	$x > 5$
$(x - 1)$	Negative	Positive	Positive
$(x - 5)$	Negative	Negative	Positive
$(x - 1)(x - 5)$	**Positive**	Negative	**Positive**

So, $f(x)$ is increasing when x is smaller than 1 or greater than 5.

17. **The correct answer is B.** For every (3 + 2) ounces of whiskey and soda, 3 ounces are whiskey. The question is asking you to find how many ounces of whiskey there are when the total of whiskey and soda together is 30 ounces. Set up and solve the following proportion:

$$\frac{3}{3 + 2} = \frac{x}{30}$$

$$\frac{3}{5} = \frac{x}{30}$$

$$3 \times 30 = 5x$$

$$x = 18$$

18. **The correct answer is C.** During the seven-year period from 2003 to 2009, including 2003 and 2009, the tennis player won 5 + 6 + 7 + 6 + 8 + 7 + 4 matches—that is, 43 of them. So, on average, he won $\frac{43}{7}$, or 6.1 (rounded to the nearest tenth), matches.

19. **The correct answer is B.** Let x be the speed of plane 1. Then, the speed of plane 2 is $x + 75$. Each of the planes travels for 4 hours. Using the formula *distance = rate × time* yields the distances traveled by each plane: plane 1 travels $4x$ miles and plane 2 travels $4(x + 75)$ miles. The sum of these distances is 1,800. This gives the equation $4x + 4(x + 75) = 1,800$. Solve for x, as follows:

$4x + 4(x + 75) = 1,800$

$8x + 300 = 1,800$

$8x = 1,500$

$x = 187.5$

So, the speed of plane 1 is 187.5 mph and the speed of plane 2 is 187.5 + 75 = 262.5 mph. Thus, their average is $\frac{187.5 + 262.5}{2} = 225$ mph.

20. **The correct answer is D.** Multiply the numerator by the reciprocal of the denominator in order to simplify the given fraction:

$$\frac{\frac{3}{4}}{\frac{5}{6}} = \frac{3}{4} \times \frac{6}{5} = \frac{3}{2} \times \frac{3}{5} = \frac{9}{10}$$

So, the reciprocal of this fraction is $\frac{10}{9}$.

21. **The correct answer is D.** First, sum the three times to get 45 minutes 72 seconds. Dividing by 3 yields 15 minutes 24 seconds. To convert this to seconds, use the fact that 1 minute = 60 seconds. Doing so yields 15 minutes 24 seconds = 15(60) + 24 seconds = 924 seconds.

22. **The correct answer is C.** Restrict attention to the second column since you are told that the customer bought vitamin water. This gives a total of 140 outcomes to consider. Of these, 30 bought a quinoa salad. So, the probability is $\frac{30}{140} = \frac{3}{14}$.

23. **The correct answer is C.** A "which of the following" question tells you to go straight to the answer choices. So, go down the list and test each choice. If two numbers are equal to each other, then their logarithms—in any base—are equal as well, and vice versa. Therefore, choices A and B present correct statements. Next, remember that $\log_a (xy) = \log_a x + \log_a y$. However, the statement in choice C is incorrect: it assumes, incorrectly, that $\log_a (xy) = \log_a x \times \log_a y$, using 6 and 8 as x and y, respectively. Thus, choice C is the correct answer. For the record, check choice D. Take 4 and 12 as factors of 48, and manipulate the equation in the question stem:

$$\ln 12^x = \ln 48$$
$$\ln 12^x = \ln (4 \times 12)$$
$$x \ln 12 = \ln 4 + \ln 12$$
$$x \ln 12 - \ln 12 = \ln 4$$
$$(\ln 12)(x - 1) = \ln 4$$

Choice D does, indeed, give a correct statement and is not the answer.

24. **The correct answer is C.** Sum the ten data values to get 190. Then, divide by 10 to conclude that the mean is $\frac{190}{10} = 19$.

25. The correct answer is D. Let P be the original price. If the current price of $20 is 20% less than the original price, then it is equal to 80% of the original price. Use this to set up and solve an equation:

$$20 = \frac{80}{100}P$$
$$20 = \frac{4}{5}P$$
$$20 \times \frac{5}{4} = P$$
$$P = 25$$

26. The correct answer is D. The range of a data set is the difference between the maximum and minimum values. Here, this is $87 - 21 = 66$.

27. The correct answer is C. The perimeter of a square is 4 times the length of one of its sides. Here, this is

$$4 \times \left(4\frac{7}{8}\right) = 4 \times \frac{39}{8} = \frac{39}{2} = 19\frac{1}{2}.$$

28. The correct answer is D. Differentiate twice, keeping in mind the derivatives of trigonometric functions:

$$f'(x) = 2\frac{d}{dx}(\cos x)$$
$$= -2\sin x$$

So, the second derivative is:

$$f''(x) = -2\frac{d}{dx}(\sin x)$$
$$= -2\cos x$$

29. The correct answer is A. The maximum and minimum temperatures are exactly 8 degrees higher and lower than $61°F$. The solutions of the absolute value equation $|x - a| = b$ are $x = a \pm b$. Applying that to this scenario with $a = 61$ and $b = 8$ yields the desired temperatures. So, the equation is $|x - 61| = 8$.

30. The correct answer is D. Solve the inequality $x^2 - 40x \geq 500$:

$$x^2 - 40x \geq 500$$
$$x^2 - 40x - 500 \geq 0$$
$$(x - 50)(x + 10) \geq 0$$

The left side is nonnegative when $x \leq -10$ and when $x \geq 50$. The first one does not help since x is a number of dozen, but we can conclude from the second inequality that Ellen must sell at least 50 dozen to make at least $500.

31. The correct answer is B. Find the indefinite integral; then evaluate it at π and at 0, subtracting the latter value from the former:

$$\int_0^\pi \sec^2 x \, dx = \tan x \Big|_0^\pi$$
$$= \frac{\sin x}{\cos x} \Big|_0^\pi$$
$$= \frac{\sin \pi}{\cos \pi} - \frac{\sin 0}{\cos 0}$$
$$= \frac{0}{1} - \frac{0}{1}$$
$$= 0$$

32. The correct answer is A. "Of" means multiply. Also, note that $\frac{1}{5} = 0.2$. So, you have:

$$(0.2\%)\frac{1}{5} = \frac{0.2}{100} \times \frac{1}{5} = \frac{1}{100}(0.2 \times 0.2) = \frac{0.04}{100} = 0.0004$$

33. The correct answer is C. If the average of a and b is 26, then

$$\frac{a+b}{2} = 26 \Rightarrow a + b = 52.$$

If the average of a and c is 18, then $\frac{a+c}{2} = 18 \Rightarrow a + c = 36$. In order to find what $b - c$ is, subtract this second equation from the first:

$$a + b = 52$$
$$-(a + c = 36)$$
$$b - c = 16$$

34. The correct answer is D. Solve the inequality:

$$3(2-p) < 3 - 2(2p+1)?$$
$$6 - 3p < 3 - 4p - 2$$
$$6 - 3p < 1 - 4p$$
$$6 + p < 1$$
$$p < -5$$

35. The correct answer is B. This problem is fairly simple. The inequality asks for what values of x a certain absolute value will be greater than a negative number. The answer is, for all of them! No matter what you let x be, the absolute value will be either zero or positive—thus, greater than -1. So, the solution of this inequality is all real numbers.

36. The correct answer is A. Solve for x, keeping in mind that $\ln e = 1$:

$$\ln e^7 = 1 - x$$
$$7 \ln e = 1 - x$$
$$7 = 1 - x$$
$$x = -6$$

37. The correct answer is A. Differentiate using the quotient rule:

$$\frac{d}{dw}\left(\frac{w-3}{2w+1}\right)$$
$$= \frac{\left[\frac{d}{dw}(w-3)\right](2w+1) - (w-3)\left[\frac{d}{dw}(2w+1)\right]}{(2w+1)^2}$$
$$= \frac{(2w+1) - (w-3)2}{(2w+1)^2}$$
$$= \frac{7}{(2w+1)^2}$$

When $w = 3$, $f'(3) = \dfrac{7}{(2 \times 3 + 1)^2} = \dfrac{1}{7}$.

38. The correct answer is D. Let x be the number of white roses, y the number of tulips, and z the number of long-stem red roses. Since a total of 250 flowers were purchased, it follows that $x + y + z = 250$. Also, the planner bought 35 more tulips than white roses, which means $y = x + 35$. Finally, multiplying the number of each type of flower purchased by the cost of one such flower and summing those three costs yields the equation $4.25x + 3.75y + 8.4z = 1,673.25$.

Solve the following 3×3 system:

$$\begin{cases} x + y + z = 250 \\ y = x + 35 \\ 4.25x + 3.75y + 8.40z = 1,673.25 \end{cases}$$

Substitute the expression for y given by the second equation into the first and third equations to get the following 2×2 system in x and z:

$$\begin{cases} 2x + z = 215 \\ 8x + 8.4z = 1,542 \end{cases}$$

To solve this system, solve the first equation for z and substitute that expression in for z in the second equation, and solve for x:

$$8x + 8.4(215 - 2x) = 1,542$$
$$8x + 1,806 - 16.8x = 1,542$$
$$-8.8x = -264$$
$$x = 30$$

So, 30 white roses, 65 tulips, and $250 - (30 + 65) = 155$ long stem red roses were purchased.

39. The correct answer is A. Two perpendicular lines have negative reciprocal slopes—that is, the slopes' product equals −1. The figure shows the equation of $f(x)$ in slope-intercept form ($y = mx + b$, where m is the slope), so you can tell that the slope of $f(x)$ is $\frac{3}{2}$. Therefore, the slope of $g(x)$ has to equal $-\frac{2}{3}$. This eliminates choices C and D. Furthermore, the figure shows that $g(x)$ goes through the point $(0,-1)$. b in $y=mx+b$ is y-intercept, so $b=-1$. Therefore, the answer must be $y=-\frac{2}{3}x-1$.

40. The correct answer is D. The vectors are already connected head-to-tail, so $v + w = u$. Therefore, $w = u - v$.

41. The correct answer is B. Since there are 20 data values, the median is the average of the 10th and 11th values, namely $\frac{10 + 15}{2} = 12.5$.

42. The correct answer is A. Let x be the probability that a civil engineering major will be class president. Then the probability that a mechanical engineering major and the probability that an electrical engineering major will be class president are both x, as well, while the probability that a chemical engineering major will be class president is $2x$. Since the class president will definitely come from one of these four disciplines, $x + x + x + 2x = 1$. Therefore, $x = \frac{1}{5}$. So, the chance that the class president will be a civil engineering major is $\frac{1}{5}$. Kathy is one of the 15 civil engineering majors, so her particular probability of being class president is $\frac{1}{5} \times \frac{1}{15} = \frac{1}{75}$.

43. The correct answer is D. Substitute $V = 6{,}500$ and $h = 30$ into the volume formula $V = \frac{1}{3}\pi r^2 h$ and solve for r:

$$6{,}500 = \tfrac{1}{3}\pi r^2(30)$$
$$\frac{6{,}500}{10\pi} = r^2$$
$$\frac{650}{\pi} = r^2$$
$$\sqrt{\frac{650}{\pi}} = r$$

So, the radius is $\sqrt{\dfrac{650}{\pi}}$ feet.

44. The correct answer is B. Note that log has base 10. Substitute pH = 7.1 into the equation and solve for [Z]:

$$7.1 = -\log_{10}[Z]$$
$$-7.1 = \log_{10}[Z]$$
$$10^{-7.1} = [Z]$$

45. The correct answer is D. Use the substitution rule. Let $u = \ln 2x = \ln 2 + \ln x$, in which case $du = \frac{1}{x}\,dx$. Then:

$$\int \frac{\ln 2x}{x}\,dx = \int u\,du = \frac{u^2}{2} + c = \frac{(\ln 2x)^2}{2} + c$$

46. The correct answer is D. The total number of campers attending the camp in year t is $f(t) + m(t)$. The portion of these that are female is $\dfrac{f(t)}{f(t) + m(t)}$.

47. **The correct answer is D.** Do not bother sketching the graph. Rather, look at the answer choices and see if you can identify it, or eliminate any choices, quickly. Indeed, you can eliminate choice C because the graph of the sine function is continuous and wave-like, while the graph in this answer is not. You can also eliminate choice B because the sine of zero equals zero, so the graph of $f(x)$ must go through the origin. Finally, you know that the sine of an angle is at most 1 and at least −1. So, twice the sine of an angle (which is what appears in the equation of function $f(x)$) must vary between −2 and 2. Only choice D satisfies this criterion, so this choice is the correct answer.

48. **The correct answer is A.** The general form of a third-degree polynomial is $ax^3 + bx^2 + cx + d$. The first three derivatives of such a function are:

$$f'(x) = 3ax^2 + 2bx + c$$

$$f''(x) = 6ax + 2b$$

$$f'''(x) = 6a$$

Now, the third derivative of the polynomial in the question equals 12 when x equals 1. Therefore:

$$6a = 12 \Rightarrow a = 2$$

The second derivative equals 10 when x equals 1. Therefore:

$$6a \times 1 + 2b = 10 \Rightarrow 12 + 2b = 10 \Rightarrow b = -1$$

The first derivative equals 11 when x equals 1. Therefore:

$$3a \times 1^2 + 2b \times 1 + c = 11 \Rightarrow 6 - 2 + c = 11 \Rightarrow c = 7$$

You have no information about d, which means that any third-degree polynomial with $a = 2$, $b = -1$, and $c = 7$ is correct. Only choice A features such a polynomial, so it is the correct answer.

APPENDIX

Pharmacy Career Options

Pharmacy Career Options

OVERVIEW

- **Pharmacy Careers**
- **Academic Pharmacist**
- **Ambulatory Care Pharmacist**
- **Community Pharmacist**
- **Consultant Pharmacist**
- **Hospital and Institutional Pharmacist**
- **Managed Care Pharmacist**
- **Nuclear Pharmacist**
- **Oncology Pharmacist**
- **Pharmacy Informaticist**
- **U.S. Public Health Service Pharmacist**

PHARMACY CAREERS

According to the US Bureau of Labor Statistics (BLS), choosing a career in pharmacy is an excellent career choice. It is a field with significant career opportunities. Although earning potential is relatively high, the down side is the working hours. Many pharmacists must work nights, weekend, and holidays. Recently, there were 270,000 pharmacists working in the United States. Employment is expected to grow by 17 percent between 2008 and 2018, which is faster than average for all occupations. The projected total by 2018 is 315,800.

Several factors are driving the demand for pharmacists. As the number of medications that patients take increases, more pharmacists will be needed for patient counseling about drug interactions and for monitoring of drug regimens. Pharmacists increasingly will find employment opportunities in outpatient care centers, nursing care facilities, and doctors' offices. In addition, the BLS projects increased employment opportunities in mail-order prescription businesses, hospitals, drugstores, grocery stores, and mass retailers like Walmart.

Median earnings in a recent year for all pharmacy occupations were $106,410. The top 10 percent of pharmacists took home $131,440 and the lowest 10 percent less than $77,390.

NOTE

For information
on your state's
licensing
procedure,
contact your
state's board of
pharmacy.

In terms of training, pharmacists take two years of prepharmacy courses at an accredited undergraduate college or university and then four years at an accredited college of pharmacy, earning a Pharm.D. (Doctor of Pharmacy) degree at graduation. A typical undergraduate program includes courses in math, chemistry, biology, and physics. Some pharmacy graduates enroll in a 1- or 2-year residency or fellowship program. To become practicing pharmacists, graduates must pass a series of exams to be licensed. All fifty states and the District of Columbia, Guam, Puerto Rico, and the U.S. Virgin Islands require the North American Pharmacist Licensure Examination (NAPLEX). Forty-four states and the District of Columbia also require the Multistate Pharmacy Jurisprudence Examination (MPJE). The other states and territories administer their own exams.

Residential mental retardation, mental health, and substance abuse facilities provide the highest wages; the hourly mean wage is $58.84, which translates into $122,380 per year. The mean hourly wage for pharmacists at general merchandise stores is $54.26, or $112,860 per year.

In terms of geographical location, the top states with the highest employment level for pharmacists are California, Texas, Florida, New York, and Pennsylvania. The top-paying states for pharmacists are Maine, California, Alaska, Alabama, and Vermont.

Many pharmacists work in community settings such as drugstores and in health-care settings such as hospitals. According to the Bureau of Labor Standards, about 65 percent of pharmacists work in retail settings such as drugstores and supermarket pharmacies. A small percentage of this group own their pharmacies. Hospitals employ the next largest group of pharmacists, about 22 percent. But there are many different work environments that employ pharmacists. The following are some of them.

ACADEMIC PHARMACIST

NOTE

Looking for a
residency? Check
the American
Society of
Health-System
Pharmacists at
www.ashp.org.

According to the American Association of Colleges of Pharmacy (AACP), there are more than 3,000 full-time faculty in colleges and schools of pharmacy. AACP also notes that "a typical pharmacy program has an average of 250 adjunct practitioner-educators." There are also a large number of faculty vacancies at any given time, most for full-time faculty. By 2004-05, the number of faculty nearing retirement over the next decade was a concern for pharmacy colleges. A shortage of faculty is driving the recruitment and development of candidates in the field of academic pharmacy. The average salary for a full professor in a recent year was $145,982, and the average salary for an instructor was $85,268, both according to AACP.

In addition to their teaching duties, pharmacy faculty conduct research and may be involved in patient care and public service. There may also be opportunities to act as consultant for a variety of domestic and international organizations involved in health care. Appointments to a pharmacy faculty are typically for nine or ten months rather than for a full year.

Pharmacy faculty teach pharmaceutical sciences; pharmacy practice and clinical sciences; and social, economic, behavioral, and administrative pharmacy. These areas cover the biological sciences, drug discovery, medicinal and natural products, and pharmacology, as well as continuing education and experiential education.

Faculty in the pharmaceutical sciences teach classes and also conduct research on drug development. Typical preparation for a career in this branch of academic pharmacy includes an undergraduate degree in a science or a Pharm.D. degree, a Ph.D. in the same discipline or in the pharmaceutical sciences, four to five years' experience as a teaching assistant, and two years of post-doctoral research.

Faculty responsible for pharmacy practice are involved in teaching, research, and patient care. Some of the research may be conducted with human subjects. Typical preparation is a Pharm.D. degree and a residency or fellowship, and may include a higher-level degree.

Social, behavioral, and administrative faculty in pharmacy colleges are involved in people, health care, and pharmacy services in a variety of environments, such as institutional and business organizations. In addition to conducting research, faculty members teach professional and graduate students. The pharmacy school faculty do not necessarily have backgrounds in pharmacy. Rather, they have training and experience in such areas as economics, epidemiology, and the social, psychological, and cultural issues related to health policy, such as the cost and effectiveness of drugs. For example, pharmacoeconomic analysis can be used to determine the best allocation of health-care dollars. Typical preparation for social, behavioral, and administrative faculty includes a Ph.D. in one of the above-mentioned fields.

AMBULATORY CARE PHARMACIST

Ambulatory care is a pharmacy specialty described by the Board of Pharmacy Specialties (BPS) as "the provision of integrated, accessible health-care services by pharmacists who are accountable for addressing medication needs, developing sustained partnerships with patients, and practicing in the context of family and community." Ambulatory care pharmacists work in institutional settings such as hospital outpatient clinics and in community-based clinics. Depending on employer, location, and experience, salaries for ambulatory care pharmacists range from the lower end of the pay scale to the average for pharmacists.

In terms of preparation, according to BPS, candidates for this specialty must be graduates of an accredited school or college of pharmacy, be currently licensed as pharmacists, and pass the Ambulatory Care Specialty Certification Examination. In addition, a candidate must complete one of three different practice experience requirements. First, the candidate may satisfy the requirement with four years of practice experience, half of which must be spent in an ambulatory care situation. Second, the candidate may complete a PGY1 (post-graduate year 1) residency and a year of practice; half of that time must be spent in an ambulatory care situation. Or, third, the candidate may complete a PGY2 residency in ambulatory care pharmacy.

In addition to being certified, ambulatory care pharmacists must be recertified after seven years as a practicing ambulatory care pharmacist. The content of the exam provides an indication of the kind of work that this specialty engages in. Half of the exam consists of questions on direct patient care; 20 percent ask questions related to practice management; 15 percent are related to retrieval, generation, interpretation, and dissemination of knowledge; 10 percent ask about patient advocacy; and 5 percent are about public health issues. One hundred hours of continuing education credits may be substituted for taking the exam.

NOTE

The American Pharmacists Association, www.pharmacist. com, was founded in 1852 and today provides a forum for debate and policy setting by and for its members.

COMMUNITY PHARMACIST

A community pharmacist may work for a chain of drugstores, may work in a pharmacy in some other type of retail store such as a supermarket, or may own his or her own pharmacy. In a recent year, there were over 23,000 independently owned pharmacies in the United States. As the National Community Pharmacists Association (NCPA) describes them, "the nation's independent pharmacists are small business entrepreneurs and multifaceted health-care providers who represent a vital part of the United States' health-care delivery system." While not entrepreneurs, those who work for chain pharmacies also represent the link between the medical profession and the patient.

Being a community pharmacist requires good interpersonal and verbal communication skills because the community pharmacist interacts with consumers as well as health-care professionals. According to AACP, the community pharmacist's role is evolving into one of "counseling and medications therapy." Instead of going to your doctor for a flu shot or a pneumonia vaccination, you can go to a pharmacist certified to give these immunizations. Through accreditation programs such as the Diabetes Accreditation Standards, pharmacists can earn credentials in helping patients manage chronic conditions such as high cholesterol, hypertension, and diabetes. Among the top services offered by independent community pharmacies are diabetes training and blood pressure monitoring. Community pharmacists may also run smoking cessation programs and lactation classes as well as help patients navigate Medicare and Medicaid changes. No longer is your local pharmacist relegated to counting out pills and labeling pill bottles.

AACP lists starting salaries as high as $75,000 for pharmacists working for chain stores. Working for a retail chain may lead to management positions if a pharmacist is interested. Depending on location—rural, suburban, or urban—owners of independent pharmacies may make more than $100,000 a year. The average independent pharmacy has sales of $4.0 million, according to NCPA.

AACP lists two factors that will drive the demand for community pharmacists in the near future: an aging population and the growing use of medication therapy by the health-care system. These two trends translate into an increasing need for community pharmacists. Some states are already experiencing a shortage of community pharmacists.

CONSULTANT PHARMACIST

According to AACP, consultant pharmacists provide "a broad spectrum of administrative, distributive, and clinical services to more than 1.7 million nursing facility residents and hundreds of thousands of others in a wide variety of care environments." The environments include adult day-care programs, community-based care facilities, long-term care facilities, nursing facilities, hospices, alcohol and drug rehabilitation facilities, industrial factories, correctional institutions, and individuals living independently.

The field has some 10,000 practitioners. In terms of preparation, no special training or licensing is required. Salaries tend toward the top range of pharmacy jobs with some topping out at around $140,000 for those employed by large care companies. The states with the most jobs in this field tend to be those with large populations of older people such as North Carolina and Florida.

As you can see from the list of environments in which consultant pharmacists work, they do not deal only with elderly patients. However, much of their practice is with older people because they work in places such as long-term care facilities and nursing homes. Consultant pharmacists can be certified in geriatric pharmacy (CGP). The certification must be renewed every five years either by passing a test or by taking 75 hours of continuing education in the field.

One factor driving the need for consultant pharmacists is the aging population, which requires more oversight of their complex medication regimens to avoid "adverse drug reactions, drug interactions, excessive use of medications, and inappropriate and duplicative drug therapy," according to AACP. Another factor is federal regulations. Nursing facilities and intermediate care facilities for the mentally retarded are required by law to have the drug regimens reviewed by a pharmacist.

HOSPITAL AND INSTITUTIONAL PHARMACIST

The hospital and institutional pharmacy occupation includes pharmacists working not only in hospitals, but in nursing homes, extended care facilities, neighborhood health centers, and health maintenance organizations (HMO), according to AACP. They are part of a team of doctors and nurses that provide direct patient care in these settings and are a major factor in assuring patient safety in terms of drug therapy.

More than 38,000 pharmacists work in hospital and institutional pharmacy positions, either full- or part-time, and AACP projects the need for an additional 65,000 pharmacists for this field by 2020. The BLS reports that the average mean salary in general medical and surgical hospitals in a recent year was $112,860. The American Society of Health-System Pharmacists (ASHP) in a survey reported that salaries ranged from $100,000 to $170,000. The size and type of hospital and institutional setting as well as area of the country affect salaries.

According to AACP, the duties of pharmacists in these institutional settings include responsibility for seeing that each patient receives "the appropriate medication, in the correct form and dosage, at the correct time" and monitoring for allergies and adverse effects of drugs. Depending on the facility, pharmacists may provide services in any or all of the following areas: adult medicine, pediatrics, oncology, ambulatory care, and psychiatry.

Larger facilities and HMOs can provide opportunities for pharmacists to move up into management positions. As the head of a pharmacy department, a pharmacy manager deals with personnel administration, workflow, and budgeting. The department head also interfaces with other departments, as well as having responsibility for negotiations over pricing with pharmaceutical companies, wholesalers, and equipment makers. Cost containment and quality control, not just drug therapy, have become important parts of a pharmacy manager's role, according to ASHP.

NOTE

For more information on this career, check the American Society of Health-System Pharmacists at www.ashp.org.

MANAGED CARE PHARMACIST

The American Pharmacists Association (APA) defines managed care as "a system designed to optimize patient care and outcomes and foster quality through greater coordination of medical services." The purpose of managed care is to reduce the cost of medical care while ensuring quality care. More than 200 million people in the United States are in managed care programs.

Pharmacists working in a managed care environment may work for a traditional managed care organization (MCO), but managed care pharmacists also work for health plans and health maintenance organizations (HMOs), preferred provider organizations (PPOs), point-of-service plans (POS), and pharmacy benefit management companies (PBMs). They are not frontline pharmacists, but administrators.

The APA lists a variety of tasks for managed care pharmacists. Depending on the employer, a managed care pharmacist may work with a team of doctors and others to determine the most effective treatments for patients, including drug therapies. Managed care pharmacists also review patient medications to ensure that patients are using the most appropriate medications and in the correct dosages, and they also participate in care management programs—disease state management—for patients most at risk of complications from certain chronic conditions such as hypertension. Educating providers and patients is also an important aspect of the job of a managed care pharmacist. At certain levels, managed care pharmacists may deal with networks of local pharmacies, pharmaceutical manufacturers, insurance companies, and some design pharmacy benefit programs and may develop and manage a plan's formulary. The focus at all levels is on cost containment, quality control, and the appropriateness of drug therapies.

In addition to a Pharm.D. degree, a residency program in managed care pharmacy is desirable for job candidates in this specialty. A recent online survey by a managed care market research firm found that the median salary was $130,000 to $139,000 for highly experienced managed care pharmacists.

NUCLEAR PHARMACIST

The Board of Pharmacy Specialties (BPS) defines nuclear pharmacy as the specialty within pharmacy that "seeks to improve and promote the public health through the safe and effective use of radioactive drugs for diagnosis and therapy." A nuclear pharmacist works as one of a health-care team and specializes in the "procurement, compounding, quality control testing, dispensing, distribution, and monitoring of radiopharmaceuticals." Work environments include nuclear pharmacies, hospitals, research organizations, academic institutions, pharmaceutical companies, and government agencies.

In terms of training, pharmacists who wish to become nuclear pharmacists must undergo specialized training, some of which is related to safe handling of radiopharmaceuticals. The specialty is certified by the BPS. To be eligible for certification, a candidate must have a pharmacy degree from an accredited school or college of pharmacy, have a current license to practice, have 4,000 hours of experience in nuclear pharmacy practice, and pass the BPS certification exam. The experience may be earned through a combination of undergraduate and graduate work, including earning a master's of science or a doctorate in nuclear pharmacy or through training and practice. Recertification is required every seven years.

The median salary is $113,000 with the mid-range of salaries between $104,000 and $125,000. Experience, employer, and geographic location impact salaries.

ONCOLOGY PHARMACIST

According to the Board of Pharmacy Specialties (BPS), oncology pharmacists "recommend, design, implement, monitor, and modify pharmacotherapeutic plans to optimize outcomes in patients with malignant diseases." Oncology pharmacy became a separate specialty in 1996.

Oncology pharmacists work in health-care teams with doctors, nurses, and other care givers to provide treatment for cancer patients, but they are the ones who prepare the appropriate medications and dosages for patients. It is their job to see that the drugs are safe, stable, and free of contaminants from the pharmacy environment.

In terms of preparation, oncology pharmacists have a Pharm.D. degree and are also board certified by BPS. To be eligible for certification, a pharmacist must have a degree from an accredited school or college of pharmacy and be currently licensed to practice. The candidate must complete four years of practice with at least half the time in oncology pharmacy or complete a PGY2 (post-graduate year 2) residency in oncology pharmacy and have spent at least half of an additional year in oncology pharmacy. As of January 1, 2013, candidates must hold a residency accredited by the American Society of Health-System Pharmacists to be eligible for certification. The last step is passing BPS's certification exam, and like its other specialties, BPS requires recertification every seven years.

Depending on years of experience, employer, and region of the country, salaries for oncology pharmacists range from around $95,000 to a high of $140,000.

PHARMACY INFORMATICIST

Health or medical informatics can be defined as "a discipline that includes all aspects of the information science of health care, from fundamental research to clinical application." Pharmacy informatics, or pharmcoinformatics, according to the American Medical Informatics Association (AMIA), involves the "intersection of informatics, technology, and medication management for efficient, beneficial patient health care." Pharmacy informatics is one of the twelve specialties listed in the field of health informatics. Others include clinical research informatics, consumer health informatics, nursing informatics, and public health/population informatics. According to the AMIA, clinical informatics relates to pharmacists when the information is used for health-care delivery.

The Healthcare Information and Management Systems Society (HIMSS) defines pharmacy informatics as "the scientific field that focuses on medication-related data and knowledge within the continuum of health-care systems—including its acquisition, storage, analysis, use, and dissemination—in the delivery of optimal medication-related patient care and health outcomes." A goal is to develop best practices and reliable systems in order to increase patient safety by decreasing medication errors.

In terms of preparation, a pharmacy informaticist typically has a Pharm.D. and has completed a residency as well as earning a second degree in information technology, health administration, or business administration. All pharmacy schools now offer informatics.

NOTE

For more on oncology pharmacy, check the Board of Pharmacy Specialties at www.bpsweb.org and the International Society of Oncology Pharmacy Practitioners at www.isopp.org.

NOTE

For more information, check the Healthcare Information and Management Systems Society at www.himss.org, the American Medical Informatics Association at www.amia.org, and the American Society of Health-System Pharmacists at www.ashp.org.

A starting salary of $40,000 to $50,000 is typical for those specializing in informatics, but it depends on specialty, degree, experience, employer, and region of the country. Because of the continuing complexity of drug therapies, this is a rapidly growing field within pharmacy. According to an HIMSS survey, the average salary for health-care IT professionals in general in a recent year was $114,176. It was $109,993 for someone working in a hospital as part of a multi-hospital system.

U.S. PUBLIC HEALTH SERVICE PHARMACIST

NOTE

For more information, check the U.S. Public Health Service at www.usphs.gov.

The United States Public Health Service (USPHS) was founded in 1798 and today provides pharmaceutical care to Native Americans on their reservations, to prisoners in federal correctional institutions, and to members of the U.S. Coast Guard, among other functions. The mission of the U.S. Public Health Service is to promote the public health by

- controlling and preventing disease.
- improving the health-care system, including the development of innovations in health care.
- assuring the safe and effective use of drugs and medical devices.
- expanding national health resources.
- responding to natural disasters, technological emergencies, and biological and chemical terrorism.
- shaping health work force, medical knowledge, technology, and other resources toward the goal of better health.

The USPHS employs more than 1,000 pharmacists in its Commissioned Corps (CC) and another 200 in the federal Civil Service (CS). USPHS pharmacists can be found across the country in all regions and in every state, and in urban and rural settings. Pharmacists in the Commissioned Corps are commissioned officers. Public health pharmacists work in the:

- Indian Health Service
- Food and Drug Administration
- Federal Bureau of Prisons
- National Institutes of Health
- Coast Guard
- Health Resources and Services Administration
- Centers for Disease Control and Prevention
- Agency for Toxic Substances and Disease Registry
- Substance Abuse and Mental Health Services Administration
- Agency for Healthcare Research and Quality
- Immigration and Naturalization Service
- Center for Medicare and Medicaid Services

The service recruits pharmacists and offers the JRCOSTEP program to help students currently in school pay for their education and offers signing bonuses for practicing pharmacists. The USPHS promises applicants "quality of practice, opportunities for professional growth, and quality of life." Pharmacists in the USPHS, depending on their jobs, "are involved in patient care, new drug approval and monitoring, medical research, health-care policy, and epidemiology." Salaries in the CC depend on officer grade and years of service and include housing and subsistence pay. After-tax monthly pay for an officer with dependents and three years or less of service is $3,820 to $5,863 monthly, or $45,840 to $69,356 annually. Without dependents, the amounts are slightly less, $3,554 to $5,390.

Pharmacists working for the USPHS have access to continuing education programs, as well as graduate programs paid for by the government. An added benefit to employment in the Public Health Service is retirement income. An officer may retire after twenty years with a pension, including cost-of-living adjustments.

NOTES

NOTES

NOTES

NOTES

NOTES

NOTES

NOTES

NOTES

NOTES

NOTES

NOTES